# ORAL AND MAXILLOFACIAL DISEASES

# ORAL AND MAXILLOFACIAL DISEASES

An illustrated guide to the diagnosis and management of diseases of the oral mucosa, gingivae, teeth, salivary glands, jaw bones and joints

## Fourth Edition

### Crispian Scully
CBE, MD, PhD, MDS, MRCS, FDSRCPS, FFDRCSI, FDSRCS, FRCPath,
FMedSci, FHEA, FUCL, DSc, DChD, DMed (HC), Dr HC
**Professor of Oral Medicine, Pathology and Microbiology**
University of London
**Professor of Special Care Dentistry, Eastman Dental Institute**
University College London
**Visiting Professor**
Universities of Bristol, Edinburgh, Granada and Helsinki
**Honorary Consultant**
University College London Hospitals, and Great Ormond Street Hospital for Children London, UK

### Stephen R Flint
MA, PhD, MBBS, FFDRCSI, FDSRCS, FICD, FTCD
**Professor and Consultant in Oral Medicine**
Dublin Dental School and Hospital, Trinity College, Dublin, Ireland

### Jose V Bagan
MD, DDS, PhD
**Professor**
Valencia University and Hospital General Universitario de Valencia, Valencia, Spain

### Stephen R Porter
MD, PhD, FDSRCS, FDSRCSE, FHEA
**Professsor of Oral Medicine**
Eastman Dental Institute, University College London
**Honorary Consultant**
University College London Hospitals, UK

### Khursheed F Moos
OBE, MB, BS, BDS, FRCS, FDSRCS, FDSRCSE, FDSRCPS
**Emeritus Professor and Honorary Consultant**
Glasgow Hospitals, University of Glasgow, UK

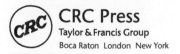

**CRC Press**
Taylor & Francis Group
Boca Raton   London   New York

CRC Press is an imprint of the
Taylor & Francis Group, an **informa** business

First published in 2010 by Martin Dunitz Ltd.
This edition published in 2010 by Informa Healthcare

CRC Press
Taylor & Francis Group
6000 Broken Sound Parkway NW, Suite 300
Boca Raton, FL 33487-2742

First issued in paperback 2019

© 2010 by Taylor & Francis Group, LLC
CRC Press is an imprint of Taylor & Francis Group, an Informa business

No claim to original U.S. Government works

ISBN-13: 978-0-367-44600-0 (pbk)
ISBN-13: 978-0-415-41494-4 (hbk)

**Visit the Taylor & Francis Web site at**
**http://www.taylorandfrancis.com**

**and the CRC Press Web site at**
**http://www.crcpress.com**

A CIP record for this book is available from the British Library.

Typeset by Exeter Premedia Services

# CONTENTS

# PREFACE TO THE FOURTH EDITION

This atlas of oral and maxillofacial pathology differs from other atlases by the inclusion of clinical detail on diseases of the oral mucosa, gingivae, teeth, salivary glands, jaw bones and joints, and of a wide range of the more obvious extraoral manifestations. It is intended primarily as a pictorial diagnostic aid, both for dental healthcare professionals, surgeons and physicians, with text that provides a concise synopsis of stomatology.

The previous editions over the past 20 years have been extremely successful and the Atlas has become increasingly popular because of the very wide coverage of oral and maxillofacial diseases and the depth of information contained. Versions have also been published in French, German and Portuguese.

This fourth edition welcomes a new author and provides one of the most comprehensively illustrated coverage of oral and maxillofacial diseases of which we are aware worldwide. The Atlas had also, however, become rather large and heavy and, therefore, it has been revised, updated and re-organized, and some new conditions included. It has been further improved to include better examples of many conditions, particularly additional examples of the more common orofacial conditions or where clinical diagnosis can be difficult because of varied presentations.

A major challenge with all books is how best to persuade publishers to afford enough pages without an excessively high price, and how best to organize and present the material. Our first edition presented conditions according to the International Classification of Diseases but this is incomplete and not always helpful in clinical diagnosis. We have here attempted to highlight the more common and/or important conditions by including more text and/or illustrations of these.

Chapter 1 summarizes the systemic disorders seen mainly in hospital practice, with some detail about the more important conditions but only a less detailed outline of the less common or less relevant disorders: further background can be found in *Medical Problems in Dentistry* (Scully C), Elsevier, London, 2010. Clearly, systemic factors may also influence conditions discussed in other chapters.

Chapters 2–11 cover the conditions which are more common and/or important in day-to-day primary care practice, and largely of local aetiology. Much more detail on aetiopathogenesis, clinical features, diagnosis and management of these conditions has been included. One can always argue as to which disease is best placed in which particular section but we trust readers will find the condition in which they are interested, somewhere.

The specific section on diagnosis and management has also been updated and continues to be presented in the clear and easy-to-use format and covers differential diagnoses by symptoms, signs and site, investigations and management of the various conditions covered in the book, the drugs used in the management of oral diseases and the oral and perioral adverse effects of drug treatment. The further reading has been fully updated.

We are grateful to our colleagues who have kindly provided some illustrations; particular thanks in addition to those acknowledged in the previous editions are to Antonio Azul (Lisbon), Drore Eisen (Cincinnatti), Catherine Flaitz (Houston), Florencio Monje Gil (Valencia), Rodney Grahame (London), Navdeep Kumar (London), Jane Luker (Bristol), Nick Rogers (Rochester), Richard Welbury (Glasgow) and Donald Winstock (London); to the publishers and our co-authors of *Dermatology of the Lips* (Scully C, Bagan JV, Eisen D, Porter S, Rogers RS) Isis Medical Media, Oxford, 2000; *A Colour Atlas of Orofacial Health and Disease* in *Children and Adolescents* (Scully C, Welbury R, Flaitz C, Almedia ODP) Martin Dunitz, London, 2001; *Orofacial Disease; an Update for the Dental Team* (Scully C, Porter SR), Elsevier Harcourt, London & Edinburgh, 2002; *Oral and Maxillofacial Medicine* (Scully C) Elsevier, London and Edinburgh, 2007; *Oral and Maxillofacial Medicine and Pathology* (Scully C, Almeida ODP, Bagan JS, Diz Dios P, Mosqueda A), Blackwell, Oxford, 2010; The oral cavity and lips (Scully C, Hegarty A) In *Rook's Textbook of Dermatology*. 8th edition. Eds: Burns DA, Breathnach SM, Cox N, Griffiths C, Blackwell Science, Oxford, 2010, and to the publishers of *British Dental Journal, British Journal of Dermatology, International Journal of Oral and Maxillofacial Surgery, Journal of Oral Pathology and Medicine, Medicina Oral, Oral Diseases, Oral Oncology* and *Oral Surgery, Oral Medicine and Oral Pathology*.

All typing and image preparation was carried out by Crispian Scully. Our thanks are to Paul Darkins and John Evans for assistance with the image scanning.

Crispian Scully
Jose-Vicente Bagan
Stephen R Flint
Stephen R Porter
Khursheed F Moos

# 1 MAXILLOFACIAL COMPLICATIONS IN SYSTEMIC CONDITIONS

A range of systemic conditions, treatments and complications can present with maxillofacial manifestations. Some of the more common or important conditions are summarised here, in alphabetic order, with their main maxillofacial manifestations. Others which also have maxillofacial manifestations are discussed elsewhere in the text.

# 1.1 CARDIOVASCULAR DISEASE

- angina pectoris
- angiomas
- anticoagulants
- congenital heart disease
- drugs
- giant cell arteritis

- hereditary haemorrhagic telangiectasia (HHT)
- hypertension
- polyarteritis nodosa
- transplantation
- Wegener granulomatosis
- Williams syndrome

## ANGINA PECTORIS

Angina pectoris—pain related to cardiac ischaemia—may be referred to the jaw rarely, mainly to the mandible. Ulcers may result from use of nicorandil (chapter 1.6). Patients with angina or acute coronary syndrome appear more likely to have a positive interleukin-1 polymorphism and severe periodontitis.

## ANGIOMAS

Angiomas (haemangiomas) may be hamartomas or acquired. Most are small but some haemangiomas are large and may result in enlargement of soft tissues and underlying bone (Klippel–Trenaunay or angioosteohypertrophy syndrome), while others may be part of more widespread disease such as the von Hippel–Lindau syndrome (involving retina, cerebellum, spinal cord, kidneys, pancreas, liver but rarely the mouth), the Dandy–Walker syndrome (associated with posterior fossa brain abnormalities), Maffucci syndrome (multiple enchondromas) or Sturge–Weber syndrome. Haemangiomas may be extensive in Sturge–Weber syndrome (Figs 1.1.1 and 1.1.2) (encephalofacial angiomatosis)—a genetic condition in which a haemangioma affects the upper face and usually extends through the facial skeleton into the brain occipital lobe, producing epilepsy and often glaucoma, hemiplegia and learning impairment and neuralgia. Radiography shows calcification intracranially in the haemangioma. The haemangioma may extend intraorally and be associated with hypertrophy of the affected jaw, macrodontia and

accelerated tooth eruption. Since the patients are often treated with phenytoin there is frequently also drug-related gingival enlargement.

Treatment for haemangiomas can include injection of sclerosants, or surgery (scalpel, laser, cryosurgery, photocoagulation or plasma knife).

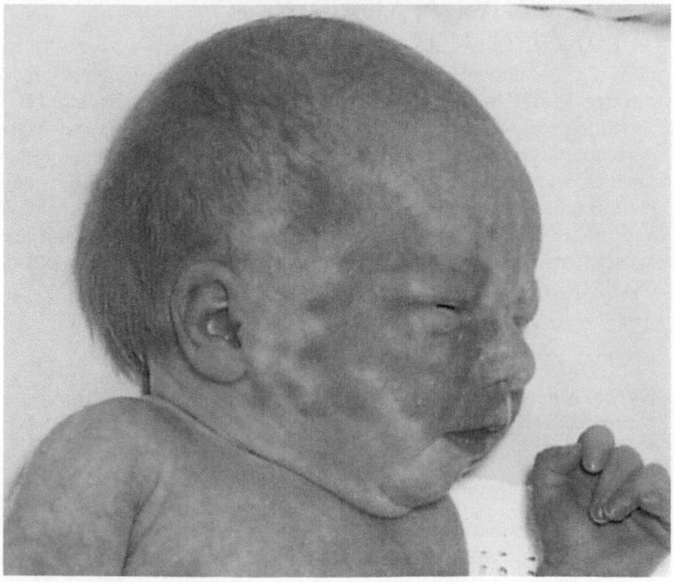

## ANTICOAGULANTS

Anticoagulants cause a bleeding tendency which may manifest with gingival bleeding or oral bruises.

## CONGENITAL HEART DISEASE

Congenital heart disease may result in central cyanosis—seen especially in the lips, tongue and other mucosae which appear purple: the teeth appear milky white in contrast (Figs 1.1.3 and 1.1.4). Tetralogy of Fallot, one of the more common of the cyanotic congenital heart diseases, consists of ventricular septal defect, pulmonary stenosis, right ventricular hypertrophy and an aorta that overrides both ventricles. Children with congenital heart disease in some studies have tended to have significantly more caries and an increased prevalence of fissured and geographic tongue.

## DRUGS

Drugs such as cardioactive or antihypertensive agents can produce gingival swelling, dry mouth, ulcers, lichenoid and other lesions (see chapter 1.6). Calcium-channel blockers, particularly nifedipine, may lead to gingival swelling (Fig. 1.1.5) (chapter 1.6) and dry mouth. Nicorandil may cause oral (chapter 1.6) as well as anal, gastrointestinal and perioral ulceration. Beta-blockers may cause lichenoid lesions or dry mouth (chapter 1.6). Angiotensin converting enzyme inhibitors may cause

*Figure 1.1.1* Sturge–Weber syndrome showing facial angioma.

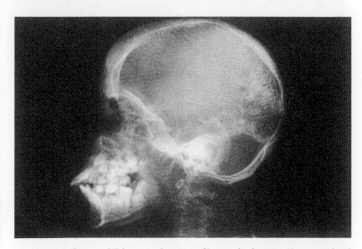

*Figure 1.1.2* Sturge–Weber syndrome radiograph showing intracerebral angioma.

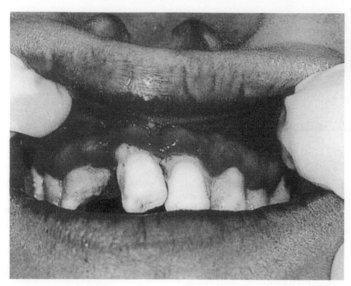

*Figure 1.1.3* Central cyanosis in Down syndrome showing purple gingivae and lips.

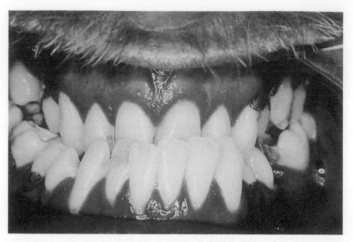

*Figure 1.1.4* Central cyanosis in congenital heart disease showing teeth appearing white against the purple gingivae.

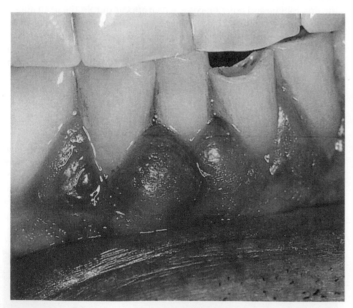

*Figure 1.1.5* Nifedipine a common cause of drug-induced gingival swelling showing interdental swellings.

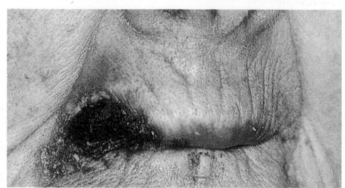

*Figure 1.1.6* Giant cell arteritis—a rare cause of lip or tongue ischaemic necrosis.

angioedema, or a burning sensation (chapter 1.6). Orolingual angioedema may be a complication of thrombolytics used in stroke victims.

## GIANT CELL ARTERITIS
Giant cell arteritis (granulomatous, cranial or temporal arteritis)—a systemic vasculitis—may present with pain, usually over the temple, and can cause retinal artery spasm and blindness, or stroke. Rarely, there can be tongue or lip pain or 'jaw claudication', or ischaemic necrosis of tongue or lip (Fig. 1.1.6). Giant cell arteritis is sometimes associated with polymyalgia rheumatica and is a medical emergency; corticosteroids are indicated to avoid the retinal damage.

## HEREDITARY HAEMORRHAGIC TELANGIECTASIA (HHT)
HHT (Osler–Rendu–Weber syndrome)—an autosomal dominant genetic disorder caused by disruption in the transforming growth factor (TGF) signalling pathway, by mutations in endoglin gene (HHT1) and activin A receptor type II-like 1 gene (HHT2)—results in blood vessel abnormalities with deficient capillaries. Telangiectases and arteriovenous malformations are found primarily in the nose, skin of the face, hands and mouth and stomach, and also in the respiratory tract, intestines, kidneys, liver and brain. The telangiectatic lesions may bleed profusely (Figs 1.1.7 and 1.1.8) and laser or cryosurgery may be indicated.

## HYPERTENSION
Hypertension—various antihypertensive drugs can cause oral complaints, especially dry mouth (chapter 1.6).

## POLYARTERITIS NODOSA
Polyarteritis nodosa—a vasculitis affecting medium-sized arteries, possibly related to a reaction to hepatitis B virus, manifests with ischaemic damage mainly to skin, heart, kidneys and nervous system. Mouth ulcers may be seen (Fig. 1.1.9).

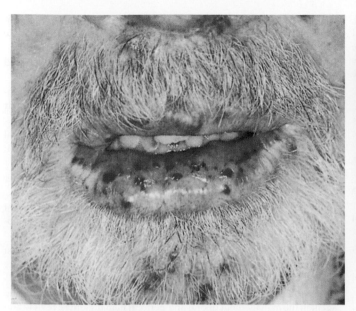

*Figure 1.1.7* Hereditary haemorrhagic telangiectasia showing multiple telangiectases.

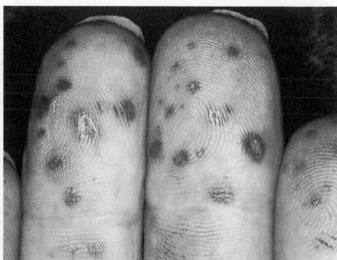

*Figure 1.1.8* Hereditary haemorrhagic telangiectasia showing cutaneous telangiectases.

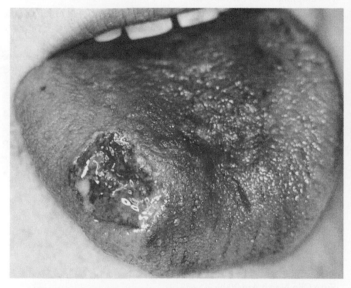

*Figure 1.1.9* Polyarteritis nodosa—causing lingual ulceration.

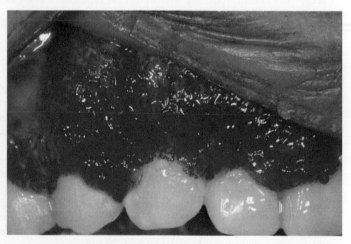

*Figure 1.1.10* Wegener granulomatosis showing almost pathognomonic strawberry appearance of gingivae.

## TRANSPLANTATION

Transplantation necessitates that the patient is T-cell immunosuppressed to prevent graft rejection (chapters 1.6 and 1.7). Oral complications are mainly those related to the immunosuppression needed to prevent graft rejection, and may include infections and neoplasms. Infections such as candidosis, herpes simplex virus-related ulceration and hairy leukoplakia may be seen. An increased susceptibility to lip cancer after transplantation is related to exposure to immunosuppressive agents and UV light. Post-transplantation patients are also prone to graft-versus-host disease (GVH), lymphoproliferative diseases, Kaposi sarcoma and some carcinomas (chapter 1.6). Drugs used after cardiac transplantation may also produce other maxillofacial adverse side-effects; the most common is gingival swelling caused by ciclosporin or nifedepine (chapter 1.6).

## WEGENER GRANULOMATOSIS

Wegener granulomatosis—a rare vasculitis characterized by necrotizing granulomatous inflammation of small- and medium-sized blood vessels, with antineutrophil cytoplasmic antibodies directed at neutrophil proteinase 3—mainly affects the respiratory tract and kidneys. Symptoms include antral pain, discoloured or bloody nasal discharge and, occasionally, nasal or oral ulcers or palatal perforation, lingual infarction or sialadenitis. Characteristic, and almost pathognomonic, is the 'strawberry' appearing gingival swelling sometimes seen (Fig. 1.1.10).

*Microscopic polyangiitis*, a systemic necrotising vasculitis that clinically and histologically affects small-sized vessels but without granulomas, may present similarly.

## WILLIAMS SYNDROME

Williams syndrome—a rare congenital disorder involving the cardiovascular system, connective tissue and central nervous system presents characteristic facial features with full prominent cheeks, wide mouth, long philtrum, small nose with depressed nasal bridge, heavy orbital ridges and medial eyebrow flare. The bony chin is deficient and the mandibular plane angle is high. Microdontia is common and nearly one half have agenesis of one or more permanent teeth. Incisors tend to be tapered or screwdriver-shaped. Molars are often taurodont.

## FURTHER READING

Angiero F, Benedicenti S, Romanos GE, Crippa R. Treatment of hemangioma of the head and neck with diode laser and forced dehydration with induced photocoagulation. Photomed Laser Surg 2008; 26: 113–18.

Axelsson S. Variability of the cranial and dental phenotype in Williams syndrome. Swed Dent J Suppl 2005; 170: 3–67.

Beil CM, Keberle M. Oral and oropharyngeal tumors. Eur J Radiol 2008; 66: 448–59.

Carter LM, Brizman E. Lingual infarction in Wegener's granulomatosis: a case report and review of the literature. Head Face Med 2008; 4: 19.

Comi AM. Pathophysiology of Sturge–Weber syndrome. J Child Neurol 2003; 18: 509–16.

Crinzi RA, Palm NV, Mostofi R, Indresano AT. Management of a dental infection in a patient with Sturge–Weber disease. J Am Dent Assoc 1980; 101: 798–800.

Dahan D, Fenichel GM, El-Said R. Neurocutaneous syndromes. Adolesc Med 2002; 13: 495–509.

Davé S, Van Dyke TE. The link between periodontal disease and cardiovascular disease is probably inflammation. Oral Dis 2008; 14: 95–101.

Egred M. Nicorandil-associated ulcerations. Eur J Gastroenterol Hepatol 2007; 19: 395–8.

Frantz MC, Frank H, von Weyhern C, Kiefer J. Unspecific parotitis can be the first indication of a developing Wegener's granulomatosis. Eur Arch Otorhinolaryngol 2008; 265: 131–4.

Friedlander AH, Yoshikawa T, Chang DS, Feliciano Z, Scully C. Atrial fibrillation: pathogenesis, medical-surgical management and dental implications. J Am Dent Assoc 2009; 140: 167–77.

Goteiner D, Ashmen R, Lehrman N, Janal MN, Eskin B. Presence and significance of interleukin-1 polymorphism in patients who present with acute coronary syndrome, angina, and chronic periodontitis: an epidemiologic pilot study. J Periodontol 2008; 79: 138–43.

Kutluhan A, Bozdemir K, Ugras S. The treatment of tongue haemangioma by plasma knife surgery. Singapore Med J 2008; 49: e312–14.

Miyazaki H, Kato J, Watanabe H, et al. Intralesional laser treatment of voluminous vascular lesions in the oral cavity. Oral Surg Oral Med Oral Pathol Oral Radiol Endod 2009; 107: 164–72.

el-Mostehy MR, Stallard RE. The Sturge–Weber syndrome: its periodontal significance. J Periodontol 1969; 40: 243–6.

Mutalik SS, Bathi RJ, Naikmasur VG. Sturge–Weber syndrome: physician's dream; surgeon's enigma. N Y State Dent J 2009; 75: 44–5.

Ottomeyer C, Hennerici MG, Szabo K, et al. Raising awareness of orolingual angioedema as a complication of thrombolysis in acute stroke patients. Cerebrovasc Dis 2009; 27: 307–8.

Radford DJ, Thong YH. Facial and immunological anomalies associated with tetralogy of Fallot. Int J Cardiol 1989; 22: 229–39.

Rai K, Supriya S, Hegde AM. Oral health status of children with congenital heart disease and the awareness, attitude and knowledge of their parents. J Clin Pediatr Dent 2009; 33: 315–18.

Scully C, Azul AM, Crighton A, et al. Nicorandil can induce severe oral ulceration. Oral Surg Oral Med Oral Pathol Oral Radiol Endod 2001; 91: 189–93.

Scully C, Roberts G, Shotts R. The mouth in heart disease. Practitioner 2001; 245: 432–7.

Scully C, Diz Dios P, Shotts R. Oral health care in patients with the most important medically compromising conditions; 4. Patients with cardiovascular problems. CPD Dent 2004; 5: 50–5.

Scully C, Diz Dios P, Shotts R. Oral health care in patients with the most important medically compromising conditions; 5. Patients at risk for endocarditis. CPD Dent 2004; 5: 75–9.

Selim H, Selim A, Khachemoune A, Metwally SA. Use of sclerosing agent in the management of oral and perioral hemangiomas: review and case reports. Med Sci Monit 2007; 13: CS114–19.

Sharathkumar AA, Shapiro A. Hereditary haemorrhagic telangiectasia. Haemophilia 2008; 14: 1269–80.

Shiboski CH, Regezi JA, Sanchez HC, Silverman Jr S. Oral lesions as the first clinical sign of microscopic polyangiitis: a case report. Oral Surg Oral Med Oral Pathol Oral Radiol Endod 2002; 94: 707–11.

Shotts RH, Scully C, Avery CM, Porter SR. Nicorandil-induced severe oral ulceration: a newly recognized drug reaction. Oral Surg Oral Med Oral Pathol Oral Radiol Endod 1999; 87: 706–7.

Stecksén-Blicks C, Rydberg A, Nyman L, Asplund S, Svanberg C. Dental caries experience in children with congenital heart disease: a case-control study. Int J Paediatr Dent 2004; 14: 94–100.

Tasioula V, Balmer R, Parsons J. Dental health and treatment in a group of children with congenital heart disease. Pediatr Dent 2008; 30: 323–8.

Thomas-Sohl KA, Vaslow DF, Maria BL. Sturge–Weber syndrome: a review. Pediatr Neurol 2004; 30: 303–10.

Turgeman Y, Atar S, Rosenfeld T. "Cyanotic blue tongue" in severe rheumatic tricuspid regurgitation. Isr Med Assoc J 2001; 3: 286–7.

Wakefield YS, Theaker ED, Pemberton MN. Angiotensin converting enzyme inhibitors and delayed onset, recurrent angioedema of the head and neck. Br Dent J 2008; 205: 553–6.

Weeda Jr LW, Coffey SA. Wegener's granulomatosis. Oral Maxillofac Surg Clin North Am 2008; 20: 643–9.

Yang Y, Sun M, Hou R, et al. Preliminary study of fibrin glue combined with pingyangmycin for the treatment of venous malformations in the oral and maxillofacial region. J Oral Maxillofac Surg 2008; 66: 2219–25.

# 1.2 ENDOCRINOLOGICAL AND METABOLIC CONDITIONS

- Addison disease
- congenital hypoparathyroidism
- congenital hypothyroidism
- Cushing syndrome
- diabetes insipidus
- diabetes mellitus
- gigantism/acromegaly
- hyperparathyroidism
- hyperthyroidism

- hypothyroidism
- multiple endocrine neoplasia (adenoma) (MEN or MEA) syndromes
- pituitary dwarfism
- precocious puberty
- pregnancy
- preterm children
- metabolic disorders

## ADDISON DISEASE

Addison disease—hypoadrenocorticism—is associated with lowered plasma cortisol levels which cause feedback increased pituitary secretion of adrenocorticotrophic hormone (ACTH) and precursor hormones with melanocyte stimulating hormone-like activity, causing mucocutaneous hyperpigmentation. Similar hyperpigmentation is also seen in Nelson syndrome (increased ACTH production after bilateral adrenalectomy).

Classically hypoadrenocorticism is of autoimmune aetiology, but the same features may be caused by adrenal neoplasms or, rarely, infections such as tuberculosis, cytomegalovirus or histoplasmosis. There are occasional associations of Addison disease with other diseases, particularly autoimmune diseases, such as the probable TASS syndrome of thyroiditis, Addison disease, Sjögren syndrome and sarcoidosis.

### Clinical features

Maxillofacial hyperpigmentation of a brown, grey or black colour, especially at sites of trauma such as the buccal mucosae or tongue, is typical (Figs 1.2.1 and 1.2.2), although most patients with oral hyperpigmentation prove to have causes other than Addison disease.

Generalised skin hyperpigmentation is also seen with particular pigmentation in the sun-exposed or traumatised sites, the areolae and the genitalia.

The patient with hypoadrenocorticism may also complain of weakness, anorexia and weight loss.

### Diagnosis

Lowered blood pressure, reduced serum cortisol and sodium, raised serum potassium, reduced 24-hour urinary cortisol levels and impaired Synacthen (synthetic ACTH) test are confirmatory. Raised serum levels of adrenocorticotropin and renin confirm the diagnosis.

### Management

Replacement hormone therapy and treatment of the underlying cause.

## CONGENITAL HYPOPARATHYROIDISM

Congenital hypoparathyroidism—due to a rare chromosome 1 genetic defect—may cause seizures, retarded growth and mental development and unusual facies, and may manifest with dental hypoplasia and delayed tooth eruption and, if there is an associated immune defect, chronic candidosis (Figs 1.2.3 and 1.2.4). Autoimmune polyendocrinopathy-candidosis-ectodermal dystrophy and Shprintzen (velocardiofacial) syndrome are discussed in chapter 1.7.

## CONGENITAL HYPOTHYROIDISM

Congenital hypothyroidism, due to thyroid deficiency at birth (sometimes because of dietary iodine deficiency), may cause retarded growth and mental development and unusual facies, and can present with macroglossia and delayed tooth eruption (Fig. 1.2.5) or salivary agenesis.

## CUSHING SYNDROME

Cushing syndrome—hypercortisolism, from excess exogenous corticosteroids—or Cushing disease (hypercortisolism arising from an ACTH-producing pituitary adenoma), can cause facial swelling, hirsutism and erythema (Fig. 1.2.6).

## DIABETES INSIPIDUS

Diabetes insipidus—a condition caused by lack of antidiuretic hormone, or resistance to it—is characterized by excessive thirst, excretion of large amounts of severely diluted urine and dry mouth. It may arise rarely from head injury, lithium treatment, Langerhans histiocytosis or neurological involvement in Behçet disease.

## DIABETES MELLITUS

Diabetes mellitus—caused by lack of insulin, or resistance to it—is characterized by excessive thirst, excretion of large amounts of severely diluted urine, dry mouth, liability to arteriosclerosis and an immune defect. It can present with periodontal disease (Figs 1.2.7 and 1.2.8), xerostomia (Fig. 1.2.8), candidosis, sialosis, burning mouth sensation or lichen planus. Oral changes may be seen mainly in severe insulin-dependent diabetics. Diabetes is characterised by hyperglycaemia and microvascular changes and phagocyte defects.

Parodontal abscesses, infections and rapid periodontal breakdown are the most obvious maxillofacial features. Dry mouth may be caused by dehydration. Other oral lesions may include candidosis such as angular stomatitis or median rhomboid glossitis, burning sensation of the tongue and other oral mucosal surfaces, and lichenoid lesions induced by hypoglycaemic drugs. Autonomic neuropathy may cause sialosis, or gustatory sweating and, with dehydration, contributes to xerostomia. Hyperglycaemic ketoacidosis may cause halitosis. The incidence of birth defects in newborns of women with diabetes including deformities of the face and palate is approximately three to five times higher than among nondiabetics.

Rare complications include rhinocerebral mucormycosis (zygomycosis; see chapter 1.8), squamous carcinoma, diabetic angiopathy presenting

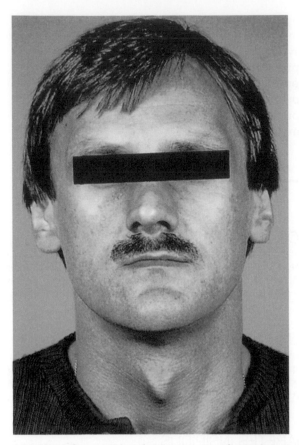

*Figure 1.2.1* Hypoadrenocorticism showing cutaneous hyperpigmentation.

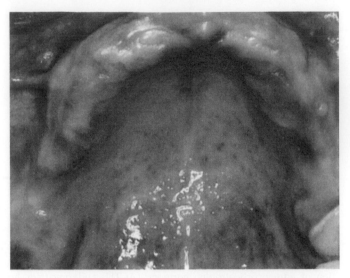

*Figure 1.2.2* Hypoadrenocorticism showing oral hyperpigmentation.

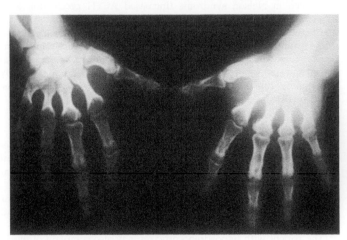

*Figure 1.2.4* Hypoparathyroidism showing shortened metacarpal bones.

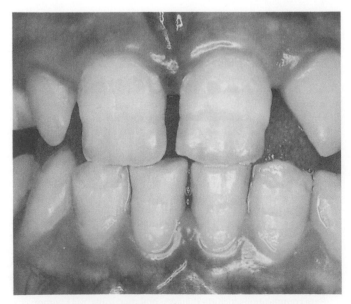

*Figure 1.2.3* Hypoparathyroidism showing hypoplastic teeth.

with palatal petechiae and acanthosis nigricans. Mononeuritis multiplex may cause facial palsy.

## GIGANTISM/ACROMEGALY

Gigantism/acromegaly—caused by excessive growth hormone, from a pituitary adenoma—lead to excessive weight and height, plus pressure effects from the tumour such as headache and visual defects. Gigantism can also manifest with spaced teeth, mandibular prognathism, macroglossia and megadontia (Fig. 1.2.9).

## HYPERPARATHYROIDISM

Hyperparathyroidism—overactivity of the parathyroid glands resulting in excess production of parathyroid hormone—disturbs calcium and bone homeostasis. This primary type causes skeletal lesions in virtually

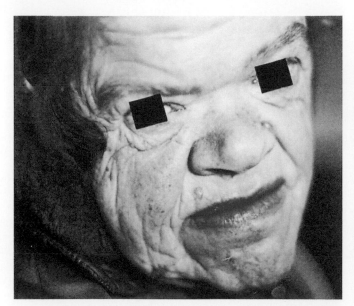

*Figure 1.2.5* Hypothyroidism—facies of congenital hypothyroidism.

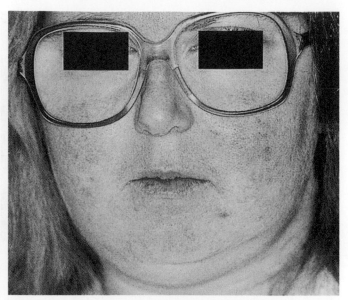

*Figure 1.2.6* Cushingoid facies (moon face).

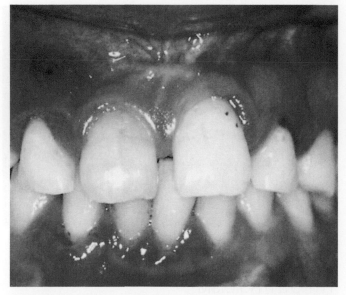

*Figure 1.2.7* Diabetes mellitus showing periodontitis and abscesses.

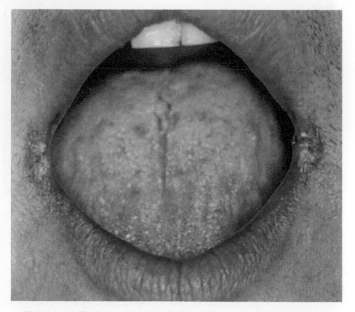

*Figure 1.2.8* Diabetes showing dry mouth and angular stomatitis.

all patients, microscopically indistinguishable from the central giant cell granuloma of bone (brown tumours).

### Clinical features

Skeletal changes in primary hyperparathyroidism typically include generalised rarefaction, and sometimes lytic lesions (osteitis fibrosa cystica), but an almost pathognomonic oral change is the loss of the lamina dura (Figs 1.2.10–1.2.12). The characteristic radiographic sign of the condition is subperiosteal bone resorption, and 'tufting' of terminal phalanges. Skull and jaw involvement are late complications.

Giant-cell granulomas are not always associated with hyperparathyroidism.

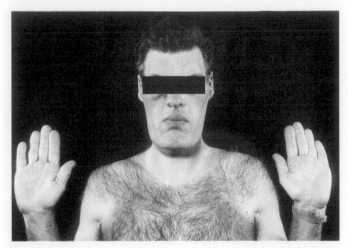

*Figure 1.2.9* Gigantism showing large hands and mandible.

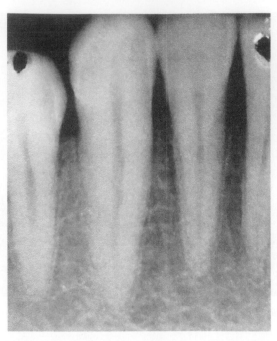

*Figure 1.2.10* Hyperparathyroidism—loss of lamina dura.

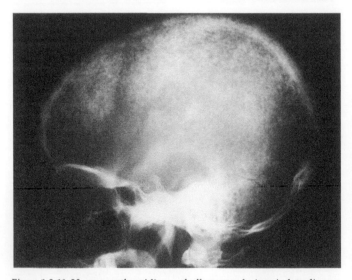

*Figure 1.2.11* Hyperparathyroidism—skull osseous lesions in late disease.

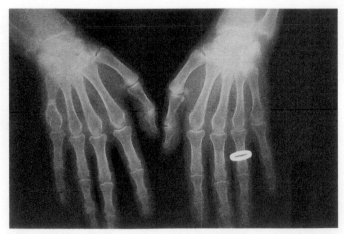

*Figure 1.2.12* Hyperparathyroidism—tufting of terminal phalanges.

**Diagnosis**
Imaging may confirm the above bone changes. Serology will reveal raised calcium, reduced phosphate and increased alkaline phosphatase levels.

**Management**
Parathyroidectomy.

## HYPERTHYROIDISM

Hyperthyroidism—excessive production of thyroid hormones—has no specific maxillofacial manifestations. Radioiodine therapy of hyperthyroidism occasionally produces hyposalivation. Some anti-thyroid drugs (e.g. carbimazole) may produce neutropenia with resultant oral ulceration. Thyroiditis may manifest with xerostomia.

## HYPOTHYROIDISM

Hypothyroidism may follow radioiodine therapy of hyperthyroidism, or treatment of laryngeal neoplasms, or removal of a lingual thyroid in the absence of normal thyroid tissue. Hypothyroidism may underlie a few cases of orofacial pain, burning mouth syndrome or periodontitis. Thyroiditis may manifest with xerostomia.

## MULTIPLE ENDOCRINE NEOPLASIA (ADENOMA) (MEN OR MEA) SYNDROMES

MEN or MEA—rare autosomal dominant conditions of multiple endocrine glands—feature tumours which can be benign or malignant (Table 1.2.1). MEN 2B can cause oral mucosal neuromas (Figs 1.2.13 and 1.2.14).

**TABLE 1.2.1** MULTIPLE ENDOCRINE NEOPLASIA (MEN) SYNDROMES

| Gene | 1 | 2A (Werner syndrome) | 2B (Sipple syndrome) | FMTC |
|---|---|---|---|---|
| | MEN1 | RET | RET | RET |
| Mucosal neuromas | − | − | + | − |
| Medullary thyroid carcinoma | − | + | + | + |
| Parathyroid hyperplasia | + | + | − | − |
| Phaeochromocytoma | − | + | ± | − |
| Pituitary adenoma; pancreatic tumours | + | − | − | − |

*Abbreviations*: FMTC, familial medullary thyroid carcinoma; RET, rearrangement during transfection.

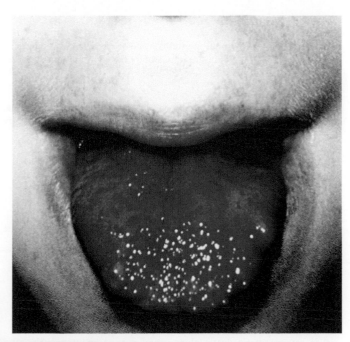

Figure 1.2.13 Multiple endocrine adenoma syndrome—mucosal neuromas.

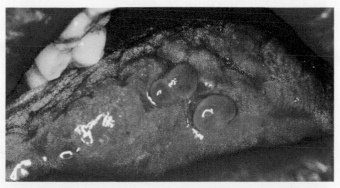

Figure 1.2.14 Multiple endocrine adenoma syndrome—mucosal neuromas.

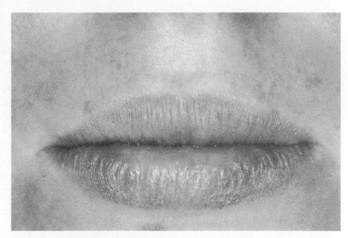

Figure 1.2.15 Pregnancy—chloasma.

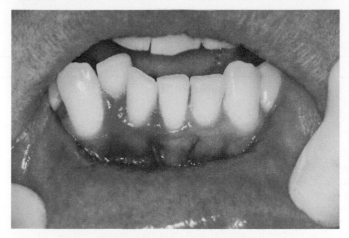

Figure 1.2.16 Pregnancy gingivitis.

## PITUITARY DWARFISM

Pituitary dwarfism—due to hypopituitarism—though rare, can present with microdontia and delayed tooth eruption.

## PRECOCIOUS PUBERTY

Precocious puberty—the onset of puberty before the age of seven to eight years—can have several causes including exposure to bisphenol A (*bis*–glycidyl methacrylate; found in some dental resins), and can cause accelerated tooth eruption (and in McCune–Albright syndrome, it is associated with fibrous dysplasia).

## PREGNANCY

Pregnancy, mainly after second month, may result in exacerbation of chronic gingivitis ('pregnancy gingivitis'). Pyogenic granulomas are also fairly common in pregnancy at the site of a particularly dense plaque accumulation and are then termed pregnancy epulides (Figs 1.2.15–1.2.17).

## Clinical features

*Pregnancy gingivitis*

A highly vascular marginal gingivitis appears at the second month of pregnancy, reaches a maximum intensity by the eighth month and then regresses.

*Pregnancy epulis*

This is a soft, red or occasionally firm, swelling of a dental papilla, usually found anteriorly. It may be asymptomatic unless traumatised by biting or toothbrushing.

## Diagnosis

- Biopsy sometimes.
- Pregnancy test occasionally.
- Differentiate
  - Pregnancy gingivitis: from Wegener granulomatosis (rarely; see chapter 1.1).
  - Pregnancy epulis: from other epulides.

## Management

- Pregnancy gingivitis: improve the oral hygiene.
- Pregnancy epulis: improve the oral hygiene.
  - If asymptomatic, leave alone—may regress spontaneously after parturition.
  - If symptomatic, excision biopsy.

## PRETERM CHILDREN

Preterm children may have enamel defects and/or palatal grooving, a higher number of malocclusion traits, more malocclusion traits per individual, a greater orthodontic treatment need and altered craniofacial morphology. The anterior cranial base tends to be significantly shorter with a less convex skeletal profile and significantly shorter maxillary length. The lower incisors are significantly more retroclined and retruded. There is a relation postulated between periodontitis and preterm births.

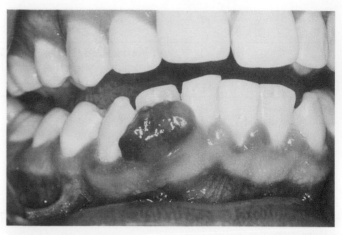

*Figure 1.2.17* Pregnancy epulis (pyogenic granuloma) and gingivitis.

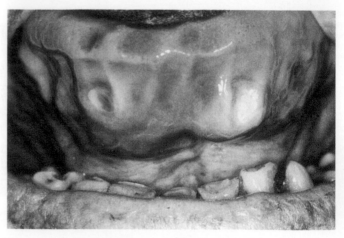

*Figure 1.2.18* Amyloid disease, causing macroglossia, resulting in impressions of the teeth and ulceration.

**TABLE 1.2.2** MAXILLOFACIAL MANIFESTATIONS IN METABOLIC DISORDERS

| Disorder | Manifestations |
| --- | --- |
| Alcaptonuria | Tooth discolouration |
| Amyloidosis | Amyloid deposits in mouth or salivary glands, enlarged tongue, purpura (Fig. 1.2.18), possible obstructive sleep apnoea |
| Autoinflammatory syndromes | Aphthous-like ulcers |
| Congenital hyperuricaemia (Lesch–Nyhan syndrome) | Self-mutilation (Fig. 1.2.19) |
| Erythropoietic porphyria | Reddish teeth, bullae/erosions, dental hypoplasia |
| Haemochromatosis | Salivary swelling, dry mouth, hyperpigmentation. Labial salivary gland biopsy may assist diagnosis |
| Hypophosphataemia | Dental hypoplasia, large pulp chambers (Fig. 1.2.20) |
| Hypophosphatasia | Loosening and loss of teeth (hypoplastic cementum) |
| Lipoid proteinosis | Mucosal lumps, gingival swelling (Figs 1.2.21 and 1.2.22), salivary swelling |
| Mucopolysaccharidoses | Spaced teeth, delayed tooth eruption, temporomandibular joint anomalies, enamel defects (Figs 1.2.23–1.2.25) |
| Niemann–Pick disease | Delayed tooth eruption, loosening of teeth, mucosal hyperpigmentation |
| Rickets (vitamin D dependent) | Dental hypoplasia, large pulp chambers |
| Trimethylaminuria | Halitosis |
| Vitamin B12 or folic acid deficiency | Ulcers, glossitis, angular cheilitis, burning mouth (Fig. 1.2.26) |
| Vitamin C deficiency (scurvy) | Gingival swelling, purpura, ulcers (Figs 1.2.27 and 1.2.28) |

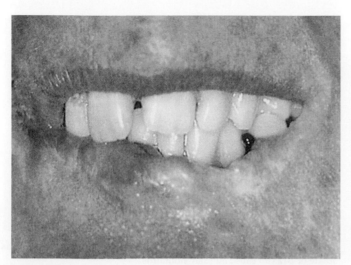

Figure 1.2.19  Lesch–Nyhan syndrome with consequent self-mutilation.

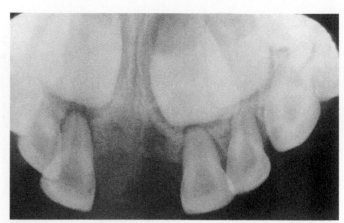

*Figure 1.2.20*  Hypophosphatasia—large pulp chambers and early loss of deciduous teeth.

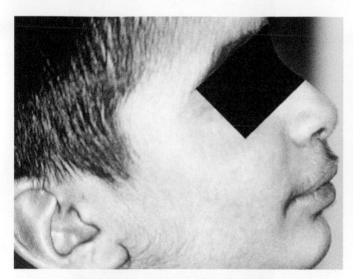

*Figure 1.2.21*  Lipoid proteinosis showing everted fissured lips.

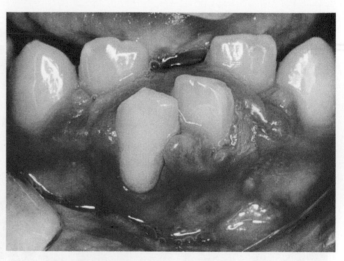

*Figure 1.2.22*  Lipoid proteinosis—gingival swelling and malocclusion.

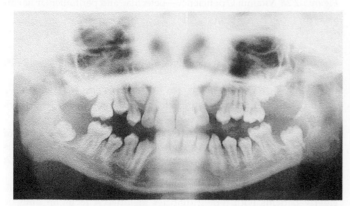

*Figure 1.2.23*  Hurler syndrome—delayed and incomplete tooth eruption and radiolucencies around crowns of second molars.

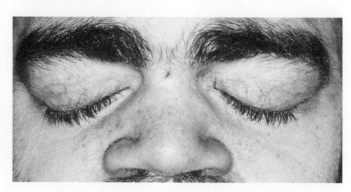

*Figure 1.2.24*  Hurler syndrome—facies and hirsutism.

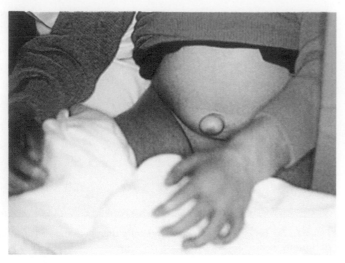

*Figure 1.2.25* Hurler syndrome—clawed hands, hepatosplenomegaly, umbilical hernia.

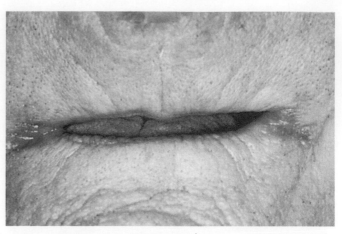

*Figure 1.2.26* Vitamin B deficiency—deficiencies of B vitamins such as folate or B12 can cause angular stomatitis.

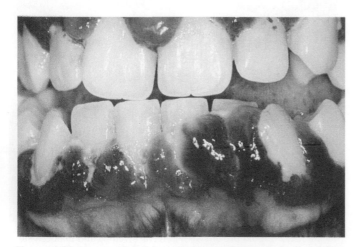

*Figure 1.2.27* Vitamin C deficiency here manifests with frank swollen, haemorrhagic and ulcerated gingivae.

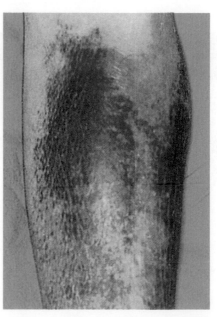

*Figure 1.2.28* Vitamin C deficiency—petechiae and perifollicular haemorrhage.

## METABOLIC DISORDERS

Other metabolic disorders can present with maxillofacial manifestations (Table 1.2.2).

## FURTHER READING

Al-Sebeih K, Karagiozov K, Jafar A. Penetrating craniofacial injury in a pediatric patient. J Craniofac Surg 2002; 13: 303–7.

Bsoul SA, Terezhalmy GT, Moore WS. Addison disease (adrenal insufficiency). Quintessence Int 2003; 34: 784–5.

Chan KC, Edelman M, Fantasia JE. Labial salivary gland involvement in neonatal hemochromatosis: a report of 2 cases and review of literature. Oral Surg Oral Med Oral Pathol Oral Radiol Endod 2008; 106: e27–30.

Chang CP, Shiau YC, Wang JJ, Ho ST, Kao CH. Decreased salivary gland function in patients with autoimmune thyroiditis. Head Neck 2003; 25: 132–7.

Changlai SP, Chen WK, Chung C, Chiou SM. Objective evidence of decreased salivary function in patients with autoimmune thyroiditis (chronic thyroiditis, Hashimoto's thyroiditis). Nucl Med Commun 2002; 23: 1029–33.

Collin HL, Niskanen L, Uusitupa M, et al. Oral symptoms and signs in elderly patients with type 2 diabetes mellitus. A focus on diabetic neuropathy. Oral Surg Oral Med Oral Pathol Oral Radiol Endod 2000; 90: 299–305.

Daniels JS. Primary hyperparathyroidism presenting as a palatal brown tumor. Oral Surg Oral Med Oral Pathol Oral Radiol Endod 2004; 98: 409–13.

Femiano F, Lanza A, Buonaiuto C, et al. Burning mouth syndrome and burning mouth in hypothyroidism: proposal for a diagnostic and therapeutic protocol. Oral Surg Oral Med Oral Pathol Oral Radiol Endod 2008; 105: e22–7.

Fukui N, Amano A, Akiyama S, Daikoku H, Wakisaka S. Oral findings in DiGeorge syndrome: clinical features and histologic study of primary teeth. Oral Surg Oral Med Oral Pathol Oral Radiol Endod 2000; 89: 208–15.

Harila V, Heikkinen T, Grön M, Alvesalo L. Open bite in prematurely born children. J Dent Child (Chic) 2007; 74: 165–70.

Jabbour SA. Cutaneous manifestations of endocrine disorders: a guide for dermatologists. Am J Clin Dermatol 2003; 4: 315–31.

Kar DK, Gupta SK, Agarwal A, Mishra SK. Brown tumor of the palate and mandible in association with primary hyperparathyroidism. J Oral Maxillofac Surg 2001; 59: 1352–4.

Kelly A, Pomarico L, de Souza IP. Cessation of dental development in a child with idiopathic hypoparathyroidism: a 5-year follow-up. Oral Surg Oral Med Oral Pathol Oral Radiol Endod 2009; 107: 673–7.

Lin CC, Sun SS, Kao A, Lee CC. Impaired salivary function in patients with noninsulin-dependent diabetes mellitus with xerostomia. J Diabetes Complications 2002; 16: 176–9.

Machuca G, Rodríguez S, Martínez M, Bullón P, Machuca C. Descriptive study about the influence of general health and socio-cultural variables on the periodontal health of early menopausal patients. Periodontology 2005; 2: 75–84.

Manfredi M, McCullough MJ, Vescovi P, Al-Kaarawi ZM, Porter SR. Update on diabetes mellitus and related oral diseases. Oral Dis 2004; 10: 187–200.

McGovern E, Fleming P, Costigan C, Dominguez M, Coleman DC. Oral health in autoimmune polyendocrinopathy candidiasis ectodermal dystrophy (APECED). Eur Arch Paediatr Dent 2008; 9: 236–44.

Moore PA, Guggenheimer J, Etzel KR, Weyant RJ, Orchard T. Type 1 diabetes mellitus, xerostomia, and salivary flow rates. Oral Surg Oral Med Oral Pathol Oral Radiol Endod 2001; 92: 281–91.

Muzzi L, Pini Prato GP, Ficarrat G. Langerhans' cell histiocytosis diagnosed through periodontal lesions: a case report. J Periodontol 2002; 73: 1528–33.

Paulsson L. Premature birth—studies on orthodontic treatment need, craniofacial morphology and function. Swed Dent J Suppl 2009; 199: 9–66.

Paulsson L, Bondemark L. Craniofacial morphology in prematurely born children. Angle Orthod 2009; 79: 276–83.

Perniola R, Tamborrino G, Marsigliante S, De Rinaldis C. Assessment of enamel hypoplasia in autoimmune polyendocrinopathy-candidiasis-ectodermal dystrophy (APECED). J Oral Pathol Med 1998; 27: 278–82.

Porter SR, Glover S, Scully C. Oral hyperpigmentation and adrenocortical hypofunction in a patient with acquired immunodeficiency syndrome. Oral Surg Oral Med Oral Pathol 1990; 70: 59–60.

Porter SR, Haria S, Scully C, Richards A. Chronic candidiasis, enamel hypoplasia, and pigmentary anomalies. Oral Surg Oral Med Oral Pathol 1992; 74: 312–14.

Rythén M, Norén JG, Sabel N, et al. Morphological aspects of dental hard tissues in primary teeth from preterm infants. Int J Paediatr Dent 2008; 18: 397–406.

Sacco G, Carmagnola D, Abati S, et al. Periodontal disease and preterm birth relationship: a review of the literature. Minerva Stomatol 2008; 57: 233–46, 246–50.

Sallai A, Hosszú E, Gergics P, Rácz K, Fekete G. Orolabial signs are important clues for diagnosis of the rare endocrine syndrome MEN 2B. Presentation of two unrelated cases. Eur J Pediatr 2008; 167: 441–6.

Scardina GA, Messina P. Modifications of interdental papilla microcirculation: a possible cause of periodontal disease in Hashimoto's thyroiditis? Ann Anat 2008; 190: 258–63.

Scully C, Diz Dios P, Shotts R. Oral health care in patients with the most important medically compromising conditions; 8. Diabetes mellitus. CPD Dent 2005; 6: 7–11.

Scully C, Hodgson T, Porter SR. Mouth conditions in the elderly; part 2. Practitioner 2000; 244: 1050–5.

Scully C, Porter SR, Hodgson T. Mouth conditions in the elderly; part 1. Practitioner 2000; 244: 938–53.

Shah SS, Oh CH, Coffin SE, Yan AC. Addisonian pigmentation of the oral mucosa. Cutis 2005; 76: 97–9.

Skamagas M, Breen TL, LeRoith D. Update on diabetes mellitus: prevention, treatment, and association with oral diseases. Oral Dis 2008; 14: 105–14.

Szymajda A, Eledrisi MS, Patel R, et al. Diabetes insipidus as a consequence of neurologic involvement in Behçet's syndrome. Endocr Pract 2003; 9: 33–5.

Taylor GW, Borgnakke WS. Periodontal disease: associations with diabetes, glycemic control and complications. Oral Dis 2008; 14: 191–203.

Wittmann AL. Macroglossia in acromegaly and hypothyroidism. Virchows Arch A Pathol Anat Histol 1977; 373: 353–60.

Zambrano M, Nikitakis NG, Sanchez-Quevedo MC, Sauk JJ, Sedano H. Oral and dental manifestations of vitamin D-dependent rickets type I: report of a pediatric case. Oral Surg Oral Med Oral Pathol Oral Radiol Endod 2003; 95: 705–9.

# 1.3 GASTROINTESTINAL AND PANCREATIC DISORDERS

- chronic pancreatitis
- coeliac disease
- Crohn disease
- cystic fibrosis
- familial adenomatous polyposis (FAP)
- gastro-oesophageal reflux disease (GORD)

- malabsorption
- neoplasms
- pernicious anaemia
- Peutz–Jegher syndrome
- short bowel syndrome
- ulcerative colitis

## CHRONIC PANCREATITIS

Chronic pancreatitis—often associated with alcoholism or autoimmunity—may have impaired salivary gland function and sialosis as a rare presentation. Occasionally, autoimmune pancreatitis is associated with Mikulicz disease (chapters 1.15 and 2.7).

## COELIAC DISEASE

Coeliac disease (gluten-sensitive enteropathy)—a reaction to gliaden, a gluten protein found in wheat, rye and barley—causes an autoimmune reaction and damage to the jejunum, causing malabsorption. Other autoimmune disorders, IgA deficiency, and dermatitis herpetiformis may be associated. Spongiosis is seen in the oral mucosa and, in severe coeliac disease, affected children may suffer ulcers, glossitis, angular stomatitis and tooth enamel defects (which can also be seen in healthy first-degree relatives).

Up to 3% of patients seen as out-patients with recurrent mouth ulcers prove to have coeliac disease (Figs 1.3.1 and 1.3.2).

Patients with dermatitis herpetiformis often also have coeliac disease.

## CROHN DISEASE

Crohn disease—and conditions such as orofacial granulomatosis (OFG), Melkersson–Rosenthal syndrome (MRS) and granulomatous cheilitis (GC)—appear related. These other conditions may well represent oligosymptomatic Crohn disease since they appear microscopically like Crohn disease to show submucosal chronic inflammation with many mononuclear, interleukin-1 producing cells and non-caseating granulomas in the submucosa and lymph nodes. Crohn disease can involve any part of the gastrointestinal tract, including the mouth.

The inflammatory response is probably mediated by factors such as tumour necrosis factor alpha. *Mycobacterium avium* subspecies *paratuberculosis* is one agent incriminated in Crohn disease, and other workers have implicated a lack of *Faecalibacterium prausnitzii*. Diet, oral contraceptives, nonsteroidal antiinflammatory drugs, isotretinoin and smoking have also been incriminated. *Mycobacterium paratuberculosis* has also been incriminated in MRS, while OFG may sometimes result from adverse reactions to various food additives, such as cinnamaldehyde or benzoates, butylated hydroxyanisole or dodecyl gallate (in margarine), or to menthol (in peppermint oil) or cobalt, though these reactions are by no means always relevant.

### Clinical features

In Crohn disease and in OFG, facial or labial swelling, mucosal tags or gingival purple granulomatous enlargements, cobblestoning of mucosa, ulcers, glossitis, angular stomatitis, and painless, persistent cervical lymphadenopathy may be seen. Ulcers classically involve the buccal sulcus where they appear as linear ulcers, often with granulomatous masses flanking them (Figs 1.3.3–1.3.14).

The regional lymph nodes are enlarged in 50% of cases. In Crohn disease, there may also be gastrointestinal symptoms, perianal tags (Fig. 1.3.15), fever and mild constitutional symptoms including headache and even visual disturbance. Pyostomatitis vegetans may also be seen, but is more usually associated with ulcerative colitis.

### Diagnosis

Thorough investigation to eliminate other causes of granulomatous disease such as sarcoidosis is essential (biopsy, full blood picture, levels of albumin, calcium, folate, iron and vitamin B12: intestinal radiology, sigmoidoscopy and colonoscopy, chest radiography, serum levels of calcium, angiotensin-converting enzyme and gallium scan).

Dietary-related cases can only be confirmed by an exclusion diet to eliminate food allergens. Skin tests may be useful.

### Management

Reactions to dietary components should be sought and possible provoking substances avoided. Elimination diets may be warranted in some patients with OFG. Conservative management has included nonsteroidal anti-inflammatory agents, antimicrobials, antimalarials, clofazimine and mast cell stabilizers, or intralesional corticosteroid injections.

Metronidazole may produce resolution in GC. Clofazimine appears effective during the early stages.

Intralesional corticosteroid injections may also reduce the swelling. The injection of triamcinolone into the lips after local analgesia may be effective. The injections may have to be repeated every four to six months once a response plateau has been reached.

Other managements which have occasionally been helpful include long-term penicillin, minocycline, erythromycin, ketotifen or immunomodulators. Systemic corticosteroids are rarely indicated; not all respond. Azathioprine, dapsone, sulphapyridine or salazopyrine may be helpful.

## CYSTIC FIBROSIS

Cystic fibrosis (chapter 1.14).

## FAMILIAL ADENOMATOUS POLYPOSIS (FAP)

FAP—an autosomal dominant condition caused by mutation in the *APC* tumour suppressor gene on chromosome 5—is characterized by the development during the second decade of life of hundreds of adenomas in the colon and rectum. These eventually cause rectal bleeding or anaemia, or develop into cancer.

A less aggressive variant—termed attenuated FAP, is characterized by fewer colorectal adenomatous polyps (usually 10–100), a later age of adenoma appearance and a lower cancer risk.

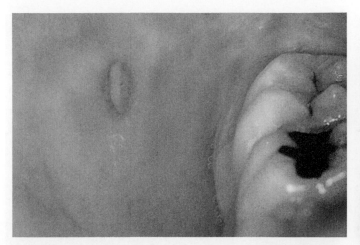

Figure 1.3.1 Coeliac disease showing aphthous-like ulceration.

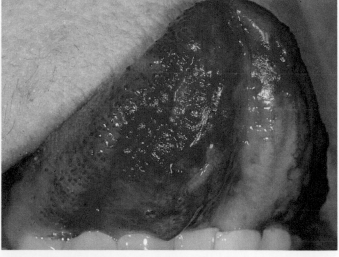

Figure 1.3.2 Coeliac disease leading to iron, B12 and folate deficiency and Moeller glossitis.

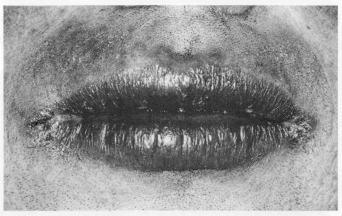

Figure 1.3.3 Orofacial granulomatosis presenting with swollen lips and angular stomatitis.

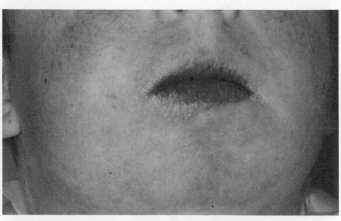

Figure 1.3.4 Orofacial granulomatosis presenting with cheek swelling.

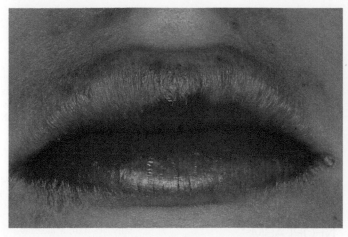

Figure 1.3.5 Crohn disease presenting with lip swelling.

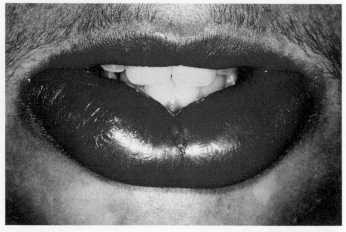

Figure 1.3.6 Crohn disease causing lip swelling to the extent there is fissuring.

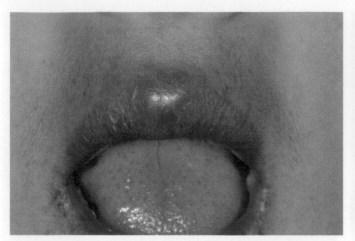

*Figure 1.3.7* Crohn disease causing upper lip swelling mainly.

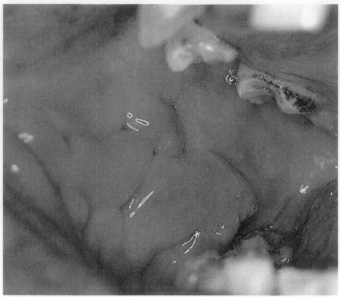

*Figure 1.3.8* Orofacial granulomatosis presenting with mucosal cobblestoning.

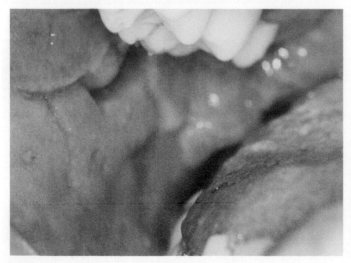

*Figure 1.3.9* Crohn disease—cobblestoning.

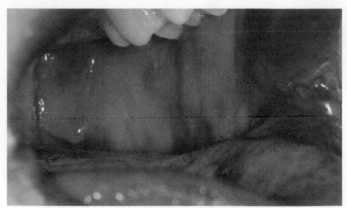

*Figure 1.3.10* Crohn disease—mucosal tag.

### Clinical features

FAP is initially symptomless but later gastrointestinal features appear. Extraintestinal manifestations may include osteomas, dental anomalies (unerupted teeth, agenesis of one or more teeth, supernumerary teeth, dentigerous cysts and odontomas), congenital hypertrophy of retinal pigment epithelium, desmoid tumours and extracolonic cancers (thyroid, liver, bile ducts and central nervous system).

Where there are skull and mandible osteomas, dental abnormalities and fibromas on scalp, shoulders, arms and back, the term Gardner syndrome is employed (Figs 1.3.16–1.3.18).

### Diagnosis

Clinical plus imaging and colonic polyp biopsy.

### Management

The intestinal polyps have a 100% risk of undergoing malignant transformation: therefore, the early identification of disease and colectomy is critical.

## GASTRO-OESOPHAGEAL REFLUX DISEASE (GORD)

GORD—a common condition where the lower oesophageal sphincter is abnormally relaxed and allows the stomach's acidic contents to flow back or 'reflux' into the oesophagus—can present with acid taste, tooth erosion and halitosis (Figs 1.3.19 and 1.3.20).

## MALABSORPTION

Malabsorption or malnutrition from any cause can present with ulcers, glossitis, burning mouth sensation and angular stomatitis (Fig. 1.3.21).

## NEOPLASMS

Neoplasms in the gastrointestinal tract may lead to aphthous-like ulcers, glossitis, angular stomatitis, occasionally jaw or other oral metastases,

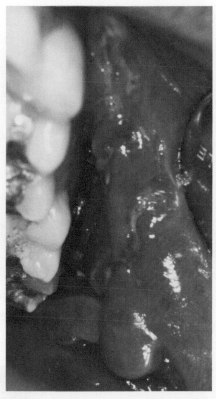

Figure 1.3.11 Crohn disease—gross cobblestoning.

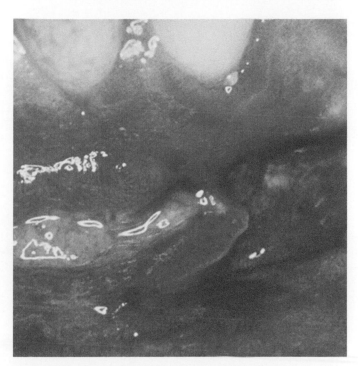

Figure 1.3.12 Crohn disease—mucosal tags.

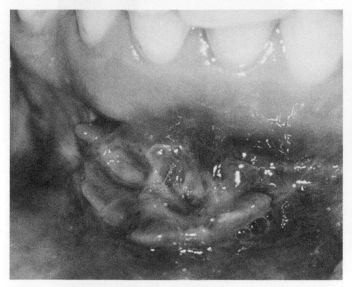

Figure 1.3.13 Crohn disease—mucosal tags.

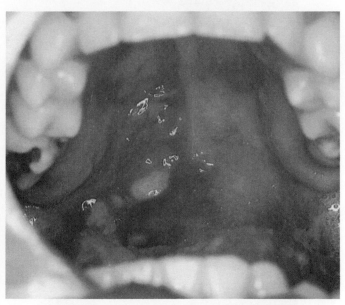

Figure 1.3.14 Crohn disease—aphthous-like ulceration.

or rarely, hyperpigmentation or acanthosis nigricans (Figs 1.3.22 and 1.3.23) (chapter 1.11).

## PERNICIOUS ANAEMIA

Pernicious anaemia—an autoimmune condition due to antibodies directed against gastric parietal cells, which then fail to produce the intrinsic factor necessary for vitamin B12 absorption in the terminal ileum—can present with ulcers, glossitis, burning mouth sensation or angular stomatitis.

## PEUTZ–JEGHER SYNDROME

Peutz–Jegher syndrome (lentigo polyposis)—an autosomal dominant disorder, due to a chromosome 19p *STK11/LKB1* (serine/threonine

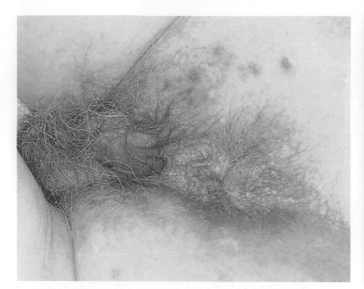

*Figure 1.3.15* Crohn disease—perianal disease.

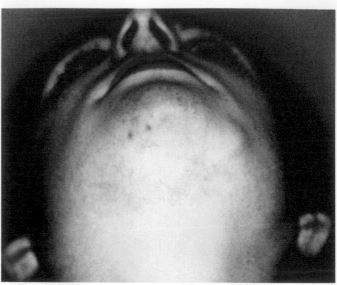

*Figure 1.3.16* Gardner syndrome—desmoid tumour.

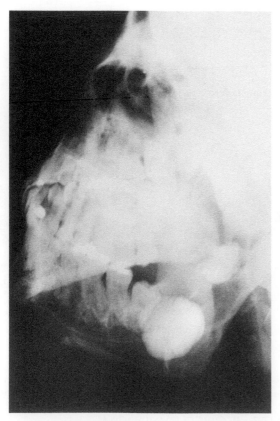

*Figure 1.3.17* Gardner syndrome—osteomas.

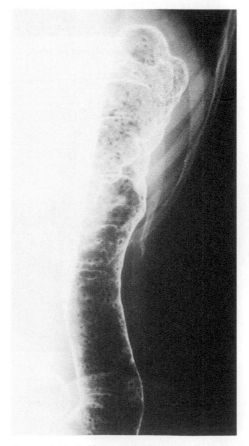

*Figure 1.3.18* Gardner syndrome; colonic polyps.

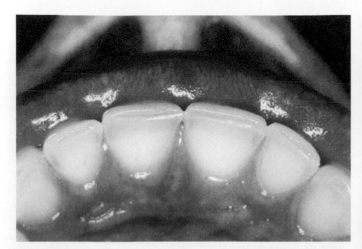

*Figure 1.3.19* Gastro-oesophageal reflux disease showing tooth erosion palatally.

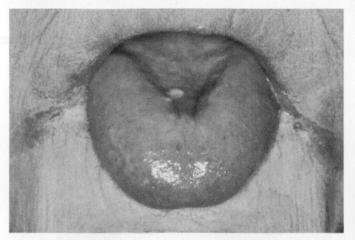

*Figure 1.3.21* Gastrointestinal neoplasm resulting in iron deficiency, glossitis and angular stomatitis.

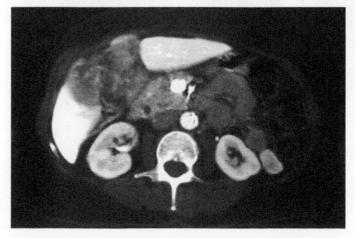

*Figure 1.3.23* Neoplasm underlying acanthosis nigricans.

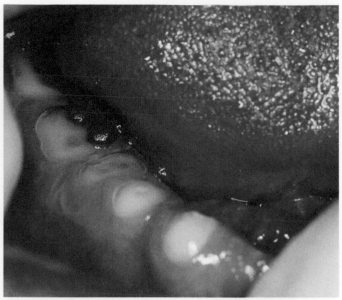

*Figure 1.3.20* Gastro-oesophageal reflux disease—severe case showing advanced erosion.

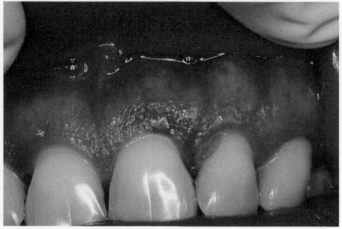

*Figure 1.3.22* Acanthosis nigricans affecting the gingiva in a patient with cholangiocarcinoma.

kinase 11) gene mutation causing a DNA repair defect—presents with circumoral melanosis and intestinal polyposis.

### Clinical features

Mucocutaneous melanotic macules are seen around the lips (Fig. 1.3.24), nose and sometimes eyes, and intraorally at any site, although rarely on the tongue or floor of mouth. The pigmentation is typically spray-like and brown and precedes detection of polyps. The polyps, mainly in the

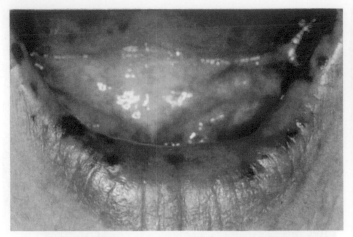

*Figure 1.3.24* Peutz–Jegher syndrome hyperpigmented macules on lips.

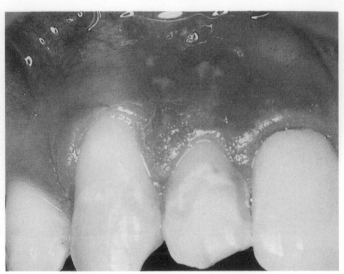

*Figure 1.3.25* Ulcerative colitis causing pyostomatitis vegetans.

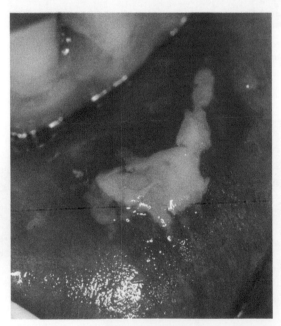

*Figure 1.3.26* Ulcerative colitis can mimic syphilis with snailtrack ulceration.

small intestine, may cause intussusception and obstruction. Almost 50% of patients with Peutz–Jegher syndrome also develop and die from cancer by age 57 years: malignant neoplasms may involve the gastrointestinal tract, ovary, cervix, testis and breast.

*Diagnosis*
Clinical and imaging.

*Management*
Gastrointestinal consultation.

## SHORT BOWEL SYNDROME

Short bowel syndrome—a malabsorption condition caused by the surgical removal of part of the small intestine—may lead to alveolar bone loss.

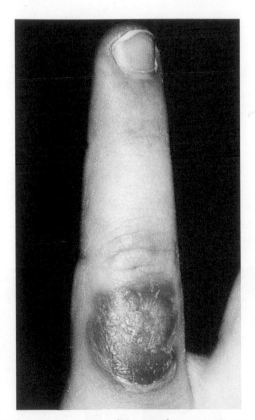

*Figure 1.3.27* Ulcerative colitis—pyoderma gangrenosum.

## ULCERATIVE COLITIS

Ulcerative colitis—an idiopathic inflammatory bowel disorder that affects the colon with ulceration and polyps—can cause oral pustules (pyostomatitis vegetans), and ulcers (Figs 1.3.25–1.3.27). Pyodermatitis–pyostomatitis vegetans is a rare vegetating, pustular, eosinophilic, mucocutaneous disorder characterized by genital, axillary and oral lesions, as well as lesions on the scalp. Ophthalmic, musculoskeletal: cutaneous lesions, together with erythema nodosum and deep vein thrombosis are features that can mimic Behçet syndrome.

## FURTHER READING

Aggarwal VR, Sloan P, Horner K, et al. Dento-osseous changes as diagnostic markers in familial adenomatous polyposis families. Oral Dis 2003; 9: 29–33.

Bartlett DW, Evans DF, Smith BG. The relationship between gastro-oesophageal reflux disease and dental erosion. J Oral Rehabil 1996; 23: 289–97.

Campisi G, Compilato D, Iacono G, et al. Histomorphology of healthy oral mucosa in untreated celiac patients: unexpected association with spongiosis. J Oral Pathol 2009; 38: 34–41.

Campisi G, Di Liberto C, Carroccio A, et al. Celiac disease: oral ulcer prevalence, assessment of risk and association with gluten free diet in children. Dig Liver Dis 2008; 40: 104–7.

Capodiferro S, Scully C, Ficcarra G, et al. Orofacial granulomatosis; report of two cases with gingival onset. Eur J Inflamm 2007; 5: 51–6.

Daley TD, Armstrong JE. Oral manifestations of gastrointestinal diseases. Can J Gastroenterol 2007; 21: 241–4.

Farrokhi F, Vaezi MF. Extra-esophageal manifestations of gastroesophageal reflux. Oral Dis 2007; 13: 349–59.

Flutter L, Mulik R. Peutz–Jegher syndrome. Arch Dis Child 2008; 93: 163.

Half E, Bercovich D, Rozen P. Familial adenomatous polyposis. Orphanet J Rare Dis 2009; 4: 22.

Hegarty AM, Barrett AW, Scully C. Pyostomatitis vegetans. Clin Exp Dermatol 2004; 28: 1–7.

Kamisawa T, Tu Y, Egawa N, et al. Salivary gland involvement in chronic pancreatitis of various etiologies. Am J Gastroenterol 2003; 98: 323–6.

Kamisawa T, Tu Y, Sasaki R, et al. The relationship of salivary gland function to elevated serum IgG4 in autoimmune pancreatitis. Intern Med 2007; 46: 435–9.

Leão JC, Hodgson T, Scully C, Porter S. Review article: orofacial granulomatosis. Aliment Pharmacol Ther 2004; 20: 1019–27.

Lo Russo L, Campisi G, Di Fede O, et al. Oral manifestations of eating disorders: a critical review. Oral Dis 2008; 14: 479–84.

Malahias T, Cheng J, Brar P, Minaya MT, Green PH. The association between celiac disease, dental enamel defects, and aphthous ulcers in a United States Cohort. J Clin Gastroenterol 2009. [Epub ahead of print].

Pastore L, Campisi G, Compilato D, Lo Muzio L. Orally based diagnosis of celiac disease: current perspectives. J Dent Res 2008; 87: 1100–7.

Pastore L, Carroccio A, Compilato D, et al. Oral manifestations of celiac disease. J Clin Gastroenterol 2008; 42: 224–32.

Pereira CM, Coletta RD, Jorge J, Lopes MA. Peutz–Jeghers syndrome in a 14-year-old boy: case report and review of the literature. Int J Paediatr Dent 2005; 15: 224–8.

Rowland M, Fleming P, Bourke B. Looking in the mouth for Crohn's disease. Inflamm Bowel Dis 2009; 16: 332–37.

Scully C. Gastroenterological diseases and the mouth. Practitioner 2001; 245: 215–22.

da Silva PC, de Almeida Pdel V, Machado MA, et al. Oral manifestations of celiac disease. A case report and review of the literature. Med Oral Patol Oral Cir Bucal 2008; 13: E559–62.

Tilakaratne WM, Freysdottir J, Fortune F. Orofacial granulomatosis: review on aetiology and pathogenesis. J Oral Pathol Med 2008; 37: 191–5.

Wijn MA, Keller JJ, Giardiello FM, Brand HS. Oral and maxillofacial manifestations of familial adenomatous polyposis. Oral Dis 2007; 13; 360–5.

# 1.4 HAEMATOLOGICAL DISEASE

- agranulocytosis
- aplastic anaemia
- bleeding tendencies
- Fanconi anaemia
- haematinic deficiency
- haematopoietic stem cell transplantation
- haemoglobinopathies
- haemolytic disease of newborn
- haemophilia
- hypereosinophilic syndrome (HES)

- hypoplasminogenaemia
- leukaemias
- leukocyte defects
- lymphomas
- multiple myeloma
- plasmacytosis
- Plummer–Vinson syndrome
- polycythaemia
- thrombocytopenia
- von Willebrand disease

## AGRANULOCYTOSIS
Agranulocytosis (see leukocyte defects).

## APLASTIC ANAEMIA
Aplastic anaemia—a rare acquired defect of all bone marrow haematopoietic blood lineages—can present with ulcers and a bleeding tendency (Fig. 1.4.1).

## BLEEDING TENDENCIES
Bleeding tendencies can result in gingival bleeding, oral purpura or haematomas (Figs 1.4.2 and 1.4.3).

## FANCONI ANAEMIA
Fanconi anaemia—an autosomal recessive disorder of short stature, skeletal anomalies and bone marrow aplasia—has an increased incidence of leukaemias and solid tumours, including oral carcinoma (Fig. 1.4.4). Microdontia and hypodontia are the main dental manifestations.

## HAEMATINIC DEFICIENCY
Haematinic deficiency (haematinics are agents such as iron, folic acid or vitamin B12 that improve the blood number of erythrocytes and/or the haemoglobin concentration) can underlie burning mouth sensation, glossitis, ulcers and angular stomatitis (Figs 1.4.5 and 1.4.6).

Glossitis is one oral manifestation which may be seen in the pre-anaemic stage as well as in anaemia. A significant proportion of patients with aphthous-like ulcers prove to be deficient in a haematinic. Angular stomatitis may be caused by haematinic deficiencies. Although deficiency of iron or other haematinics such as folate or vitamin B12 can cause sore tongue with atrophic glossitis, many haematinic-deficient patients with a sore tongue have no obvious glossitis.

### Clinical features
The tongue may appear completely normal but causes discomfort or burning sensation, or there may be:

- linear or patchy red lesions—especially in vitamin B12 deficiency,
- depapillation with erythema—in deficiencies of iron, folic acid or B vitamins,
- depapillation begins at the tip and margins of the dorsum but later involves the whole dorsum,
- pallor—in iron deficiency,
- ulceration and/or
- angular stomatitis.

Rare types of deficiency affect the tongue. They are as follows:

- Riboflavin: lingual papillae enlarge initially but are later lost,
- Niacin: red, swollen, enlarged "beefy" tongue and
- Pyridoxine: swollen, purplish tongue.

Deficiencies of vitamins of the B group other than B12 are an occasional cause of glossitis—mainly seen in chronic alcoholics or in those with malabsorption.

### Diagnosis
As sore tongue can be the initial symptom of a deficiency of iron, folate or vitamin B12 and can precede any fall in the haemoglobin level, a full blood picture with assays of iron, vitamin B and folate are essential in management. Biopsy is rarely indicated. Differentiate from erythema migrans, lichen planus and acute candidosis.

### Management
Replacement therapy *after* underlying cause of deficiency is established and rectified.

## HAEMATOPOIETIC STEM CELL TRANSPLANTATION
Haematopoietic stem cell transplantation necessitates that the patient is T-cell immunosuppressed to prevent graft rejection. Orofacial complications are mainly those related to the cytotoxic agents and immunosuppression used to prevent graft rejection, and may include mucositis, xerostomia, infections such as candidosis, herpes simplex virus (HSV)-related ulceration and hairy leukoplakia, and graft-versus-host disease (GVHD). HSV-1 oral shedding before transplantation is associated with a decreased survival rate in allograft patients. Lichenoid lesions, superficial mucoceles and sicca features may be

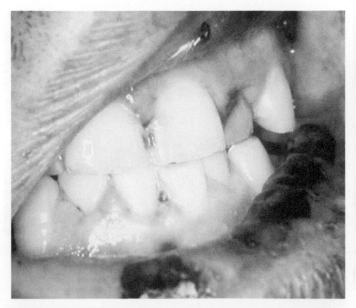

*Figure 1.4.1* Aplastic anaemia—spontaneous purpura and ecchymoses.

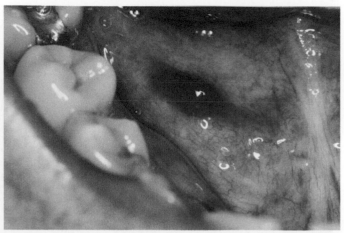

*Figure 1.4.2* Haematoma.

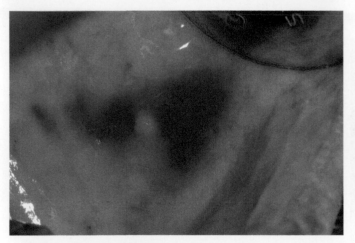

*Figure 1.4.3* Haematoma.

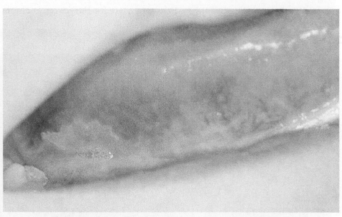

*Figure 1.4.4* Fanconi anaemia—pallor and leukoplakia.

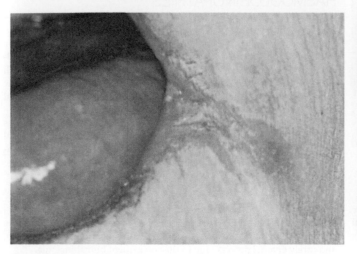

*Figure 1.4.5* Iron deficiency anaemia—glossitis and angular stomatitis.

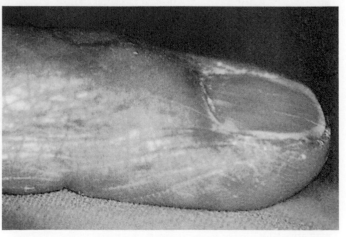

*Figure 1.4.6* Iron deficiency anaemia—koilonychia (spooned nails).

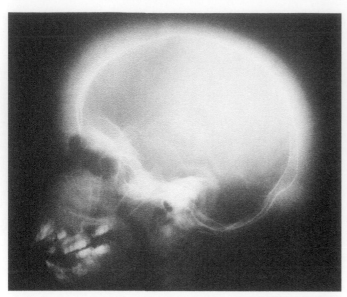

*Figure 1.4.7* Haemoglobinopathy—hair on end appearance from bone marrow hyperplasia attempting to compensate for the severe anaemia.

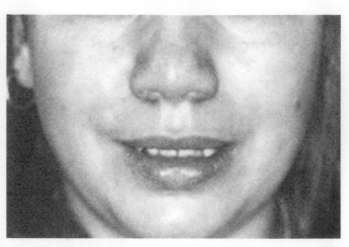

*Figure 1.4.8* Haemoglobinopathy—maxillary enlargement from bone marrow hyperplasia.

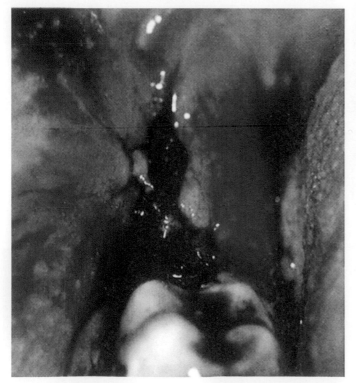

*Figure 1.4.9* Haemophilia—post-extraction bleeding.

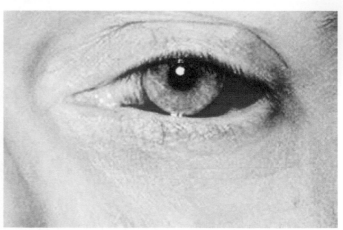

*Figure 1.4.10* Haemophilia—spontaneous bleeding into tissues.

## HAEMOGLOBINOPATHIES

Haemoglobinopathies—such as sickle cell anaemia and thalassaemias—may present with oral pallor, and maxillary hyperplasia owing to marrow expansion (Figs 1.4.7 and 1.4.8). There can be a radiographic stepladder appearance of the alveolar bone, and delayed dental development. *Thalassaemia major* may present with spiky-shaped short tooth roots, taurodont teeth, attenuated lamina dura, enlarged bone marrow spaces, small maxillary sinuses, absence of the inferior alveolar canal and thin mandibular cortex.

*Sickle cell anaemia* may also present with bone changes, and features related to infarcts, stroke and facial palsy, paraesthesia of the mental nerve, maxillofacial pain, pulpal necrosis and enamel hypomineralisation or occasionally with infections such as osteitis.

## HAEMOLYTIC DISEASE OF NEWBORN

Haemolytic disease of newborn (erythroblastosis fetalis)—an autoimmune reaction against erythrocytes—is a rare cause of tooth pigmentation, and rarely enamel defects, due to the consequent bilirubinaemia.

seen in GVHD. Drugs used after transplantation may also produce other maxillofacial adverse side-effects; the most common is gingival swelling caused by ciclosporin or nifedepine (chapter 1.6). Neoplasms may arise later.

## HAEMOPHILIA

Haemophilia—mainly due to a genetic defect of a blood coagulation factor—produces a bleeding tendency. Haemophilia A (classic haemophilia—due to deficient factor VIII) is 10 times as common as haemophilia B (Christmas disease) where factor IX is deficient. These defects of blood coagulation factors, or acquired haemophilia, unlike thrombocytopenia, rarely predispose to spontaneous gingival haemorrhage, oral petechiae or ecchymoses. Tooth eruption and exfoliation are usually uneventful but, occasionally, there can be a small bleed into the follicle. Any breach of the mucosa, however, especially tooth extraction, can lead to persistent bleeding (Figs 1.4.9–1.4.11) that is occasionally fatal. Bleeding into tissues causes aesthetic problems but, more importantly joint damage and a main danger is that haemorrhage into the fascial spaces, especially from surgery in the lower molar region, can track into the neck and embarrass the airway.

## HYPEREOSINOPHILIC SYNDROME (HES)

HES is a rare disorder characterised by persistent and marked eosinophilia and a poor prognosis because of end-organ damage (particularly endomyocardial fibrosis), or because of associated myeloid leukaemia or T-cell lymphoma. Oral mucosa ulceration can be seen early especially in the myeloproliferative form.

## HYPOPLASMINOGENAEMIA

Hypoplasminogenaemia is an unusual cause of gingival swelling and ulceration and ligneous conjunctivitis (Figs 1.4.12 and 1.4.13).

## LEUKAEMIAS

Leukaemias are malignant disorders of leukocytes, in which the leukocytes are dysfunctional and there is also anaemia and thrombocytopenia.

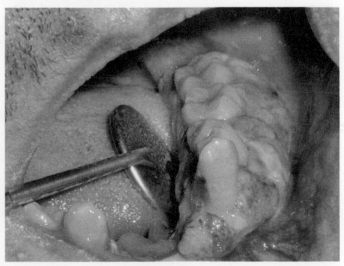

*Figure 1.4.12* Hypoplasminogenaemia (plasminogen deficiency) presents with swollen ulcerated gingivae.

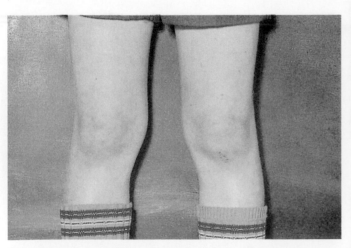

*Figure 1.4.11* Haemophilia—spontaneous bleeding into joints (haemarthrosis) can be crippling.

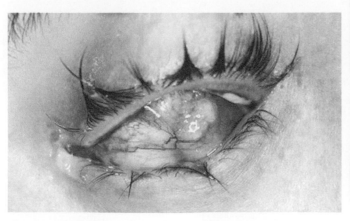

*Figure 1.4.13* Hypoplasminogenaemia can cause ligneous conjunctivitis.

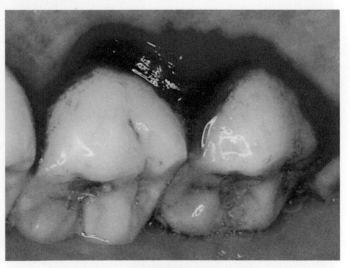

*Figure 1.4.14* Leukaemia—predisposes to spontaneous gingival haemorrhage.

There is thus a predisposition to oral infections, ulcers, bleeding tendency, gingival swelling mainly in myelomonocytic leukaemia and cervical lymph node enlargement (Figs 1.4.14–1.4.22). Spontaneous gingival haemorrhage is common and can be so profuse as to dissuade the patient from oral hygiene, but this simply aggravates the problem as the

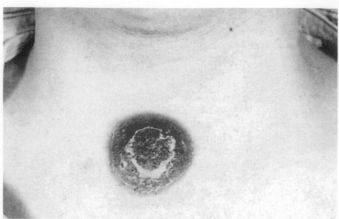

*Figure 1.4.16* Leukaemia—deposit of leukaemic cells (chloroma) in a very pale child.

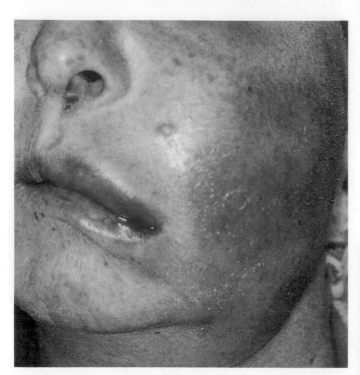

*Figure 1.4.15* Leukaemia—spreading odontogenic infection.

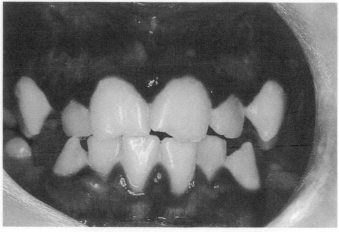

*Figure 1.4.18* Leukaemia—gingival swelling.

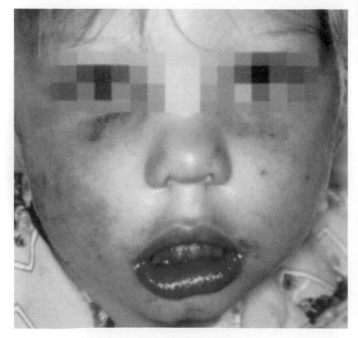

*Figure 1.4.17* Leukaemia—showing facial pallor, herpes and bruising.

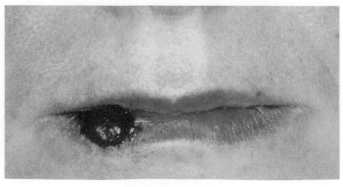

*Figure 1.4.19* Leukaemia—herpes complicated by bleeding tendency.

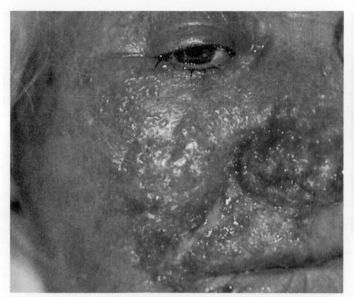

Figure 1.4.20 Leukaemia—maxillary zoster (shingles).

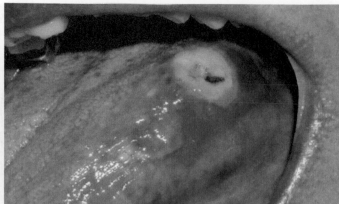

Figure 1.4.21 Leukaemia causing oral ulceration.

Leukaemic deposits may uncommonly appear in the mouth, or on the face and neck. Leukaemic deposits in the gingivae occasionally cause swelling of variable degree in the gingivae, a feature especially of myelomonocytic leukaemia (a variant of acute myeloid leukaemia).

## LEUKOCYTE DEFECTS

Leukocyte defects affecting the neutrophils can manifest with ulcers and infections predominantly pyogenic bacterial, gingivitis, rapidly destructive periodontal disease and oral ulceration. Recurrent mouth ulcers are sometimes due to viral infections such as intra-oral herpes simplex recurrences, or cytomegalovirus (CMV), and candidosis (Figs 1.4.23–1.4.26). Zygomycoses are rare, invasive fungal infections which mainly occur in immunocompromised patients, especially during prolonged neutropenia (chapter 1.4). Typically there is, as in agranulocytosis, only a minimal red inflammatory halo around the ulcers. Gangrene may be seen in patients with neutropenia.

*Chronic benign neutropenia* may result in oral ulceration, severe periodontitis and antral infections.

*Cyclic neutropenia* manifests with recurring oral ulceration and severe periodontitis.

*Chediak-Higashi syndrome* typically presents with cervical lymph node enlargement, oral ulceration and periodontitis.

*Chronic granulomatous disease* manifests with cervical lymph node enlargement and suppuration, candidosis, enamel hypoplasia, acute gingivitis and oral ulceration.

## LYMPHOMAS

Lymphomas—cancers that arise in lymphocytes and present as solid tumours of lymphoid cells—can cause cervical lymphadenopathy, oral ulcers or swellings (Figs 1.4.27–1.4.36) especially in the fauces, soft palate or gingiva. Patients with lymphocytic lymphomas are also predisposed to develop squamous carcinomas of the head and neck, possibly owing at least partly to the chemotherapy.

Non-Hodgkin lymphoma often appears in the fauces or gingiva. T/natural killer cell lymphomas (formerly termed lethal midline granulomas) usually present as a diffuse painless palatal swelling that eventually ulcerates and may produce considerable destruction. Sino-nasal types often express T-cell intracellular antigen 1 (TIA-1), perforin and granzyme B. Plasmablastic lymphomas are seen particularly in HIV

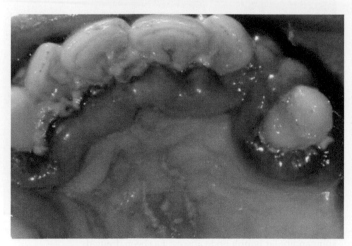

Figure 1.4.22 Leukaemia causing gingival swelling and ulceration.

gingivae then become inflamed, more hyperaemic and bleed more profusely. Oral purpura is also common, particularly where there is trauma, such as the suction exerted by an upper denture. The immune defects lead to a liability to infection: candidosis is extremely common, but Aspergillus and Mucor are rare opportunists. Of the viral infections, recurrent herpes simplex is common; the lesions can be extensive and because of the thrombocytopenia, there is often bleeding into the lesion. Zoster is also common in leukaemic patients and hairy leukoplakia may rarely be seen. Bacterial infections are uncommon but a wide range of organisms may be involved, including *Staphylococcus aureus*, *Pseudomonas aeruginosa*, *Klebsiella pneumoniae*, *Staphylococcus epidermidis*, *Escherichia coli*, enterococci and septicaemia may originate from oral lesions. Simple odontogenic infections can spread widely and be difficult to control.

Mouth ulcers in leukaemia are common, often lack an inflammatory halo and may result from cytotoxic therapy, infections or can be non-specific.

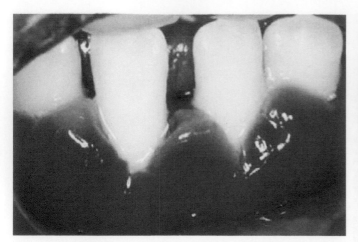

*Figure 1.4.23* Leukocyte disorders—neutropenia.

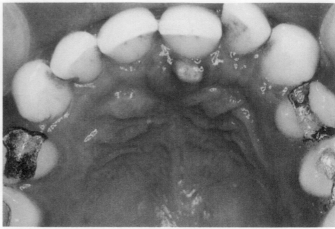

*Figure 1.4.24* Leukocyte disorders—neutropenia causing ulceration.

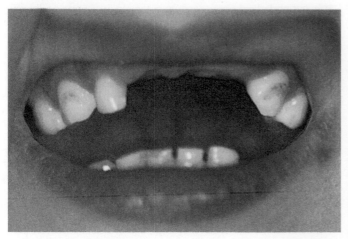

*Figure 1.4.25* Leukocyte disorders—chronic granulomatous disease and enamel hypoplasia from childhood infections.

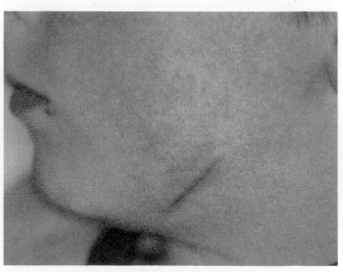

*Figure 1.4.26* Leukocyte disorders—chronic granulomatous disease; a submandibular lymph node abscess has been drained.

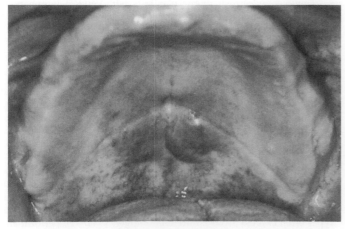

*Figure 1.4.27* Lymphoma.

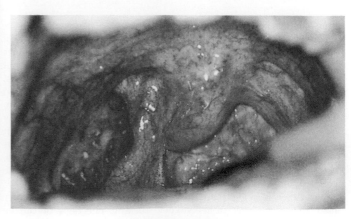

*Figure 1.4.28* Lymphoma.

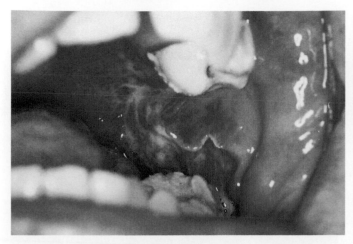

*Figure 1.4.29* Lymphoma.

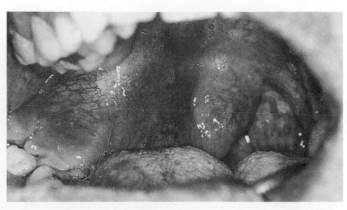

*Figure 1.4.30* Lymphoma.

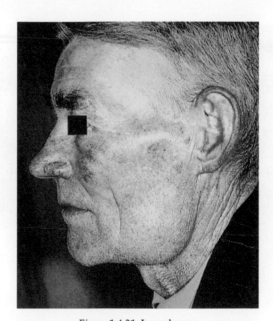

*Figure 1.4.31* Lymphoma.

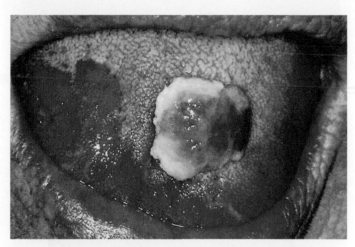

*Figure 1.4.32* Mycosis fungoides—a T-cell lymphoma causing a lingual swelling. This patient coincidentally has erythema migrans.

disease and may be associated with Epstein–Barr virus (EBV) and/or Kaposi sarcoma herpesvirus.

African Burkitt lymphoma is associated with EBV and typically affects children before the age of 12 to 13 years. The jaws, particularly the mandible, are common sites of presentation (Fig. 1.4.36). Massive swelling, which ulcerates in the mouth, may be seen. Radiographically, the teeth may appear to be 'floating in air'. Discrete radiolucencies in the lower third molar region, destruction of lamina dura and widening of the periodontal space may be seen on radiography. The disease may also cause oral pain, paraesthesia or increasing tooth mobility. The jaws are less frequently involved in non-African Burkitt lymphoma, the association with EBV is tenuous, and the disease is less common.

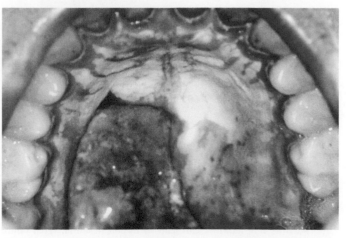

*Figure 1.4.33* T/natural killer cell lymphoma causing palatal ulceration.

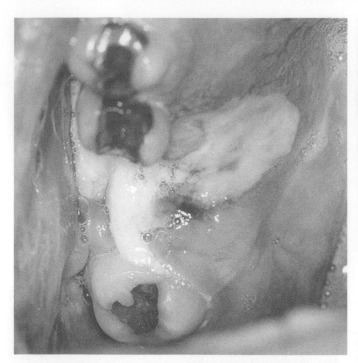

*Figure 1.4.34* Lymphoma presenting as ulceration.

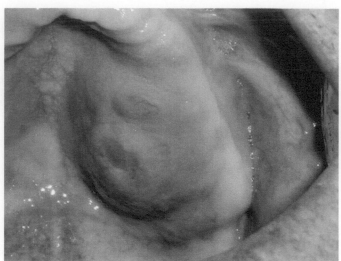

*Figure 1.4.35* Lymphoma presenting as swelling.

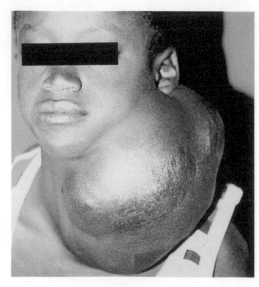

*Figure 1.4.36* Burkitt lymphoma.

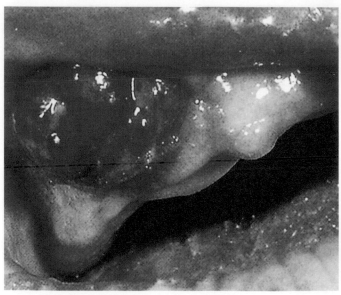

*Figure 1.4.37* Myeloma—soft tissue lesion.

## MULTIPLE MYELOMA

Multiple myeloma *(myelomatosis: Kahler disease)*—characterised by clonal expansion of malignant plasma cells in the bone marrow—presents with bone pain, and with anaemia, neutropenia and/or thrombocytopaenia as a consequence of loss of abnormal bone marrow function. Plasma cells release cytokines and abnormal immunoglobulins. Cytokines such as interleukin-1 can lead to hypercalcaemia, renal failure, suppression of haematopoiesis and many other effects.

### Clinical features

Most commonly found in males over 50 years of age, myelomatosis particularly affects the bone marrow of the skull and axial skeleton, with pain, swelling and pathological fractures, while vertebral destruction also gives rise to neurological sequelae. Abnormal immunoglobulins (paraproteins) with defective antibody activity predispose to infection, including recurrent varicella zoster virus infection. The paraproteins may also cause plasma hyperviscosity with Raynaud-type phenomena, a clotting or bleeding tendency, neurological sequelae, renal dysfunction and ultimately, there may be circulatory impairment, or amyloidosis.

The jaws and skull may develop multiple areas of radiolucency (Figs 1.4.37–1.4.41), but soft tissue lesions are rare (Fig. 1.4.42). Mental paraesthesia or hypoaesthesia can occur, and deposits of amyloid can arise intra-orally.

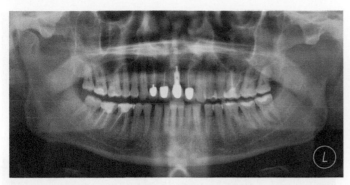

Figure 1.4.38 Myeloma—symptomless left mandibular condylar radiolucency.

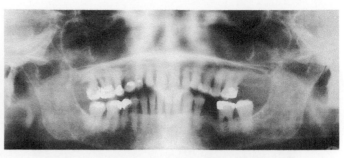

Figure 1.4.39 Myeloma—multiple jaw radiolucencies.

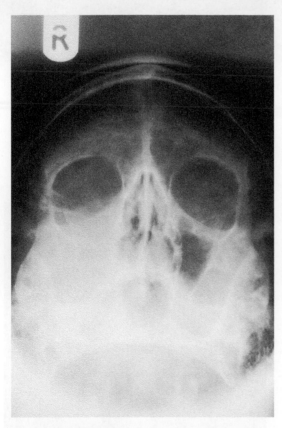

Figure 1.4.40 Myeloma—skull and jaw radiolucencies.

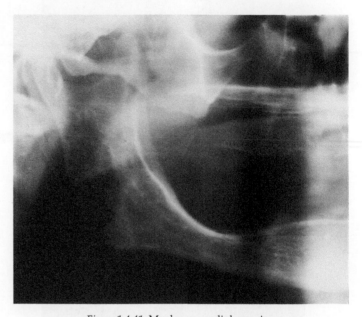

Figure 1.4.41 Myeloma—radiolucencies.

Intravenous bisphosphonates, frequently used in the treatment of myeloma, may predispose to osteochemonecrosis of the jaws (chapters 1.6 and 2.8).

### Diagnosis

Early on, abnormal immunoglobulins [an M-type (monoclonal) plasma protein] appear in plasma with a raised erythrocyte sedimentation rate (ESR), and light chains spillover into the urine (Bence–Jones proteinuria). Bone marrow biopsy is confirmatory. Radiography in later stages shows multiple punched-out radiolucencies, especially in the skull and jaws; scanning shows multiple hot spots.

### Management

Management is with radiotherapy and cytotoxic chemotherapy. Thalidomide and new analogues are now considered of benefit in the treatment.

## PLASMACYTOSIS

Plasmacytosis—an unusually large proportion of plasma cells in tissues—may cause gingival swelling (Fig. 1.4.43).

## PLUMMER–VINSON SYNDROME

Plummer–Vinson syndrome—also called Paterson–Brown–Kelly syndrome or sideropenic dysphagia—presents as a triad of iron deficiency anaemia, dysphagia caused by an oesophageal web, glossitis and predisposition to oral and post-cricoid carcinoma (Fig. 1.4.44).

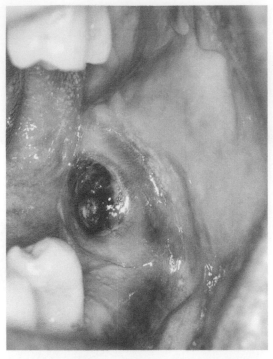

*Figure 1.4.42* Plasmacytoma.

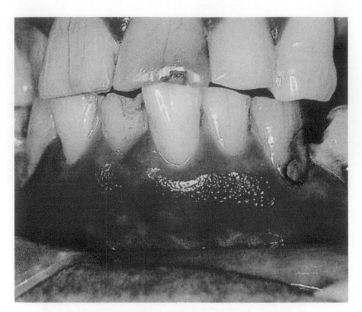

*Figure 1.4.43* Plasmacytosis.

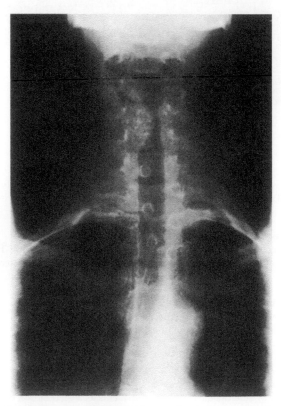

*Figure 1.4.44* Plummer–Vinson syndrome showing post-cricoid web on radiography.

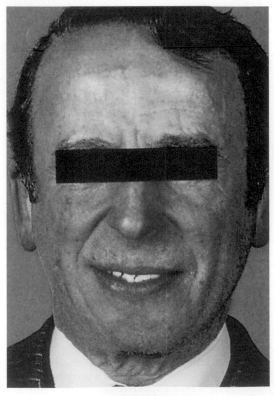

*Figure 1.4.45* Polycythaemia showing plethoric facies.

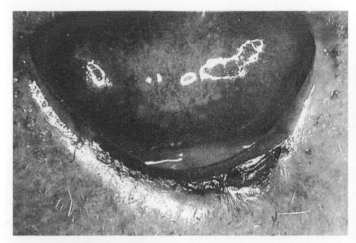

*Figure 1.4.46* Polycythaemia—viral ulceration and bleeding.

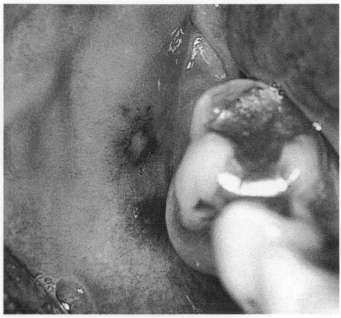

*Figure 1.4.47* Thrombocytopenia.

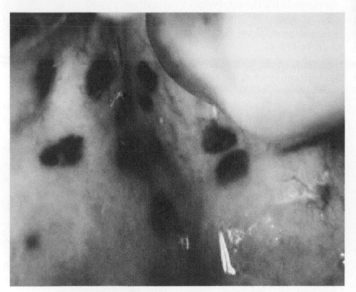

*Figure 1.4.48* Thrombocytopenia.

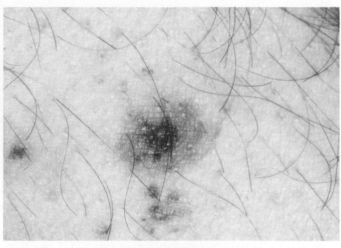

*Figure 1.4.49* Thrombocytopenia.

## POLYCYTHAEMIA

Polycythaemia (raised erythrocyte count) may be secondary to hypoxia or primary—a myeloproliferative disorder. Either type may cause cyanosis (Figs 1.4.45 and 1.4.46).

## THROMBOCYTOPENIA

Thrombocytopenia—a reduction in blood platelets—is usually due to bone marrow failure or autoimmune destruction. The latter (primary or idiopathic thrombocytopenic purpura) is the main form, but immune thrombocytopenia can also be secondary to drugs; or to disease such as autoimmune disorders (e.g. systemic lupus erythematosus, antiphospholipid antibody syndrome, immune thyroid disease, or Evans syndrome), lymphoproliferative diseases (e.g. chronic lymphocytic leukemia or large granular T-lymphocyte lymphocytic leukaemia) or chronic infections (e.g. *Helicobacter pylori*, HIV or hepatitis C virus). Sudden and severe thrombocytopenia may occur after acute infections with EBV, CMV or varicella zoster virus, or after vaccination for measles, mumps and rubella. Palatal petechiae, especially at the junction of the hard and soft palate, are almost pathognomonic of infectious mononucleosis, but can be seen in other infections such as HIV or rubella.

Spontaneous gingival or post-extraction bleeding may be an early feature of thrombocytopenia. Oral petechiae and ecchymoses may appear (Figs 1.4.47–1.4.49) mainly at sites of trauma and thus are seen mainly in the buccal mucosa, on the lateral margin of the tongue, and at the junction of hard and soft palates.

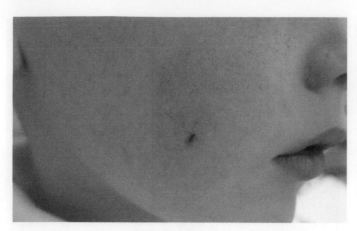

*Figure 1.4.50* von Willebrand disease showing bruising.

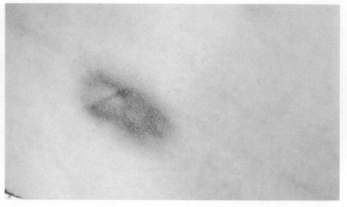

*Figure 1.4.51* von Willebrand disease—periumbilical haematoma in sister of patient in Figure 1.4.50.

## VON WILLEBRAND DISEASE

von Willebrand disease (pseudohaemophilia), the most common inherited bleeding disorder, is caused by a deficiency of, or defect in, von Willebrand factor, leading to a low blood factor VIII concentration and a platelet function defect. Unlike haemophilia A and B, von Willebrand disease affects females as well as males. The common pattern is of bleeding from mucous membranes, with gingival haemorrhage and purpura of mucous membranes and the skin, and post-extraction bleeding (Figs 1.4.50 and 1.4.51).

## FURTHER READING

Al-Wahadni A, Qudeimat MA, Al-Omari M. Dental arch morphological and dimensional characteristics in Jordanian children and young adults with beta-thalassaemia major. Int J Paediatr Dent 2005; 15: 98–104.

de Araujo MR, de Oliveira Ribas M, Koubik AC, et al. Fanconi's anemia: clinical and radiographic oral manifestations. Oral Dis 2007; 13: 291–5.

Avivi I, Avraham S, Koren-Michowitz M, et al. Oral integrity and salivary profile in myeloma patients undergoing high-dose therapy followed by autologous SCT. Bone Marrow Transplant 2009; 43: 801–6.

Balasubramaniam R, Alawi F, DeRossi S. Superficial mucoceles in chronic graft-versus-host disease: a case report and review of the literature. Gen Dent 2009; 57: 82–8.

Brennan MT, Sankar V, Baccaglini L, et al. Oral manifestations in patients with aplastic anemia. Oral Surg Oral Med Oral Pathol Oral Radiol Endod 2001; 92: 503–8.

Burke VP, Startzell JM. The leukemias. Oral Maxillofac Surg Clin North Am 2008; 20: 597–608.

Chehal H, Cohen DM, Bhattacharyya I. AAOMP case challenge: multiple red plaques with severe burning and soreness on the tongue. J Contemp Dent Pract 2009; 10: 96–100.

Cines DB, Liebman H, Stasi R. Pathobiology of secondary immune thrombocytopenia. Semin Hematol 2009; 46(1 Suppl 2): S2–14.

Field EA, Speechley JA, Rugman FR, Varga E, Tyldesley WR. Oral signs and symptoms in patients with undiagnosed vitamin B12 deficiency. J Oral Pathol Med 1995; 24: 468–70.

Flint SR, Sugerman P, Scully C, Smith JG, Smith MA. The myelodysplastic syndromes. Case report and review. Oral Surg Oral Med Oral Pathol 1990; 70: 579–83.

da Fonseca M, Oueis HS, Casamassimo PS. Sickle cell anemia: a review for the pediatric dentist. Pediatr Dent 2007; 29: 159–69.

Gómez-Moreno G, Cutando A, Arana C, Scully C. Hereditary blood coagulation disorders. Management and dental treatment. J Dent Res 2005; 84: 978–85.

Graells J, Ojeda RM, Muniesa C, Gonzalez J, Saavedra J. Glossitis with linear lesions: an early sign of vitamin B12 deficiency. J Am Acad Dermatol 2009; 60: 498–500.

Guimaraes AL, Gomes CC, da Silva LM, et al. Association between oral HSV-1 and survival in allogeneic hematopoietic stem cell transplanted patients. Med Oral Patol Oral Cir Bucal 2009; 14: E62–8.

Hazza'a AM, Al-Jamal G. Dental development in subjects with thalassemia major. J Contemp Dent Pract 2006; 7: 63–70.

Hazza'a AM, Al-Jamal G. Radiographic features of the jaws and teeth in thalassaemia major. Dentomaxillofac Radiol 2006; 35: 283–8.

Ionescu MA, Murata H, Janin A. Oral mucosa lesions in hypereosinophilic syndrome—an update. Oral Dis 2008; 14: 115–22.

Isaacson PG. The current status of lymphoma classification. Br J Haematol 2000; 109: 258–66.

Janin A, Murata H, Leboeuf C, et al. Donor-derived oral squamous cell carcinoma after allogeneic bone marrow transplantation. Blood 2009; 113: 1834–40.

Kavadia-Tsatala S, Kolokytha O, Kaklamanos EG, Antoniades K, Chasapopoulou E. Mandibular lesions of vasoocclusive origin in sickle cell hemoglobinopathy. Odontology 2004; 92: 68–72.

Kurtulus I, Gokbuget A, Efeoglu A, et al. Hypoplasminogenemia with ligneous periodontitis: a failed local therapeutic approach. J Periodontol 2007; 78: 1164–75.

Lehman JS, Bruce AJ, Rogers RS. Atrophic glossitis from vitamin B12 deficiency: a case misdiagnosed as burning mouth disorder. J Periodontol 2006; 77: 2090–2.

Lu SY, Wu HC. Initial diagnosis of anemia from sore mouth and improved classification of anemias by MCV and RDW in 30 patients. Oral Surg Oral Med Oral Pathol Oral Radiol Endod 2004; 98: 679–85.

Mori T, Hasegawa K, Okabe A, et al. Efficacy of mouth rinse in preventing oral mucositis in patients receiving high-dose cytarabine for allogeneic hematopoietic stem cell transplantation. Int J Hematol 2008; 88: 583–7.

Patel RS, Harman KE, Nichols C, Burd RM, Pavord S. Acquired haemophilia heralded by bleeding into the oral mucosa in a patient with bullous pemphigoid, rheumatoid arthritis, and vitiligo. Postgrad Med J 2006; 82: e3.

Patton LL. Hematologic abnormalities among HIV-infected patients: associations of significance for dentistry. Oral Surg Oral Med Oral Pathol Oral Radiol Endod 1999; 88: 561–7.

Porter SR, Diz Dios P, Kumar N, et al. Oral plasmablastic lymphoma in previously undiagnosed HIV disease. Oral Surg Oral Med Oral Pathol Oral Radiol Endod 1999; 87: 730–4.

Porter SR, Matthews RW, Scully C. Chronic lymphocytic leukaemia with gingival and palatal deposits. J Clin Periodontol 1994; 21: 559–61.

Rafaniello Raviele P, Pruneri G, Maiorano E. Plasmablastic lymphoma: a review. Oral Dis 2009; 15: 38–45.

Schalk E, Mohren M, Jentsch-Ullrich K, et al. Oral graft-versus-host disease. Dent Clin North Am 2008; 52: 79–109.

Scully C, Diz Dios P, Shotts R. Oral health care in patients with the most important medically compromising conditions; 1. Platelet disorders. CPD Dent 2004; 5: 3–7.

Scully C, Diz Dios P, Shotts R. Oral health care in patients with the most important medically compromising conditions; 2. Congenital coagulation disorders. CPD Dent 2004; 5: 8–11.

Scully C, Diz Dios P, Shotts R. Oral health care in patients with the most important medically compromising conditions; 3. Anticoagulated patients. CPD Dent 2004; 5: 47–9.

Scully C, Eveson JW, Witherow H, et al. Oral presentation of lymphoma: case report of T-cell lymphoma masquerading as oral Crohn's disease, and review of the literature. Eur J Cancer B Oral Oncol 1993; 29B: 225–9.

Scully C, Gokbuget A, Kurtulus I. Hypoplasminogenaemia, gingival swelling and ulceration. Oral Dis 2007; 13; 515–18.

Scully C, Gokbuget AY, Allen C, et al. Oral manifestations indicative of plasminogen deficiency (hypoplasminogenemia). Oral Surg Oral Med Oral Pathol 2001; 91: 344–7.

Scully C, Watt-Smith P, Dios RD, Giangrande PL. Complications in HIV-infected and non-HIV-infected haemophiliacs and other patients after oral surgery. Int J Oral Maxillofac Surg 2002; 31: 634–40.

Scully C, Wolff A. Oral surgery in patients on anticoagulant therapy. Oral Surg Oral Med Oral Pathol Oral Radiol Endod 2002; 94: 57–64.

Sharathkumar AA, Shapiro A. Hereditary haemorrhagic telangiectasia. Haemophilia 2008; 14: 1269–80.

Stevenson H, Boardman C, Chu P, Field A. Mental nerve anaesthesia; a complication of sickle cell crisis during childbirth. Dent Update 2004; 31: 486–7.

Tekcicek M, Tavil B, Cakar A, et al. Oral and dental findings in children with Fanconi anemia. Pediatr Dent 2007; 29: 248–52.

Vaisman B, Medina AC, Ramirez G. Dental treatment for children with chronic idiopathic thrombocytopaenic purpura: a report of two cases. Int J Paediatr Dent 2004; 14: 355–62.

Van Dis ML, Langlais RP. The thalassemias: oral manifestations and complications. Oral Surg Oral Med Oral Pathol 1986; 62: 229–33.

Yalçin SS, Unal S, Gümrük F, Yurdakök K. The validity of pallor as a clinical sign of anemia in cases with beta-thalassemia. Turk J Pediatr 2007; 49: 408–12.

# 1.5 HEPATOLOGICAL DISEASE

- cirrhosis
- hepatitis
- jaundice

- primary biliary cirrhosis
- transplantation

## CIRRHOSIS

Cirrhosis is a common chronic liver disorder, which can present with a bleeding tendency, halitosis, jaundice, telangiectasia, sialosis (Figs 1.5.1–1.5.3) and maxillofacial features of alcoholism (tooth erosion, and sequelae of trauma and oral hygiene neglect). Drinking excess alcohol can lead to fatty liver, hepatitis and cirrhosis, as well as trauma, gastritis, pancreatitis, mental health problems including depression and anxiety, sexual difficulties such as impotence, myopathies, cardio-myopathy, hypertension, encephalopathy, addiction and some cancers (oral, oesophageal, liver, colon and breast).

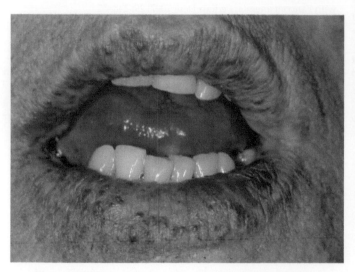

*Figure 1.5.1* Liver alcoholic cirrhosis and facial telangiectasia.

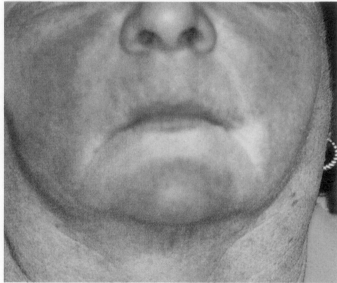

*Figure 1.5.2* Liver cirrhosis presenting with sialosis.

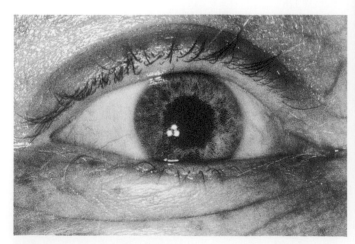

*Figure 1.5.3* Liver alcoholic cirrhosis causing jaundice showing mainly as icteric sclerae.

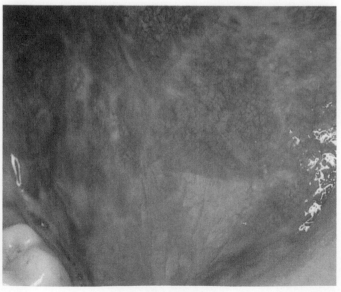

*Figure 1.5.4* Hepatitis C virus can underlie lichenoid lesions (or sicca syndrome).

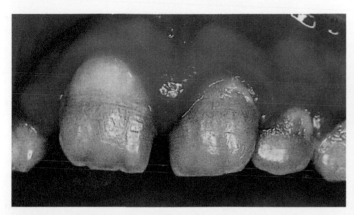

Figure 1.5.5 Biliary atresia after liver transplantation—the part of the teeth developing after transplantation are normal color.

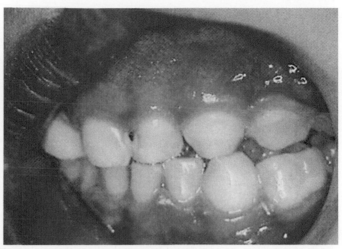

Figure 1.5.6 Biliary staining of teeth.

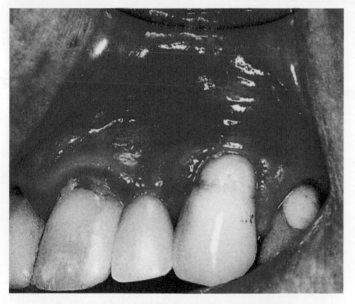

Figure 1.5.7 Primary biliary cirrhosis—telangiectasia.

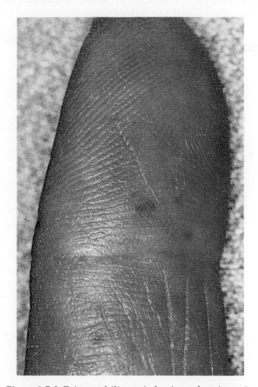

Figure 1.5.8 Primary biliary cirrhosis—telangiectasia.

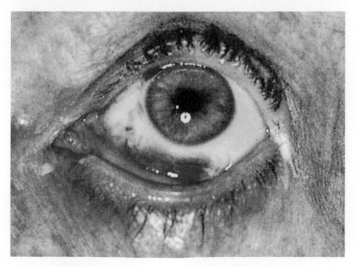

Figure 1.5.9 Primary biliary cirrhosis—telangiectasia.

## HEPATITIS

Hepatitis from any cause (drugs, alcohol and viruses) can cause a bleeding tendency and jaundice. Oral hyperpigmentation has been described. Hepatitis C virus (HCV) infection can cause jaundice, bleeding tendency, lichen planus (Fig. 1.5.4) and a sicca syndrome. HCV co-infected patients are more prone than HIV mono-infected patients to develop oral lesions.

Hepatitis B virus infection can cause jaundice, bleeding tendency and may influence the pattern of oral keratin expression.

## JAUNDICE

Jaundice in infants with conjugated hyperbilirubinaemia from rhesus incompatibility or biliary atresia can cause tooth staining (Figs 1.5.5 and 1.5.6).

## PRIMARY BILIARY CIRRHOSIS

Primary biliary cirrhosis—an autoimmune disease of the liver in which there is slow progressive destruction of the small bile ducts—can cause jaundice, telangiectasia, Sjögren syndrome and lichen planus (Figs 1.5.7–1.5.9).

## TRANSPLANTATION

Transplantation necessitates that the patient is T-cell immunosuppressed to prevent graft rejection. Oral complications are mainly those related to the immunosuppression used to prevent graft rejection, and may include infections such as candidosis, herpes simplex virus-related ulceration and hairy leukoplakia. An increased susceptibility to lip cancer after transplantation is related to exposure to immunosuppressive agents, and UV light. Post-transplantation patients are also prone to lymphoproliferative diseases, Kaposi sarcoma and some carcinomas (chapter 1.6).

Drugs used after liver transplantation may also produce other maxillofacial adverse side-effects; the most common is gingival swelling caused by ciclosporin or nifedepine (chapter 1.6).

## FURTHER READING

Carrozzo M. Oral diseases associated with hepatitis C virus infection. Part 1. Sialadenitis and salivary glands lymphoma. Oral Dis 2008; 14: 123–30.

Carrozzo M. Oral diseases associated with hepatitis C virus infection. Part 2: lichen planus and other diseases. Oral Dis 2008; 14: 217–28.

Fang F, Liu P, Wang H, et al. Studies of keratins in tongue coating samples of hepatitis B patients by mass spectrometry. Rapid Commun Mass Spectrom 2009; 23: 1703–9.

Guggenheimer J, Close JM, Eghtesad B. Sialadenosis in patients with advanced liver disease. Head Neck Pathol 2009; 3: 100–5.

Guggenheimer J, Eghtesad B, Close JM, Shay C, Fung JJ. Dental health status of liver transplant candidates. Liver Transpl 2007; 13: 280–6.

Modi AA, Liang TJ. Hepatitis C: a clinical review. Oral Dis 2008; 14: 10–14.

Richards A, Rooney J, Prime S, Scully C. Primary biliary cirrhosis. Sole presentation with rampant dental caries. Oral Surg Oral Med Oral Pathol 1994; 77: 16–18.

Shiboski CH, Krishnan S, Besten PD, et al. Gingival enlargement in pediatric organ transplant recipients in relation to tacrolimus-based immunosuppressive regimens. Pediatr Dent 2009; 31: 38–46.

# 1.6 IATROGENIC CONDITIONS

- haematopoietic stem cell transplantation
- graft-versus-host disease
- organ transplantation
- pharmacotherapy
- chemotherapy
- immunosuppressive agents
- tetracyclines
- other drugs

- osteonecrosis of the jaws (ONJ; osteochemonecrosis)
- radiotherapy
- osteoradionecrosis
- surgery
- dry socket (alveolar osteitis)
- oroantral fistula
- oronasal fistula
- dental materials

---

A range of procedures, drugs and materials can produce maxillofacial changes.

## HAEMATOPOIETIC STEM CELL TRANSPLANTATION

The procedure of haematopoietic stem cell transplantation (HSCT) (bone marrow transplantation) typically involves the ablation of recipient bone marrow cells by high-dose chemotherapy with drugs such as cyclophosphamide and total (whole) body irradiation (TBI) followed by the transfusion of bone marrow aspirate from a donor who has been stimulated with growth factors. This regimen inevitably results in profound immunosuppression until the donor graft takes and, in about 60% of cases, graft-versus-host disease (GVHD) results.

Oral complications of HSCT are common, can be a major cause of morbidity and include:

- Mucositis—typically begins around 5 days post-HSCT but, by around 9–14 days post-HSCT it resolves (Fig. 1.6.1). Apart from the measures discussed below, it may be ameliorated by use of glutamine and interleukin-11.
- Ulceration—usually a consequence of granulocytopenia, this typically resolves by around 9–14 days post-HSCT, when the neutrophils rise >500 cells/ml.
- Xerostomia.
- Bleeding.
- Infections—are frequent, mainly caused by candidosis, human papillomaviruses (HPV) or by herpesviruses when they may cause ulceration. Mucormycosis is a rare but serious complication. Septicaemia is also rare and serious, but 25–75% of septicaemias arise from the oral flora.

GVHD may ensue. Lymphoproliferative syndromes [post-transplant lymphoproliferative disorder (PTLD)] and lymphomas are rare complications.

## GRAFT-VERSUS-HOST DISEASE

Acute GVHD appears between 10 and 100 days post-HSCT, and affects about 60% of survivors. Chronic GVHD may follow, or may arise ab initio and it occurs after 100 days post-HSCT and affects around 50% of patients after HSCT.

*Acute GVHD* affects mainly the liver, gastrointestinal tract and mucocutaneous tissues, and can be lethal. The oral lesions are difficult or impossible to differentiate from mucositis and consist of:

- painful mucosal desquamation and ulceration (Figs 1.6.2–1.6.13)
- cheilitis

- xerostomia
- infections
- purpura and bleeding (Figs 1.6.2–1.6.13).

*Chronic GVHD* is severe and involves multiple organs, mainly the liver, gastrointestinal tract, eyes and mucocutaneous tissues including, in 80% of cases, the mouth coincidentally with the skin, and lesions include:

- erythema
- lichenoid lesions
- ulceration
- xerostomia and taste abnormalities
- infections
- hairy leukoplakia
- sclerodermatous syndrome.

Pyogenic granulomas have also been reported.

### Diagnosis
Diagnosis of GVHD is from the history and clinical features and a mucosal or labial salivary gland biopsy which show mononuclear cell infiltrates.

### Management
Prophylactic immunosuppressive therapy usually using methotrexate and ciclosporin is often used for the first 100 days post-HSCT to try to prevent GVHD. Acute GVHD is treated with high-dose immunosuppressive therapy. Oral lesions are best treated with use of:

- oral hygiene measures
- analgesics (morphine or hydromorphone)
- topical azathioprine or ciclosporin
- non-alcoholic chlorhexidine mouth rinses
- nystatin mouth washes or fluconazole
- pilocarpine or cevimeline
- xylitol chewing gum
- artificial saliva and moisturizing gels
- growth factors.

## ORGAN TRANSPLANTATION

Following solid organ transplantation, all patients are placed on immunosuppressive drugs for life to prevent T-cell alloimmune rejection. Each transplant programme uses various combinations of agents slightly differently.

*Induction immunotherapy* usually consists of a short course of IL-2 receptor-blocking antibodies such as daclizumab and basiliximab.

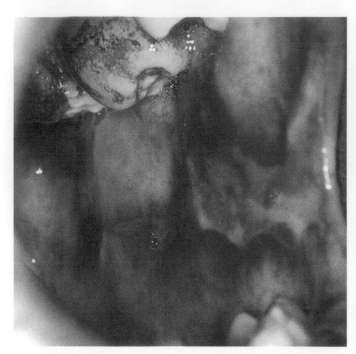

*Figure 1.6.1* Haematopoietic stem cell transplant. Mucositis.

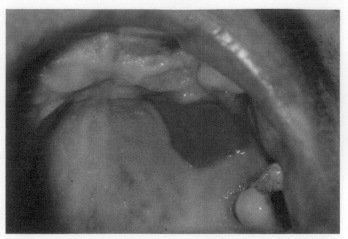

*Figure 1.6.2* Haematopoietic stem cell transplant. Graft-versus-host-disease causing palatal herpetic ulcer.

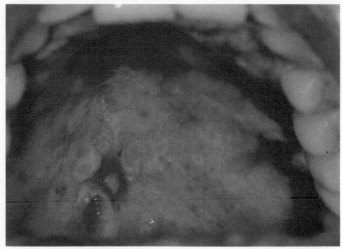

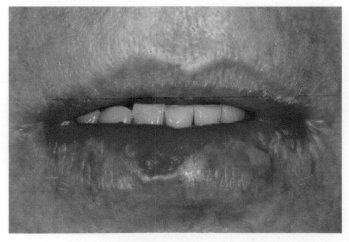

*Figure 1.6.4* Haematopoietic stem cell transplant. Graft-versus-host-disease causing mucositis.

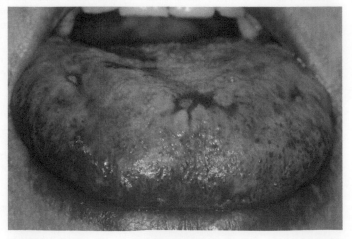

*Figure 1.6.3* Haematopoietic stem cell transplant. Graft-versus-host-disease causing severe dysplasia of lip.

*Maintenance immunosuppression* is usually based on a calcineurin inhibitor (e.g. ciclosporin, tacrolimus or sirolimus), and/or corticosteroids, sometimes combined with corticosteroid-sparing agents such as azathioprine, ciclosporin, newer antimetabolites such as mycophenolate mofetil or antiproliferative agents such as rapamycin.

### Complications

Immunosuppressive therapy leads to liability to infections—especially with mycobacteria, viruses and fungi—which may spread rapidly, and can be clinically silent or atypical, and leads to a liability to develop neoplasms (Figs 1.6.14–1.6.17).

*Figure 1.6.5* Haematopoietic stem cell transplant. Graft-versus-host-disease.

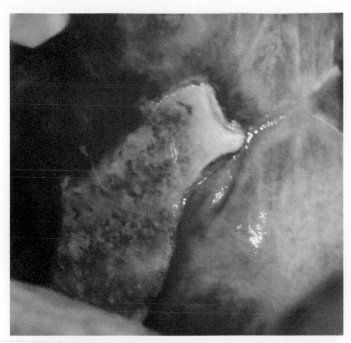

Figure 1.6.6 Haematopoietic stem cell transplant. Graft-versus-host-disease.

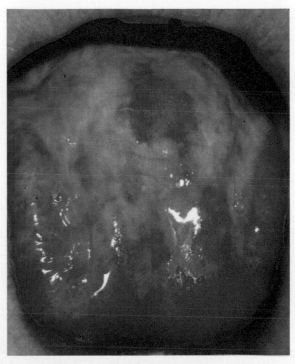

Figure 1.6.7 Haematopoietic stem cell transplant. Graft-versus-host-disease (GVHD). Chronic GVHD on tongue.

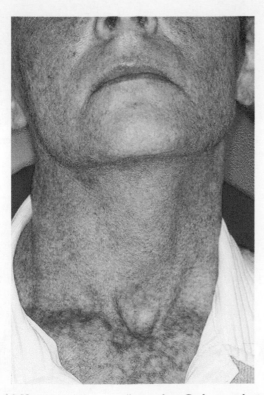

Figure 1.6.8 Haematopoietic stem cell transplant. Graft-versus-host-disease.

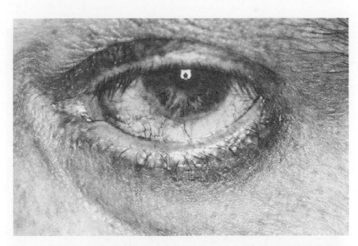

Figure 1.6.9 Haematopoietic stem cell transplant. Graft-versus-host-disease.

*Bacterial infection* is the most common cause of deaths occurring during the first post-operative months. Mycobacterial infection is a rare but important complication of transplantation. Frank or latent TB infection and infection with non-tuberculous mycobacteria such as *Mycobacterium avium* complex or *M. chelonei*, including unusual species such as *Mycobacterium abscessus*, *M. genavense*, *M. gordonae* and *M. xenopi* may be seen. Transplant patients have significantly increased mean periodontal probing depths than healthy controls.

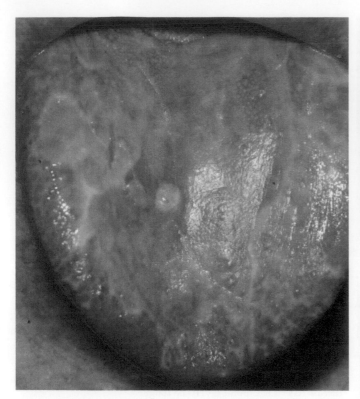

*Figure 1.6.10* Haematopoietic stem cell transplant. Graft-versus-host-disease (GVHD). Chronic GVHD.

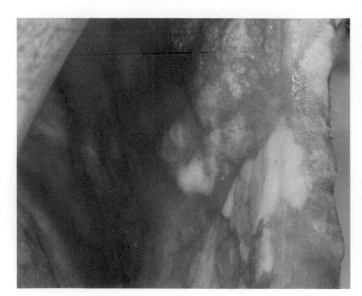

*Figure 1.6.12* Haematopoietic stem cell transplant. Graft-versus-host-disease (cGVHD). Chronic GVHD of commissure.

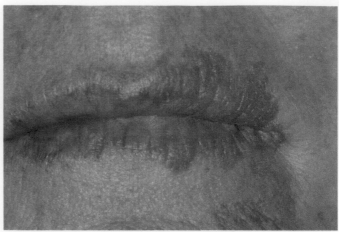

*Figure 1.6.11* Haematopoietic stem cell transplant. Graft-versus-host-disease (GVHD). Chronic GVHD periorally.

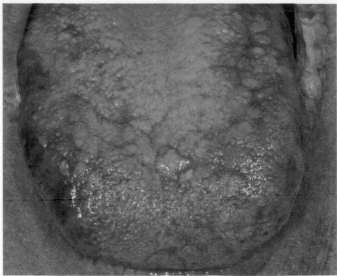

*Figure 1.6.13* Haematopoietic stem cell transplant. Graft-versus-host-disease (GVHD). Chronic GVHD on tongue.

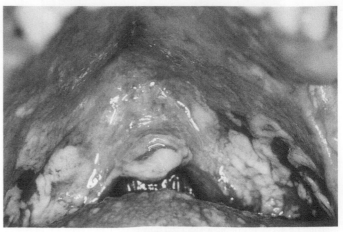

*Figure 1.6.14* Transplantation—candidosis.

*Viral infections* account for substantial morbidity and mortality. Herpes simplex virus (HSV) infections are common and usually treated with a 10–14-day course of aciclovir or famciclovir. Varicella zoster virus infections may appear, especially herpes zoster and usually treated with aciclovir or famciclovir. Cytomegalovirus (CMV) infection is one of the

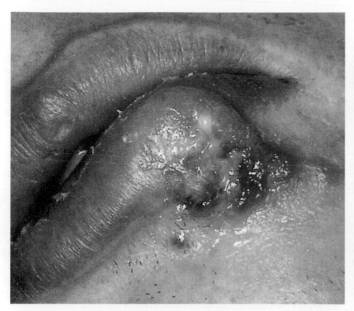

*Figure 1.6.15* Transplantation—herpes.

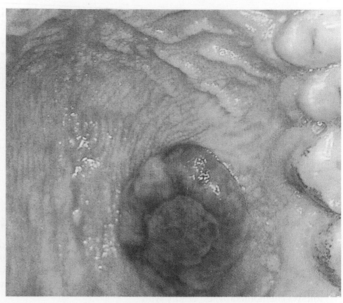

*Figure 1.6.16* Transplantation—Kaposi sarcoma.

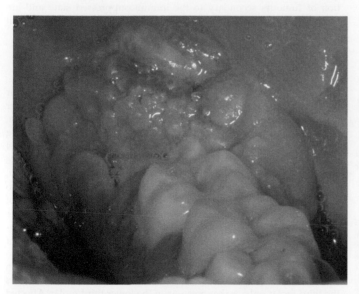

*Figure 1.6.17* Transplantation—lymphoma.

other most common infections, and usually appears 3 or more weeks after transplantation, presenting with fever, leukopenia and malaise. Patients with systemic CMV infections are treated with ganciclovir.

*Fungal infections* can cause severe local or even systematically invasive infections. Candidal infections are the most common, can be systemic and typically involve *Candida albicans*, but *C. kruseii* and many others species may be implicated. *Cryptococcus neoformans* infections may cause pulmonary, CNS and disseminated cutaneous disease in immunosuppressed patients. *Aspergillus niger, flavus* or *fumigatus* infections may infect the lungs, upper respiratory tract (including the maxillary antrum), skin, soft tissues and CNS. *Mucor* and *Rhizopus* infections (zygomycosis; phycomycosis) are rarely encountered but can cause destructive CNS, sinus or soft tissue infections. Rhinocerebral zygomycosis is usually seen after renal or liver transplantation. *Pneumocystis* infections are common. Antifungal and antiviral prophylaxis may be appropriate since even mild mycotic infections can be a serious threat.

*Malignant neoplasms*, including melanoma, basal cell carcinoma, Kaposi sarcoma, lymphomas and squamous cell carcinomas of the skin and lip, and carcinoma of the cervix, external genitalia and perineum can be complications in transplant recipients. Several of these tumours have a viral aetiology. Post-transplant lymphoproliferative disease (PTLD) is relatively uncommon after solid organ and allogeneic bone marrow transplantation, but the more intense the immunosuppression used, the higher the incidence, and the earlier it appears. PTLD is a group of B-cell proliferations, associated with EBV infection (either from virus reactivation or primary post-transplant infection). The heterogeneous tumours range from B-cell hyperplasia to malignant immunoblastic lymphoma but all PTLD, irrespective of histology, are potentially, and frequently, fatal. Risk factors that have been identified as predictive of PTLD include recipient pre-transplant EBV seronegativity and donor EBV seropositivity.

PTLDs typically develop within 1 year of transplantation but they may appear from 1 month to 14 years. Clinical presentation varies from aggressive disease with diffuse involvement starting early in the post-transplantation period and with polyclonal lesions developing over days or weeks, to localised lesions that are indolent and slow-growing over many months. The most common sites involved are lymph nodes, liver, lung, kidney, bone marrow, small intestine, spleen, CNS, large bowel, tonsils and salivary glands. T-cell PTLD not associated with EBV infection tends to affect extranodal sites. Whether PTLD is localised or disseminated, the tumours are progressive and mortality rates may reach 60–100%.

Fever, weight loss, an infectious mononucleosis-like syndrome (anorexia, lethargy, sore throat and lymphadenopathy), gastrointestinal symptoms (diarrhea and abdominal pain), pulmonary symptoms (dyspnoea) and CNS or neurological symptoms are common. PTLD is diagnosed by having a high index of suspicion in a patient who has recently undergone transplantation and presents with unexplained fever, weight loss, lymphadenopathy, hepatosplenomegaly and positive histopathology, and EBV–DNA, RNA or viral protein on biopsy.

Treatment of PTLD is to reduce or withdraw immunosuppression, and to treat EBV infection with ganciclovir and, since lowering immunosuppression carries the risk of allograft rejection, additional treatment modalities are indicated (rituximab—an anti-CD20 monoclonal antibody; interferon alfa—a proinflammatory and antiviral agent; intravenous immunoglobulin; immunoglobulin and cytotoxic T-lymphocytes; surgical excision; localised radiation or combination chemotherapy).

## PHARMACOTHERAPY

A range of drugs can occasionally produce maxillofacial lesions. Chemotherapy is very frequently associated with maxillofacial complications.

## CHEMOTHERAPY

The adverse effects of chemotherapy can include the following:

- Mucositis is widespread oral erythema, ulceration and soreness, and sometimes bleeding, common after chemo- or radiotherapy. Sometimes called *mucosal barrier injury*, it is common during the treatment of cancer but also in the conditioning prior to HSCT. Mucositis invariably follows chemotherapy; especially with
  o Cisplatin
  o Etoposide
  o Fluorouracil
  o Melphalan

Also with

- Doxorubicin
- Methotrexate
- Taxanes
- Vinblastine

Less with

- Asparaginase
- Carmustine

Mucositis may affect some two-thirds of patients (Fig. 1.6.18) and appears 3–15 days after cancer treatment. The impaired mucosal barrier

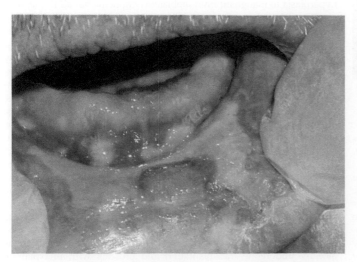

*Figure 1.6.18* Chemotherapy—mucositis.

predisposes to life-threatening septic complications. Management aims at pain relief, hastening healing and preventing infections. However, prophylaxis is the goal.

Pain relief is usually achieved with opioids. Attempts to aid healing can include medications to reduce salivation and thus exposure of the mucosa to chemotherapeutic drugs that are secreted in saliva; anti-inflammatory medications; cytokines such as interleukin (IL)-1, IL-11, TGF-beta3, keratinocyte growth factor, granulocyte-macrophage-colony-stimulating factor and granulocyte colony-stimulating factor; thalidomide: an angiogenesis-inhibiting drug; and amifostine, a cytoprotector.

- Infections—especially candidal, HSV and HPV.
- Pain—related not only to mucositis or infections, but possibly to drugs such as vinca alkaloids and doxorubicin.
- Bleeding—thrombocytopenia increases the liability to gingival and oral bleeding.
- Xerostomia.
- Damage to developing maxillofacial and dental tissues (microdontia, hypodontia, root abnormalities, abnormal enamel and delayed eruption).

## IMMUNOSUPPRESSIVE AGENTS

Immunosuppressive regimes are increasingly used for an ever-widening range of disorders including allograft receipt, autoimmune disease and tumour therapy. Maxillofacial complications may be a direct consequence of the immunosuppressive agent, or reflect opportunistic infection or tumours secondary to the immunosuppressed state and are fundamentally the same as those seen in HIV/AIDS and other T-cell immune defects.

## TETRACYCLINES

Generalised intrinsic tooth staining of a significant brown or grey colour may be caused by tetracyclines given to a pregnant or lactating mother or to children under the age of 8 years. Tetracyclines cross the placenta, enter breast milk and are taken up by dentine in the child's developing teeth, and by bone. Tetracyclines diffuse through dentine to the enamel interface, chelating calcium ions and incorporating into hydroxyapatite as a stable orthophosphate complex. When the affected teeth first erupt, they have a bright-yellow band-like appearance but upon exposure to sunlight, the colour gradually changes to grey or red-brown. Bands of yellow and brown are most obvious at the tooth necks where the thinner enamel allows the colour of the stained dentine to show through. Staining is greater in light-exposed anterior teeth, and with larger doses of tetracyclines, and is worse with, for example, tetracycline than oxytetracycline. Even in older children, tetracyclines cause staining but by then most tooth crowns have been formed. The staining then usually affects the third molar only or the roots—as in the lower third molar. Affected teeth may fluoresce bright yellow under ultraviolet light and this helps to distinguish tetracycline staining from dentinogenesis imperfecta. Fluorescence is also seen in undecalcified sections viewed under ultraviolet light (Figs 1.6.19–1.6.22).

Minocycline can lead to a green-grey or blue-grey intrinsic staining during and after the complete formation and eruption of teeth. Minocycline may act by binding to iron ions. Doxycycline and nitrofurantoin have also been reported to cause tooth discolouration.

## OTHER DRUGS

A range of drugs can occasionally produce maxillofacial complications (Table 1.6.1; Figs 1.6.23–1.6.45).

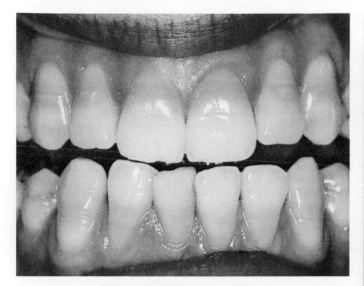

*Figure 1.6.19* Tetracycline stain.

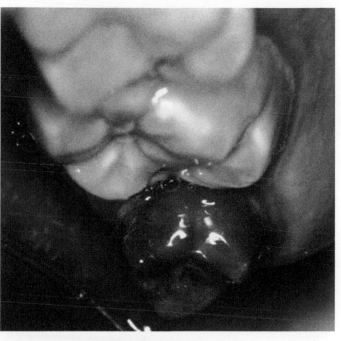

*Figure 1.6.20* Tetracycline stain.

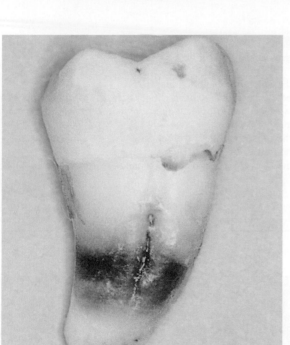

*Figure 1.6.21* Tetracycline stain.

# OSTEONECROSIS OF THE JAWS (ONJ; OSTEOCHEMONECROSIS)

Jaw osteonecrosis is an important condition that can be caused by exposure to:

- Red phosphorus.
- Heavy metals.
- Toxic endodontic materials.
- Corticosteroids.

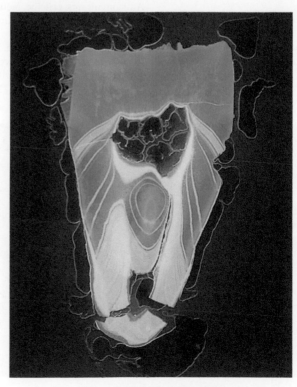

*Figure 1.6.22* Tetracycline stain.

**TABLE 1.6.1** MAXILLOFACIAL DRUG-INDUCED LESIONS (SEE ALSO SECTION 3.5)

| Lesions | Main drugs implicated |
| --- | --- |
| Abnormal facial movements (dyskinesias) | Phenothiazines and metoclopramide |
| Angioedema | Angiotensin-converting enzyme inhibitors, aldesleukin (human recombinant IL-2), interferon (IFN)-alpha and many others |
| Burning sensation | Angiotensin-converting enzyme inhibitors and protease inhibitors |
| Candidosis | Broad spectrum antimicrobials, corticosteroids, other immunosuppressants or cytotoxic drugs |
| Dental hypoplasia | Cytotoxic drugs |
| Dry mouth | Tricyclic antidepressants, calcium channel blockers, phenothiazines, antihypertensives, lithium and many other drugs. Taste can also thus be disturbed by bisphosphonates, metronidazole or penicillamine |
| Erythema multiforme | Barbiturates, sulfonamides and very many other drugs |
| Gingival swelling | Phenytoin, ciclosporin or calcium channel blockers such as nifedipine |
| Halitosis | Solvent misuse, amyl nitrites, nitrates, phenothiazine, amphetamines, cytotoxic drugs, disulfiram, melatonin, nicotine lozenges, mycophenolate sodium and aztreonam |
| Herpesvirus infections | Corticosteroids, other immunosuppressants or cytotoxic drugs |
| Hyperpigmentation | Tobacco, betel, amlodipine, antimalarials, adrenocorticotrophic hormone, minocycline |
| Human papillomaviruses | Immunosuppressive agents |
| Lichenoid lesions | A range of drugs, especially NSAIDs |
| Maxillofacial developmental defects | Alcohol, anticonvulsants, cytotoxic drugs |
| Mucositis | Cytotoxic agents |
| Osteonecrosis of the jaws | Bisphosphonates, bevacizumab, denosumab |
| Pain | Vinca alkaloids, doxorubicin |
| Potentially malignant disorders and oral carcinoma | Alcohol, betel, khat, tobacco, immunosuppressant agents |
| Sensory changes | Carmustine infusion, capsaicin, articaine, labetalol, prilocaine, sulthiame. |
| Sialorrhoea | Quetiapine, aripiprazole, clozapine, benzodiazepines, neuroleptics, cholinesterase inhibitors and pilocarpine |
| Sialosis | Alcohol, valproic acid, sympathomimetic agents such as isoprenaline, phenylbutazone, isoprenaline, anti-thyroid drugs and phenothiazines, methyl dopa |
| Taste disturbance | Any drug causing dry mouth, and busulphan, ketoconazole and other drugs |
| Tics | Anticonvulsants, caffeine, methylphenidate, antiparkinsonian drugs |
| Tooth discolouration | Intrinsic from use of tetracyclines, or extrinsic (superficial) and caused by chlorhexidine, some antibiotics and iron preparations |
| Tooth root anomalies | Cytotoxic drugs or phenytoin. |
| Ulcers | Many drugs (e.g. NSAIDs, nicorandil, alendronate, sirolimus, tacrolimus), any drug that induces neutropenia or agranulocytosis (e.g. carbimazole, deferiprone) and especially cytotoxic drugs used in chemotherapy |

*Abbreviation*: NSAIDs, non-steroidal anti-inflammatory drugs.

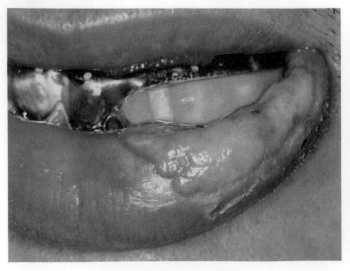

*Figure 1.6.23* Drug-induced burn.

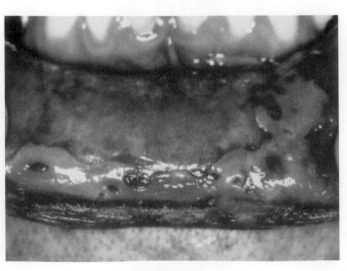

*Figure 1.6.24* Drug-induced burn.

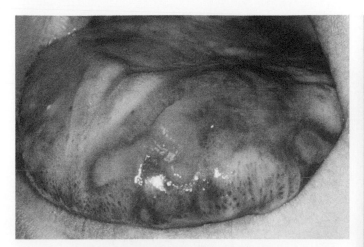

Figure 1.6.25 Drug-induced lichenoid reaction.

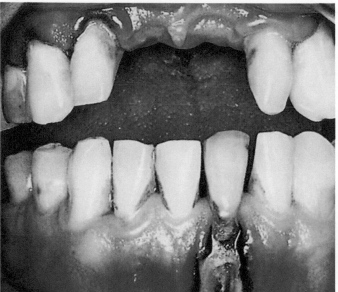

Figure 1.6.26 Bismuth lines.

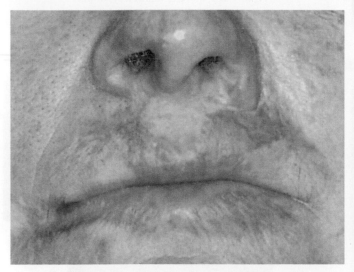

Figure 1.6.27 Pigmentation from phenytoin use in epilepsy.

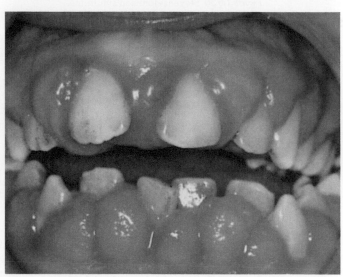

Figure 1.6.28 Gingival swelling from phenytoin.

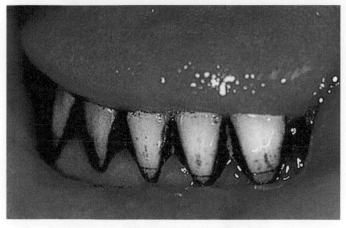

Figure 1.6.29 From stain.

- Severe herpes zoster or other infections, particularly in patients who have been irradiated in the head and neck or who are immunocompromised.
- bisphosphonates—powerful osteoclast inhibitors—especially when used intravenously. Bisphosphonates suppress bone turnover to the point that the repair of physiological microdamage is abolished and some such as nitrogen-containing bisphosphonates which also have antiangiogenic activity are especially liable to cause this complication. Bisphosphonates are remarkably persistent drugs, being incorporated in the skeleton without being degraded for years.

Exodontia is the main precipitant. Over 90% of patients developing bisphosphonate-related osteonecrosis of the jaws (BRONJ or ONJ) have received *intravenous* bisphosphonates (pamidronate and/or zoledronic acid) and very few cases have followed the use of oral bisphosphonates

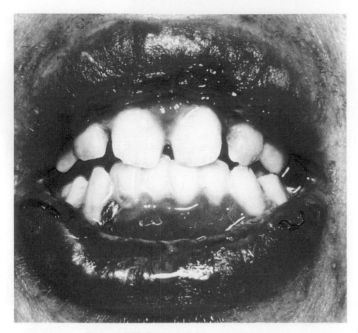

*Figure 1.6.30* Stevens–Johnson syndrome.

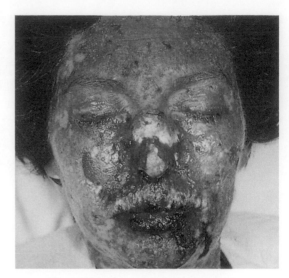

*Figure 1.6.31* Stevens–Johnson syndrome.

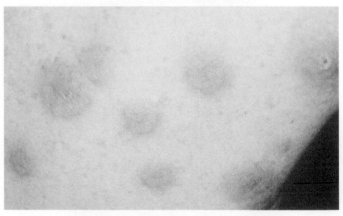

*Figure 1.6.33* Stevens–Johnson syndrome.

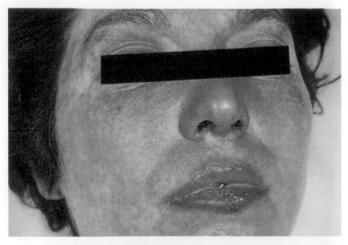

*Figure 1.6.32* Stevens–Johnson syndrome.

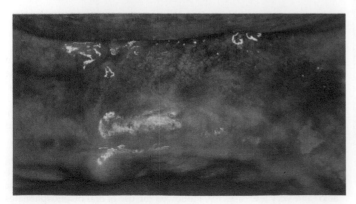

*Figure 1.6.34* Amalgam tattoo.

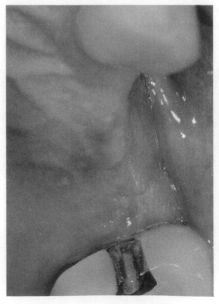

*Figure 1.6.35* Amalgam tattoo.

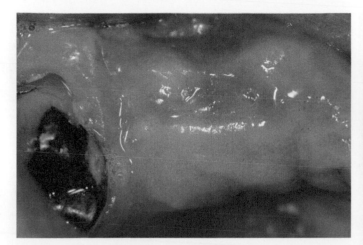

*Figure 1.6.36* Amalgam tattoo.

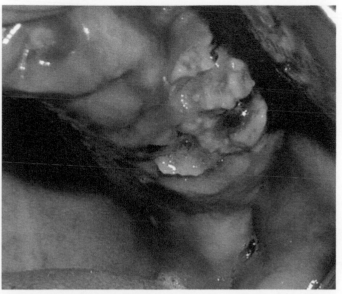

*Figure 1.6.37* Bisphosphonate related osteonecrosis.

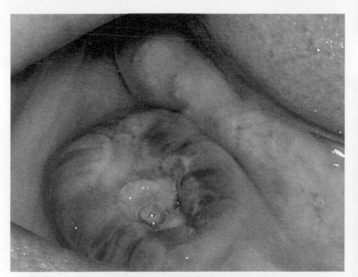

*Figure 1.6.38* Bisphosphonate related osteonecrosis.

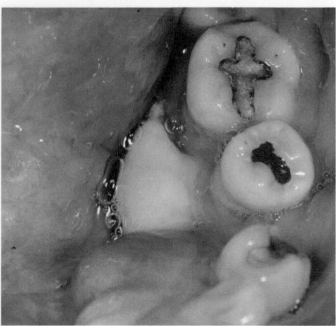

*Figure 1.6.39* Bisphosphonate related osteonecrosis.

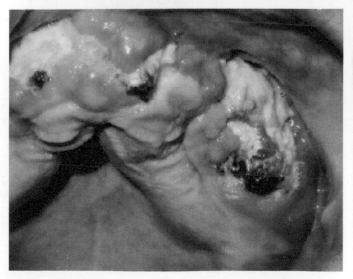

*Figure 1.6.40* Bisphosphonate related osteonecrosis.

(e.g. alendronate and ibandronate). Acquired factors for BRONJ also include use of other anti-angiogenic agents, advanced age, diabetes and dental trauma. Genetic factors, such as polymorphisms on *CYP2C8* gene may be a risk factor.

- Bevacizumab or denosumab or sunitinib may also predispose to osteonecrosis.

### Clinical features
Patients usually present after a history of dental extraction with painful, exposed and necrotic bone, primarily of the mandible.

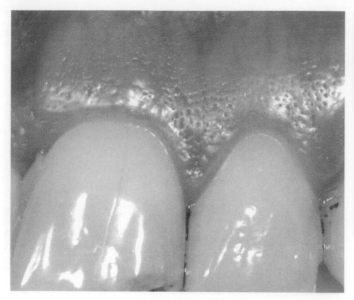

*Figure 1.6.41* Minocycline causing bone staining.

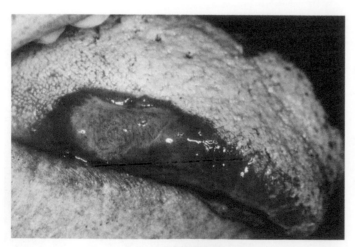

*Figure 1.6.43* Drug-induced ulceration.

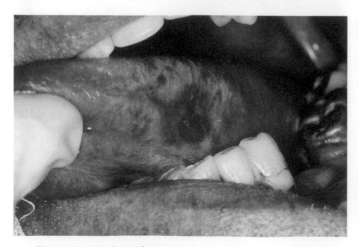

*Figure 1.6.45* Lichenoid reaction to an antihypertensive agent.

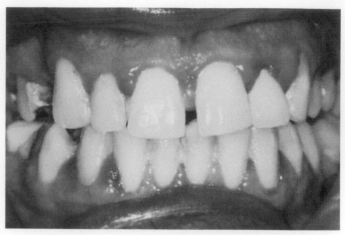

*Figure 1.6.42* Gingival swelling with anticonvulsants.

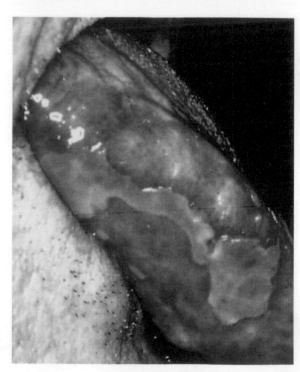

*Figure 1.6.44* Drug-induced lichenoid erosions.

### Diagnosis

The diagnosis is clinically supported by imaging. The bone has a moth-eaten appearance similar to that of osteoradionecrosis (ORN).

### Management

Minimal interference is recommended; antimicrobials and analgesics may help. Provision of preventative care together with any necessary surgical dentistry prior to bisphosphonate therapy may be the most advantageous strategy of preventing BRONJ.

## RADIOTHERAPY

Radiotherapy involving the mouth and salivary glands invariably produces mucositis (Figs 1.6.46–1.6.65) which is dose-dependent and seen

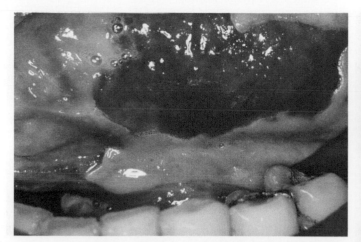

*Figure 1.6.46* Radiation injury—mucositis.

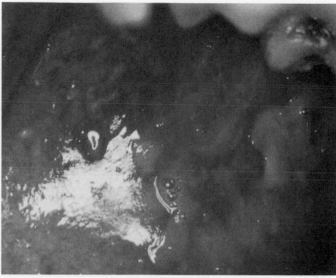

*Figure 1.6.47* Radiation injury—mucositis.

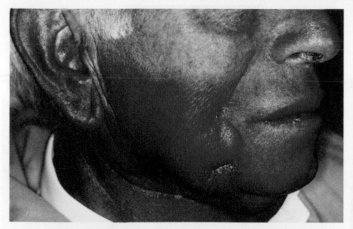

*Figure 1.6.48* Radiation injury—cutaneous erythema.

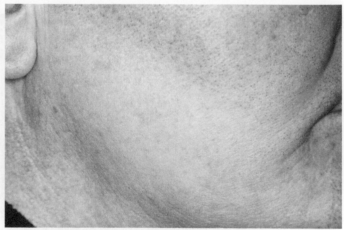

*Figure 1.6.49* Radiation injury—hair loss.

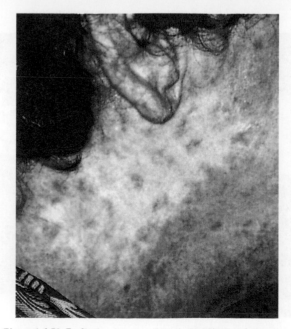

*Figure 1.6.50* Radiation injury—depigmentation and scarring.

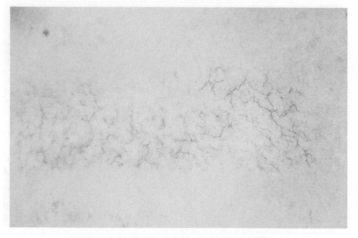

*Figure 1.6.51* Radiation injury—pigmentation.

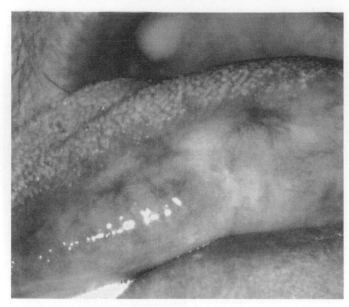

*Figure 1.6.52*  Radiation injury—scarring.

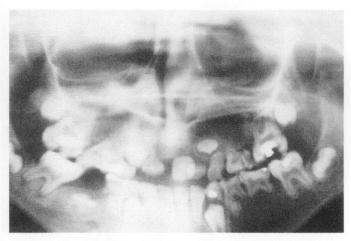

*Figure 1.6.53*  Radiation injury—disrupted odontogenesis.

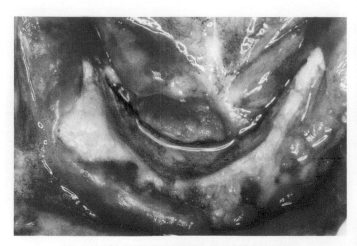

*Figure 1.6.54*  Radiation injury—osteoradionecrosis.

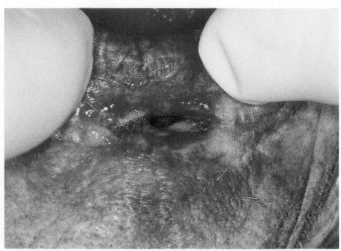

*Figure 1.6.55*  Radiation injury—osteoradionecrosis.

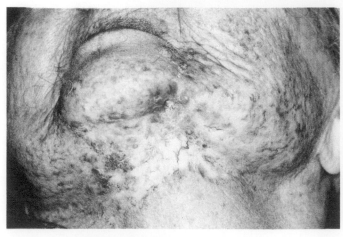

*Figure 1.6.56*  Radiation injury—scarring.

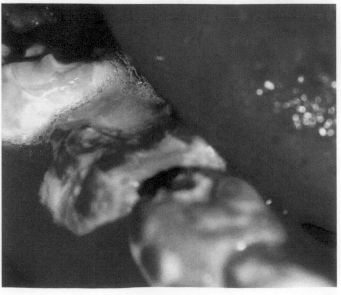

*Figure 1.6.57*  Radiation injury—calculus and caries.

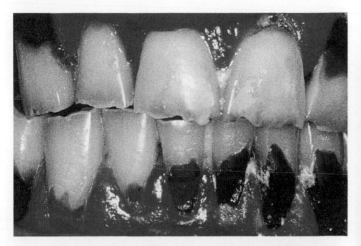

Figure 1.6.58 Radiation injury—xerostomia and caries.

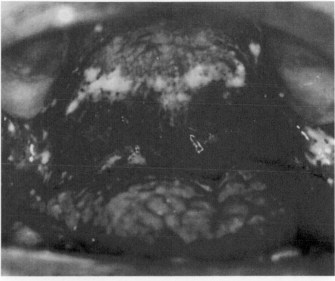

Figure 1.6.59 Radiation injury—candidosis.

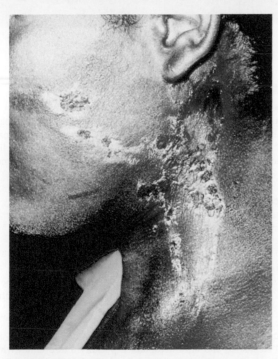

Figure 1.6.60 Radiation injury—a radiation accident that resulted in fatalities and burns as here.

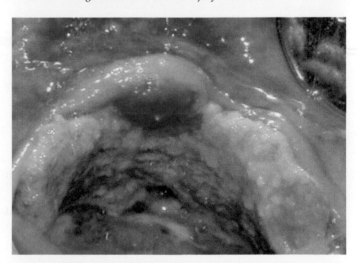

Figure 1.6.61 Radiation injury—osteoradionecrosis.

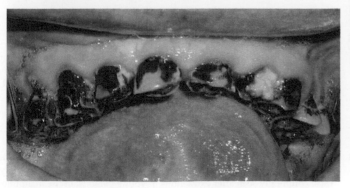

Figure 1.6.62 Radiation injury.

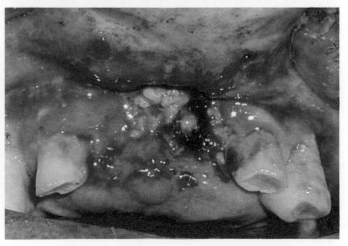

Figure 1.6.63 Radiation injury—osteoradionecrosis.

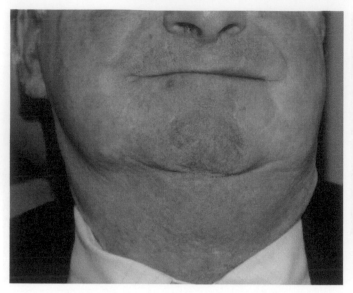

*Figure 1.6.64* Radiation injury—lymphoedema.

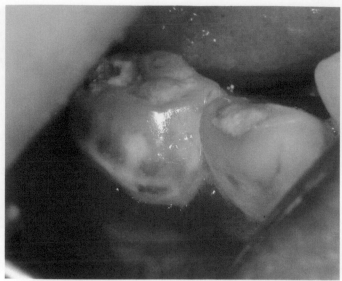

*Figure 1.6.65* Radiation injury—caries.

especially after external beam radiotherapy involving the maxillofacial tissues. It is also common in upper mantle head and neck radiation, and particularly in TBI. Mucositis is especially seen with chemoradiotherapy regimens, such as those involving:

- cisplatin and fluorouracil
- cisplatin, epirubicin, bleomycin
- carboplatin.

Mucositis is invariable where radiation involves the oral mucosa but can be reduced by using:

- minimising doses and field of radiation and intensity modulated radio therapy (IMRT) or image guided radio therapy (IGRT)
- mucosa-sparing blocks
- amifostine before therapy
- betametasone mouthwashes.

Ionising radiation also predisposes to xerostomia, taste loss and to endarteritis obliterans which can lead to trismus and ORN. Longer term consequences of radiotherapy include skin scarring, and telangiectasia develop on skin and mucosa.

Irradiation also predisposes to subsequent neoplasia: for example, radiotherapy to oropharyngeal neoplasms predisposes to subsequent salivary neoplasms. Irradiation of the mandibular condyle, or other growth areas, can result in facial deformity. Irradiation of developing teeth can produce microdontia, hypodontia, root abnormalities, abnormal enamel and retarded tooth eruption.

## OSTEORADIONECROSIS

The risk of ORN is greatest:

- when radiation dose exceeds 60 Gy
- from 10 days before to several years after radiotherapy (particularly at 3–12 months)
- in the malnourished or immunoincompetent.

The initiating factor is often trauma, such as tooth extraction, or oral infection or ulceration from an appliance. The mandible, a compact bone with high density and poor vascularity, is more prone than the maxilla to ORN. With the advent of plesiotherapy and other improved radiotherapeutic techniques such as IMRT or IGRT, ORN is now less common.

### Clinical features
Presentation is of exposed bone in an irradiated mouth, with or without external sinuses, pain and pathological fracture.

### Diagnosis
Apart from the history and clinical features, imaging shows the 'moth-eaten' appearance of the jaw and sometimes a pathological fracture.

### Management
Local cleansing, and antimicrobials, especially tetracycline (which has high bone penetrance) long-term are indicated; hyperbaric oxygen and sequestrectomy may assist.

## SURGERY
Bleeding and bruising (Figs 1.6.66–1.6.78) can follow any trauma or surgery. Few maxillofacial procedures leave significant deformities but cancer surgery can be an exception.

Infections of oral wounds may be seen, including dry socket and, rarely, osteomyelitis (Chapter 2.8).

## DRY SOCKET (ALVEOLAR OSTEITIS)
If the blood clot in a tooth extraction socket breaks down, presumably from the action of fibrinolysins, then the socket becomes 'dry'. This is typically most commonly seen after extractions in young persons; in the mandible;

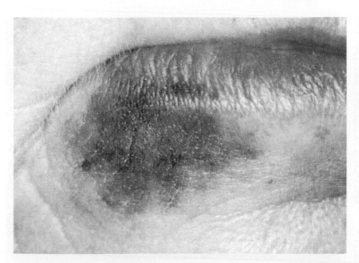

Figure 1.6.66 Surgery—trauma.

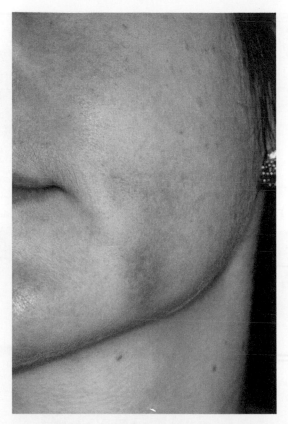

Figure 1.6.67 Ecchymosis after trauma.

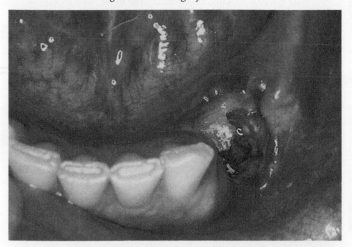

Figure 1.6.68 Alveolar osteitis.

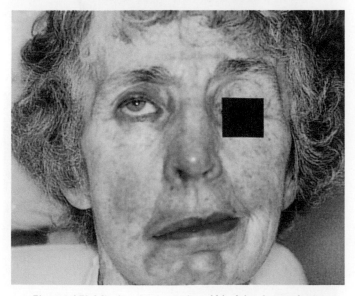

Figure 1.6.70 Misplaced inferior dental block local anaesthesia.

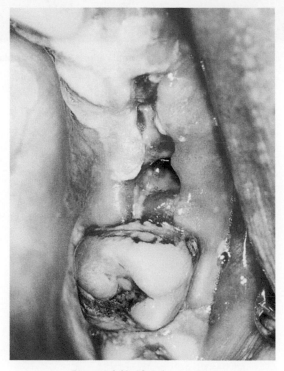

Figure 1.6.69 Alveolar osteitis.

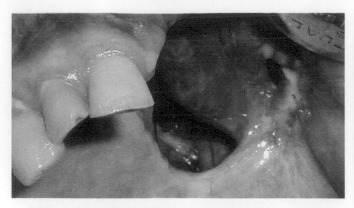

*Figure 1.6.71* Surgery complication—oroantral communication.

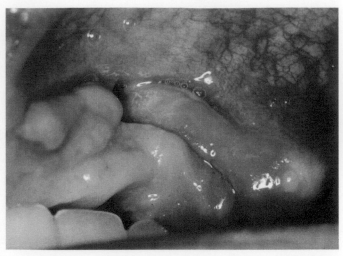

*Figure 1.6.72* Oroantral fistula (due to retained roots).

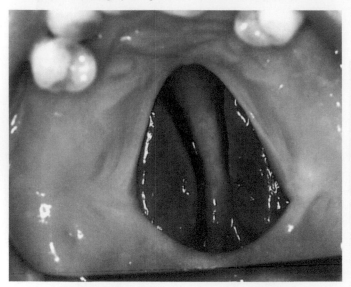

*Figure 1.6.73* Surgery complication—oronasal fistula.

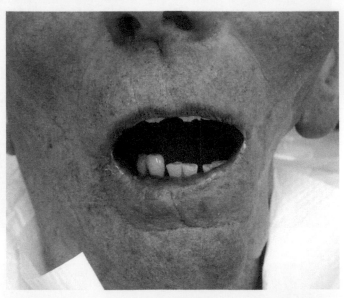

*Figure 1.6.74* Surgery—deformity and scarring.

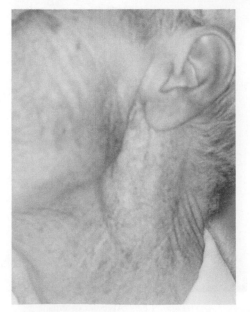

*Figure 1.6.75* Surgery complication—deformity and scarring.

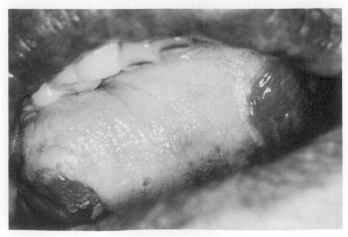

*Figure 1.6.76* Skin graft.

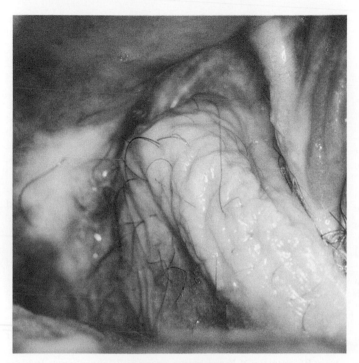

*Figure 1.6.77* Skin graft.

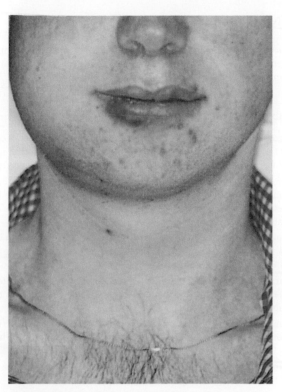

*Figure 1.6.78* Surgery complication—bruising.

in the molar region; after extractions under local anaesthesia; and after traumatic extractions. Smoking and oral contraceptive use predispose to dry socket as do any immunocompromising conditions or bone disorders such as Paget disease of bone and use of bisphosphonates.

### Clinical features
Dry socket manifests with the onset of fairly severe pain 2–4 days after extraction, bad taste in the mouth and halitosis. The socket has no clot and the surrounding mucosa is inflamed and the area is tender to any palpation.

### Diagnosis
The diagnosis is clinical but imaging may be indicated to exclude other causes of post-operative pain such as pathology associated with another tooth or a jaw fracture.

### Management
Healing of a dry socket is aided if debris is irrigated away and the socket dressed. Systemic antimicrobial therapy is rarely warranted.

## OROANTRAL FISTULA
Oroantral fistula (OAF) is almost invariably traumatic in aetiology, usually following extraction of an upper molar or premolar tooth, occasionally following violence or surgery. Rarely a fistula may arise as a consequence of malignancy (e.g. carcinoma, lymphoma or Wegener granulomatosis), osteochemonecrosis or infections [e.g. zygomycosis (mucormycosis), or aggressive periodontitis in HIV disease].

### Clinical features
Fluid passes from the mouth into the maxillary sinus (antrum) and may enter the nose. Occasionally, the antral lining becomes infected or prolapses through an OAF.

### Diagnosis
The diagnosis is initially clinical test with a dental mirror which may show the OAF or blow air *across* the OAF, when the sound is altered. The sound from a sucker is also altered. Nose-blowing should be avoided but shows intra-oral bubbling.

Sterile silver probing may confirm the OAF, and imaging may be confirmatory and may be required to establish the cause of the fistula and determine the degree of any chronic sinusitis.

### Management
If the OAF >4 mm diameter, an antral regimen of decongestants; avoidance of nose-blowing; and surgical repair is usually indicated.

## ORONASAL FISTULA
Oronasal fistulae may be caused by trauma, or surgery, such as the removal of a palatal neoplasm. Oronasal fistulae may also arise with tertiary syphilis, mucormycosis, 'crack' cocaine use and nasal-type natural killer or T-cell lymphomas.

## DENTAL MATERIALS

Dental materials may occasionally be responsible for burns, allergies or tattoos (e.g. amalgam tattoos). Nerve palsy can arise from a misplaced dental local anaesthetic injection. Articaine and prilocaine can be neurotoxic.

## FURTHER READING

Aragon-Ching JB, Ning YM, Chen CC, et al. Higher incidence of osteonecrosis of the Jaw (ONJ) in patients with metastatic castration resistant prostate cancer treated with anti-angiogenic agents. Cancer Invest 2009; 27: 221–6.

Bagan J, Scully C, Sabater V, Jimenez Y. Osteonecrosis of the jaws in patients treated with intravenous bisphosphonates (BRONJ): a concise update. Oral Oncol 2009; 45: 551–4.

Bagan JV, Jimenez Y, Diaz JM, et al. Osteonecrosis of the jaws in intravenous bisphosphonate use: proposal for a modification of the clinical classification. Oral Oncol 2009; 45: 645–6.

Bagan JV, Jimenez Y, Murillo J, et al. Jaw osteonecrosis associated with bisphosphonates: multiple exposed areas and its relationship to teeth extractions. Study of 20 cases. Oral Oncol 2006; 42: 327–9.

Bagan JV, Murillo J, Jimenez Y, et al. Avascular jaw osteonecrosis in association with cancer chemotherapy: series of 10 cases. J Oral Pathol Med 2005; 34: 120–3.

Bagan JV, Thongprasom K, Scully C. Adverse oral reactions associated with the Cox-2 inhibitor rofecoxib. Oral Dis 2004; 10: 401–3.

Bhansali A, Bhadada S, Sharma A, et al. Presentation and outcome of rhino-orbital-cerebral mucormycosis in patients with diabetes. Postgrad Med J 2004; 80: 670–4.

Dios PD, Scully C. Adverse effects of antiretroviral therapies: focus on orofacial effects. Expert Opin Drug Saf 2002; 1: 304–17.

Ellis PE, Benson PE. Potential hazards of orthodontic treatment–what your patient should know. Dent Update 2002; 29: 492–6.

Erbagci Z. Amlodipine associated hyperpigmentation. Saudi Med J 2004; 25: 103–5.

Femiano F, Scully C, Gombos F. Linear IgA dermatosis induced by a new angiotensin-converting enzyme inhibitor. Oral Surg Oral Pathol Oral Med 2003; 95: 169–73.

Fernández A, Vázquez S, Rodríguez-González L. Tongue hyperpigmentation resulting from peginterferon alpha-2a and ribavirin treatment in a Caucasian patient with chronic hepatitis C. J Eur Acad Dermatol Venereol 2008; 22: 1389–91.

Gittinger FS, Raible A, Kempf VA. Non-tuberculous mycobacterial infection of the parotid gland in an immunosuppressed adult. J Med Microbiol 2008; 57(Pt 4): 536–9.

Giuliani M, Lajolo C, Sartorio A, et al. Oral lesions in HIV and HCV co-infected individuals in HAART era. J Oral Pathol Med 2008; 37: 468–74.

Giuliani M, Lajolo C, Sartorio A, et al. Oral lichenoid lesions in HIV-HCV-coinfected subjects during antiviral therapy: 2 cases and review of the literature. Am J Dermatopathol 2008; 30: 466–71.

Greuter S, Schmid F, Ruhstaller T, Thuerlimann B. Bevacizumab-associated osteonecrosis of the jaw. Ann Oncol 2008; 19: 2091–2.

Haresaku S, Hanioka T, Tsutsui A, Watanabe T. Association of lip pigmentation with smoking and gingival melanin pigmentation. Oral Dis 2007; 13: 71–6.

Hillerup S. Iatrogenic injury to the inferior alveolar nerve: etiology, signs and symptoms, and observations on recovery. Int J Oral Maxillofac Surg 2008; 37: 704–9.

Holty JE, Gould MK, Meinke L, Keeffe EB, Ruoss SJ. Tuberculosis in liver transplant recipients: a systematic review and meta-analysis of individual patient data. Liver Transplant 2009; 15: 894–906.

Holty JE, Sista RR. Mycobacterium tuberculosis infection in transplant recipients: early diagnosis and treatment of resistant tuberculosis. Curr Opin Organ Transplant 2009; 14: 613–18.

Ioannidou E, Kao D, Chang N, Burleson J, Dongari-Bagtzoglou A. Elevated serum interleukin-6 (IL-6) in solid-organ transplant recipients is positively associated with tissue destruction and IL-6 gene expression in the periodontium. J Periodontol 2006; 77: 1871–8.

Imanguli MM, Alevizos I, Brown R, Pavletic SZ, Atkinson JC. Oral graft-versus-host disease. Oral Dis 2008; 14: 396–412.

Kaste SC, Goodman P, Leisenring W, et al. Impact of radiation and chemotherapy on risk of dental abnormalities: a report from the Childhood Cancer Survivor Study. Cancer 2009. [Epub ahead of print].

Kissel SO, Hanratty JJ. Periodontal treatment of an amalgam tattoo. Compend Contin Educ Dent 2002; 23: 930–2, 934, 936.

Ko C, Citrin D. Radiotherapy for the management of locally advanced squamous cell carcinoma of the head and neck. Oral Dis 2009; 15: 121–32.

Leão JC, Duart A, Gueiros LA , et al. Severe oral epithelial dysplasia in a patient receiving adalimumab therapy. J Oral Pathol Oral Med 2005; 34: 447–8.

Logan RM. Advances in understanding of toxicities of treatment for head and neck cancer. Oral Oncol 2009; 45: 844–8.

Marx RE, Sawatari Y, Fortin M, Broumand V. Bisphosphonate-induced exposed bone (osteonecrosis/osteopetrosis) of the jaws: risk factors, recognition, prevention, and treatment. J Oral Maxillofac Surg 2005; 63: 1567–75.

Mauz PS, Mörike K, Kaiserling E, Brosch S. Valproic acid-associated sialadenosis of the parotid and submandibular glands:diagnostic and therapeutic aspects. Acta Otolaryngol 2005; 125: 386–91.

Owens BM, Johnson WW, Schuman NJ. Oral amalgam pigmentations (tattoos): a retrospective study. Quintessence Int 1992; 23: 805–10.

Ozcelik O, Haytac MC, Akkaya M. Iatrogenic trauma to oral tissues. J Periodontol 2005; 76: 1793–7.

Peltekis G, Palaskas D, Samanidou M, et al. Severe migratory angioedema due to ACE inhibitors use. Hippokratia 2009; 13: 122–4.

Porter SR, Scully C. Adverse drug reactions in the mouth. Clin Dermatol 2000; 18: 525–32.

Razonable RR. Nontuberculous mycobacterial infections after transplantation: a diversity of pathogens and clinical syndromes. Transpl Infect Dis 2009; 11: 191–4.

Rosenthal DI, Trotti A. Strategies for managing radiation-induced mucositis in head and neck cancer. Semin Radiat Oncol 2009; 19: 29–34.

Sarasquete ME, González M, San Miguel JF, García-Sanz R. Bisphosphonate-related osteonecrosis: genetic and acquired risk factors. Oral Dis 2009; 15: 382–7.

Scully C. Discoloured tongue; a new cause? Br J Dermatol 2001; 144: 1293–4.

Scully C, Azul A, Crighton A, et al. Nicorandil can induce severe oral ulceration. Oral Surg Oral Med Oral Pathol 2001; 91: 189–93.

Scully C, Bagan JV. Adverse drug reactions in the orofacial region. Crit Rev Oral Biol Med 2004; 15: 221–39.

Scully C. Cannabis; adverse effects from an oromucosal spray. Br Dent J 2007; 203: 336–7.

Scully C, Dios PD. HIV topic update; orofacial effects of antiretroviral therapies. Oral Dis 2001; 7: 205–10.

Scully C, Diz Dios P, Shotts R. Oral health care in patients with the most important medically compromising conditions; 6. Patients undergoing radiotherapy. CPD Dentistry 2004; 6: 80–4.

Scully C, Diz Dios P, Shotts R. Oral health care in patients with the most important medically compromising conditions; 7. Patients undergoing chemotherapy. CPD Dentistry 2005; 6: 03–06.

Scully C, Epstein J, Sonis S. Oral mucositis: a challenging complication of radiotherapy, chemotherapy, and radiochemotherapy: part 1, pathogenesis and prophylaxis of mucositis. Head and Neck 2003; 25: 1057–70.

Scully C, Epstein J, Sonis, S. Oral mucositis; a challenging complication of radiotherapy, chemotherapy, and radiochemotherapy: part 2, diagnosis and management of mucositis. Head and Neck 2004; 26: 77–84.

Scully C, Porter S. Orofacial disease: update for the dental clinical team: 4. Red, brown, black and bluish lesions. Dent Update 1999; 26: 169–73.

Scully C, Porter S. ABC of oral health. Swellings and red, white, and pigmented lesions. BMJ 2000; 321: 225–8.

Scully C, Porter S. Orofacial disease: update for the dental clinical team: 4. Red, brown, black and bluish lesions. Dent Update 1999; 26: 169-73.

Scully C, Sonis S, Diz Dios P, Oral mucositis. Oral Dis 2006; 12: 229–241.

Seward GR. Amalgam tattoo. Br Dent J 1998; 184: 470–1.

Shiboski CH, Krishnan S, Besten PD, et al. Gingival enlargement in pediatric organ transplant recipients in relation to tacrolimus-based immunosuppressive regimens. Pediatr Dent 2009; 31: 38–46.

Soysa NS, Samaranayake LP, Ellepola ANB. Antimicrobials as a contributory factor in oral candidosis – a brief overview. Oral Dis 2008; 14: 138–43.

Stopeck A, Body JJ, Fujiwara Y, et al. Denosumab versus zoledronic acid for the treatment of breast cancer patients with bone metastases: results of a randomized phase 3 study. Eur J Cancer Suppl 2009; 7: 2, abstract 2LBA.

Telang GH, Ditre CM. Blue gingiva, an unusual oral pigmentation resulting from gingival tattoo. J Am Acad Dermatol 1994; 30: 125–6.

Tewari S, Sharma RK, Abrol P, Sen R. Necrotizing stomatitis: a possible periodontal manifestation of deferiprone-induced agranulocytosis. Oral Surg Oral Med Oral Pathol Oral Radiol Endod 2009; 108: e13–19.

Tredwin C, Naik S, Lewis NJ, Scully C. Hydrogen peroxide tooth-whitening (bleaching) products: review of adverse effects and safety issues. Br Dent J 2006; 200: 371–6.

Tredwin C, Scully C, Bagan JV. Drug-induced dental disorders. Adverse Drug React Bull 2005; 232: 891–4.

Tredwin C, Scully C, Bagan JV. Drug-induced disorders of teeth. J Dent Res 2005; 84: 596–602.

Treister N, Sheehy N, Bae EH, et al. Dental panoramic radiographic evaluation in bisphosphonate-associated osteonecrosis of the jaws. Oral Dis 2009; 15: 88–92.

Watson CJ, Gimson AE, Alexander GJ, et al. A randomized controlled trial of late conversion from calcineurin inhibitor (CNI)-based to sirolimus-based immunosuppression in liver transplant recipients with impaired renal function. Liver Transplant 2007; 13: 1694–702.

Watt-Smith S, Mehta K, Scully C. Mefloquine-induced trigeminal sensory neuropathy. Oral Surg Oral Med Oral Pathol 2001; 92: 163–5.

Woo MH, Ippoliti C, Bruton J, et al. Headache, circumoral paresthesia, and facial flushing associated with high-dose carmustine infusion. Bone Marrow Transplant 1997; 19: 845–7.

# 1.7 IMMUNODEFICIENCIES

- acatalasia
- ataxia telangiectasia
- chronic mucocutaneous candidosis
- autoimmune polyendocrinopathy–candidosis–ectodermal dystrophy
- common variable immunodeficiency
- di George syndrome
- hereditary angioedema
- human immunodeficiency virus disease and acquired immune deficiency syndrome
- hyper-IgM syndromes
- leukocyte defects
- myeloperoxidase deficiency
- neutropenias
- Papillon–Lefevre syndrome
- selective IgA deficiency
- severe combined immunodeficiency
- sex-linked agammaglobulinaemia
- T-cell immune defects
- Wiskott–Aldrich syndrome

## ACATALASIA

Acatalasia (Takahara disease)—a rare neutrophil defect of the enzyme catalase, seen mainly in Japan, Korea, Israel and Switzerland—may present with gangrene.

## ATAXIA TELANGIECTASIA

Ataxia telangiectasia (Louis Bar syndrome)—a rare neurodegenerative disease characterised by telangiectasis and ataxia, with immunodeficiency—may present with recurrent sinusitis, oral ulceration, facial and oral telangiectasia, and cervical lymphomas. The ataxia telangiectasia mutated (ATM) gene plays a role in DNA damage response and may be overexpressed in oral potentially malignant disorders and oral carcinoma, but there is no known association of the most common ATM gene mutation with risk for oral carcinoma.

## CHRONIC MUCOCUTANEOUS CANDIDOSIS

Chronic mucocutaneous candidosis (CMC) is a complex group of familial and non-familial conditions, which predispose to chronic candidosis. Familial forms can be autosomal dominant or autosomal recessive, with or without endocrinopathies. All types manifest with chronic candidosis affecting especially the nails and mucosae (Figs 1.7.1 and 1.7.2) and up to one half suffer from endocrine dysfunction (Fig. 1.7.3; Candida-endocrinopathy syndrome). One familial dominant type is associated with deficiency of intracellular adhesion molecule-1 and nail candidosis.

## AUTOIMMUNE POLYENDOCRINOPATHY–CANDIDOSIS–ECTODERMAL DYSTROPHY

Autoimmune polyendocrinopathy–candidosis–ectodermal dystrophy, caused by mutations in the autoimmune regulator gene, and seen especially in Finns, Sardinians and Iranian Jews, is characterised by CMC and autoimmune damage to endocrine organs, presenting mainly with hypoparathyroidism, Addison disease and diabetes. Other manifestations may include parietal cell atrophy, gonadal failure, and there may be a liability to oral carcinoma (Figs 1.7.4 and 1.7.5). There is a higher prevalence of periodontal disease, caries, dental erosion and enamel defects compared with controls. One familial recessive type is associated with hyperimmunoglobulinaemia E and features which include abnormal facies, palate and tongue (*Job syndrome*) (Figs 1.7.6 and 1.7.7).

## COMMON VARIABLE IMMUNODEFICIENCY

Common variable immunodeficiency results in recurrent sinusitis and candidosis (including CMC).

## DI GEORGE SYNDROME

Di George syndrome (Velocardiofacial syndrome, Shprintzen syndrome, conotruncal anomaly face syndrome, congenital thymic aplasia, Strong syndrome, Sedlackova syndrome)—due to a chromosome 22 deletion—manifests with a cardiac abnormality (especially fallot tetralogy), abnormal facies, thymic aplasia, cleft palate and hypocalcaemia (CATCH 22). Abnormal facies, CMC, viral infections, and bifid uvula (submucous cleft) or overt cleft palate are the main maxillofacial anomalies but there is also a range of psychiatric complications.

## HEREDITARY ANGIOEDEMA

Hereditary angioedema (HANE)—C1 esterase inhibitor (C1-INH) deficiency—is associated with activation of kinin-like substances, increased capillary permeability and autoactivation of C1 with consumption of C4 and C2. Thus C4 plasma level falls but C3 levels are usually normal.

### Clinical features

HANE may not present until later childhood or adolescence and about half of the affected patients have no family history of angioedema. HANE can mimic allergic angioedema (Chapter 2.1; Figs 1.7.8 and 1.7.9). Abdominal pain, nausea or vomiting, diarrhoea, rashes and peripheral oedema sometimes herald an attack. Skin and visceral organs (respiratory and gastrointestinal) may be involved by typically massive local oedema without concomitant pruritus, often affecting the lips, mouth, face and neck region (Figs 2.1.99 and 2.1.100). Oedema may persist for many hours and the airway is threatened.

There are several known triggers, including trauma (especially dental trauma), anxiety, menstruation, infection, exercise, alcohol consumption and stress. Medications (e.g. oestrogen, ACE inhibitors and angiotensin II type 1 receptor antagonists) and pregnancy have also been shown to induce attacks. However, attacks can occur in the absence of any identifiable initiating event.

There is a range of types of HANE, but clinical features are identical in all.

### Diagnosis

Plasma C1 esterase levels are reduced (Type 1 HANE) but in 15% the enzyme is present but dysfunctional (Type 2 HANE). Plasma C4 level falls but C3 levels are normal. Quantitative and functional analyses of C1 INH (both antigenic and functional C1-INH), C4 and C1q should be performed when angioedema is suspected.

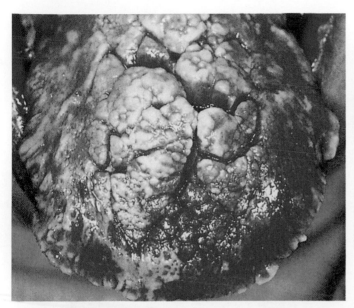

Figure 1.7.1 Chronic mucocutaneous candidosis—candidosis of tongue.

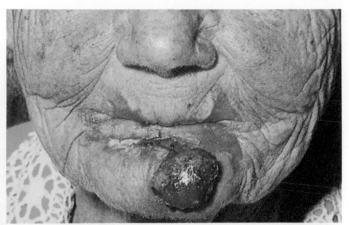

Figure 1.7.2 Chronic mucocutaneous candidosis with candidal granuloma.

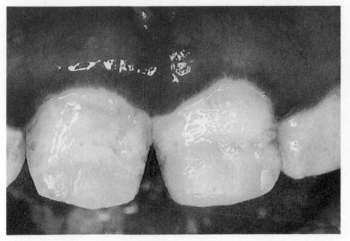

Figure 1.7.3 Chronic mucocutaneous candidosis with gingival candidosis and enamel hypoplasia.

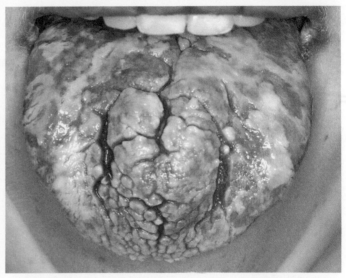

Figure 1.7.4 Autoimmune polyendocrinopathy–candidosis–ectodermal dystrophy with lingual candidosis.

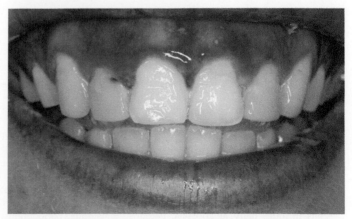

Figure 1.7.5 Autoimmune polyendocrinopathy–candidosis–ectodermal dystrophy with hypoparathyroidism and Addison disease.

Analysis of C1q can help differentiate between HANE and acquired angioedema caused by C1-INH deficiency.

## Management

C1 esterase concentrates are available for replacement of the missing C1-INH. Acute exacerbations should be treated with intravenous purified, virus-inactivated, human plasma-derived C1-INH concentrate or recombinant human C1-INH. Drugs such as ecallantide, a potent kallikrein inhibitor; and icatibant, a bradykinin 2 receptor antagonist, may also be helpful. Intravenous fresh frozen plasma may also be useful in acute HANE but occasionally exacerbates symptoms. Attenuated androgens (e.g. danazoland stanzolol) or antifibrinolytic agents are now less commonly used. Corticosteroids, antihistamines and epinephrine can be useful adjuncts but are rarely efficacious in aborting acute attacks.

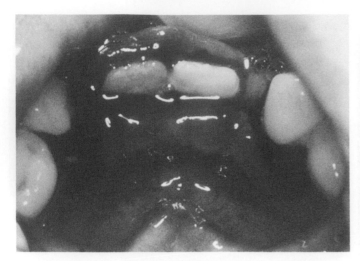

*Figure 1.7.6* Job syndrome.

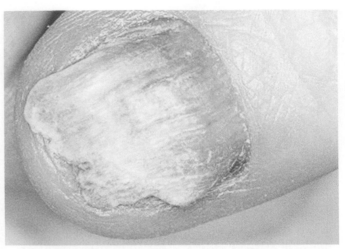

*Figure 1.7.7* Job syndrome.

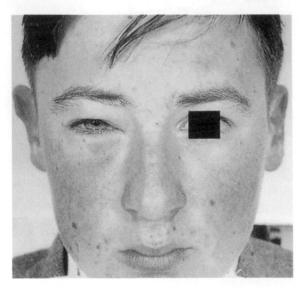

*Figure 1.7.8* Hereditary angioedema during attack.

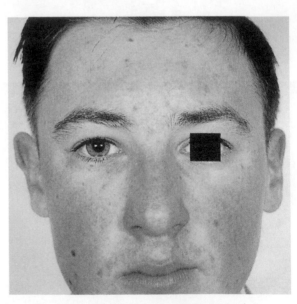

*Figure 1.7.9* Hereditary angioedema after attack.

## HUMAN IMMUNODEFICIENCY VIRUS DISEASE AND ACQUIRED IMMUNE DEFICIENCY SYNDROME

Human immunodeficiency virus (HIV) disease and acquired immune deficiency syndrome (AIDS) presents mainly with infections and neoplasms. Cervical lymphadenopathy is an almost invariable feature of HIV disease and AIDS.

HIV infection eventually leads to HIV disease and then AIDS and most patients with HIV disease develop head and neck and oral manifestations. Oral features are now classified as strongly, less commonly or possibly, associated with HIV/AIDS (Table 1.7.1).

Infections include particularly herpetic, candidal and papillomaviruses; neoplasms are mainly Kaposi sarcoma and lymphoma. A range of other lesions includes hairy leukoplakia, parotitis, xerostomia, periodontitis, aphthous-like ulcers, cranial nerve lesions, or purpura (Figs 1.7.10–1.7.49). Lesions are most likely when the CD4 cell count is low and HCV

**TABLE 1.7.1**   MAXILLOFACIAL MANIFESTATIONS IN HIV/AIDS

| Common | Less common | Rare |
|---|---|---|
| Cervical lymphadenopathy | Herpes simplex | Mycobacterial ulcers |
| Candidosis | Herpes zoster | Cryptococcal ulcers |
| Hairy leukoplakia | Cytomegalovirus | Histoplasmal ulcers |
| Kaposi sarcoma | Human papillomavirus | Addisonian pigmentation |
| | Periodontitis and gingivitis | Osteomyelitis |
| | Recurrent ulcers | Cranial neuropathies |
| | Lymphoma | Other infections |
| | Parotitis | Salivary gland neoplasms |
| | Xerostomia | |

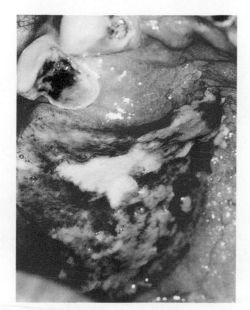

Figure 1.7.10 HIV infection—blastomycosis.

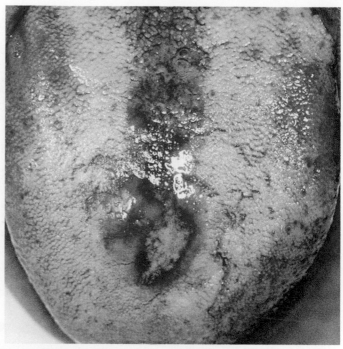

Figure 1.7.11 HIV infection—cytomegalovirus infection.

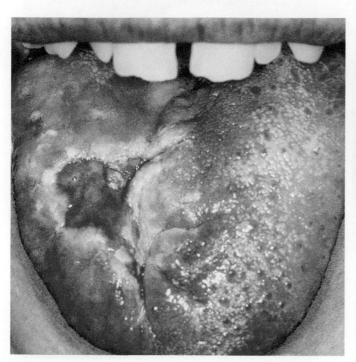

Figure 1.7.12 HIV infection—cytomegalovirus infection.

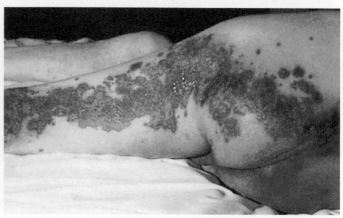

Figure 1.7.13 HIV infection—zoster.

### Fungal infections

Oral levels of *Candida albicans* and other yeasts are increased. Oral candidosis is common, often an early or the initial manifestation of HIV/AIDS, and frequently associated with oesophageal candidosis. Oral candidosis is:

- the most common opportunistic infection in HIV-infected persons;
- often the initial manifestation of symptomatic HIV infection;
- seen at some point in at least 90% of HIV-infected patients;
- seen in all groups at risk, especially HIV-infected intravenous drug users; and
- a predictor of liability to systemic opportunistic infections.

Oral candidosis is more frequent with:

- increasing severity of HIV disease and lower CD4 and/or CD4/CD8 ratios

co-infected patients are more prone than HIV mono-infected patients to develop oral lesions. Lesions are often controlled, at least temporarily, by anti-retroviral treatment.

The possibility of a diagnosis of HIV/AIDS is heightened where there are additional suggestive lesions or where there is clear high risk of HIV infection such as in an intravenous drug user.

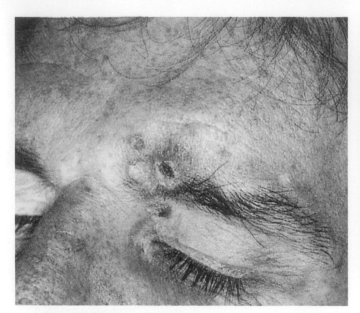

*Figure 1.7.14* HIV infection—varicella zoster virus infection.

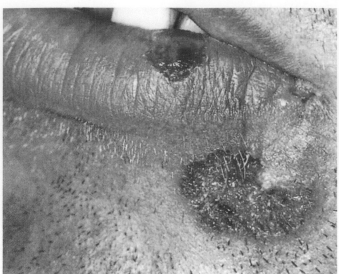

*Figure 1.7.15* HIV infection—herpes simplex virus infection.

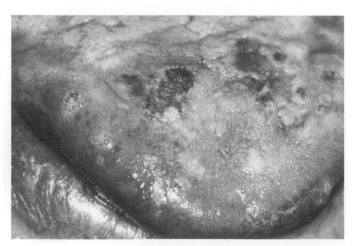

*Figure 1.7.16* HIV infection—herpes simplex virus infection.

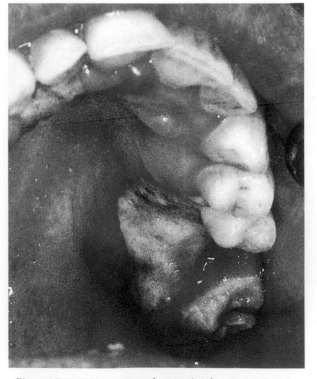

*Figure 1.7.17* HIV infection—herpes simplex virus infection.

- xerostomia
- smoking
- antimicrobial use.

Up to 25% of HIV-infected patients with candidosis have *C. albicans* plus other species.

Thrush (pseudomembranous candidosis) is one of the most obvious lesions. Erythematous candidosis may be a common early oral manifestation of HIV infection and presents as pink or red macular or mixed red and white lesions, typically on the palate or tongue, or median rhomboid glossitis and often with white lesions. Other types of candidosis also seen may include:

- angular stomatitis (cheilitis) and
- hyperplastic candidiasis.

Infections with non-albicans species are increasing, coincident with increasing use of chronic antifungal therapy. *C. krusei* and *Torulopsis glabrata* particularly are becoming a problem since they are less likely to respond to fluconazole. New species closely related to *C. krusei*, such as *C. inconspicua*, have emerged and are often fluconazole-resistant. New organisms such as *C. dubliniensis*, related to *C. albicans*, have appeared, but at least at present remain largely fluconazole-sensitive.

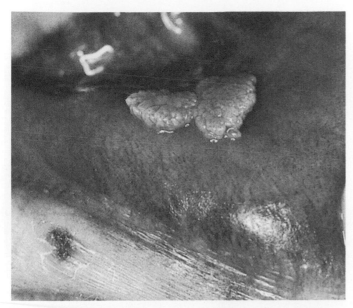

Figure 1.7.18 HIV infection—human papillomavirus infection.

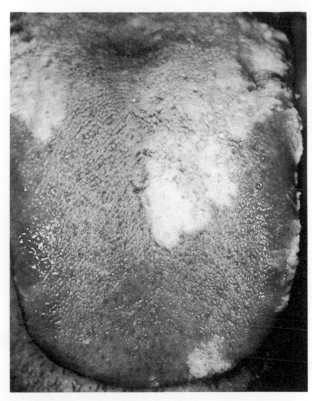

Figure 1.7.19 HIV infection—Epstein–Barr virus infection (hairy leukoplakia).

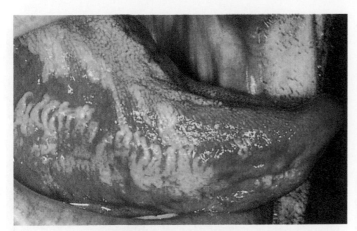

Figure 1.7.20 HIV infection—Epstein–Barr virus infection (hairy leukoplakia).

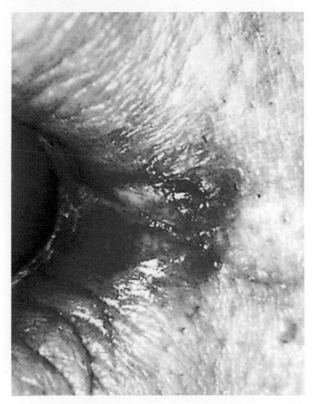

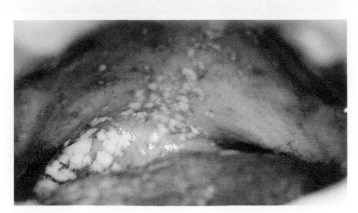

Figure 1.7.21 HIV infection—candidosis.

Figure 1.7.22 HIV infection—candidosis.

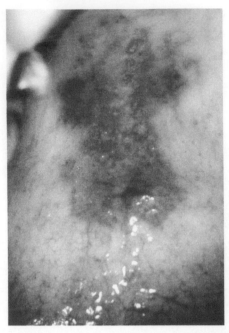

*Figure 1.7.23* HIV infection—candidosis showing thumbprint pattern.

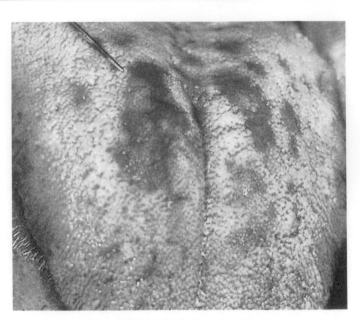

*Figure 1.7.24* HIV infection—candidosis.

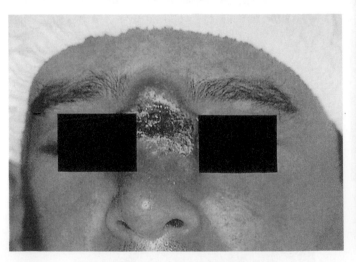

*Figure 1.7.25* HIV infection—histoplasmosis.

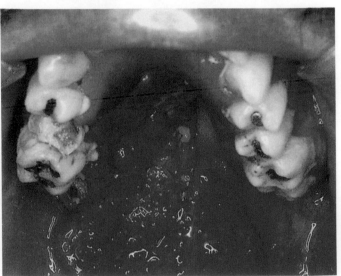

*Figure 1.7.26* HIV infection—histoplasmosis.

Diagnosis of oral candidosis is mainly clinical. Early treatment is warranted, because of the discomfort and also because foci may act as reservoirs for spread, particularly to the oesophagus. Predisposing factors such as smoking and xerostomia should be controlled. Anti-retroviral treatment of HIV infection may aid resolution. Conventional antifungal treatment is indicated initially, and although fluconazole may be required especially if there is oesophageal infection, azole resistance is an increasing problem. Antifungal prophylaxis should also be considered.

Oral histoplasmosis and cryptococcosis are rare.

### Viral infections

Common infections are as follows:

- Human papillomaviruses (HPV) causing warts, papillomas or condylomas (Chapter 1.8).
- Herpes simplex virus (HSV), usually perioral or intraoral, sometimes severe and persistent but rarely disseminate—they usually respond well to aciclovir or valaciclovir.
- Varicella zoster virus (VZV), may cause severe herpes zoster, especially in highly active antiretroviral therapy (HAART).

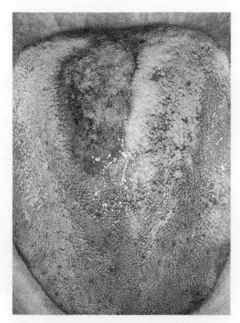

*Figure 1.7.27* HIV infection—histoplasmosis.

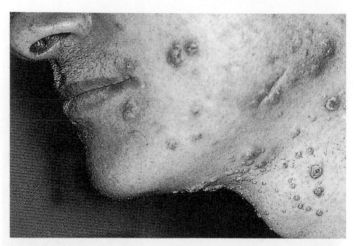

*Figure 1.7.28* HIV infection—molluscum contagiosum.

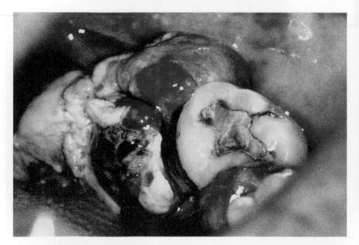

*Figure 1.7.29* HIV infection—epithelioid angiomatosis.

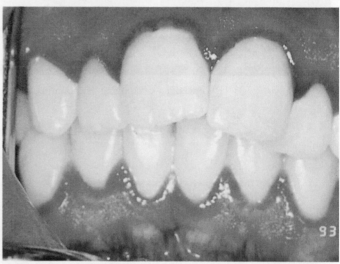

*Figure 1.7.30* HIV infection—linear gingival erythema.

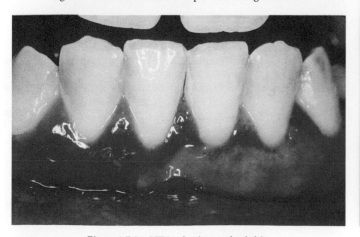

*Figure 1.7.31* HIV infection—gingivitis.

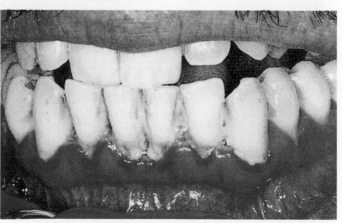

*Figure 1.7.32* HIV infection—necrotizing gingivitis.

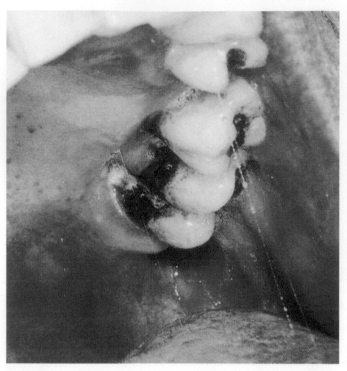

*Figure 1.7.33* HIV infection—necrotizing periodontitis.

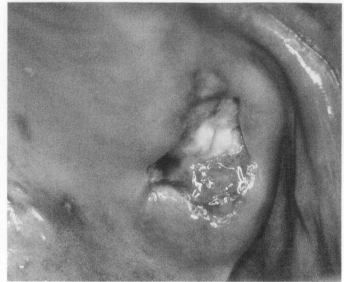

*Figure 1.7.34* HIV infection—osteitis.

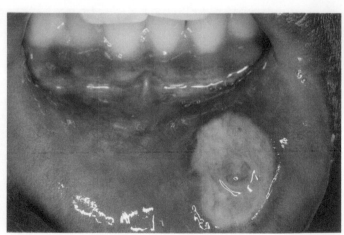

*Figure 1.7.36* HIV infection—aphthous-like ulceration.

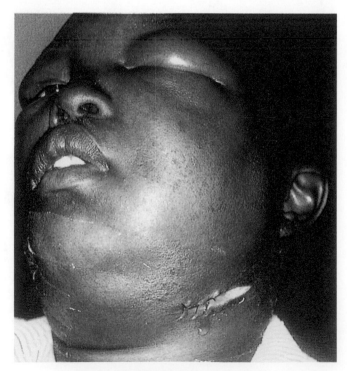

*Figure 1.7.35* HIV infection—osteomyelitis.

- Cytomegalovirus (CMV) may cause mouth ulcers.
- Hairy leukoplakia (Chapters 1.8, 2.3) may be Epstein–Barr virus (EBV)-related.
- Kaposi sarcoma (KS) is caused by Kaposi sarcoma herpesvirus (KSHV).
- Oral and salivary gland lymphomas may be EBV- and/or KSHV (herpes virus 8) -related. Lymphomas are often:
  o non-Hodgkin lymphomas
  o part of widespread disease
  o seen in the maxillary gingivae/fauces
  o fairly resistant to therapy.

Diagnosis must be confirmed by biopsy examination. Management is with chemotherapy.

- Parvovirus may be associated with salivary gland lesions.

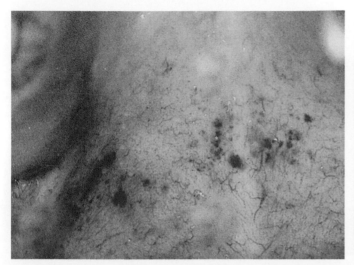

Figure 1.7.37 HIV infection—petechiae.

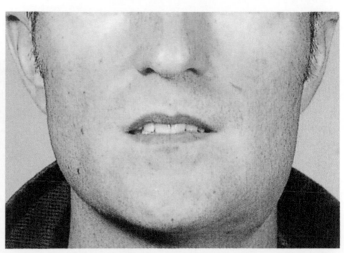

*Figure 1.7.38* HIV salivary gland disease.

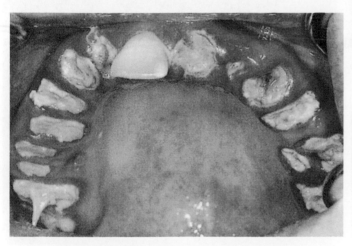

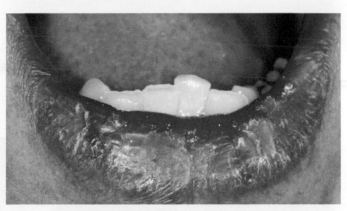

*Figure 1.7.40* HIV infection—cheilitis.

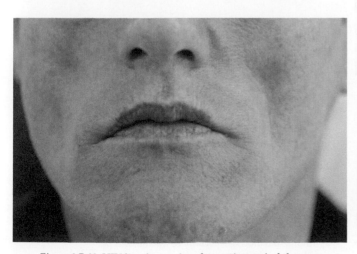

*Figure 1.7.39* HIV infection—xerostomia and caries.

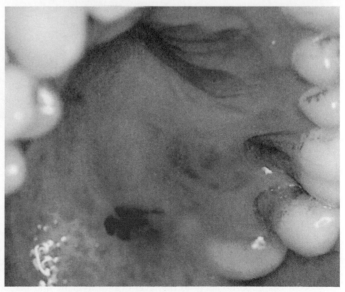

*Figure 1.7.41* HIV lipodystrophy after antiretroviral therapy.

*Figure 1.7.42* HIV infection—Kaposi sarcoma.

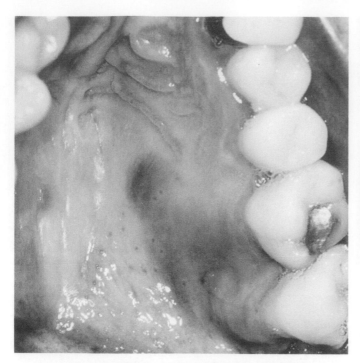

Figure 1.7.43  HIV infection—Kaposi sarcoma.

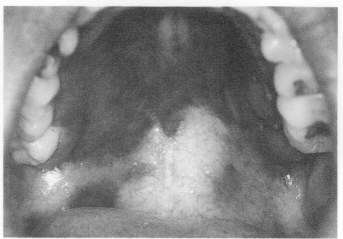

Figure 1.7.44  HIV infection—Kaposi sarcoma.

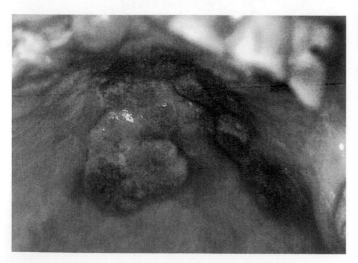

Figure 1.7.45  HIV infection—Kaposi sarcoma.

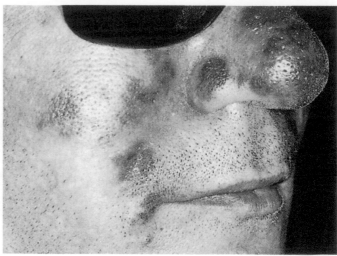

Figure 1.7.46  HIV infection—Kaposi sarcoma.

o are painful
o are localised
o cause rapid alveolar bone loss.
- post-extraction infections; osteomyelitis after jaw fractures
- cancrum oris (noma)
- Epithelioid angiomatosis—caused by the bacterium *Bartonella* (*Rochalimaea*) *henselae* or *quintana* that clinically and histologically mimics KS but responds well to antibiotics.

### Other possibly infective lesions

Chronic parotitis is seen mainly in children with HIV infection and may be associated with xerostomia.

Mouth ulcers in HIV disease may be unrelated to the HIV infection, or may be related to:

- aphthous-like ulcers, especially of the major type
- neoplasms such as Kaposi sarcoma or lymphoma

### Bacterial infections

Bacterial infections include:

- mycobacterial
- sinusitis; chronic sinusitis may be related to bacteria (or, increasingly, to fungi such as aspergillosis or zygomycosis)
- gingivitis or periodontitis. Necrotizing ulcerative gingivitis and periodontitis can be features of HIV infection, and typically:
  o occur disproportionately to the level of oral hygiene and plaque control

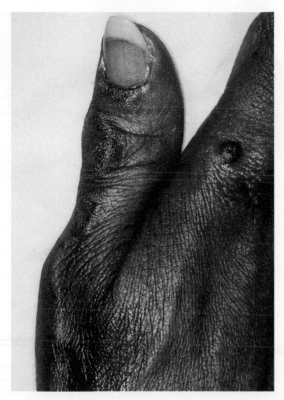

*Figure 1.7.47* HIV infection—Kaposi sarcoma.

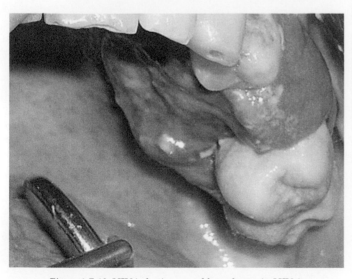

*Figure 1.7.49* HIV infection—oral lymphoma in HIV-1.

- opportunistic pathogens such as the herpesviruses, fungi (e.g. histoplasmosis or cryptococcosis), mycobacteria (e.g. tuberculosis or non-tuberculous mycobacteria) or protozoa (e.g. leishmaniasis)
- recreational drug use.

Ulcers may be part of disseminated disease, such as CMV infection, cryptococcosis or lymphoma, and thus a physician should be consulted. Diagnosis can be difficult and biopsy with microbial DNA

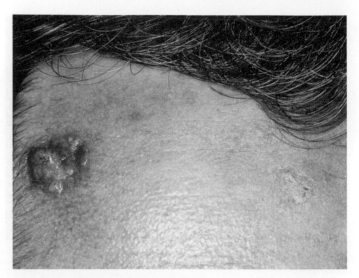

*Figure 1.7.48* HIV infection—basal cell carcinoma and Kaposi sarcoma.

studies may well be indicated. Management depends on the aetiology. Chlorhexidine and topical analgesics can be helpful but antimicrobials or other specific therapies are often indicated, depending on the cause. Granulocyte colony stimulating factors or thalidomide may be helpful in aphthous-like ulceration.

### Other maxillofacial lesions

A wide spectrum of other maxillofacial lesions can be seen in HIV/AIDS, including:

- Xerostomia (HIV-salivary gland disease), seen particularly in HIV-infected children.
- Cystic salivary lesions are increasingly recognised and there is an increase in salivary gland neoplasms.
- Cranial neuropathies, such as facial palsy, pain or sensory loss.
- Adverse effects of anti-retroviral drugs, such as lipodystrophy, burning mouth, dry mouth, taste disturbance or erythema multiforme.

### Immune reconstitution inflammatory syndrome (IRIS)

IRIS, which may follow HAART, may be accompanied by oral candidosis, viral infections (Kaposi sarcoma, papillomavirus infections, zoster) or parotitis.

## HYPER-IgM SYNDROMES

Hyper-IgM syndromes may be associated with leukopenia or hypoimmunoglobulinaemia. Mouth ulceration is a common feature.

## LEUKOCYTE DEFECTS

Leukocyte defects (Chapter 1.4).

## MYELOPEROXIDASE DEFICIENCY

Myeloperoxidase (MPO) deficiency—a common defect in the enzyme MPO in neutrophils—may be symptomless or manifest with chronic candidosis (including CMC).

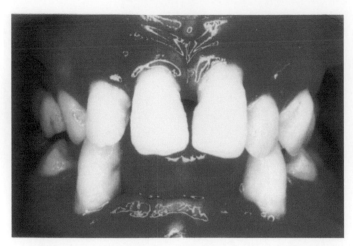

*Figure 1.7.50* Early tooth loss in Papillon–Lefevre syndrome.

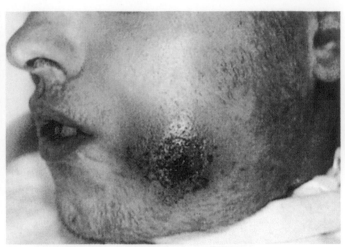

*Figure 1.7.51* Noma.

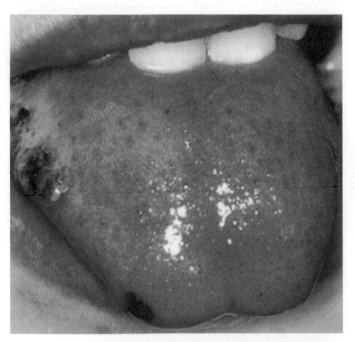

*Figure 1.7.52* Wiskott–Aldrich syndrome showing petechiae.

## NEUTROPENIAS

Neutropenias (Chapter 1.4).

## PAPILLON–LEFEVRE SYNDROME

Papillon–Lefevre syndrome and the related Haim–Munk syndrome are allelic mutations in cathepsin C in neutrophils, manifesting with accelerated periodontitis and tooth loss in both dentitions, and hyperkeratosis of palms and soles of feet appear in the first few years of life (palmoplantar hyperkeratosis) (Fig. 1.7.50).

## SELECTIVE IgA DEFICIENCY

Selective IgA deficiency—the most common primary (genetically determined) immune defect—can cause tonsillar hyperplasia, oral ulceration, viral infections and parotitis. Some patients are healthy but those who also lack $IgG_2$ suffer recurrent respiratory infection, autoimmune disorders and atopy. Mouth ulcers, and a reduced protection against dental caries are the main oral features but sialadenitis may also occur.

## SEVERE COMBINED IMMUNODEFICIENCY

Severe combined immunodeficiency—where there are both T- and B-lymphocyte defects—presents typically with candidosis (including CMC), viral infections, oral ulceration, absent tonsils and recurrent sinusitis.

## SEX-LINKED AGAMMAGLOBULINAEMIA

Sex-linked agammaglobulinaemia (Bruton disease)—where there are low levels or lack of all serum immunoglobulin classes—may present with cervical lymph node enlargement, oral ulceration, recurrent sinusitis and absent tonsils.

## T-CELL IMMUNE DEFECTS

T-cell immune defects predispose to infections, oral ulceration, periodontitis and malignant neoplasms (rarely). Complications may include gangrenous stomatitis (noma) (Fig. 1.7.51).

### Infections

- Fungal infections:
  - Candidosis (see Chapter 1.8).
  - *Aspergillus* spp. may infect the paranasal sinuses, palate or other sites by direct extension and haematogenously. Diagnosis is by demonstration of hyphae in a smear, serology and biopsy. Intravenous amphotericin may be effective.
  - Mucormycosis (zygomycosis: phycomycosis) is infection by *Mucor* or *Rhizopus* spp., mainly of the paranasal sinuses and nose of immunosuppressed or poorly controlled diabetic or leukaemic

patients. Diagnosis is by biopsy and culture: treatment is by control of underlying disease, debridement and intravenous amphotericin.

- Bacterial infections:
  o Mycobacterioses.
  o Odontogenic infections—which can be lifethreatening, and broad-spectrum antimicrobials are needed (such as penicillin plus gentamicin).
- Viral infections:
  o HSV or VZV infections; antivirals such as acyclovir, valaciclovir or famciclovir are indicated for severe HSV infections.
  o EBV infections resulting in hairy leukoplakia or lymphoma.
  o HPV infections (Chapter 1.8).
  o KSHV infections.

### Neoplasms

Neoplasms, at least some of which are virally related, may include Kaposi sarcoma; lymphomas, and squamous cell carcinomas of the skin and of the lip. Some patients develop oral white lesions (keratoses).

## WISKOTT–ALDRICH SYNDROME

Wiskott–Aldrich syndrome—a rare x-linked combined immune defect due to lack of Wiskott–Aldrich syndrome protein—manifests with thrombocytopenia, immunodeficiency and eczema (TIE syndrome) and can present with candidosis, viral infections and purpura (Fig. 1.7.52).

## FURTHER READING

Aldous JA, Olson GJ, Parkin MJ. Dental observations of hyper IgE disorder. J Clin Pediatr Dent 2007; 32: 69–72.

Al-Otaibi LM, Ngui SL, Scully C, Porter SR, Teo CG. Salivary human herpesvirus 8 shedding in renal allograft recipients with Kaposi's sarcoma. J Med Virol 2007; 79: 1357–65.

Atkinson JC, O'Connell A, Aframian D. Oral manifestations of primary immunological diseases. J Am Dent Assoc 2000; 131: 345–56.

Beyari MM, Hodgson TA, Kondowe W, et al. Herpesvirus 8 virus (Kaposi's sarcoma-associated herpesvirus) in urine: monotypy and compartmentalisation . J Clin Microbiol 2004; 42: 3313–16.

Beyari MM, Hodgson TA, Kondowe W, et al. Inter- and intra-person cytomegalovirus infection in Malawian families. J Med Virol 2005; 75: 575–82.

Beyari MM, Hodgson TA, Cook RD, et al. Multiple human herpesvirus 8 infection. J Infect Dis 2003; 188: 678–89.

Freeman AF, Domingo DL, Holland SM. Hyper IgE (Job's) syndrome: a primary immune deficiency with oral manifestations. Oral Dis 2009; 15: 2–7.

Frezzini C, Leao JC, Porter S. Current trends of HIV disease of the mouth. J Oral Pathol Med 2005; 34: 513–31.

He Y, Chen Q, Li B. ATM in oral carcinogenesis: association with clinicopathological features. J Cancer Res Clin Oncol 2008; 134: 1013–20.

Kumar N, McLean K, Inoue N, et al. Herpesvirus 8 genoprevalence in people at disparate risks of Kaposi's sarcoma. J Med Virol 2006; 79: 52–9.

Leao JC, Ferreira AMC, Martins S, et al. Cheilitis glandularis; an unusual presentation in a patient with HIV infection. Oral Surg Oral Med Oral Pathol Oral Radiol Endod 2003; 95: 142–4.

Leao JC, Kumar N, McLean KA, et al. Effect of human immunodeficiency virus-1 protease inhibitors on the clearance of human herpesvirus 8 from blood of human Immunodeficiency virus-1-infected patients. J Med Virol 2000; 62: 416–20.

Leao JC, Ribeiro CM, Carvalho AA, Frezzini C, Porter S. Oral complications of HIV disease. Clinics (Sao Paulo) 2009; 64: 459–70.

Liu X, Hua H. Oral manifestation of chronic mucocutaneous candidiasis: seven case reports. Oral Pathol Med 2007; 36: 528–32.

Mbopi-Keou FX, Belec L, Teo CG, Scully C, Porter S. Synergism between HIV and other viruses in the mouth. Lancet Infect Dis 2002; 2: 416–24.

Mbopi-Keou FX, Legoff J, Picketty C, et al. Salivary production of IgA and IgG to human herpes virus 8 latent and lytic antigens by patients in whom kaposi's sarcoma has regressed. AIDS 2004; 18: 338–40.

McGovern E, Fleming P, Costigan C, et al. Oral health in autoimmune polyendocrinopathy candidiasis ectodermal dystrophy (APECED). Eur Arch Paediatr Dent 2008; 9: 236–44.

Milian MA, Bagan JV, Jimenez Y, Perez A, Scully C. Oral leishmaniasis in an HIV-positive patient. Report of a case involving the palate. Oral Dis 2002; 8: 59–61.

Nikfarjam J, Pourpak Z, Shahrabi M, et al. Oral manifestations in selective IgA deficiency. Int J Dent Hyg 2004; 2: 19–25.

Porter SR, Scully C. Orofacial manifestations in the primary immunodeficiency disorders. Oral Surg Oral Med Oral Pathol 1994; 78: 4–13.

Scully C, Greenspan J. Human immunodeficiency virus (HIV) transmission in dentistry. J Dent Res 2006; 85: 794–800.

Scully C, Porter SR. HIV topic update; oro-genital transmission of HIV. Oral Dis 2000; 6: 92–8.

Scully C, Watt-Smith P, Dios P, Giangrande PLF. Complications in HIV-infected and non-HIV-infected hemophiliacs and other patients after oral surgery. Int J Oral Maxillofac Surg 2002; 31: 634–40.

Shebl FM, Bhatia K, Engels EA. Salivary gland and nasopharyngeal cancers in individuals with acquired immunodeficiency syndrome in United States. Int J Cancer 2009; Oct 6. [Epub ahead of print].

Shprintzen RJ. Velo-cardio-facial syndrome: 30 years of study. Dev Disabil Res Rev 2008; 14: 3–10.

Spyridonidou S, Yapijakis C, Nkenke E, et al. A common 9 bp deletion in the ataxia-telangiectasia-mutated gene is not associated with oral cancer. Anticancer Res 2009; 29: 3191–3.

Szczawinska-Poplonyk A, Gerreth K, Breborowicz A, Borysewicz-Lewicka M. Oral manifestations of primary immune deficiencies in children. Oral Surg Oral Med Oral Pathol Oral Radiol Endod 2009; Jul 11. [Epub ahead of print].

Tar I, Kiss C, Maródi L, Márton IJ. Oral and dental conditions of children with selective IgA deficiency. Pediatr Allergy Immunol 2008; 19: 33–6.

Teo J, Codarini M. Fevers and mouth ulcers. J Paediatr Child Health 2001; 37: 507–9.

Tsang CSP, Samaranayake LP. Immune reconstitution inflammatory syndrome after highly active antiretroviral therapy: a review. Oral Dis 2010; 16: 248–56.

Zhang X, Reichart PA, Song Y. Oral manifestations of HIV/AIDS in China: a review. Oral Maxillofac Surg 2009; 13: 63–8.

# 1.8 INFECTIONS

- aspergillosis
- blastomycosis
- candidosis
- cat scratch disease
- Coxsackie and ECHO
- cytomegalovirus (CMV)
- Epstein–Barr virus (EBV)
- gonorrhoea
- herpes simplex virus (HSV)
- herpes varicella zoster
- histoplasmosis
- hiv
- human herpesvirus 6 (HHV-6)
- human papillomavirus (HPV)

- impetigo
- Kaposi sarcoma herpesvirus (KSHV)
- Kawasaki disease
- leishmaniasis
- leprosy
- Lyme disease
- measles
- mucormycosis
- mumps
- paracoccidioidomycosis
- rubella
- syphilis
- toxoplasmosis
- tuberculosis

## ASPERGILLOSIS

Aspergillosis is a rare mycotic cause (Aspergillus species such as *Aspergillus fumigatus*) of ulcers (especially in immune defects) (Figs 1.8.1 and 1.8.2) or sinus infections.

## BLASTOMYCOSIS

Blastomycosis is a rare mycotic cause (*Blastomyces dermatitidis*) of ulcers and pulmonary disease (especially in immune defects) (Fig. 1.8.3).

## CANDIDOSIS

Candidosis may present with white lesions, red lesions or angular stomatitis (Fig. 1.8.4).

## CAT SCRATCH DISEASE

Cat scratch disease is a bacterial infection (*Bartonella henselae*) that can cause cervical lymph node enlargement (Chapter 2.6).

## COXSACKIE AND ECHO

Coxsackie and ECHO are enterovirus infections that may present with ulcers in hand, foot and mouth disease and herpangina (Figs 1.8.5–1.8.8).

*Hand, foot and mouth disease* (vesicular stomatitis with exanthem) is caused by Coxsackie virus A16 mainly, but A5, A7, A9 and A10 or viruses of the B9 group, ECHOviruses or other enteroviruses may be responsible.

It is seen in schoolchildren and their contacts. The incubation period is up to a week. A rash is not always present or may affect more proximal parts of the limbs or buttocks. The vesicles usually heal spontaneously in about 1 week. Small painful vesicles surrounded by an inflammatory halo are seen especially on the dorsum and lateral aspect of the fingers and toes. Small ulcers, surrounded by an inflammatory halo affect the tongue or buccal mucosa.

Reports of other manifestations such as encephalitis are very rare, except in enterovirus 71 infection.

Diagnosis is clinical. There are no specific antiviral agents available, so treatment consists mainly of adequate fluid intake, especially in children. Treatment is indicated particularly to reduce fever and control pain. Antipyretics/analgesics, such as paracetamol/acetaminophen elixir, help relieve pain and fever. A soft bland diet is needed, as the mouth can be very sore. Local antiseptics (0.2% aqueous chlorhexidine mouthwashes) may aid resolution.

*Herpangina* is usually caused by Coxsackie viruses A1–A6, A8, A10, A12 or A22, but similar syndromes can be caused by Coxsackie B and echoviruses. Herpangina Zahorsky, caused by Coxsackie virus A4, particularly affects infants and small children. The infection has an incubation period of up to a week. Most herpangina is seen in schoolchildren and their contacts. Herpangina, presents with fever, malaise, headache and a sore throat caused by an ulcerating vesicular eruption in the oropharynx, mainly on the fauces and soft palate. The vesicles rupture to leave painful, shallow, round ulcers which heal spontaneously in 7–10 days.

Faucial ulcers with a rash and aseptic meningitis are characteristics of echovirus 16 infection. Lesions resembling Koplik spots along with a rash and aseptic meningitis may be seen in echovirus 9 infections.

Diagnosis and management are as for hand, foot and mouth disease.

## CYTOMEGALOVIRUS (CMV)

CMV infection can cause a glandular fever syndrome (Paul–Bunnell negative glandular fever), and is a rare cause of ulcers (especially in immune defects) (Chapter 1.7).

## EPSTEIN–BARR VIRUS (EBV)

EBV infection presents with glandular fever syndrome [in infectious mononucleosis (IM): Paul–Bunnell positive glandular fever], sore throat, tonsillar exudate, palatal petechiae and cervical lymph node enlargement. More common in teenagers and young adults, the incubation of 30–50 days is followed by fever, sore throat and lymph node enlargement. Mouth ulcers (Figs 1.8.9–1.8.12) may be seen together with faucial oedema and tonsillar exudate, which can be severe and can potentially obstruct the airway. Palatal petechiae, especially at the junction of the hard and soft palate, are almost pathognomonic of IM, but can be seen in other infections such as HIV. A rare presentation of IM is an isolated

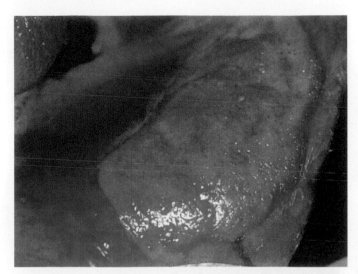

Figure 1.8.1 Aspergillus infection causing a mucosal lesion.

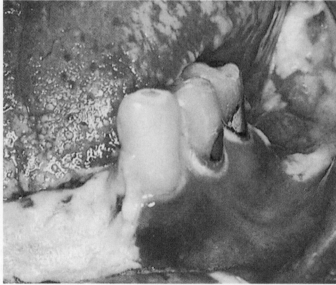

Figure 1.8.2 Aspergillus infection of the maxillary antrum.

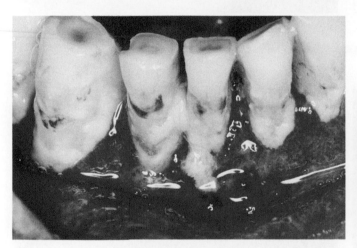

Figure 1.8.3 Blastomycosis causing gingival lesions that clinically mimic carcinoma.

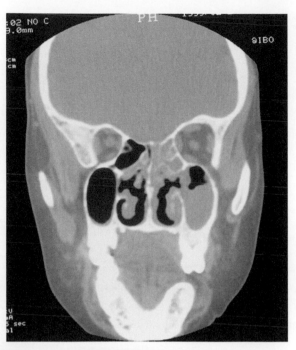

Figure 1.8.4 Candidosis; acute pseudomembranous candidosis in a renal transplant patient.

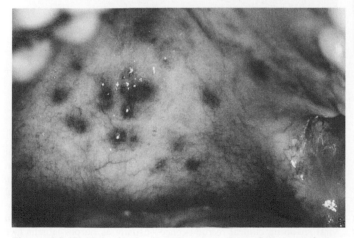

Figure 1.8.5 Hand, foot and mouth disease—a Coxsackie virus infection.

lower motor neurone facial palsy. Some develop sicca syndrome. A feature that may suggest IM is the occurrence of a rash if the patient is given ampicillin or amoxicillin (this may also be seen in lymphoid leukaemias). A few patients develop a maculopapular often morbilliform rash even if they are not taking synthetic penicillins.

EBV may also cause persistent malaise, recurrent parotitis, possibly in children and has associations with Duncan disease (X-linked lymphoproliferative syndrome), post-transplant lymphoproliferative disease,

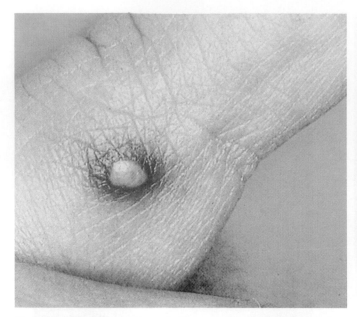

*Figure 1.8.6* Hand, foot and mouth disease—a Coxsackie virus infection.

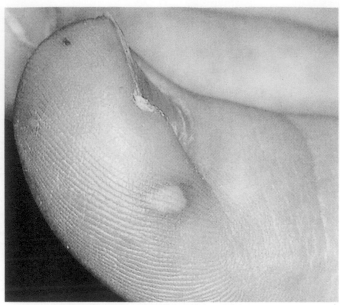

*Figure 1.8.7* Hand, foot and mouth disease—a Coxsackie virus infection.

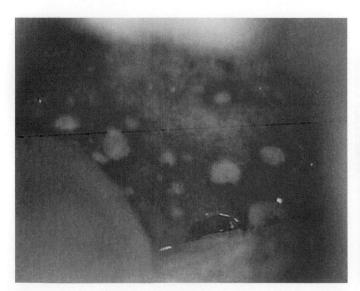

*Figure 1.8.8* Herpangina—a Coxsackie virus infection causing palatal ulceration.

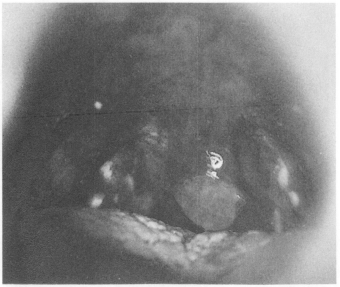

*Figure 1.8.9* Infectious mononucleosis (infection with Epstein–Barr virus) causing faucial ulceration, candidosis, sloughs and oedema.

hairy leukoplakia, Burkitt lymphoma and lymphomas in immunocompromised persons, nasopharyngeal carcinoma and other neoplasms.

## GONORRHOEA

Gonorrhoea is a sexually transmitted bacterial infection with *Neisseria gonorrhoea* that can cause pharyngitis, occasionally gingivitis and rarely temporomandibular arthritis.

## HERPES SIMPLEX VIRUS (HSV)

HSV infection causes stomatitis. It is usually caused by HSV-1, but sometimes HSV-2. HSV must contact mucosae or abraded skin when HSV surface glycoproteins mediate cell attachment and penetration. HSV is neuroinvasive and neurotoxic and infects neurones of dorsal root and autonomic ganglia. HSV remains latent thereafter in the ganglion, usually the trigeminal ganglion, but can be reactivated to result in viral shedding clinical recrudescence—usually as herpes labialis (see below, and also Bell palsy and erythema multiforme).

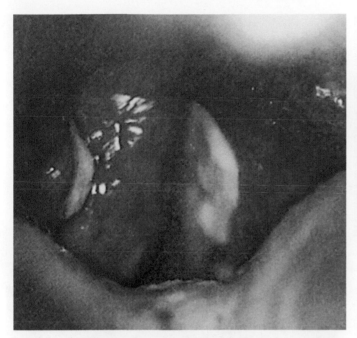

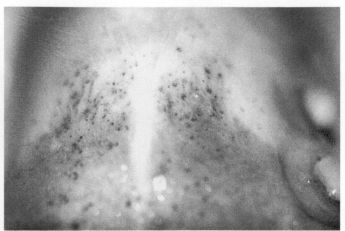

*Figure 1.8.11* Infectious mononucleosis (infection with Epstein–Barr virus) manifesting with palatal petechiae.

*Figure 1.8.10* Infectious mononucleosis (infection with Epstein–Barr virus) causing faucial oedema and tonsillar sloughs.

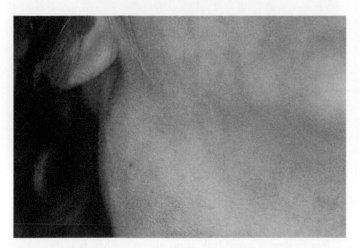

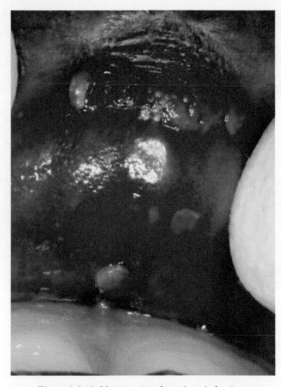

*Figure 1.8.12* Infectious mononucleosis (infection with Epstein–Barr virus) with pronounced cervical lymphadenopathy.

*Figure 1.8.13* Herpes simplex virus infection.

Typically an infection between ages 2–4 years, an increasing number of adults are now affected and can be severely ill, with malaise, fever and cervical lymph node enlargement. After an incubation period of approximately 6–7 days, gingival oedema, erythema, vesiculation and ulceration (Figs 1.8.13–1.8.30) are prominent features of primary infection. Widespread vesicles break down to leave pin-point ulcers that enlarge and fuse to produce irregular painful oral ulcers. The tongue is often coated and there is halitosis. Rarely, acute ulcerative gingivitis follows. Additionally, the saliva is heavily infected with HSV which may cause lip and skin lesions and is a source for cross-infection.

Rare complications of HSV infection include encephalitis and mononeuropathies, including facial palsy. Primary infection of the finger by

HSV can cause a painful whitlow. This was an occupational hazard for non-immune dental, medical or paramedical personnel when they did not wear protective gloves.

Herpetic stomatitis should be differentiated from other causes of mouth ulcers, especially herpangina, hand, foot and mouth disease, chickenpox and shingles, erythema multiforme and leukaemia. Diagnosis is largely clinical. Viral studies occasionally used for diagnosis can include:

- Polymerase chain reaction detection of HSV-DNA—sensitive and rapid but expensive.
- Electron microscopy—not always available.

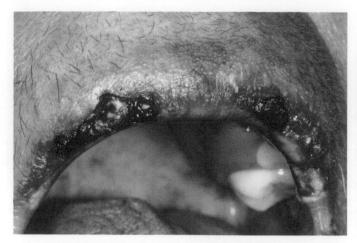

Figure 1.8.14 Herpes simplex virus infection.

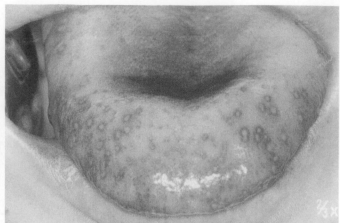

Figure 1.8.15 Herpes simplex virus infection.

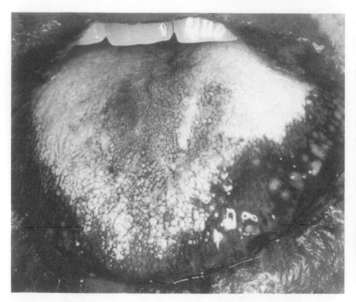

Figure 1.8.16 Herpes simplex virus infection.

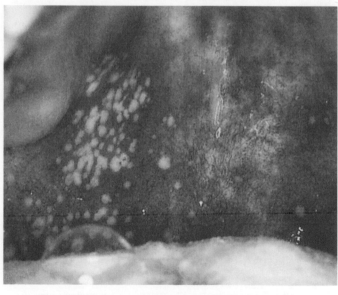

Figure 1.8.17 Herpes simplex virus infection in an adult.

- Culture—takes days to give a result.
- Immunodetection—conventional enzyme-linked immunosorbent assays for serum antibodies have poor sensitivity and specificity, while newer assays based on glycoprotein G-1 HSV glycoproteins are comparable with Western blot assays. A rising titre of serum antibodies is confirmatory, but only gives the diagnosis retrospectively.
- Smears for viral damaged cells—rarely used.

Treatment is indicated particularly to reduce fever and control pain. Aciclovir or valaciclovir orally or parenterally is useful in the otherwise apparently healthy patient if seen early in the course of the disease, and in immunocompromised patients. Antivirals do not, however, reduce the frequency of subsequent recurrences. Antiviral resistance is becoming a significant problem to immunocompromised persons, especially those with severe immune defects. Alternative therapies include foscarnet, n-docosanol, idoxuridine and tromantadine hydrochloride.

Reactivation of latent HSV is mainly on the lips as herpes labialis (Chapters 1.8 and 2.1). HSV infection at sites other than mucocutaneous junctions can simulate herpes zoster.

Recurrent intraoral herpes in normal patients tends to affect the tongue, hard palate or gingiva and heals within 1–2 weeks. It is rare intraorally but may follow the trauma of a local anaesthetic injection or may be seen in immunocompromised patients.

Immunocompromised patients may develop chronic, often dendritic, HSV reactivation ulcers—the so-called 'geometric herpetic stomatitis'—seen, for example, in HIV disease or leukaemia. Diagnosis of recurrent intraoral HSV in healthy patients is mainly from zoster. Diagnosis of recurrent intraoral HSV in immunocompromised patients can be difficult since the lesions can mimic many other causes of oral ulceration.

Diagnosis is largely clinical and viral studies are rarely used. Clinical diagnosis tends to underestimate the frequency of these lesions and viral studies may be needed—particularly since there may be CMV co-infection.

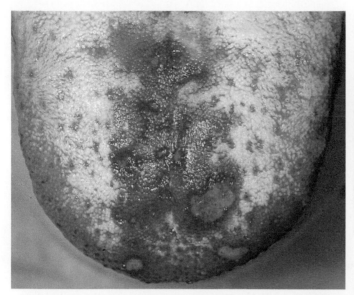

Figure 1.8.18 Herpes simplex virus infection.

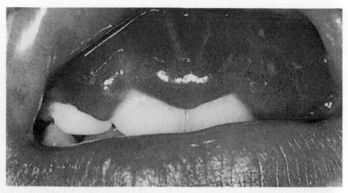

Figure 1.8.19 Herpes simplex virus infection causing gingivitis.

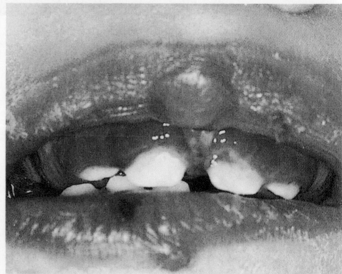

Figure 1.8.21 Herpes simplex virus infection; stomatitis with extraoral lesions.

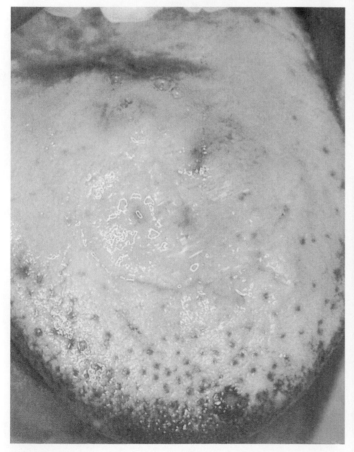

Figure 1.8.20 Herpes simplex virus infection with pronounced tongue coating.

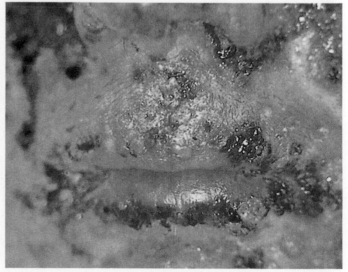

Figure 1.8.22 Herpes simplex virus infection in eczema (Kaposi varicelliform eruption).

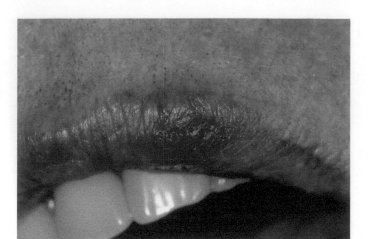

*Figure 1.8.23* Herpes simplex virus recurrence (herpes labialis).

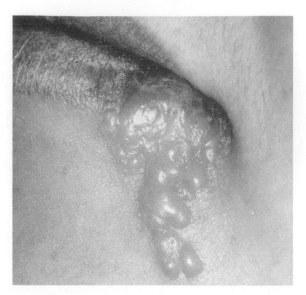

*Figure 1.8.24* Herpes simplex virus recurrence (herpes labialis).

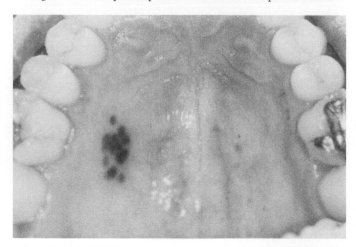

*Figure 1.8.25* Herpes simplex virus recurrence intraorally.

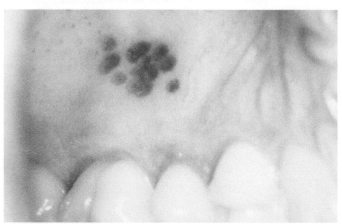

*Figure 1.8.26* Herpes simplex virus recurrence intraorally.

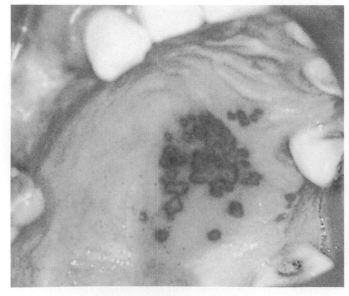

*Figure 1.8.27* Herpes simplex virus recurrence intraorally.

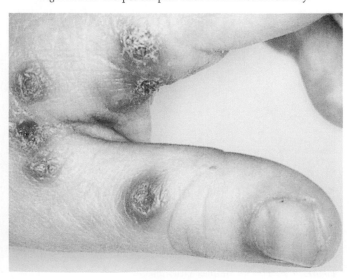

*Figure 1.8.28* Herpes simplex virus extraorally.

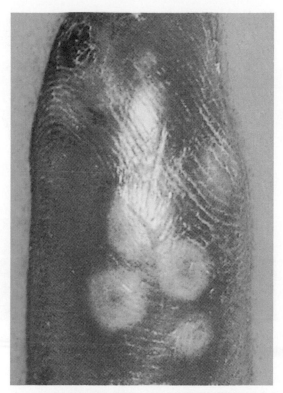

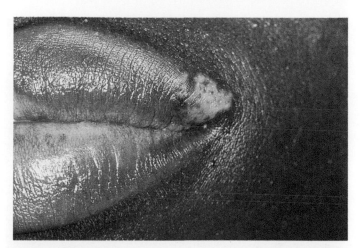

*Figure 1.8.30* Impetigo complicating herpes simplex virus infection.

*Figure 1.8.29* Herpes simplex virus infection extraorally in a dental professional who worked without protective gloves.

Antivirals (systemic aciclovir or other antivirals such as valaciclovir or famciclovir) will achieve maximum benefit only if given early in the disease, but may be indicated in:

- patients who have severe, widespread or persistent lesions; and
- immunocompromised persons.

Recurrent intraoral herpes in healthy patients can be managed with symptomatic treatment with a soft diet and adequate fluid intake, antipyretics/analgesics (paracetamol elixir) and local antiseptics (0.2% aqueous chlorhexidine mouthwashes).

Recurrent intraoral herpes in immunocompromised patients is difficult to manage and systemic aciclovir or valaciclovir or other antivirals may well be needed. A soft diet and adequate fluid intake, antipyretics/analgesics (paracetamol elixir) and local antiseptics (0.2% aqueous chlorhexidine mouthwashes) may help. Antiviral resistance is becoming a significant problem to immunocompromised persons, especially those with a severe immune defect. Alternative therapies then include foscarnet, *n*-docosanol, idoxuridine and tromantadine hydrochloride.

## HERPES VARICELLA ZOSTER

Herpes varicella zoster virus (VZV) infection causes varicella (chickenpox) and zoster (shingles).

*Chickenpox* is a highly contagious typically childhood infection between ages 2–4 years, but an increasing number of adults are now affected and can be severely ill, with widespread lesions affecting skin and mucosae. After an incubation period of 2–3 weeks, a variably dense rash appears, concentrated mainly on the trunk and head and neck (Figs 1.8.31–1.8.43). The typical rash goes through macular, papular, vesicular

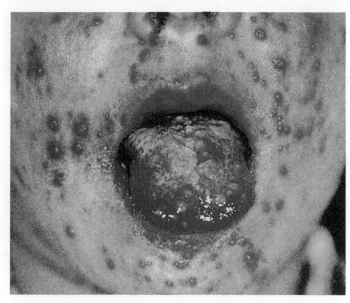

*Figure 1.8.31* Varicella zoster virus infection; chickenpox.

and pustular stages before crusting. The rash crops in waves over 2–4 days, so that lesions at different stages are typically seen.

The oral mucosa is commonly involved with vesicles, especially in the palate, which rupture to produce painful round or ovoid ulcers with an inflammatory halo.

The diagnosis is on clinical grounds. A rising antibody titre is confirmatory. Differentiation is from other mouth ulcers, especially herpes simplex and other viral infections.

Most patients will have spontaneous remission within 1 week to 10 days.

Antivirals such as aciclovir or valaciclovir if given early in the disease can be beneficial. Antivirals and immune globulins are used in most immunocompromised patients with chickenpox.

Management is otherwise symptomatic.

A vaccine against chickenpox is now available and increasingly widely used.

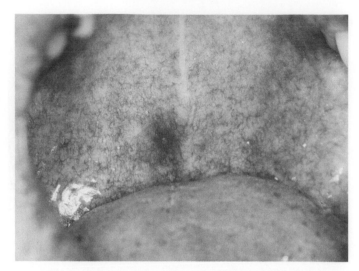

*Figure 1.8.32* Varicella zoster virus infection; chickenpox.

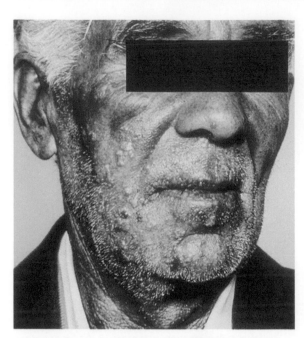

*Figure 1.8.33* Varicella zoster virus infection recurrence (shingles) of the mandibular division of the trigeminal nerve .

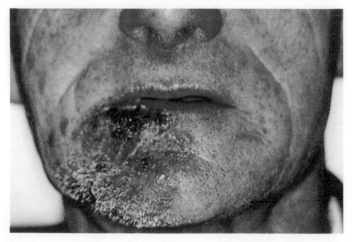

*Figure 1.8.34* Varicella zoster virus infection recurrence (shingles) of the mandibular division of the trigeminal nerve.

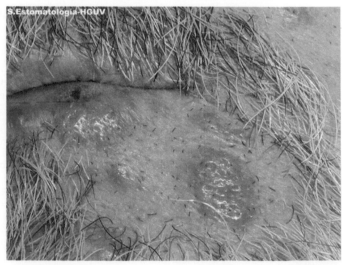

*Figure 1.8.35* Varicella zoster virus infection recurrence (shingles) of the mandibular division of the trigeminal nerve.

*Herpes zoster (shingles)* is caused by reactivation of VZV latent in dorsal root ganglia and, rarely, by reinfection. It has a bimodal distribution affecting a group of young adults who appear perfectly healthy otherwise, and also typically the elderly.

There is an increased prevalence of zoster in persons with immunocompromised cellular immunity, including those with HIV infection, malignancy, following bone marrow transplantation and in people on immunosuppressive therapies. Radiotherapy, chemotherapy and some drugs also reactivate VZV. Zoster has become a fairly common feature, for example, in the immune reconstitution syndrome in HIV-infected patients treated with active retroviral therapy.

Zoster causes pain and a rash restricted to a dermatome. Zoster most typically affects thoracic dermatomes, or occasionally other dermatomes, such as cervical dermatomes. When zoster affects cranial nerves, involvement of the central nervous system is common, and meningeal signs and symptoms are frequent. Trigeminal zoster of the

- ophthalmic division threatens sight, with the possibility of corneal ulceration, or panophthalmitis. Ophthalmic zoster also produces chemosis and periorbital oedema which may become bilateral.

- maxillary division causes a rash and periorbital oedema and ulceration of the ipsilateral palate and vestibule mainly but the eye is not involved.
- mandibular division causes ipsilateral oral ulceration in the distribution.

Zoster causes pain and a rash restricted to a dermatome with ipsilateral oral ulceration in the distribution of an affected trigeminal nerve. Mandibular and maxillary zoster may simulate toothache—the pain may precede the rash. The rash of zoster resembles that of varicella and occasionally pocks are seen beyond the affected dermatome. Occasionally, oral lesions appear in the absence of a rash.

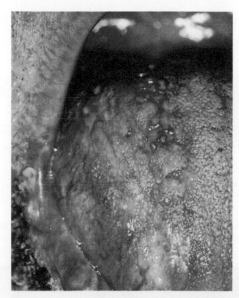

Figure 1.8.36 Varicella zoster virus infection recurrence (shingles) of the mandibular division of the trigeminal nerve.

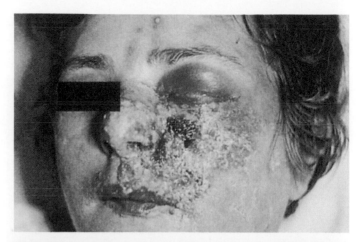

Figure 1.8.37 Varicella zoster virus infection recurrence (shingles) of the maxillary division of the trigeminal nerve.

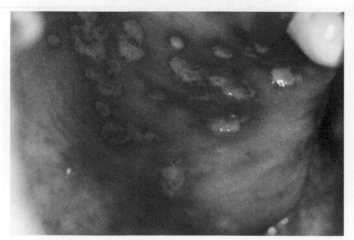

Figure 1.8.38 Varicella zoster virus infection recurrence (shingles) of the maxillary division of the trigeminal nerve.

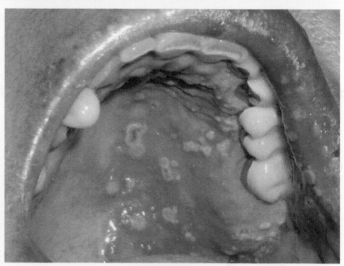

Figure 1.8.39 Varicella zoster virus infection recurrence (shingles) of the maxillary division of the trigeminal nerve.

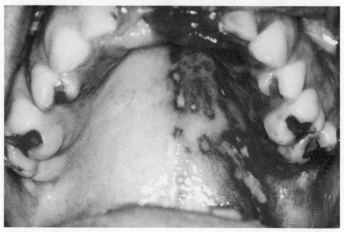

Figure 1.8.40 Varicella zoster virus infection recurrence (shingles) of the maxillary division of the trigeminal nerve.

Healing is usually uneventful, but rarely there may be scarring, bone necrosis, tooth loss or hypoplasia of developing teeth. Tissue destruction and severe post-herpetic neuralgia are more common in those who are immunocompromised. Infection of zoster lesions with *Staphylococcus aureus* can lead to a form of impetigo with delayed healing, greater scarring of the zoster lesions and dissemination of the bacterial lesions.

Diagnosis is clinical; differentiation from toothache and other causes of ulcers, especially HSV, is important. Management is with analgesics. Aciclovir or valaciclovir (high dose) orally or parenterally may help pain and healing and prevent post-herpetic neuralgia. Systemic corticosteroids may have a similar effect.

In ophthalmic zoster, an early ophthalmological opinion is important, since there can be corneal ulceration.

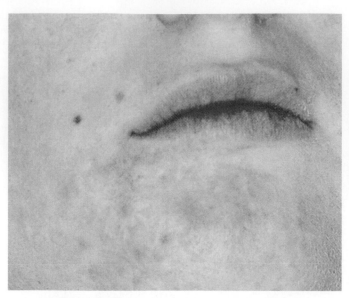

*Figure 1.8.41* Varicella zoster virus infection recurrence (shingles) of the mandibular division of the trigeminal nerve that has scarred.

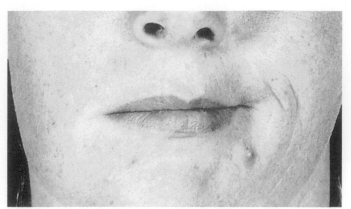

*Figure 1.8.42* Varicella zoster virus infection recurrence affecting the facial nerve (Ramsay Hunt syndrome).

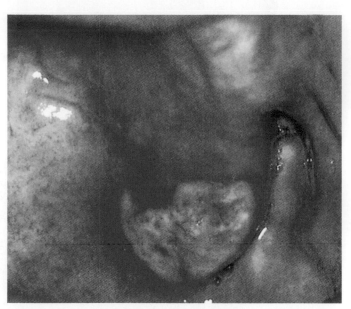

*Figure 1.8.44* Histoplasmosis.

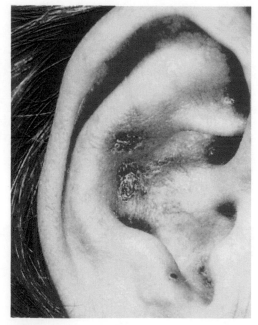

*Figure 1.8.43* Varicella zoster virus infection recurrence affecting the facial nerve (Ramsay Hunt syndrome).

## HISTOPLASMOSIS

Histoplasmosis is a rare mycotic cause (*Histoplasma capsulatum*) of ulcers and pulmonary disease (especially in immune defects) (Fig. 1.8.44).

## HIV

HIV can result in various lesions (Chapter 1.7).

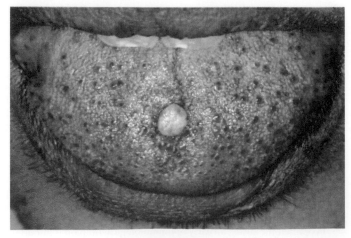

*Figure 1.8.45* Human papillomavirus infection.

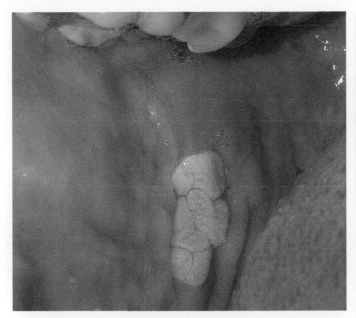

*Figure 1.8.46* Human papillomavirus infection—papilloma.

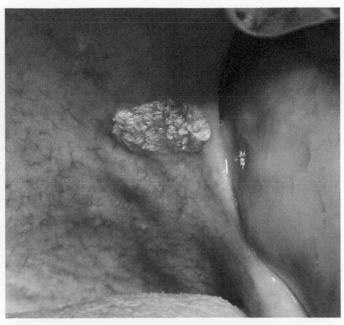

*Figure 1.8.47* Human papillomavirus infection—papilloma.

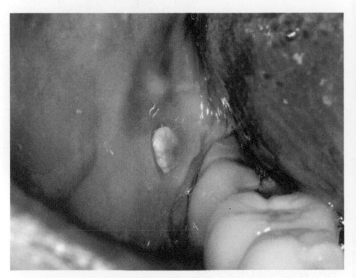

*Figure 1.8.48* Human papillomavirus infection—papilloma.

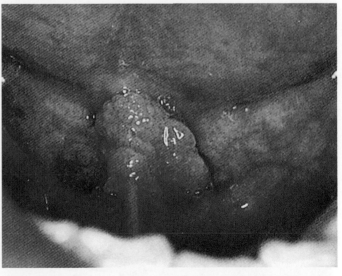

*Figure 1.8.49* Human papillomavirus infection—genital wart (condyloma acuminatum).

## HUMAN HERPESVIRUS 6 (HHV-6)

HHV-6 infection may cause cervical lymph node enlargement, glandular fever syndrome or a drug-induced hypersensitivity syndrome (Chapter 1.8).

## HUMAN PAPILLOMAVIRUS (HPV)

HPV infection causes warts, papillomas, condylomas or carcinomas (Figs 1.8.45–1.8.50).

## IMPETIGO

Impetigo is a highly contagious bacterial infection caused by staphylococcus or rarely by the streptococcus, and affects mainly young children, with golden-coloured blisters and vesicles (Fig. 1.8.51).

## KAPOSI SARCOMA HERPESVIRUS (KSHV)

KSHV (HHV-8) causes Kaposi sarcoma, as well as Castleman disease, and primary effusion lymphomas.

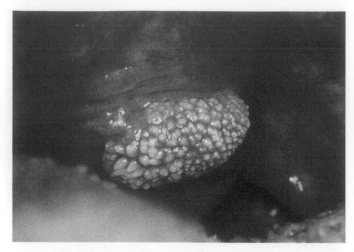

*Figure 1.8.50* Human papillomavirus infection—genital wart (condyloma acuminatum).

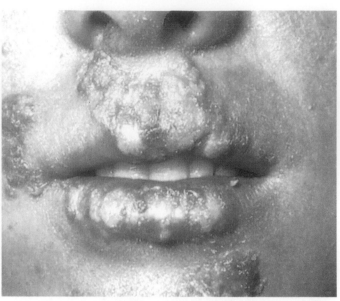

*Figure 1.8.51* Impetigo.

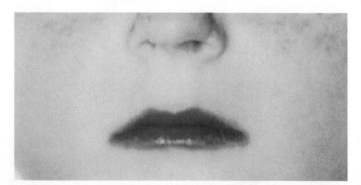

*Figure 1.8.52* Kawasaki disease.

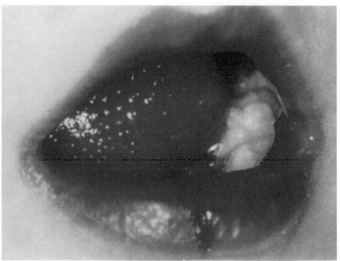

*Figure 1.8.53* Kawasaki disease.

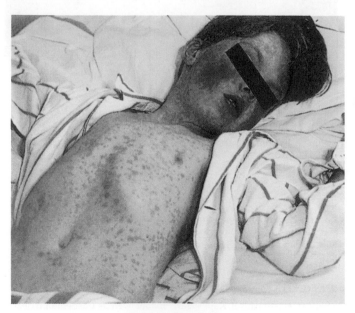

*Figure 1.8.54* Measles.

## KAWASAKI DISEASE

Kawasaki disease (mucocutaneous lymph node syndrome, infantile polyarteritis) is a vasculitis of uncertain, possibly infectious cause that can result in fever, cardiac aneurysms, conjunctival erythema, erythema and swelling of hands and feet, cervical lymph node enlargement, strawberry tongue and cheilitis (Figs 1.8.52 and 1.8.53).

## LEISHMANIASIS

Leishmaniasis is a rare parasitic cause (genus Leishmania) mainly of ulcers (especially in immune defects).

## LEPROSY

Leprosy is a bacterial infection (*Mycobacterium leprae*) that may produce facial nodules or ulceration and cranial nerve palsies.

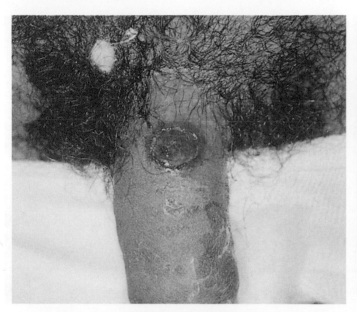

*Figure 1.8.55* Syphilis—primary (Hunterian) chancre.

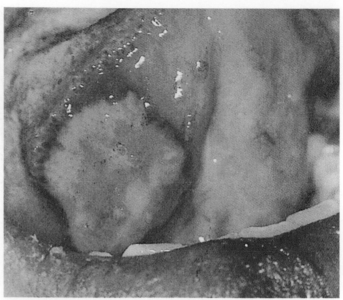

*Figure 1.8.56* Syphilis—primary (Hunterian) chancre.

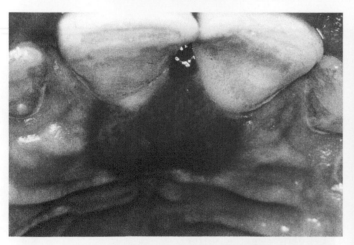

*Figure 1.8.57* Syphilis—primary (Hunterian) chancre.

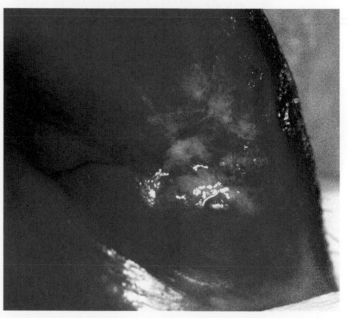

*Figure 1.8.58* Syphilis—secondary stage.

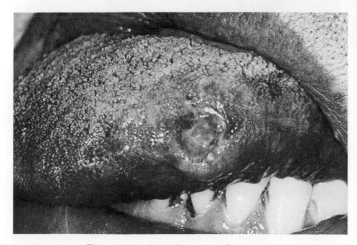

*Figure 1.8.59* Syphilis—secondary stage.

## LYME DISEASE

Lyme disease is a bacterial infection (*Borrelia burgdorferii*) that may cause facial palsy, rash and arthritis.

## MEASLES

Measles is an acute contagious infection with a paramyxovirus.

### Clinical features

The incubation of 7–10 days is followed by fever, rhinitis, cough, conjunctivitis (coryza) and then a red maculopapular rash (Fig. 1.8.54)

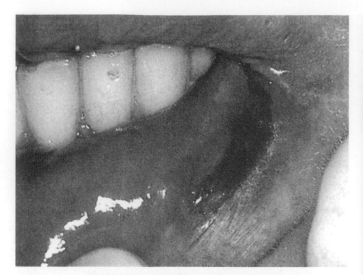

*Figure 1.8.60* Syphilis—secondary stage.

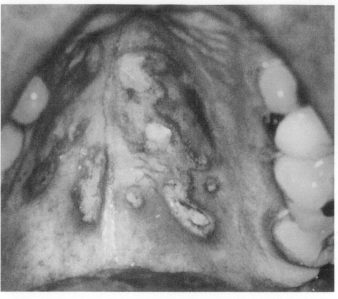

*Figure 1.8.61* Syphilis—secondary stage—snail track ulceration.

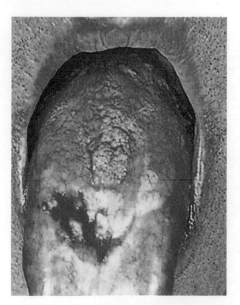

*Figure 1.8.62* Syphilis—tertiary stage.

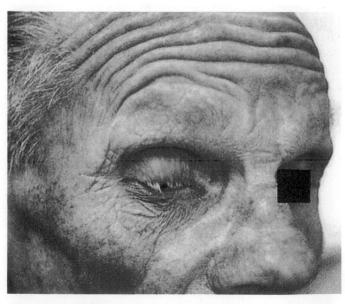

*Figure 1.8.63* Syphilis—tertiary stage showing ptosis in neurosyphilis.

initially on the forehead and behind the ears, then spreading over the whole body. It is less immediately obvious in a dark-skinned patient.

### Diagnosis
The rash is fairly characteristic. Mucosal lesions include conjunctivitis and Koplik spots. These are small, whitish, necrotic lesions, said to resemble grains of salt found in the buccal mucosa and occasionally also in the conjunctiva or genitalia, preceding the rash by 1–2 days and are pathognomonic.

### Management
This is symptomatic; fluids plus analgesics/antipyretics.

## MUCORMYCOSIS
Mucormycosis (zygomycosis) is a rare opportunistic mycotic cause (Mucorales) of ulcers and sinus infections, mainly affecting patients with immune defects in diabetes mellitus, immunodeficiency and malignancies.

## MUMPS
Mumps virus typically causes painful major salivary gland swelling (sialadenitis) (Chapter 2.7).

## PARACOCCIDIOIDOMYCOSIS
Paracoccidioidomycosis is a rare mycotic cause (*Paracoccidioides brasiliensis*) of ulcers and pulmonary disease (especially in immune defects).

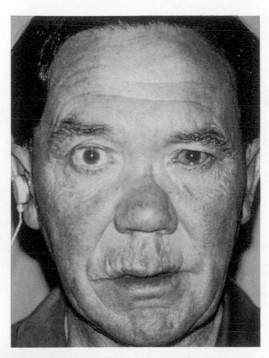

Figure 1.8.64 Syphilis—congenital showing osteitis.

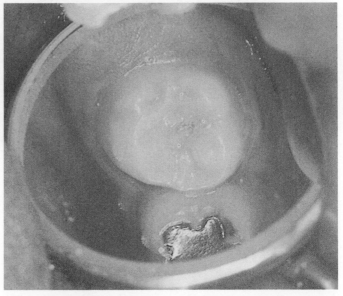

*Figure 1.8.65* Syphilis—congenital showing Hutchinson triad (dental anomalies plus interstitial keratitis and nerve deafness).

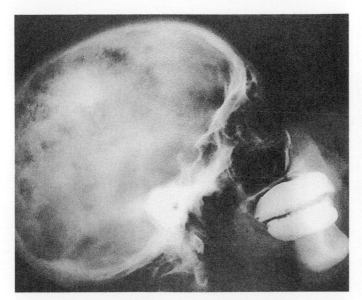

Figure 1.8.66 Syphilis—congenital showing Hutchinson incisors.

## RUBELLA

Rubella virus infection can cause cervical lymph node enlargement and oral purpura (Forchheimer spots).

## SYPHILIS

Syphilis is a sexually transmitted bacterial infection (*Treponema pallidum*), that can present with chancre, mucous-patches, ulcers, gummas, pain from neurosyphilis, leukoplakia and lymph node enlargement. Hutchinson teeth and Moon molars may be seen in congenital syphilis (Figs 1.8.55–1.8.67).

## TOXOPLASMOSIS

Toxoplasmosis is a parasitic infection (*Toxoplasma gondii*), often arising from cats, that can cause a glandular fever syndrome, with lymph node enlargement.

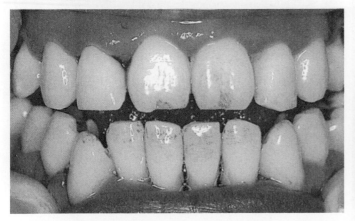

*Figure 1.8.67* Syphilis—congenital showing hypoplastic molars (Moon or mulberry molars).

## TUBERCULOSIS

Tuberculosis is a bacterial infection with *Mycobacterium tuberculosis* (occasionally *M. bovis, M. africanum, M. microti, M. canetti*) that can manifest with ulcers, lumps and cervical lymph node enlargement and pulmonary disease (Figs 1.8.68–1.8.74). Atypical mycobacteria (*M. avium* complex and *M. scrofulaceum, M. ulcerans, M chelonae, M. kansasii, M. xenopi* and others), also termed nontuberculous

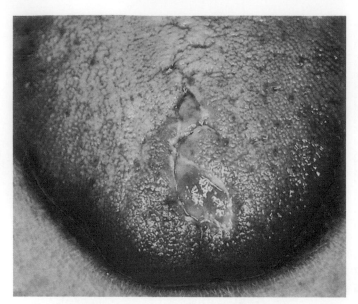

*Figure 1.8.68* Tuberculosis showing oral ulceration.

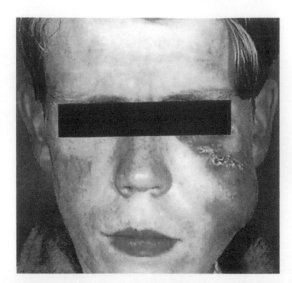

*Figure 1.8.69* Tuberculosis showing osteomyelitis.

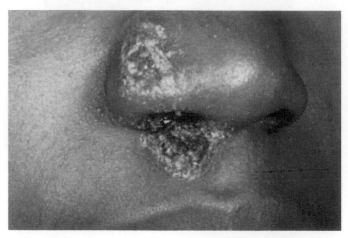

*Figure 1.8.70* Tuberculosis showing skin infection (lupus vulgaris).

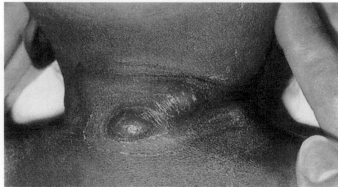

*Figure 1.8.71* Tuberculosis showing cervical lymph node abscesses (scrofula).

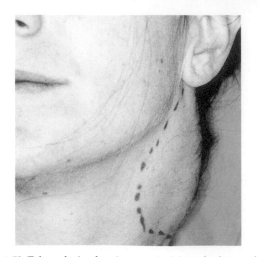

*Figure 1.8.72* Tuberculosis showing cervical lymphadenopathy from lung tuberculosis.

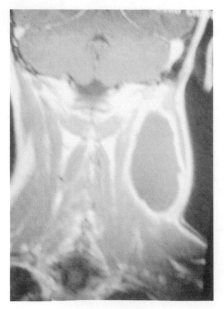

*Figure 1.8.73* Tuberculosis showing cervical lymphadenopathy from lung tuberculosis.

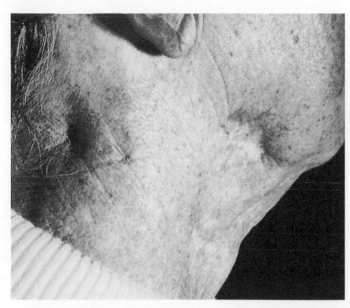

*Figure 1.8.74* Tuberculosis showing scarring from cold abscess.

mycobacteria, environmental mycobacteria and mycobacteria other than tuberculosis—can cause similar manifestations.

## FURTHER READING

Al-Karawi ZM, Manfredi M, Waugh ACW, et al. Molecular characterization of Candida spp. isolated from the oral cavity of patients from diverse clinical settings. Oral Microbiol Immunol 2002; 17: 44–9.

Almeida ODP, Jacks J, Scully C. Paracoccidioidomycosis of the mouth; an emerging deep mycosis. Crit Rev Oral Biol Med 2003; 14: 377–83.

Almeida ODP, Scully C. Fungal infections of the mouth. Brazilian J Oral Sci 2002; 1: 19–26.

Arduino PG, Porter SR. Oral and perioral herpes simplex virus type 1 (HSV-1) infection: review of its management. Oral Dis 2006; 12: 254–70.

Arduino PG, Porter SR. Herpes simplex virus type 1 infection: overview on relevant clinico-pathological features. J Oral Pathol Med 2008; 37: 107–21.

Campisi G, Panzarella V, Giuliani M, et al. Human papillomavirus: its identity and controversial role in oral oncogenesis, premalignant and malignant lesions (review). Int J Oncol 2007; 30: 813–23.

Colella G, Borriello C, Scully C. Maxillary osteonecrosis in visceral leishmaniasis. Oral Biosci Med 2004; 1: 145–8.

Dahlén G. Bacterial infections of the oral mucosa. Periodontol 2000 2009; 49: 13–38.

Femiano F, Gombos S, Scully C. Recurrent herpes labialis; efficacy of topical therapy with penciclovir compared with acyclovir (aciclovir). Oral Dis 2001; 7: 31–2.

Femiano F, Gombos S, Scully C. Recurrent herpes labialis; pilot study of the efficacy of zinc therapy. J Oral Pathol Oral Med 2005; 34: 423–5.

Fenton SJ, Unkel JH. Viral infections of the oral mucosa in children: a clinical review. Pract Periodontics Aesthet Dent 1997; 9: 683–90.

Figueiral MH, Azul A, Pinto E, et al. Denture-related stomatitis: identification and characterization of aetiological and predisposing factors—a large cohort. J Oral Rehab 2007; 34: 448–55.

Frezzini C, Leao JC, Porter S. Current trends of HIV disease of the mouth. J Oral Pathol Med 2005; 34: 513–31.

Frydenberg A, Starr M. Hand, foot and mouth disease. Aust Fam Physician 2003; 32: 594–5.

He YX, Fu D, Cao DZ, et al. Critical care and therapy based different illness state of 80 patients with severe hand-foot-and-mouth disease seen in Shenzhen. Zhonghua Er Ke Za Zhi 2009; 47: 338–43.

Kushner D, Caldwell BD. Hand-foot-and-mouth disease. J Am Podiatr Med Assoc 1996; 86: 257–9.

Leao JC, Caterino-De-Araujo A, Porter SR, Scully C. Human herpesvirus 8 (HHV-8) and the etiopathogenesis of Kaposi's sarcoma. Rev Hosp Clin Fac Med Sao Paulo 2002; 57: 175–86.

Leao JC, Porter SR, Scully C. Human herpesvirus 8 and oral health care: an update. Oral Surg Oral Med Oral Pathol Oral Radiol Endod 2000; 90: 694–704.

Milillo L, Lo Muzio L, Carlino P, et al. Candida-related denture stomatitis: a pilot study of the efficacy of an amorolfine antifungal varnish. Int J Prosthodont 2005; 18: 55–9.

Mustafa MB, Arduino PG, Porter SR. Varicella zoster virus: review of its management. J Oral Pathol Med 2009. [Epub ahead of print].

Nunez-Marti JM, Bagan JV, Scully C, Peñarrocha M. Leprosy: dental and periodontal status of the anterior maxilla in 76 patients. Oral Dis 2004; 10: 19–21.

Ord R, Coletti D. Cervico-facial necrotizing fasciitis. Oral Dis 2009; 15: 133–41.

Porter SR. Viral infection of the oral cavity. In: Wilson M, ed. Food Constituents and Oral Health: Current Status and Future Prospects. Cambridge, UK: Woodhead Publishing, 2009: 19–50.

Sällberg M. Oral viral infections of adults. Periodontol 2000 2009; 49: 87–95.

Samaranayake LP, Keung Leung W, Jin L. Oral mucosal fungal infections. Periodontol 2000 2009; 49: 39–59.

Slots J. Oral viral infections of adults. Periodontol 2000 2009; 49: 60–86.

Smith AJ, Bagg J, Ironside JW, Will RG, Scully C. Prions and the oral cavity. J Dent Res 2003; 82: 769–75.

# 1.9 MENTAL DISEASE

- anorexia nervosa
- anxiety states
- attention deficit hyperactivity disorders
- autism
- bulimia
- depression

- Down syndrome
- learning impairment
- Munchausen syndrome
- obsessive compulsive disorder
- schizophrenia
- substance abuse

## ANOREXIA NERVOSA

Anorexia nervosa—an eating disorder characterized by body image distortion, leading to the patient striving to keep weight low through starvation, exercise or medication—may manifest with oral ulcers or abrasions caused by fingers or other objects used to induce vomiting or Russell sign—abrasions on the back of the hand or fingers caused by using the hand to touch the throat to induce vomiting. Erosion of teeth (perimylolysis) may result from repeated vomiting and is most pronounced on lingual, palatal and occlusal surfaces (Fig. 1.9.1). Parotid enlargement (sialosis) and angular cheilitis may develop, as in other forms of starvation.

## ANXIETY STATES

Anxiety states and phobias can be accompanied by prominent linea alba, cheek biting and bruxism (Figs 1.9.2–1.9.10), and the effects of avoiding dental care.

## ATTENTION DEFICIT HYPERACTIVITY DISORDERS

Attention deficit hyperactivity disorders may lead to dental trauma.

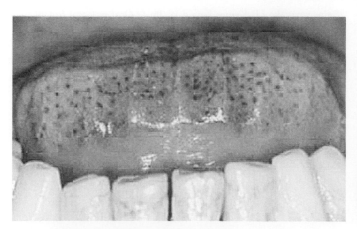

Figure 1.9.1 Erosion of teeth in anorexia nervosa.

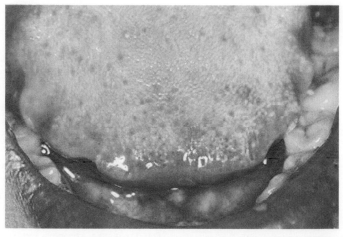

Figure 1.9.2 Stress manifesting as lingual crenation.

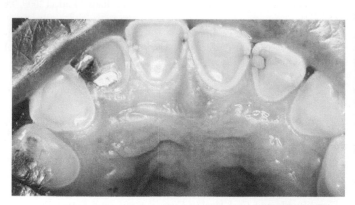

Figure 1.9.3 Stress manifesting as lingual crenation.

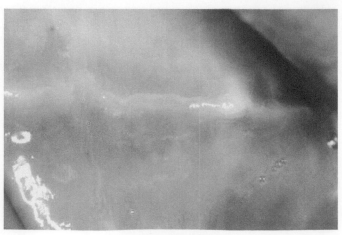

Figure 1.9.4 Stress manifesting as linea alba.

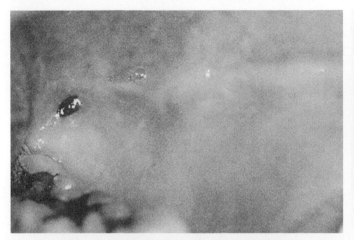

*Figure 1.9.5* Stress manifesting as linea alba.

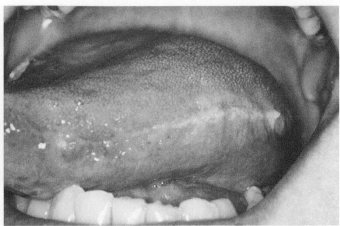

*Figure 1.9.6* Stress manifesting as linea alba.

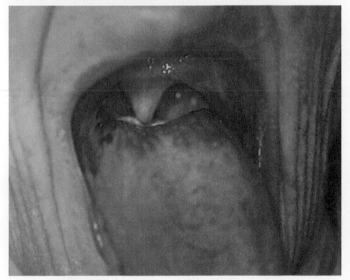

*Figure 1.9.7* Stress manifesting as overenthusiastic exhibition of the pharynx.

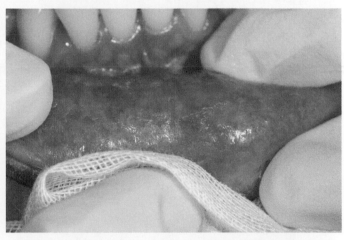

*Figure 1.9.8* Stress manifesting with lip chewing (morsicatio buccarum).

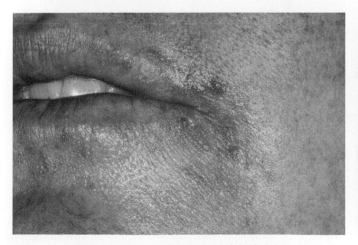

*Figure 1.9.9* Stress manifesting with lip licking.

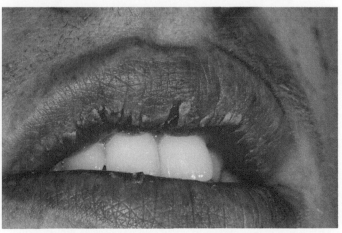

*Figure 1.9.10* Stress manifesting as exfoliative cheilitis.

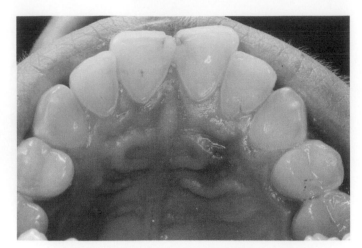

Figure 1.9.11 Erosion in bulimia.

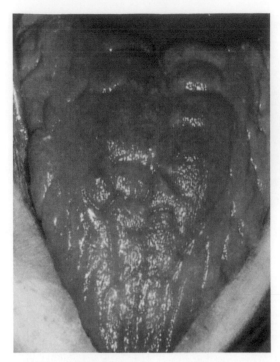

Figure 1.9.12 Depression with a dry mouth and glossitis.

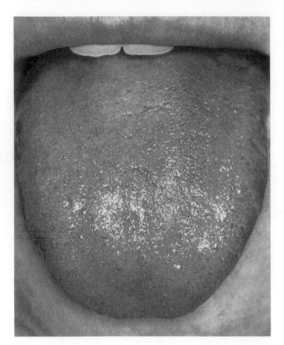

Figure 1.9.13 Burning mouth syndrome—clinically healthy tongue.

## AUTISM

Autism has no specific oral manifestations but bruxism and oral neglect can be seen.

## BULIMIA

Bulimia—an eating disorder characterized by recurrent binging and purging—may result in tooth erosion from gastric contents (Fig. 1.9.11).

## DEPRESSION

Depression can present with various complaints such as artifactual ulcers, dry mouth, discharges, pain, disturbed taste and sensation or drug reactions (Figs 1.9.12–1.9.15). There are often multiple complaints.

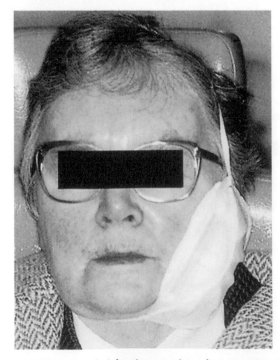

Figure 1.9.14 Idiopathic facial pain—wearing of an attention-seeking device.

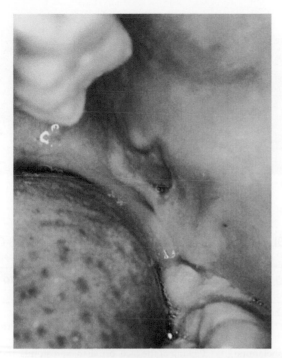

*Figure 1.9.15* Psychosis—self-mutilation.

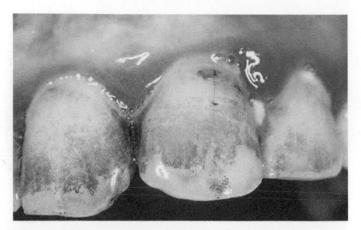

*Figure 1.9.16* Learning impairment—tooth staining.

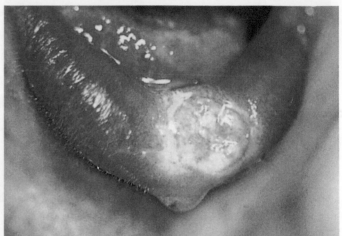

*Figure 1.9.18* Lip ulceration in psychosis.

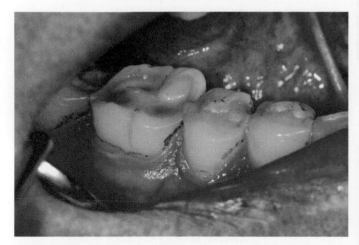

*Figure 1.9.17* Psychosis—severe attrition from tooth grinding.

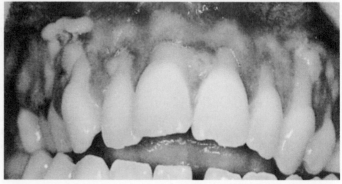

*Figure 1.9.19* Trauma—self-mutilation of gingivae achieved by using fingernails.

## DOWN SYNDROME

Down syndrome (see Chapter 1.13).

## LEARNING IMPAIRMENT

Learning impairment can be associated with bruxism, attrition, poor oral hygiene and its sequelae (gingivitis, periodontitis caries). Self-mutilation (oral artifactual disease) may be seen. Oral self-inflicted lesions are often bizarre, typically destructive, and may involve hard or soft tissues (Figs 1.9.16–1.9.19). The lesions are typically in sites that can be readily reached by the dominant hand; for example, gingival lesions may be seen in the right labial aspect of the maxilla.

## MUNCHAUSEN SYNDROME

Munchausen syndrome is a rare psychological and behavioural condition characterized by the fabrication or induction of symptoms of illness, such as lying about symptoms and also about other aspects of their life, manipulating test results and sometimes actually inflicting symptoms on themselves. Patients often 'doctor-shop' (Figs 1.9.20 and 1.9.21).

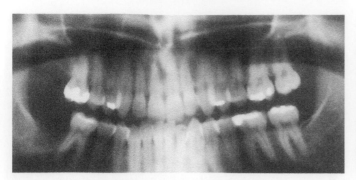

*Figure 1.9.20* Munchausen syndrome.

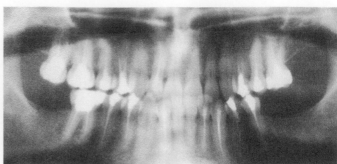

*Figure 1.9.21* Munchausen syndrome 5 years later.

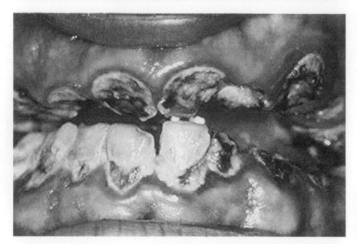

*Figure 1.9.22* Psychosis—oral neglect with caries and periodontitis.

The causes of Munchausen's syndrome are unknown. Most people with the condition refuse to accept psychiatric treatment.

Munchausen's syndrome differs from hypochondria, where the patient actually believes they are ill, but do not manipulate test results, and from malingering where the patient pretends to be ill to gain some sort of benefit, such as avoiding work, or trying to obtain compensation.

## OBSESSIVE COMPULSIVE DISORDER
Obsessive compulsive disorder—characterized by intrusive thoughts that produce anxiety, by repetitive behaviours aimed at reducing anxieties—may, where there is focus on the mouth, result in tooth abrasion from over-enthusiastic brushing, or damage from dental flossing.

## SCHIZOPHRENIA
Schizophrenia—a disorder of thought characterized by abnormalities in the perception or expression of reality—has no specific maxillofacial manifestations but neglect (Fig. 1.9.22) and drug reactions to anti-psychotics, such as dyskinesias, may be seen.

## SUBSTANCE ABUSE
The drugs most commonly abused include alcohol, amphetamine/amfetamines, barbiturates, benzodiazepines, cannabis, cocaine, ecstasy,

**TABLE 1.9.1** MAXILLOFACIAL CONSEQUENCES OF USE OF SPECIFIC RECREATIONAL DRUGS

| Drug | Possible complications in addition to oral neglect and halitosis |
|---|---|
| Alcohol | Leukoplakia, carcinoma, tooth erosion, glossitis/oral ulcers/angular stomatitis from malnutrition, sialosis, fetal alcohol syndrome |
| Amphetamine | Picking at the face, bruxism, xerostomia and increased caries incidence. 'Meth mouth' is the term given to the neglect and poor oral hygiene seen in methamphetamine users |
| Barbiturates | Facial pain, bullous reaction |
| Betel | Submucous fibrosis, leukoplakia, carcinoma |
| Cannabis | White lesions (burns), dry mouth, possible leukoplakia, carcinoma |
| Cocaine | Temporarily numbness of lips and tongue, gingival erosions, dry mouth, bruxism dental erosion. Caries and periodontal disease, especially acute necrotising gingivitis, are more frequent. Cocaine may precipitate cluster headaches. Oronasal fistulae |
| Ecstasy | Tooth clenching, bruxism, temporomandibular joint dysfunction, dry mouth, attrition, dental erosion, mucosal burns or ulceration, circumoral paraesthesiae and periodontitis |
| Khat | Leukoplakia, carcinoma |
| Nicotine | Due to tobacco—leukoplakia, carcinoma, necrotising gingivitis, periodontitis, impaired wound healing and implant success |
| Opium alkaloids | Dry mouth |
| Solvents | Perioral dermatitis, fetal gasoline/petrol syndrome |

methaqualone, nicotine and opium alkaloids. Assaults, theft and prostitution are often used to fund the drug habit and thus maxillofacial injuries, sexually transmitted and other infectious diseases are common consequences. Intravenous injection is frequently used for misuse of drugs, often with sharing of needles or syringes with the risk of blood-borne infections such as HIV, viral hepatitis (particularly B, C, D and others) and chronic liver disease.

Maxillofacial lesions may result from trauma or from oral hygiene neglect, or may be a consequence of specific drug effects (Table 1.9.1).

# FURTHER READING

Avsar A, Akbaş S, Ataibiş T. Traumatic dental injuries in children with attention deficit/hyperactivity disorder. Dent Traumatol 2009; 25: 484–9. [Epub 2009 Jun 1].

Batista LR, Moreira EA, Rauen MS, Corso AC, Fiates GM. Oral health and nutritional status of semi-institutionalized persons with mental retardation in Brazil. Res Dev Disabil 2009; 30: 839–46. [Epub 2008 Dec 4].

Binkley CJ, Haugh GS, Kitchens DH, Wallace DL, Sessler DI. Oral microbial and respiratory status of persons with mental retardation/intellectual and developmental disability: an observational cohort study. Oral Surg Oral Med Oral Pathol Oral Radiol Endod 2009; 108: 722–31.

Geier DA, Kern JK, Geier MR. A prospective study of prenatal mercury exposure from maternal dental amalgams and autism severity. Acta Neurobiol Exp (Wars) 2009; 69: 189–97.

Jain M, Mathur A, Sawla L, et al. Oral health status of mentally disabled subjects in India. J Oral Sci 2009; 51: 333–40.

Johnson D, Hearn A, Barker D. A pilot survey of dental health in a group of drug and alcohol abusers. Eur J Prosthodont Restor Dent 2008; 16: 181–4.

Khocht A, Schleifer SJ, Janal MN, Keller S. Dental care and oral disease in alcohol-dependent persons. J Subst Abuse Treat 2009; 37: 214–18. [Epub 2009 Jan 15].

Lo Russo L, Campisi G, Di Fede O, et al. Oral manifestations of eating disorders: a critical review. Oral Dis 2008; 14: 479–84.

Loo CY, Graham RM, Hughes CV. Behaviour guidance in dental treatment of patients with autism spectrum disorder. Int J Paediatr Dent 2009; 19: 390–8. [Epub 2009 Jul 9].

Oosterink FM, de Jongh A, Hoogstraten J. Prevalence of dental fear and phobia relative to other fear and phobia subtypes. Eur J Oral Sci 2009; 117: 135–43.

Scully C. Fragile X (Martin-Bell) syndrome. Dent Update 2002; 29: 196–8.

Scully C, Eveson JW. Sialosis and necrotising sialometaplasia in bulimia; a case report. Int J Oral Maxillofac Surg 2004; 33: 808–10.

Scully C, Van Bruggen W, Dios PD, Porter SR, Davison M. Down syndrome; lip lesions and *Candida albicans*. Br J Dermatol 2002; 147: 37–40.

Stanfield M, Scully C, Davison MF, Porter SR. The oral health of clients with learning disability: changes following relocation from hospital to community. Br Dent J 2003; 194: 271–7.

# 1.10 MUCOSAL, CUTANEOUS AND MUCOCUTANEOUS DISEASE

- acanthosis nigricans
- allergies
- Behçet syndrome (BS)
- Darier disease
- dermatitis herpetiformis
- dermatomyositis
- dyskeratosis congenita
- ectodermal dysplasia
- eosinophilic ulcer (EU)
- epidermolysis bullosa

- erythema multiforme
- Gorlin syndrome
- lichen sclerosis
- lichen planus (LP)
- linear IgA disease (LAD)
- pachyonychia congenita
- pemphigoid
- pemphigus
- psoriasis
- white sponge naevus

## ACANTHOSIS NIGRICANS

Acanthosis nigricans is a rare brown to black, poorly defined, velvety hyperpigmentation affecting the skin, important because some cases underlie endocrinopathies such as diabetes, or malignancy—when oral mucosal involvement is common (Figs 1.10.1 and 1.10.2).

## ALLERGIES

Allergies can present with maxillofacial features; oedema is a feature in angioedema (Quincke oedema; Figs 1.10.3–1.10.5; Chapter 2.1).

There may also be an allergic component to mucocutaneous disorders such as lichenoid lesions and erythema multiforme (EM), and possibly to orofacial granulomatosis (Chapters 1.3 and 2.1) (Figs 1.10.6 and 1.10.7).

## BEHÇET SYNDROME (BS)

BS (Behçet disease) is a chronic multisystem potentially lethal disorder. BS does not appear to be infectious or contagious. A viral aetiology (e.g. herpes simplex) has been proposed but remains to be proven. BS is found worldwide, but is most common in the Eastern Mediterranean countries and in eastern Asia, China, Korea and Japan, along the Silk route taken by Marco Polo. This together with an association with human leukocyte antigen (HLA) -B5 and especially HLA-B51 (B5101) suggest a genetic predisposition. As in RAS, heat shock proteins (hsp) have been implicated but patients with BS have circulating lymphocytes reactive with a different peptide of hsp 65-60. The many immunological findings in BS include various T-lymphocyte abnormalities (especially T-suppressor cell dysfunction), and increased polymorphonuclear leukocyte motility. There is also decreased T-helper (CD4): T-suppressor (CD8) ratio; antibody-dependent cellular cytotoxicity to oral epithelial cells and evidence of disturbance of natural killer cell activity. Circulating autoantibodies are found against intermediate filaments found in mucous membranes, cardiolipin and neutrophil cytoplasm. Circulating immune complexes are found and there is immunoglobulin and complement deposition within and around blood vessel walls with vasculitis, usually leukocytoclastic vasculitis, as in immune complex diseases, and raised levels of acute phase proteins. Hypercoagulability is a feature of the condition.

### Clinical features

- Mouth ulceration clinically identical to aphthous stomatitis is seen in 90–100% of cases, and is the usual initial manifestation of BS. HLA and immunological findings may help differentiate from RAS.

- Recurrent painful genital ulcers that tend to heal with scars are seen in 64–88% of cases.
- Ocular lesions can include uveitis with conjunctivitis (early) and hypopyon (late), retinal vasculitis (posterior uveitis), iridocyclitis and optic atrophy. The most common ocular manifestation is relapsing iridocyclitis. Both eyes are eventually involved and blindness may result.
- Central nervous system (CNS) lesions can include meningoencephalitis, cerebral infarction, psychosis, cranial nerve palsies, cerebellar and spinal cord lesions, hemi- and quadriparesis.
- Skin lesions can include erythema nodosum, papulopustular lesions and acneiform nodules. Venepuncture is, in some patients, followed by pustulation but this phenomenon (*pathergy*), said to be characteristic of BS may be dependent upon the technique used and the ethnic origins of the patient.
- The epididymis, joints, heart, intestinal tract and most other systems may also be involved in BS (Figs 1.10.8–1.10.14).

Major criteria for diagnosis include:

1. Recurrent mouth ulcers
2. Genital ulcers
3. Ocular lesions
4. CNS lesions
5. Skin lesions.

Minor criteria for diagnosis are:

1. Arthralgia: large joint arthropathies that are subacute, non-migratory, self-limiting and non-deforming.
2. Superficial or deep migratory thrombophlebitis, especially of lower limbs. Thromboses of large veins such as the dural sinuses or venae cavae can be life-threatening.
3. Intestinal lesions: inflammatory bowel disease with discrete ulcerations.
4. Lung disease: pneumonitis.
5. Renal disease: haematuria and proteinuria.

### Diagnosis

BS is rare and symptoms overlap those of other diseases, and thus it can be difficult to diagnose. The diagnosis is made on clinical grounds alone on the basis of recurrent mouth ulcers plus two or more of the following:

- Recurrent genital ulceration
- Eye lesions
- Skin lesions

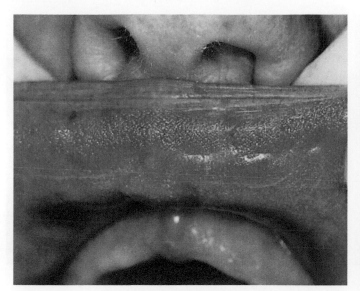

*Figure 1.10.1* Acanthosis nigricans.

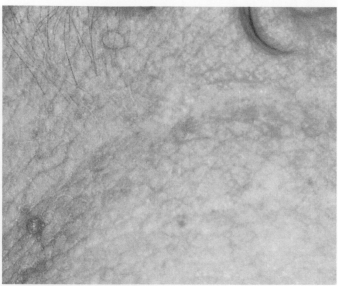

*Figure 1.10.2* Acanthosis nigricans—cutaneous lesions.

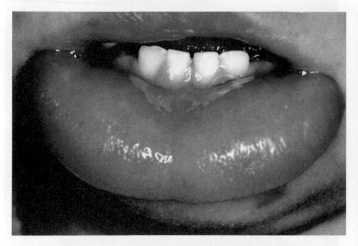

*Figure 1.10.3* Drug allergy causing labial oedema.

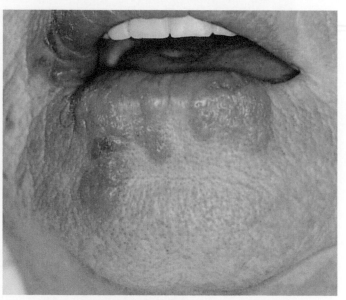

*Figure 1.10.4* Drug allergy to eugenol.

- Pathergy—this is a >2 mm diameter erythematous nodule or pustule forming 24–48 hours after sterile subcutaneous puncture of the forearm skin.

Findings of HLA-B5101, raised serum IgD and antibodies to cardiolipin and neutrophil cytoplasm are supportive of a diagnosis of BS. Serum levels of acute phase proteins and antibodies to intermediate filaments are both raised in active BS.

### Management
Patients with suspected BS warrant early specialist advice.

- Topical tetracycline mouthwash and topical corticosteroids are the drugs of choice for controlling the mouth ulcers.

- Colchicine is often the main treatment.
- Corticosteroids, azathioprine, ciclosporin, chlorambucil, cyclophosphamide, dapsone, interferon (IFN)-alpha or thalidomide may be used. Specific anti-tumour necrosis factor-alpha (TNF-α) agents have also been suggested to be of benefit.

## DARIER DISEASE
Darier disease—an autosomal dominant condition due to a defect in the ATP2A2 gene—is characterized by dark crusty patches on the

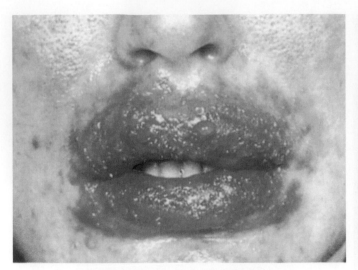

*Figure 1.10.5* Drug allergic cheilitis.

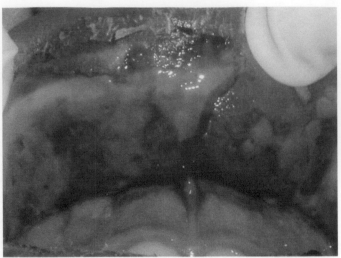

*Figure 1.10.6* Erythema multiforme is often a drug reaction.

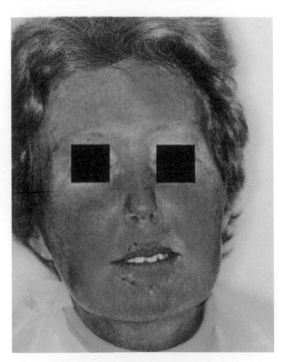

*Figure 1.10.7* Allergy to rubber dam.

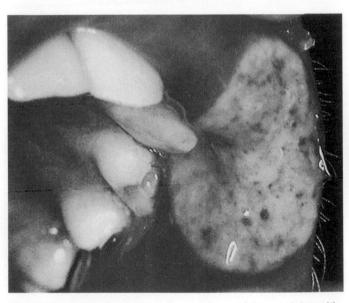

*Figure 1.10.8* Behçet disease typically manifests with large aphthous-like ulcers.

## DERMATOMYOSITIS

Dermatomyositis—an inflammatory myopathy, characterized by chronic muscle inflammation and a rash that precedes or accompanies progressive weakness—may be associated with connective tissue or autoimmune diseases, such as lupus. A patchy, bluish-purple or red, heliotrope rash characteristically develops on the eyelids and over muscles used to extend or straighten joints, such as knuckles, elbows, heels and toes. Calcium deposits may appear as hard bumps beneath the skin or in the muscle (calcinosis) (Figs 1.10.22–1.10.27).

## DYSKERATOSIS CONGENITA

Dyskeratosis congenita (Zinsser–Engman–Cole syndrome)—a rare, heterogeneous disorder associated with telomerase dysfunction and

skin (keratosis follicularis) and can present with oral white lesions, especially in the palate (Figs 1.10.15 and 1.10.16).

## DERMATITIS HERPETIFORMIS

Dermatitis herpetiformis—an immune-mediated sub-epithelial blistering disease—manifests with a pruritic rash, oral blisters, ulcers and desquamative gingivitis (Figs 1.10.17–1.10.21). Coeliac disease is a common accompaniment.

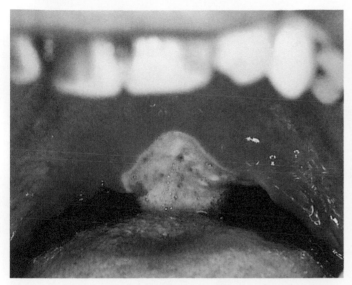

*Figure 1.10.9* Behçet disease typically manifests with large aphthous-like ulcers as here in the palate.

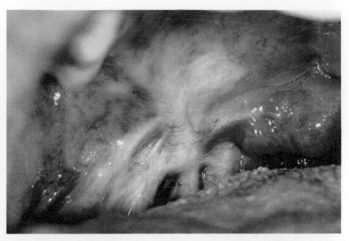

*Figure 1.10.10* Behçet disease typically manifests with large aphthous-like ulcers which scar on healing.

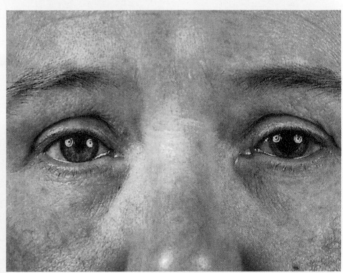

*Figure 1.10.12* Behçet disease.

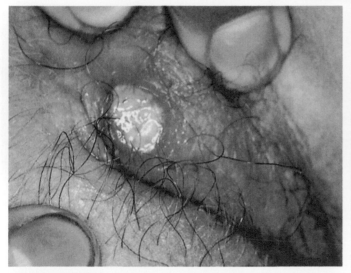

*Figure 1.10.11* Behçet disease typically manifests with aphthous-like genital ulcers.

ribosome deficiency—manifests with progressive bone marrow failure, reticulated skin hyperpigmentation, nail dystrophy and oral leukoplakia (Figs 1.10.28 and 1.10.29).

## ECTODERMAL DYSPLASIA

Ectodermal dysplasia—a group of inherited disorders (almost 200 related conditions) deriving from abnormalities of ectodermal structures defined by primary defects in the development of two or more tissues (skin, hair, nails, eccrine glands and teeth)—can present with hypodontia, dental anomalies (peg-shaped teeth and taurodontism) and thinned hair (Figs 1.10.30–1.10.35).

## EOSINOPHILIC ULCER (EU)

EU is a non-healing traumatic ulcer microscopically characterized by a diffuse, pseudoinvasive, mixed inflammatory reaction that includes large mononuclear cells, numerous eosinophils and T-cells.

Riga–Fede disease is a form of EU that develops in infants and usually occurs on the anterior ventrum of the tongue as a result of chronic trauma from the teeth usually in association with breastfeeding, sometimes drug-related (Fig. 1.10.36).

## EPIDERMOLYSIS BULLOSA

Epidermolysis bullosa—a group of rare genetic disorders caused by a mutation in the keratin gene—manifests mainly with skin and oral blisters, erosions and scarring, and dental hypoplasia (Figs 1.10.37–1.10.44). Some epidermolysis bullosa subtypes are at risk for bone marrow, musculoskeletal, heart and renal disease, and for development of squamous cell carcinoma, basal cell carcinoma (BCC) or malignant melanoma.

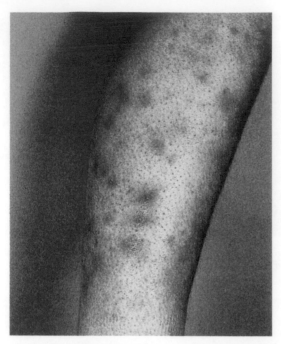

*Figure 1.10.13* Behçet disease may present with acneiform or pustular rashes.

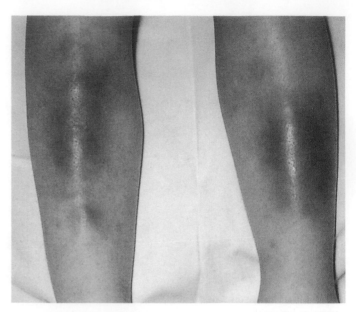

*Figure 1.10.14* Behçet disease, like other immune complex disorders may present with erythema nodosum.

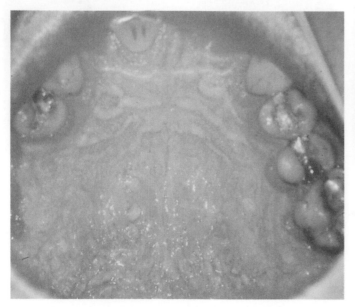

*Figure 1.10.15* Darier disease—oral white lesions similar to stomatitis nicotina.

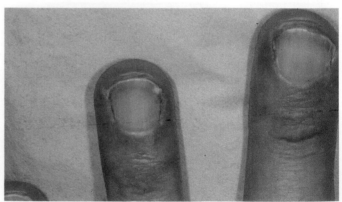

*Figure 1.10.16* Darier disease can cause nail lesions.

EM may be triggered by

- *infective agents* such as herpes simplex virus [herpes-associated EM (HAEM)] in most cases, or mycoplasma;
- *drugs* such as sulphonamides, cephalosporins, barbiturates, non-steroidal anti-inflammatory drugs or hydantoin (although the list of potential causative drugs ever increases); and
- *food additives* such as benzoates.

## Clinical features

Affected patients are often males, typically adolescents or young adults, and there are periods of remission from the disease.

- EM *minor* affects typically the skin of the back and palms and sometimes the anterior oral mucosa.
- EM *major* (sometimes termed Stevens–Johnson syndrome) affects any mucosae, skin and other sites. Conjunctivitis, stomatitis, genital

## ERYTHEMA MULTIFORME

EM appears to be an immunological reaction in which cytotoxic effector cells (CD8 T-lymphocytes) infiltrate the epithelium, inducing keratinocyte apoptosis and satellite cell necrosis. A genetic background is likely, with various HLA associations.

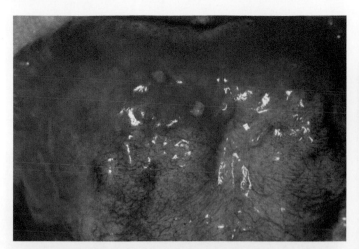

Figure 1.10.17 Dermatitis herpetiformis can present with oral ulceration.

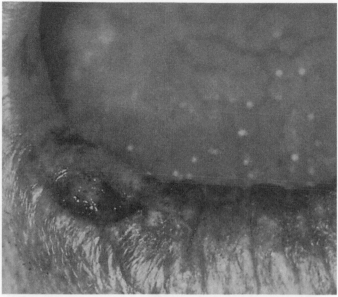

Figure 1.10.18 Dermatitis herpetiformis—ulceration.

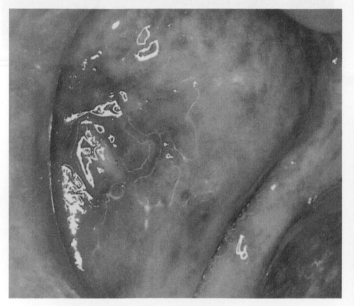

Figure 1.10.19 Dermatitis herpetiformis—ulceration.

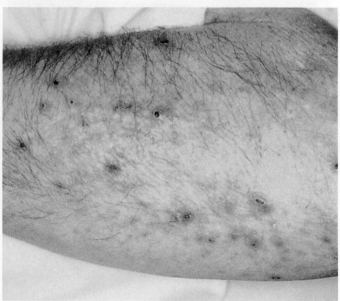

Figure 1.10.20 Dermatitis herpetiformis itchy vesicular rash on elbows and other extensor surfaces.

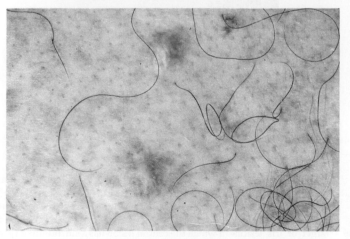

Figure 1.10.21 Dermatitis herpetiformis skin lesions.

lesions, fever and rash constitute the main manifestations. The ocular changes resemble those of mucous membrane pemphigoid—dry eyes and symblepharon may result. The typical genital lesions include balanitis, urethritis and vulval ulcers. Bronchopulmonary and renal involvement may also be seen.

The virtually pathognomonic feature of either form of EM is swollen, blood-stained or crusted lips (Figs 1.10.45–1.10.51). Oral lesions progress through macules to blisters and ulceration, typically most pronounced in the anterior parts of the mouth. Early lesions may be macular and

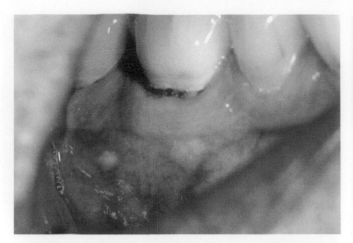

*Figure 1.10.22* Dermatomyositis lesions can be lichenoid.

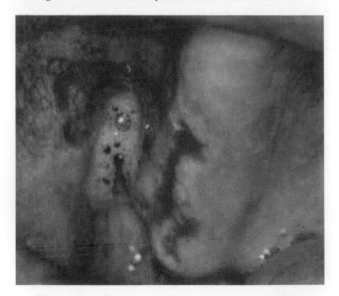

*Figure 1.10.24* Dermatomyositis—alveolar ridge erosions.

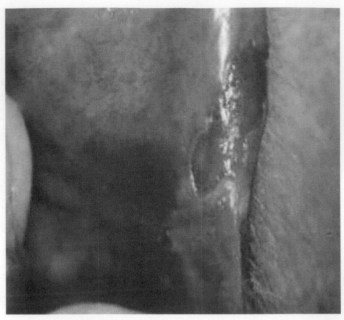

*Figure 1.10.23* Dermatomyositis—erosions at commissure.

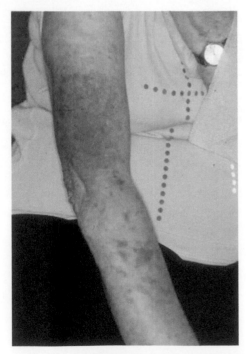

*Figure 1.10.25* Dermatomyosistis—photosensitivity.

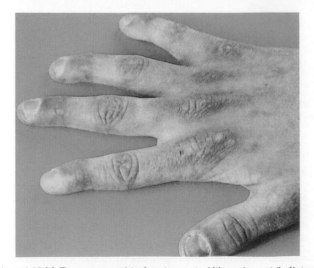

*Figure 1.10.26* Dermatomyositis showing typical lilac coloured (heliotrope) rash over knuckles and round nails.

develop the appearance of an archery target (target lesions). Extensive oral ulceration may eventually be seen. Most patients have oral lesions only but, in some, other squamous epithelia are involved. Rashes of various types (hence 'EM') are seen. The characteristic rash consists of 'target' or 'iris' lesions in which the central lesion has a surrounding ring of erythema.

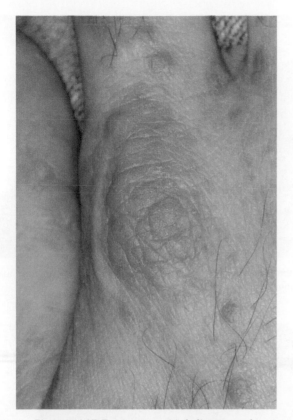

*Figure 1.10.27* Dermatomyositis heliotrope rash.

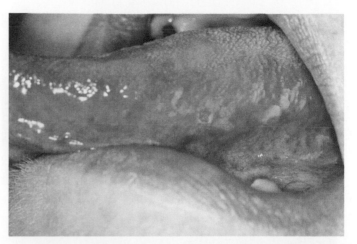

*Figure 1.10.28* Dyskeratosis congenita—oral leukoplakia.

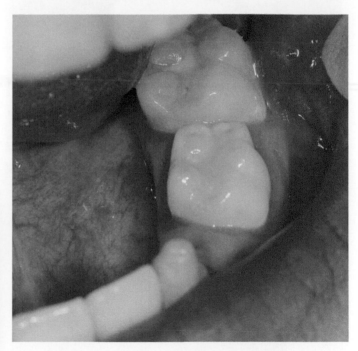

*Figure 1.10.30* Ectodermal dysplasia—dental anomalies.

### Diagnosis

The diagnosis is mainly clinical; the Nikolsky sign is negative. It may be helpful to undertake serology for *Mycoplasma pneumoniae* or herpes simplex virus, or other micro-organisms that could be implicated in the aetiology. Biopsy of perilesional tissue with immunostaining and histological examination may help but often there are few specific histopathological features.

### Management

Spontaneous healing can be slow—up to 2–3 weeks in minor EM and up to 6 weeks in EM major. Treatment is thus indicated but controversial, since no specific treatment is available.

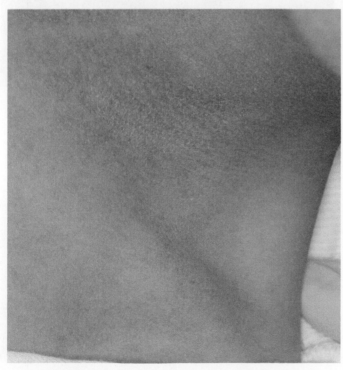

*Figure 1.10.29* Dyskeratosis congenita—skin lesions.

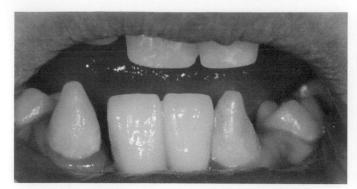

*Figure 1.10.31* Ectodermal dysplasia—hypodontia.

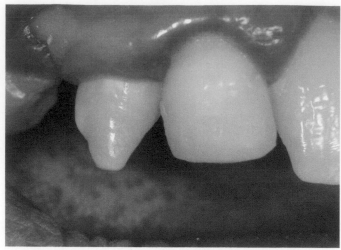

*Figure 1.10.32* Ectodermal dysplasia—hypodontia and morphological changes.

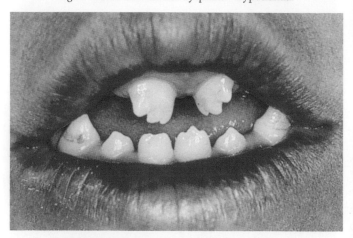

*Figure 1.10.33* Ectodermal dysplasia—hypodontia and morphological changes.

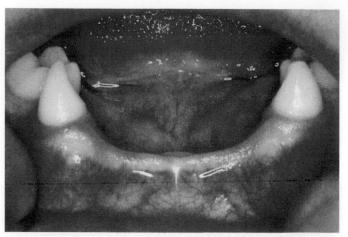

*Figure 1.10.34* Ectodermal dysplasia—hypodontia.

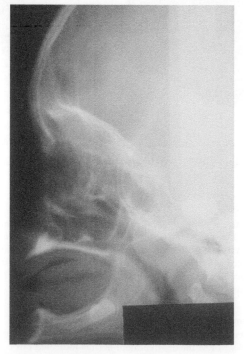

*Figure 1.10.35* Ectodermal dysplasia—hypodontia.

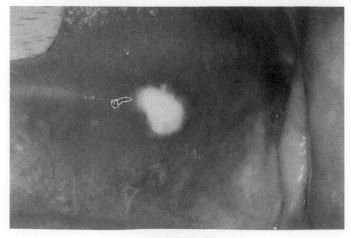

*Figure 1.10.36* Eosinophilic ulcer.

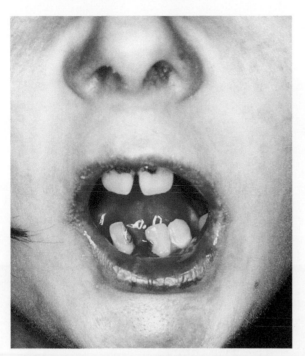

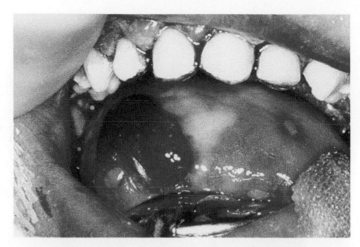

*Figure 1.10.38* Epidermolysis bullosa blistering.

*Figure 1.10.37* Epidermolysis bullosa—restricted oral opening, caries and periodontal disease.

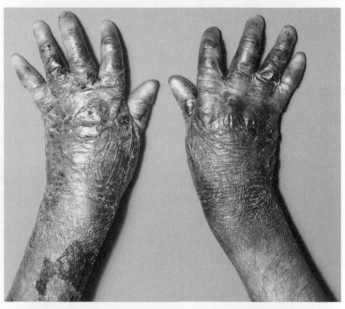

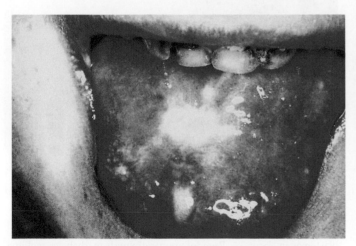

*Figure 1.10.40* Epidermolysis bullosa can affect skin and nails.

*Figure 1.10.39* Epidermolysis bullosa blistering and scarring.

- Major EM should be treated with systemic corticosteroids and/or azathioprine or other immunomodulatory drugs. Levamisole and thalidomide have occasionally been used to some effect.
- Minor EM may respond to symptomatic treatment and topical corticosteroids, but systemic corticosteroids may still be required.

- Precipitating factors, when identified, should be treated.
- Oral hygiene should be improved with 0.2% aqueous chlorhexidine mouthbaths.
- Aciclovir or valaciclovir may be indicated for treatment (and prevention) in HAEM.
- Tetracycline is indicated in EM related to *M. pneumoniae*.

In addition,

- Patients with major EM such as the Stevens–Johnson syndrome may need in-patient hospital care. Plasmapheresis possibly has a place in the management of severe disease.

## GORLIN SYNDROME

Gorlin syndrome (Gorlin–Goltz syndrome, multiple basal cell naevi syndrome; naevoid basal cell carcinoma syndrome) —an autosomal dominant condition related to chromosome 9q22.3-q31 and associated with *patched* gene (PTCH) mutations and deletions—consists mainly of multiple BCCs, keratocystic odontogenic tumours (KCOTs; odontogenic keratocyst), vertebral and rib anomalies and temporoparietal bossing with broad nasal root, calcification of the falx cerebri and abnormal sella turcica (Figs 1.10.52–1.10.59).

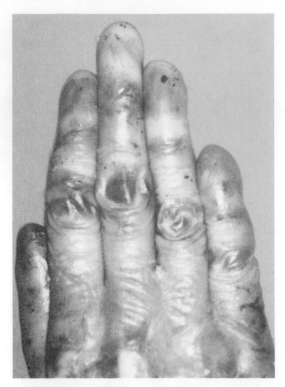

*Figure 1.10.41* Epidermolysis bullosa can affect skin and nails.

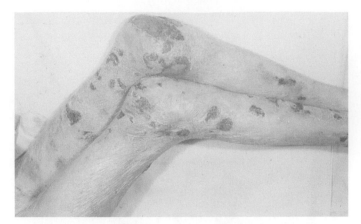

*Figure 1.10.42* Epidermolysis bullosa can affect skin.

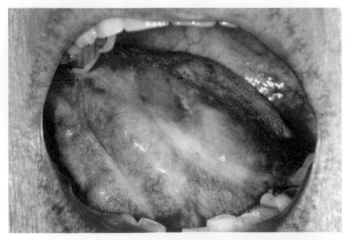

*Figure 1.10.43* Epidermolysis bullosa can affect mucosa with blistering and ulceration followed by scarring.

Multiple BCC over the nose, eyelids, cheeks and elsewhere are often an early sign. There may also be pitting of the palms or soles, and BCC can originate there.

KCOTs are seen in 75–90% of patients.

Anomalies of the vertebrae and ribs and other bones include frontal and temporoparietal bossing, a broad nasal root, prominent supra-orbital ridges and a degree of mandibular prognathism. Short fourth metacarpals are common.

Calcification of the falx cerebri is pathognomonic. There can be learning impairment in about 5% or cerebral tumours, particularly medullo-

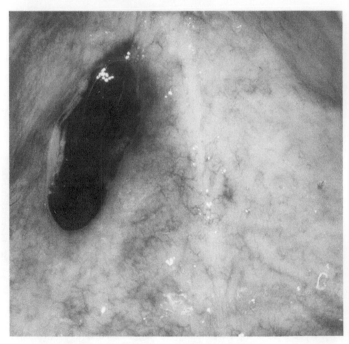

*Figure 1.10.44* Epidermolysis bullosa acquisita.

blastomas in about 5%. Pseudohypoparathyroidism, diabetes mellitus, cardiac or ovarian fibromas, lymphomesenteric cysts and congenital malformations such as cleft lip and/or palate, polydactyly, congenital ocular anomaly (cataract, microphthalmos and coloboma) may be seen.

Diagnosis is strongly suggested by the major criteria:

- positive family history
- more than one BCC
- KCOTs (first sign in 75%) mainly in the mandible during the first 30 years of life
- palmar or plantar pits
- calcified falx cerebri (in 80%).

Main differential diagnoses include Bazex syndrome (a rare acral psoriasiform dermatosis associated with internal malignancy), trichoepithelioma papulosum multiplex (an autosomal dominant disorder of multiple trichoepitheliomas) and Torre's syndrome

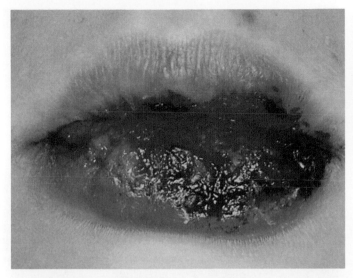

Figure 1.10.45 Erythema multiforme showing typical blood-stained serosanguinous crusting of lips.

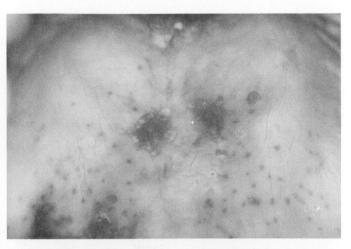

Figure 1.10.46 Erythema multiforme oral lesions.

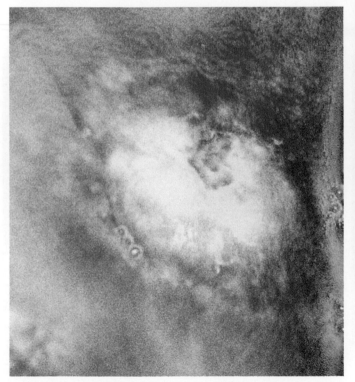

Figure 1.10.47 Erythema multiforme oral target lesions.

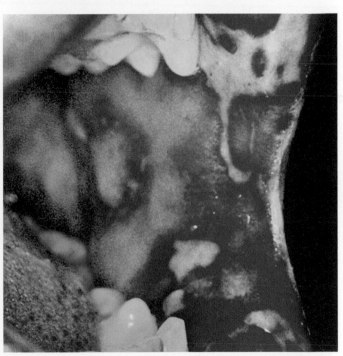

Figure 1.10.48 Erythema multiforme diffuse ulcerations.

## LICHEN SCLEROSIS

Lichen sclerosis—an idiopathic skin condition that mainly affects middle aged women—affects the vulva in women and the penis in men, rarely the oral mucosa (Fig. 1.10.60).

## LICHEN PLANUS (LP)

LP is idiopathic but there is a chronic T-lymphocyte infiltrate beneath the affected epithelia causing basal cell liquefaction. The appearance of antigen-processing cells (Langerhans cells) is one of the first observable changes though the antigen(s) that may be responsible is unknown. One hypothesis is that molecular mimicry between cytochrome p450 CYP2D6, in particular CYP2D6*4, and common oral pathogens

(Muir–Torre syndrome: association of skin sebaceous tumours with internal malignancy).

Large or prominent basal cell naevae are treated prophylactically by cryosurgery or Moh's surgery and established basal cell carcinomata by resection. Jaw cysts may be more aggressive than sporadic KCOT but are treated similarly. Potentially affected family members require genetic counselling.

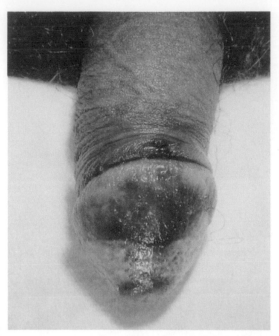

Figure 1.10.49 Erythema multiforme penile lesions.

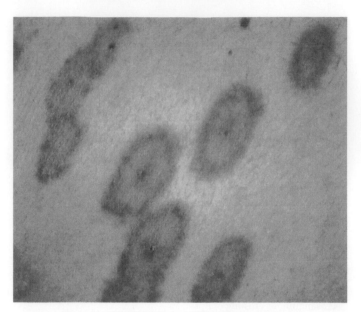

Figure 1.10.50 Erythema multiforme target lesions.

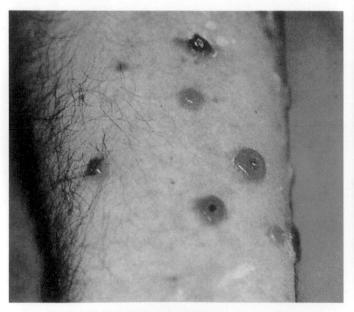

Figure 1.10.51 Erythema multiforme—skin lesions.

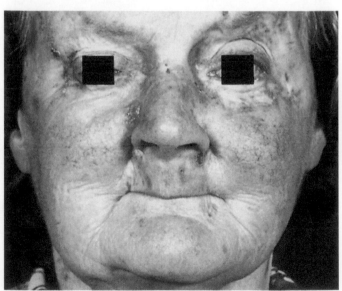

Figure 1.10.52 Gorlin syndrome showing multiple basal cell naevi and typical facies.

such as candida or herpes simplex virus may be involved in the pathogenesis.

A band-like dense mononuclear inflammatory cell infiltrate of TCD8+ cells mainly, appears in the upper lamina propria, representing a cell-mediated immunological response. Epithelial basal cells undergo flattening and hydropic changes and intercellular spaces appear, with splitting of epithelium away from the basement membrane—basal cell liquefaction—representing apoptosis (programmed cell death), caused by the T-cell production of cytokines such as TNF-α and IFN-γ. Atrophy

and even erosions can appear—leading to discomfort and the appearance of red lesions and/or ulceration.

Degeneration and premature cell death of these basal keratinocytes leads to the appearance of round or ovoid 'colloid bodies' (also termed cytoid, globular, hyaline, Civatte and Sabouraud bodies) in the epithelial spinous layer and in the lamina propria. Immune deposits (typically fibrin and sometimes IgM) are seen in colloid bodies and at the basement membrane zone (BMZ), but they probably represent non-specific exudation and not autoantibodies. The rest of the epithelium appears to react with thickening of the spinous layer (acanthosis) and granular cell

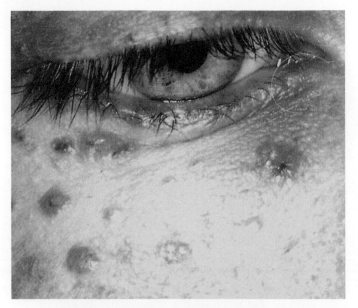

*Figure 1.10.53* Gorlin syndrome—basal cell naevi.

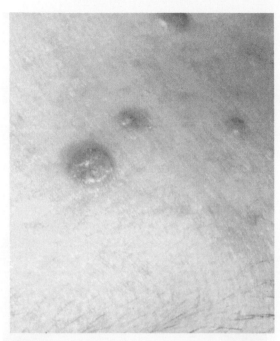

*Figure 1.10.54* Gorlin syndrome—basal cell naevi.

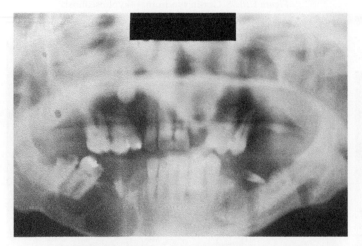

*Figure 1.10.55* Gorlin syndrome—keratocystic odontogenic tumours.

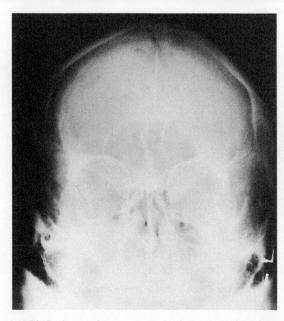

*Figure 1.10.56* Gorlin syndrome—typical calcification of the falx cerebri.

layer (hyperparakeratosis) or hyperorthokeratosis—which accounts for the clinical white lesions.

Lesions that resemble LP clinically and histologically may be induced by various identifiable factors. These lesions are termed 'lichenoid lesions' and may be caused by

- Drugs
  - antihypertensives
  - oral hypoglycaemics
  - non-steroidal anti-inflammatory agents and a range of other drugs
  - many others
- Metal restorative materials used in dentistry
- Viral infections
  - HIV disease
  - hepatitis C virus (HCV) in some populations
- Chronic graft-versus-host disease.

LP has occasional overlaps with other disorders such as pemphigoid, lichen sclerosus or lupus erythematosus, and occasional associations with other diseases, especially with diabetes mellitus and autoimmune disorders, and possibly other hepatitis viruses.

**Clinical features**

LP is common, mostly asymptomatic and bilateral. Oral white lesions are the typical features (Figs 1.10.61–1.10.97). Six clinical types of oral LP have been reported:

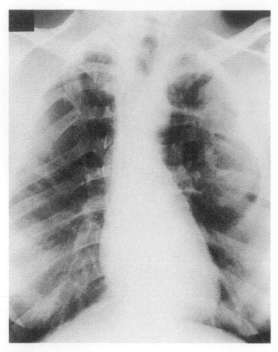

*Figure 1.10.57* Gorlin syndrome—bifid ribs and other skeletal anomalies may be seen.

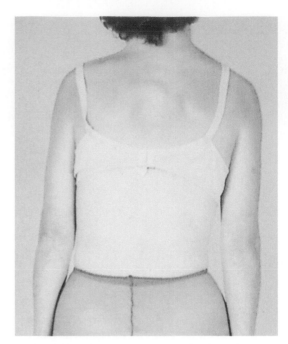

*Figure 1.10.58* Gorlin syndrome—kyphoscoliosis.

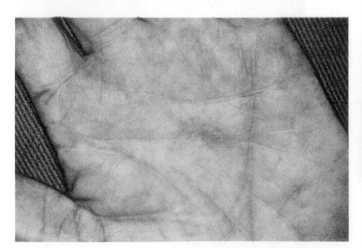

*Figure 1.10.59* Gorlin syndrome—palmar pits.

- reticular—a network of raised white lines or striae (reticular pattern)
- papular—white papules
- plaque-like—simulating leukoplakia
- erosive—red atrophic areas. LP is one of the most common causes of desquamative gingivitis
- ulcerative—erosions that are persistent, irregular and painful, with a yellowish slough (this type is less common)
- bullous—but this probably represents superficial mucoceles.

White lesions are usually asymptomatic; mild oral discomfort or burning sensations are the most common complaints in symptomatic cases, usually from atrophic areas of thin, red mucosa or erosions.

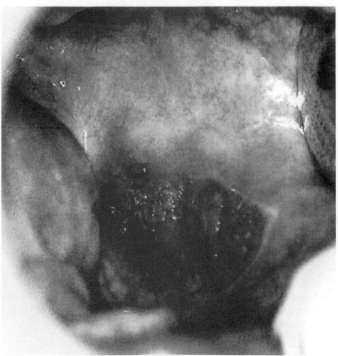

*Figure 1.10.60* Lichen sclerosis et atrophicus.

LP lesions are:

- mostly in the posterior buccal mucosa bilaterally
- occasionally on the dorsum and/or ventrum of the tongue where they may be reticular, papular or plaque-like and associated with red atrophic or erosive areas

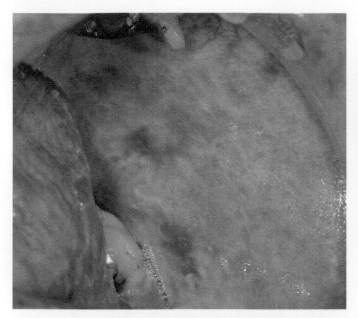

*Figure 1.10.61* Lichen planus—buccal lesions.

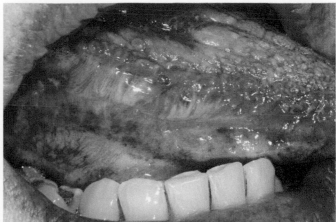

*Figure 1.10.62* Lichen planus—lingual lesions.

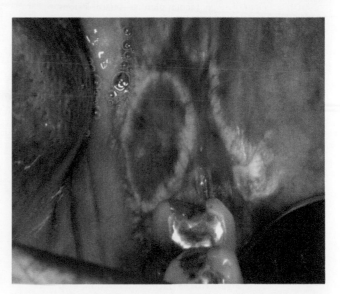

*Figure 1.10.64* Lichen planus—buccal lesions.

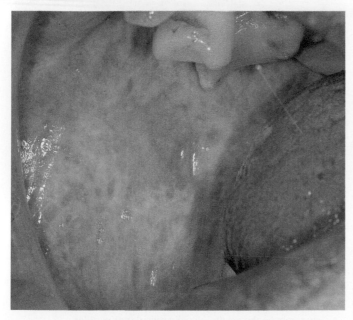

*Figure 1.10.63* Lichen planus—buccal lesions.

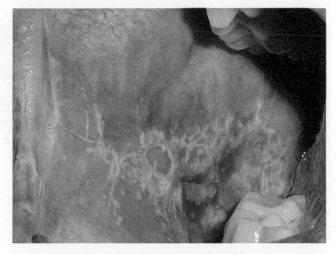

*Figure 1.10.65* Lichen planus—buccal lesions.

○ front (flexor surface) of the wrists
○ lower back
○ ankles and shins.

Trauma may induce new skin lesions (Koebner phenomenon). Lesions may also affect:

- Skin appendages: in 10% of cases there is nail involvement, usually a minor change, but occasionally resulting in shedding or destruction of the nail. The scalp is uncommonly affected, but permanently bald patches may develop.

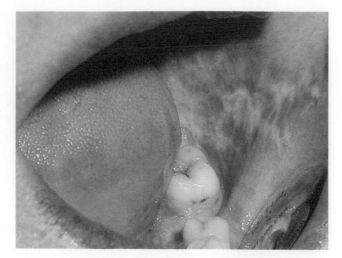

Figure 1.10.66 Lichen planus—buccal lesions.

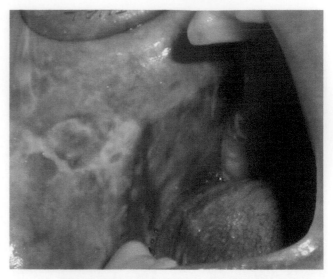

Figure 1.10.67 Lichen planus—buccal lesions.

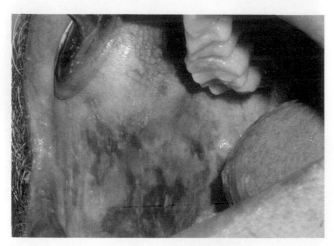

Figure 1.10.68 Lichenoid reaction.

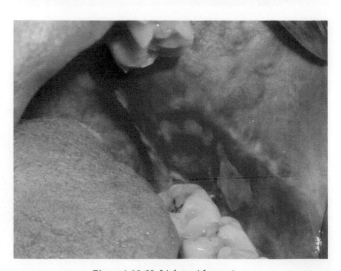

Figure 1.10.69 Lichenoid reaction.

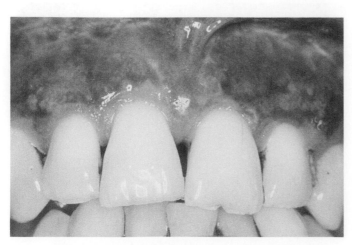

Figure 1.10.70 Lichen planus showing gingival lesions.

- occasionally on the gingiva, as a white lacework of fine white lines and papules or, in 25%, as a 'desquamative gingivitis'
- rarely on the lips—usually reticular or papular
- very rarely on the palate—usually reticular or papular.

Oral lesions of LP are often persistent and typically persist for many years. Some forms of LP, especially erosive, atrophic and other non-reticular types may be potentially malignant in <3% of cases though some of these may represent associated lichenoid dysplasia or erythroplasia.

LP may also cause lesions elsewhere, including:

- Skin: rash characterized by lesions which are
  - purple
  - polygonal
  - pruritic (itchy)
- papules—often crossed by fine white lines (Wickham striae) and is most often seen on the following:

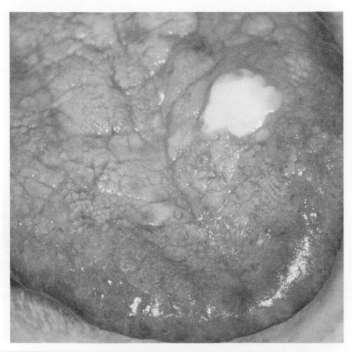

Figure 1.10.71 Lichen planus showing plaque-like lesions.

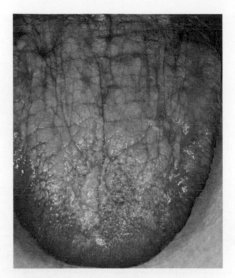

Figure 1.10.72 Lichen planus showing plaque-like lesions.

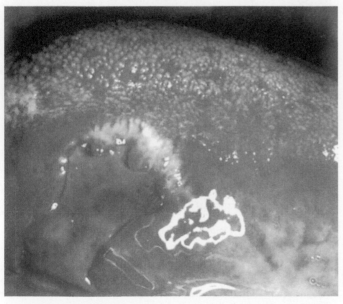

Figure 1.10.73 Lichen planus showing erosive lesions.

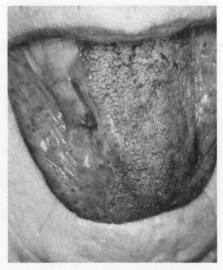

Figure 1.10.74 Lichen planus showing erosive lesions.

### Diagnosis

LP is often fairly obviously diagnosed from the clinical features but, as it can closely simulate other conditions such as lupus erythematosus, chronic ulcerative stomatitis, keratosis or even carcinoma it is, therefore, best supported by biopsy examination.

### Management

Predisposing factors should be corrected:

- It may be wise to consider removal of dental amalgams if the lesions are closely related to these, or unilateral. Unfortunately, no tests such as patch tests will reliably indicate which patients may benefit from this.
- The physician should be consulted if there is a likely systemic background, or if drugs are implicated.

- Genital mucosae:
  - The 'vulvovaginal–gingival syndrome' (Pelise syndrome) is the association of oral LP with vulvovaginal lesions of LP. This is fairly common and there is coincident onset of gingival and genital lesions in about half the reported patients, the remainder developing lesions at both sites within 2 years. The oral lesions mainly affect the labial gingivae.
  - The peno-gingival syndrome is less common and less incapacitating.

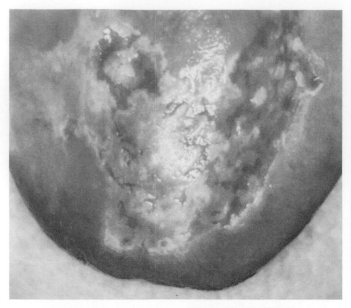

*Figure 1.10.75* Lichen planus showing erosive lesions.

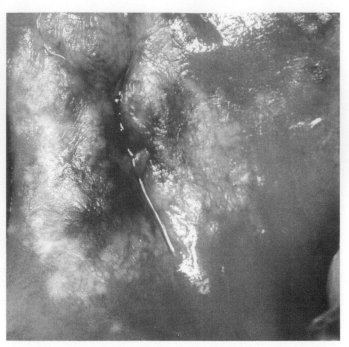

*Figure 1.10.76* Lichen planus.

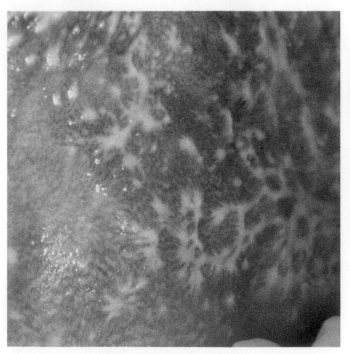

*Figure 1.10.77* Lichen planus.

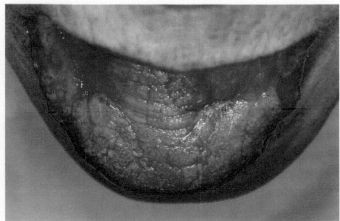

*Figure 1.10.78* Lichen planus.

fluticasone may initially be employed and should then be changed to a lower potency drug (e.g. hydrocortisone hemisuccinate, triamcinolone acetate or fluocinolone). Aloe vera may help. Topical creams or pastes can be applied in a suitable customized tray or veneer to be worn at night. In severe LP in multiple sites, patients may require systemic corticosteroids, azathioprine, cyclophosphamide, hydroxychloroquine, acitretin, thalidomide or ciclosporin. Dapsone is occasionally effective.

- Other therapies for LP include retinoids, low molecular weight heparin, efalizumab and many others, but either their efficacy has not been well proven or they have unacceptable adverse effects.

Patients, particularly those with non-reticular LP, should be monitored to exclude development of carcinoma, and tobacco and alcohol use should be minimized.

- Improvement in oral hygiene may result in some subjective benefit. Thus good oral hygiene should be maintained. Chlorhexidine or triclosan mouthwashes may help.
- Symptoms can often be controlled with topical medication such as topical corticosteroids and topical tacrolimus or even hyaluronic acid. Antifungals may help, especially where there is candidal superinfection. High potency corticosteroids such as clobetasol, fluocinonide or

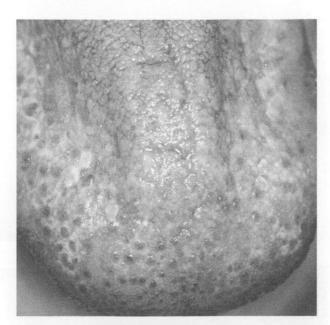

*Figure 1.10.79* Lichen planus.

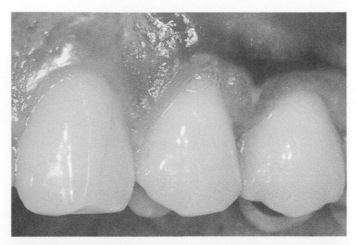

*Figure 1.10.80* Lichen planus showing gingival lesions.

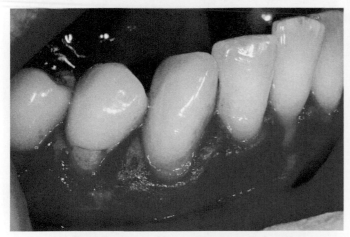

*Figure 1.10.81* Lichen planus showing gingival lesions.

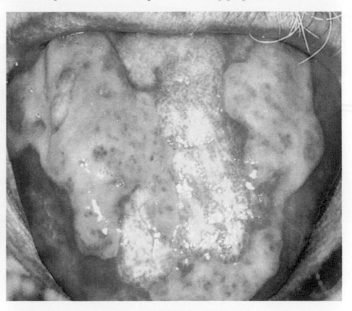

*Figure 1.10.82* Lichen planus.

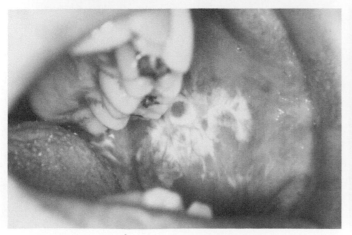

*Figure 1.10.83* Lichen planus.

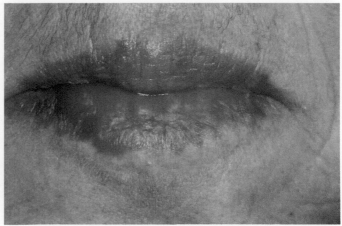

*Figure 1.10.84* Lichen planus.

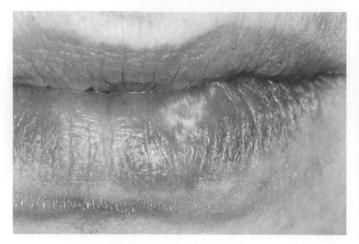

*Figure 1.10.85*  Lichen planus.

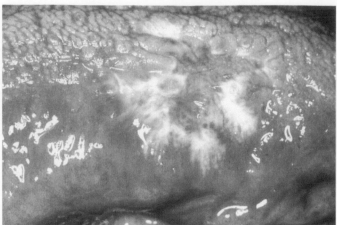

*Figure 1.10.86*  Lichen planus.

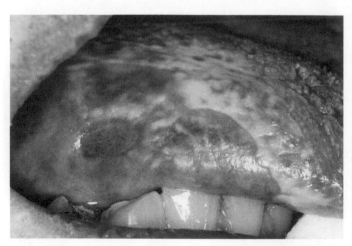

*Figure 1.10.87*  Lichen planus.

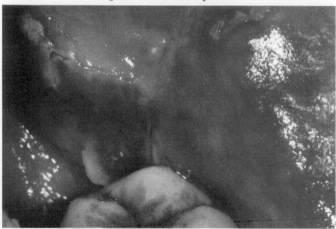

*Figure 1.10.88*  Lichen planus.

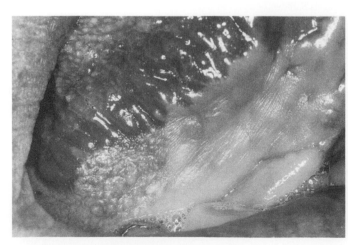

*Figure 1.10.89*  Lichen planus.

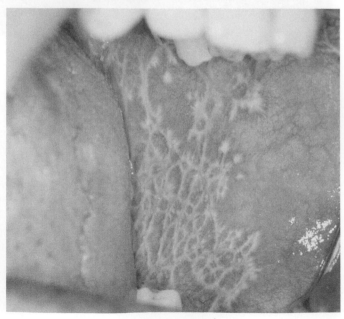

*Figure 1.10.90*  Lichen planus.

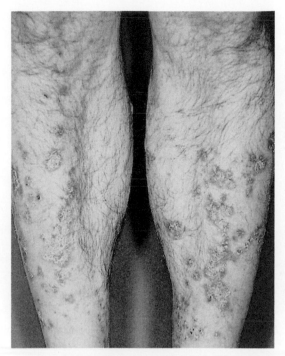

*Figure 1.10.91*  Lichen planus showing rash on shins.

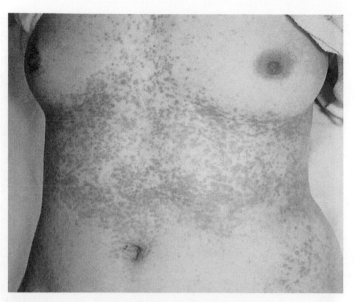

*Figure 1.10.92*  Lichen planus.

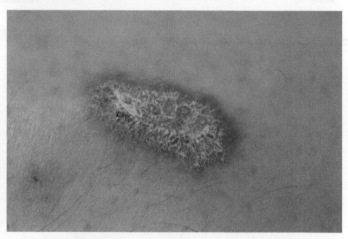

*Figure 1.10.94*  Lichen planus showing cutaneous lesions.

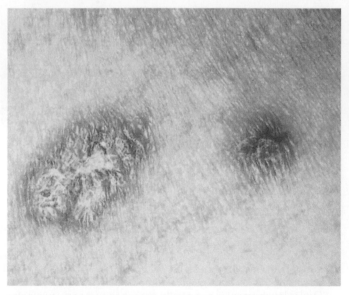

*Figure 1.10.93*  Lichen planus showing skin lesions with Wickham striae.

*Chronic ulcerative stomatitis* is a rare disorder in which lesions appear clinically similar to erosive LP but prove, on immunostaining, to be associated with stratified squamous epithelium specific antinuclear antibodies. Of note, however, these antibodies have also been observed in patients with oral LP plus HCV infection.

## LINEAR IgA DISEASE (LAD)

LAD—a sub-epithelial immune-mediated blistering disease identical to chronic bullous disease of childhood—presents before puberty with an abrupt onset of blistering in the genital region, later affecting hands, feet and face. In adults with LAD, the limbs are more often the first sites, although any area of the body may be affected later. LAD may present with oral blisters, ulcers and desquamative gingivitis (Figs 1.10.98–1.10.101).

## PACHYONYCHIA CONGENITA

Pachyonychia congenita—a rare form of autosomal dominant hereditary palmoplantar keratoderma—primarily affects nails and skin and sometimes the mouth (Fig. 1.10.102).

## PEMPHIGOID

Pemphigoid (mucous membrane previously termed cicatricial pemphigoid) is a sub-epithelial immune-mediated blistering disease, a disorder of

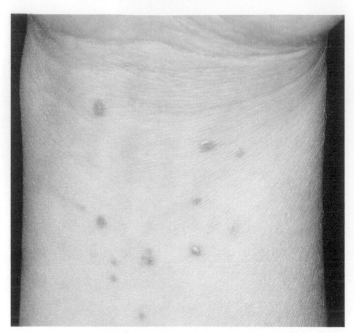

*Figure 1.10.95* Lichen planus showing cutaneous lesions.

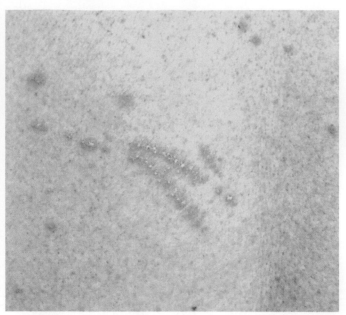

*Figure 1.10.96* Lichen planus showing Koebner phenomenon.

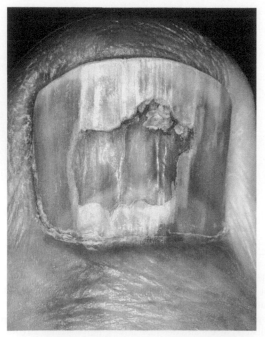

*Figure 1.10.97* Lichen planus showing nail lesions.

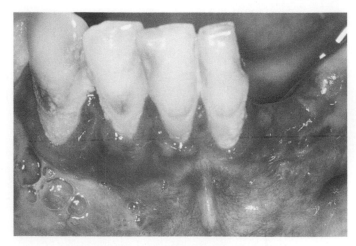

*Figure 1.10.98* Linear IgA disease—oral lesions.

stratified squamous epithelia in which there are usually IgG autoanti-bodies against epithelial BMZ. Although typically arising idiopathically and seen especially in middle-aged or older patients, mucous membrane pemphigoid may be drug-induced, particularly by penicillamine.

### Clinical features
Mucous membrane pemphigoid often affects the buccal mucosa, palate, and gingivae, causing vesicles or bullae which eventually break down to leave irregular ulcers or erosions (Figs 1.10.103–1.10.112). It is a frequent cause of desquamative gingivitis, which presents with patches of sore erythema. In contrast to marginal gingivitis, in desquamative gingivitis the interdental papillae and gingival margins may appear normal. Occasionally there is frank gingival ulceration.

Ocular involvement is potentially serious since it may culminate in blindness. Conjunctival involvement may lead to scarring and to sym-blepharon, or ankyloblepharon. The eyes are dry and the cornea becomes opaque. Other squamous epithelia may be involved; genital or laryngeal involvement may lead to stenosis. Skin lesions are uncom-mon, but vesicles, bullae and erosions may be seen. The vesicles and bullae of pemphigoid tend to be more tense than those of pemphigus and are seen most often on the abdomen, groin, axillae and flexures. Bullous pemphigoid is occasionally drug-induced, or secondary to ultraviolet light exposure. Brunsting–Perry disease is a mild variant of bullous pemphigoid.

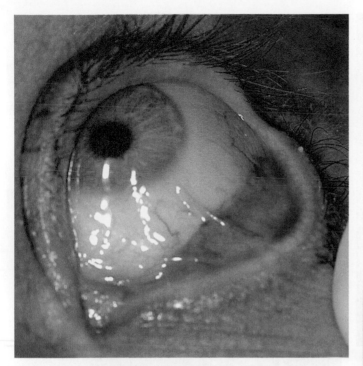

Figure 1.10.99  Linear IgA disease—ocular lesions.

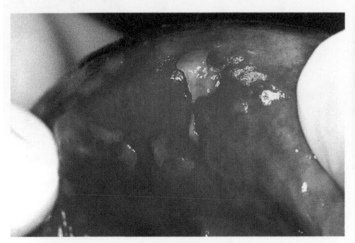

Figure 1.10.101  Linear IgA disease causing ulceration.

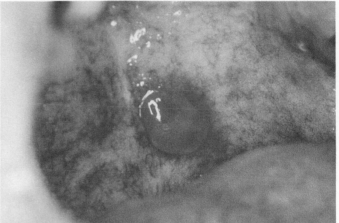

Figure 1.10.100  Linear IgA disease causing blistering.

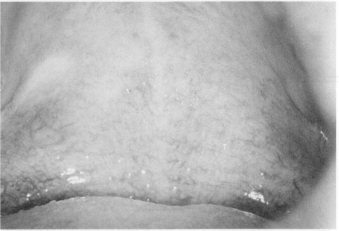

Figure 1.10.102  Pachyonychia congenita.

## Diagnosis

The oral lesions of pemphigoid may be confused clinically with pemphigus, angina bullosa haemorrhagica, dermatitis herpetiformis and LAD or, occasionally, erosive LP, acquired epidermolysis bullosa, toxic epidermal necrolysis or EM. Furthermore, the pemphigoid variants are indistinguishable clinically, by light microscopy and conventional immunostaining, one from another.

Therefore, biopsy of perilesional tissue, with histological and immunostaining examination can be essential to the diagnosis. The incisional biopsy specimen exhibits sub-epithelial clefting following staining with haematoxylin and eosin. Direct immunostaining is required to reveal the presence of BMZ immune deposits. Indirect immunofluorescence is frequently negative and the levels of serum antibody, when detected with conventional techniques, are rarely of diagnostic significance (Table 1.10.1).

Salt-split epithelial substrates (ssIIF) detect the circulating autoantibodies from patients with pemphigoid and epidermolysis bullosa acquisita binding to the roof and the base of the substrates, respectively, thus distinguishing these two diseases. In mucous membrane pemphigoid, circulating autoantibodies can bind to the roof, base, or both, corresponding to the heterogeneity of the target antigens recognized by these autoantibodies. Immunoblotting is used to check bands at 180–230 kDa or to see if any other target antigen might be detected. ELISA anti-BP180 is usually more specific than immunoblotting.

## Management

Since pemphigoid rarely spontaneously remits, treatment is usually indicated.

- Systemic manifestations must be given attention. Patients should be questioned about the presence of other mucosal symptoms, which might indicate genital or ocular involvement. Ocular manifestations affect up to 20% of patients and can lead to blindness thus an ophthalmological consultation is advised.

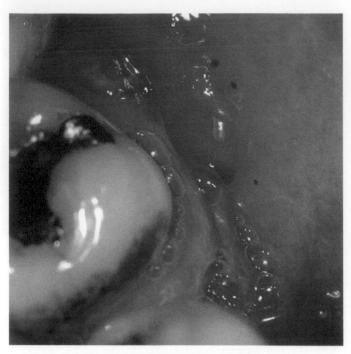

*Figure 1.10.103* Pemphigoid—blister.

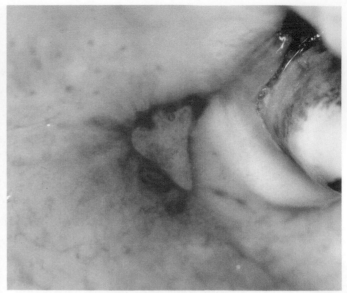

*Figure 1.10.104* Pemphigoid—erosion in a common site.

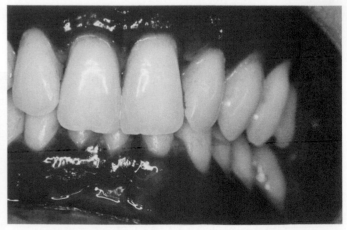

*Figure 1.10.106* Pemphigoid—desquamative gingivitis.

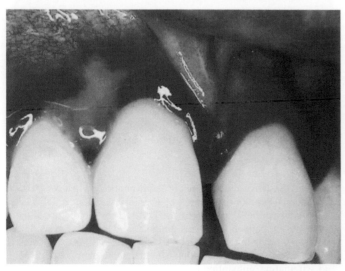

*Figure 1.10.105* Pemphigoid—desquamative gingivitis.

- Most patients with pemphigoid respond well to topical corticosteroids or tacrolimus.
- The management of desquamative gingivitis can be helped by corticosteroids used in a vacuum-formed custom tray or veneer worn during sleep and should also include oral hygiene improvement, as secondary infection may inhibit healing.
- Severe pemphigoid may need treatment with dapsone, or immunosuppression using azathioprine or systemic corticosteroids, but these are of variable benefit and/or can give rise to serious adverse effects.

## PEMPHIGUS

Pemphigus is the term given to a group of potentially lethal mucocutaneous disorders seen especially in the middle-aged or older patients, particularly in patients of Middle Eastern or Asian descent. There are a number of pemphigus variants, all characterized by autoantibodies directed against intercellular substance of stratified squamous epithelium. The autoantibodies are usually IgG. Occasional cases of pemphigus are paraneoplastic, or drug-related (e.g. to penicillamine or rifampicin).

Pemphigus vulgaris is the most common type of pemphigus involving the mouth, although still an uncommon disease. Pemphigus vegetans may involve the mouth but oral lesions of the foliaceus and erythematosus types of pemphigus are very rare.

### Clinical features

Oral lesions commonly precede skin manifestations and the vesicles or blisters are rarely seen intact since they break down rapidly to superficial irregular erosions. Initially red these later become ulcers covered

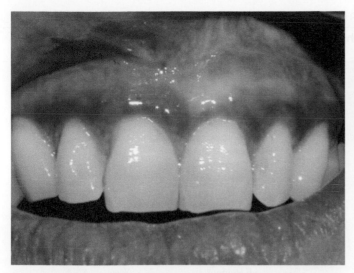

*Figure 1.10.107* Pemphigoid—desquamative gingivitis.

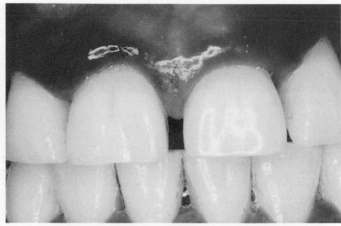

*Figure 1.10.108* Pemphigoid—desquamative gingivitis.

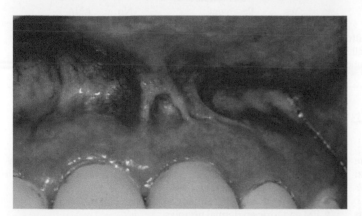

*Figure 1.10.109* Pemphigoid—desquamative gingivitis and scarring.

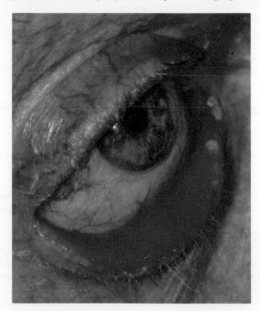

*Figure 1.10.110* Pemphigoid—conjunctival lesions.

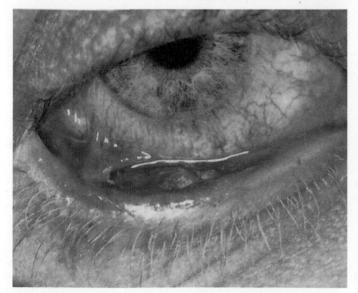

*Figure 1.10.111* Pemphigoid conjunctival lesions with symblepharon.

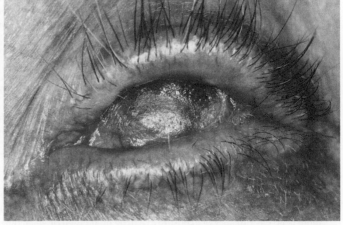

*Figure 1.10.112* Pemphigoid conjunctival lesions with ankyloblepharon.

**TABLE 1.10.1** DIFFERENTIATION OF THE MORE IMPORTANT ORAL VESICULOBULLOUS DISORDERS

| Disease | Clinical features | Main antigen | Histopathology | DIF | Epithelial location | IIF | Antibody class[a] |
|---|---|---|---|---|---|---|---|
| Pemphigus vulgaris | | Desmoglein | Acantholysis | Yes | Intercellular | Yes | IgG |
| Paraneoplastic pemphigus | | Desmoplakin | | Yes | Intercellular[b] | Yes | IgG |
| IgA pemphigus | | Desmocollin | | Yes | Intercellular | Yes | IgA |
| Bullous pemphigoid | | BP1 | Sub-epithelial bullae | Yes | Basement membrane area | Yes | IgG |
| Mucous membrane pemphigoid | | BP2 | | Yes | Basement membrane area | ± | IgG |
| Angina bullosa haemorrhagica | | None | | No | None | No | None |
| Dermatitis herpetiformis | | Trans-glutaminase | | Yes | Basement membrane area | No | IgA |
| Linear IgA disease | | Laminin | | Yes | Basement membrane area | No | IgA |
| Systemic lupus erythematosus | | NR | Vasculitis | Yes | Basement membrane area | Yes | ANA |
| Chronic discoid lupus erythematosus | | NR | | Yes | Basement membrane area | No | ANA |
| Lichen planus | | ? | T-cell infiltrate, basal cell | Often | Basement membrane area | No | (Usually fibrin) |
| Chronic ulcerative stomatitis | | ? | liquefaction | Yes | Basal cell layer nuclei | No | IgG/ANA |

[a]Usually with complement deposits.
[b]Transitional epithelium.
*Abbreviations*: NR, not relevant; BP, bullous pemphigoid; ANA, antinuclear antibody; DIF, direct immunofluorescence; IIF, indirect immunofluorescence.

with a fibrin slough. Widespread lesions may be seen, especially where the mucosa is traumatized in the buccal mucosa, palate or gingiva, and gingival involvement can lead to a form of desquamative gingivitis (Figs 1.10.113–1.10.125).

Pemphigus can affect other stratified squamous epithelium such as the nasal mucosa, conjunctivae and skin—where blisters tend to be flaccid, appear at sites of trauma (Nikolsky sign) and break down to leave extensive scabbed lesions. Rarely, the nail beds are involved.

Pemphigus vegetans (Neumann type) follows a similar course to pemphigus vulgaris, whereas the Hallopeau type is more benign but either type often presents initially in the mouth and, even in those with initial skin lesions, the mouth is usually eventually involved. White serpiginous lesions, pustules or sometimes vegetations are the main manifestations. The commissures are the sites most commonly affected and the tongue may be affected and sometimes described as a 'cerebriform tongue'.

Paraneoplastic pemphigus typically presents first on the lips, but may result in oral erosions or lichenoid lesions.

Intraepidermal IgA pustulosis may manifest with oral blisters and erosions described in the few patients with this recently disease in which there is acantholysis with intercellular IgA deposits.

Benign pemphigus (Hailey–Hailey disease) only rarely presents with oral lesions and these are indistinguishable clinically from those of pemphigus vulgaris.

## Diagnosis

- Diagnosis of an autoimmune bullous disease should be suspected when there is no clear history of exposure to a drug or allergen or when other studies for infectious origins, such as herpes or impetigo, are negative.

- The differential diagnosis includes pemphigus variants such as pemphigus foliaceus and erythematosus and pemphigus vegetans, which only rarely affect the oral mucosae, and
  o pemphigoid and other sub-epithelial blistering disorders
  o EM and toxic epidermal necrolysis
  o pyostomatitis vegetans
  o paraneoplastic pemphigus
  o IgA pemphigus (intraepithelial IgA pustulosis)
  o pemphigus associated with inflammatory bowel disease.
- To differentiate these bullous diseases, a careful history and physical examination are important, but biopsy is mandatory.
- Biopsy of perilesional tissue, with histological and immunostaining examination are essential (Table 1.10.1).
- Serum should be collected for titres of antibody to epithelial intercellular cement, which may help guide treatment. Serum autoantibodies to desmoglein are best detected using both normal human skin and monkey oesophagus by enzyme-linked immunosorbent assay.
  o The titre of circulating autoantibodies corresponds to the severity of disease.

In addition to binding to squamous epithelial cell surfaces (e.g. skin, oesophagus substrates), circulating autoantibodies from patients with paraneoplastic pemphigus also label transitional epithelium (e.g. rat bladder).

## Management

Pemphigus vulgaris is a life-threatening disorder, though current treatment, largely based on systemic immunosuppression has significantly reduced the mortality to about 10%. Physician involvement and patient information are thus important.

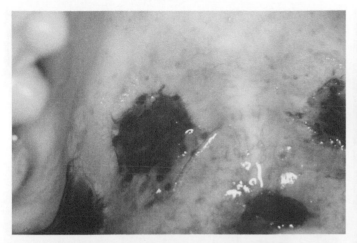

Figure 1.10.113  Pemphigus—palatal lesions.

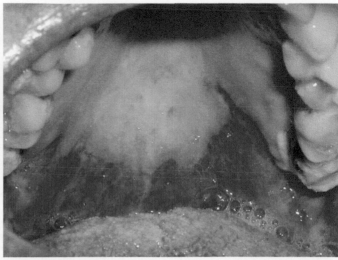

Figure 1.10.114  Pemphigus—early lesions.

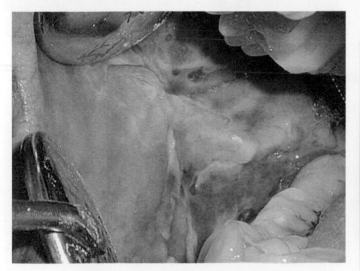

Figure 1.10.115  Pemphigus—oral erosions.

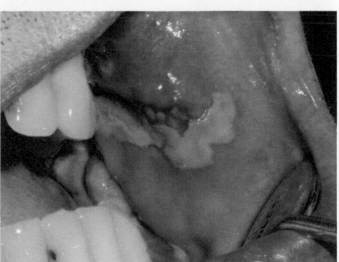

Figure 1.10.116  Pemphigus—erosions.

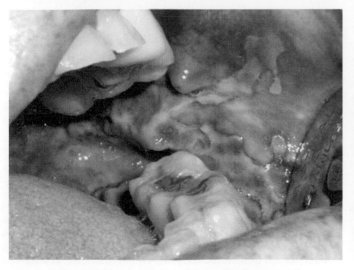

Figure 1.10.117  Pemphigus—erosions.

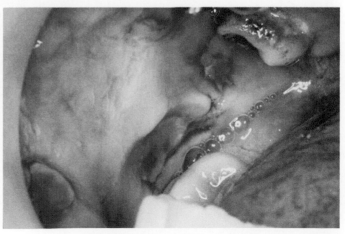

Figure 1.10.118  Pemphigus—erosions.

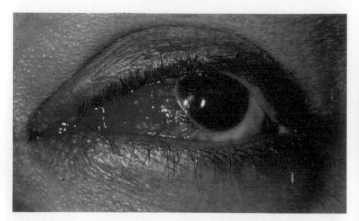

*Figure 1.10.119* Pemphigus—conjunctival involvement.

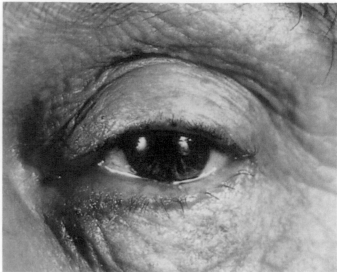

*Figure 1.10.120* Pemphigus—ocular lesions.

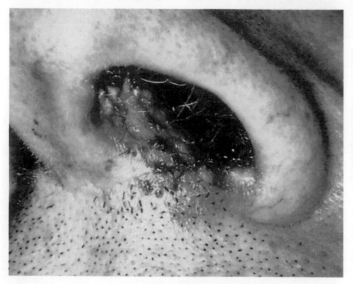

*Figure 1.10.121* Pemphigus—nasal lesions.

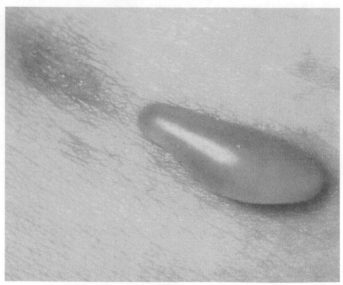

*Figure 1.10.122* Pemphigus—flaccid skin blisters.

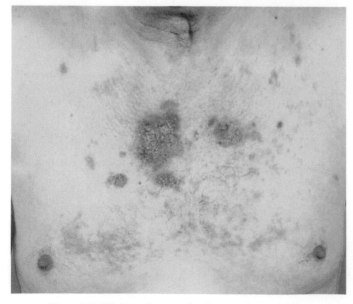

*Figure 1.10.123* Pemphigus—skin lesions after scabbing.

Patients with severe oral lesions may have lesions of other mucosae and thus should be referred to

- a pulmonary specialist—especially those patients with paraneoplastic pemphigus, and particularly if the patients have symptoms or signs suggestive of respiratory difficulty.
- a gastroenterologist—to detect possible oesophageal involvement.

Systemic therapy, often with corticosteroids (e.g. prednisolone) is essential, unless there are only localized oral lesions, when topical corticosteroids or intralesional corticosteroids may suffice for a time. Once under control, the dosage of prednisolone can be tapered or adjuncts added. It is possible to eventually induce complete and durable remissions in most patients, permitting systemic therapy to be safely discontinued without a flare in disease activity. The proportion of patients in whom this can be achieved increases steadily with time, and therapy can be discontinued in approximately 75% of patients after 10 years.

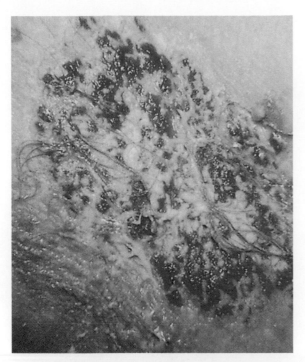

*Figure 1.10.124* Pemphigus—skin lesions.

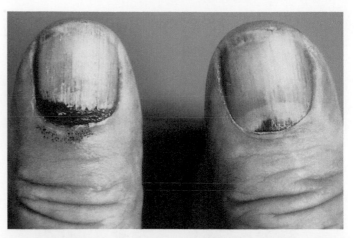

*Figure 1.10.125* Pemphigus—nail lesions.

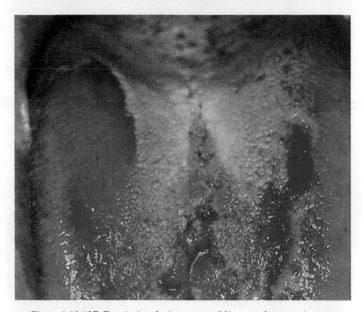

*Figure 1.10.127* Psoriasis—lesions resembling erythema migrans.

- others, such as gold, dapsone, chlorambucil, levamisole, immunoglobulins, anti-TNF-α agents (e.g. infliximab, adalumimab) or anti-CD20 agents (e.g. rituximab).

Oral lesions, however, can be persistent, and often recalcitrant even when cutaneous lesions are controlled.

## PSORIASIS

Psoriasis—a chronic, non-contagious autoimmune disease that affects the skin, joints and nails—commonly causes red, scaly patches over the elbows in particular, and rarely causes oral lesions which mimic erythema migrans (Figs 1.10.126–1.10.129).

## WHITE SPONGE NAEVUS

White sponge naevus (pachyderma oralis: white folded gingivostomatitis)— a rare autosomal dominant defect of keratins 13 or 4 (but family history may be sometimes be negative)—often affects the mouth.

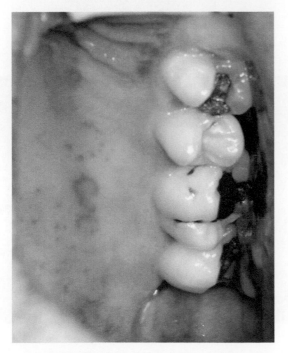

*Figure 1.10.126* Psoriasis—circinate lesions.

Adjuncts or alternatives include:

- azathioprine
- mycophenolate mofetil
- ciclosporin
- cyclophosphamide

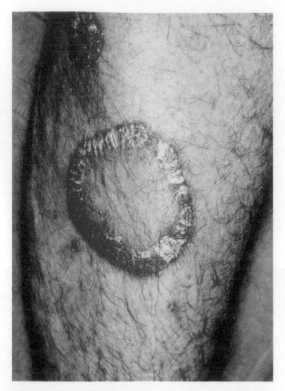

*Figure 1.10.128* Psoriasis skin plaque in a common site.

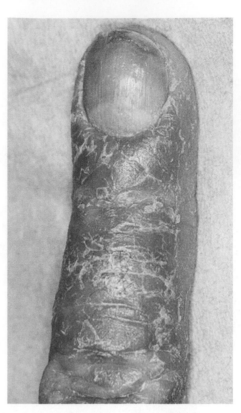

*Figure 1.10.129* Psoriasis cutaneous and nail lesions.

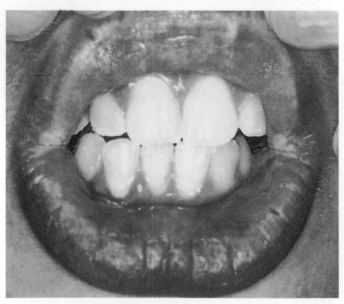

*Figure 1.10.130* White sponge naevus.

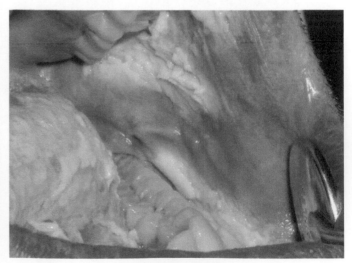

*Figure 1.10.131* White sponge naevus.

### Clinical features

The oral mucosa is almost invariably involved from birth with symptomless bilateral, white, shaggy or folded or wrinkled lesions typically seen in the buccal mucosa, sometimes in other oral sites especially the tongue, or floor of mouth, or in oesophageal, nasal, vaginal or anal mucosa. Rare cases have iris coloboma (Figs 1.10.130 and 1.10.131).

### Diagnosis

The family history and examination are usually adequate to make the diagnosis but there may be confusion with other white lesions (Chapter 2.2) when a biopsy can be indicated. Histologically, the lesion typically consists of hyperplastic epithelium in which gross oedema causes a basket-weave appearance.

## Management

Reassurance is all that is required. There are reports that tetracyclines may reduce the lesions, but these are contraindicated in children.

## FURTHER READING

Al-Johani KA, Fedele S, Porter SR. Erythema multiforme and related disorders. Oral Surg Oral Med Oral Pathol Oral Radiol Endod 2007; 103: 642–54.

Al-Otaibi L, Porter SR, Poate TWJ. Behcet's disease—a review. J Dent Res 2005; 84: 209–22.

Aziz SR, Tin P. Spontaneous angioedema of oral cavity after dental impressions. N Y State Dent J 2002; 68: 42–5.

Bagan J, Lo Muzio L, Scully C. Mucosal disease series. Number III. Mucous membrane pemphigoid. Oral Dis 2005; 11: 197–218.

Bagan J, Lo Muzio L, Scully C. Mucous membrane pemphigoid. Oral Dis 2005; 11: 197–218.

Bez C, Hallet R, Carrozzo M, et al. Lack of association between hepatotropic transfusion transmitted virus infection and oral lichen planus in British and Italian populations. Br J Dermatol 2001; 145: 990–3.

Bidarra M, Buchanan J, Scully C, Moles DR, Porter SR. Oral lichen planus; a condition with more persistence and extraoral involvement than suspected? J Oral Pathol Med 2008; 37: 582–6.

Black M, Mignogna MD, Scully C. Number II. Pemphigus vulgaris. Oral Dis 2005; 11: 119–30.

Carbone M, Arduino PG, Carrozzo M, et al. Topical clobetasol in the treatment of atrophic-erosive oral lichen planus: a randomized controlled trial to compare two preparations with different concentrations. J Oral Pathol 2009; 38: 227–33.

Carbone M, Arduino PG, Carrozzo M, et al. Course of oral lichen planus: a retrospective study of 808 northern Italian patients. Oral Dis 2009; 15: 235–43.

Carrozzo M, Brancatello F, Dametto E, et al. Hepatitis C virus-associated oral lichen planus: is the geographical heterogeneity related to HLA-DR6? J Oral Pathol Med 2005; 34: 204–8.

Carrozzo M, Thorpe RJ. Update on oral lichen planus. Expert Rev Dermatol 2009; 4: 483–94.

Challacombe SJ, Setterfield J, Shirlaw P, et al. Immunodiagnosis of pemphigus and mucous membrane pemphigoid. Acta Odontol Scand 2001; 59: 226–34.

Escudier M, Bagan J, Scully C. Behcets syndrome; (Adamantiades syndrome). Oral Dis 2006; 12: 78–84.

Farthing P, Bagan J, Scully C. Erythema multiforme. Oral Dis 2005; 11: 261–67.

Femiano F, Gombos F, Nunziata M, Esposito V, Scully C. Pemphigus mimicking aphthous stomatitis. J Oral Pathol Med 2005; 34: 508–11.

Femiano F, Gombos F, Scully C. Pemphigus vulgaris with oral involvement; evaluation of two different systemic corticosteroid therapeutic protocols. J Eur Acad Dermatol Venereol 2002; 16: 353–6.

Femiano F, Gombos F, Scully C. Oral erosive/ulcerative lichen planus: preliminary findings in an open trial of sulodexide compared with cyclosporine (ciclosporin) therapy. Int J Dermatol 2003; 42: 308–11.

Femiano F, Scully C. Oral lichen planus: clinical and histological evaluation in an open trial using a low molecular weight heparinoid (sulodexide). Int J Dermatol 2006; 45: 986–9.

Fine JD, Mellerio JE. Extracutaneous manifestations and complications of inherited epidermolysis bullosa: part II. Other organs. J Am Acad Dermatol 2009; 61: 387–402.

Gonzalez-Moles M, Scully C. Vesiculo-erosive oral mucosal disease. Management with topical corticosteroids: 1. Fundamental principles and specific agents available. J Dent Res 2005; 84: 294–301.

Gonzalez-Moles M, Scully C. Vesiculo-erosive oral mucosal disease. Management with topical corticosteroids: 2. Protocols, monitoring of effects and adverse reactions, and the future. J Dent Res 2005; 84: 302–8.

Gonzalez-Moles MA, Scully C, Gil-Montoya JA. Oral lichen planus: controversies surrounding malignant transformation. Oral Dis 2008; 14: 229–43.

Horie N, Kawano R, Inaba J, et al. Angina bullosa hemorrhagica of the soft palate: a clinical study of 16 cases. J Oral Sci 2008; 50: 33–6.

Ingafou M, Leao JC, Porter SR, Scully C. Oral lichen planus: a retrospective study of 690 British patients. Oral Dis 2006; 12: 463–8.

Jimenez Y, Bagan JV, Milian MA, Gavalda C, Scully C. Lichen sclerosus et atrophicus manifesting with localized loss of periodontal attachment. Oral Dis 2002; 8: 311–14.

Kragelund C, Hansen C, Reibel J, et al. Polymorphic drug metabolizing CYP-enzymes—a pathogenic factor in oral lichen planus? J Oral Pathol 2009; 38: 63–71.

Leao JC, Ingafou M, Khan A, Scully C, Porter SR. Desquamative gingivitis; retrospective analysis of disease associations of a large cohort. Oral Dis 2008; 14: 556–60.

Lodi G, Carrozzo M, Harris K, et al. Hepatitis G virus-associated oral lichen planus; no influence from hepatitis G virus co-infection. J Oral Pathol Med 2000; 29: 39–42.

Lodi G, Scully C, Carrozzo M, et al. Current controversies in oral lichen planus: report of an international consensus meeting. Part 1. Viral infections and etiopathogenesis. Oral Surg Oral Med Oral Pathol Oral Radiol Endod 2005; 100: 40–51.

Lodi G, Scully C, Carrozzo M, et al. Current controversies in oral lichen planus: report of an international consensus meeting. Part 2. Clinical management and malignant transformation. Oral Surg Oral Med Oral Pathol Oral Radiol Endod 2005; 100: 164–78.

Martelli Jr H, Pereira SM, Rocha TM, et al. White sponge nevus: report of a three-generation family. Oral Surg Oral Med Oral Pathol Oral Radiol Endod 2007; 103: 43–7.

Mattingly G, Rodu B, Alling R. Quincke's disease: nonhereditary angioneurotic edema of the uvula. Oral Surg Oral Med Oral Pathol 1993; 75: 292–5.

Petti FP, Bagan JV, Chaparro N, Scully C. Malignant transformation of oral lichen planus: presentation of three new documented cases and analysis of possible causes. Acta Otorrinolaringol Esp 2004; 55: 41–4.

Scully C. The mouth in dermatological disorders. Practitioner 2001; 245: 942–52.

Scully C, Bagan JV. Oral mucosal diseases: erythema multiforme. Br J Oral Maxillofac Surg 2008; 46: 90–5.

Scully C, Bagan JV, Black M, et al. Epithelial biology. Oral Dis 2005; 11: 58–71.

Scully C, Carrozzo M. Oral mucosal disease: lichen planus. Br J Oral Maxillofac Surg 2008; 46: 15–21.

Scully C, Challacombe SJ. Pemphigus vulgaris: update on etiopathogenesis, oral manifestations and management. Crit Rev Oral Biol Med 2002; 13: 397–408.

Scully C, Eisen D, Bagan JV. The diagnosis and management of oral lichen planus; a consensus approach. Oral Biosci Med 2004; 1: 21–8.

Scully C, Eisen D, Carrozzo M. Management of oral lichen planus. Am J Clin Dermatol 2000; 1: 287–306.

Scully C, Lo Muzio L. Oral mucosal diseases: mucous membrane pemphigoid. Br J Oral Maxillofac Surg 2008; 46: 358–66.

Scully C, Mignogna M. Oral mucosal disease: pemphigus. Br J Oral Maxillofac Surg 2008; 46: 272–7.

Segura S, Pujol RM. Eosinophilic ulcer of the oral mucosa: a distinct entity or a non-specific reactive pattern? Oral Dis 2008; 14: 287–95.

Solomon LW. Chronic ulcerative stomatitis. Oral Dis 2008; 14: 383–9.

Stephenson P, Scully C, Prime SS, Daly HM. Angina bullosa haemorrhagica: lesional immunostaining and haematological findings. Br J Oral Maxillofac Surg 1987; 25: 488–91.

Torgerson RR, Davis MD, Bruce AJ, Farmer SA, Rogers 3rd RS. Contact allergy in oral disease. J Am Acad Dermatol 2007; 57: 315–21.

Wongwatana S, Leao JC, Porter SR, Scully C. Oxpentifylline is not effective for symptomatic oral lichen planus. J Oral Pathol Med 2005; 34: 106–8.

# 1.11 NEOPLASTIC DISEASE

- bone neoplasms
- Langerhans histiocytosis
- leukaemia
- lipoma
- lymphoma
- melanoma
- metastases
- myxoma
- neuroblastoma

- neurofibroma
- neuroma
- odontogenic neoplasms
- oral carcinoma
- osteoma
- paraneoplastic syndromes
- salivary neoplasms
- sarcomas

## BONE NEOPLASMS
Bone neoplasms may affect the jaws (Chapters 1.11 and 2.8).

## LANGERHANS HISTIOCYTOSIS
Langerhans histiocytosis—a group of rare idiopathic disorders characterized by proliferation of bone marrow-derived Langerhans cells and mature eosinophils—can cause jaw or oral lesions. The disorders form a spectrum from an acute, fulminant, disseminated disease (Letterer–Siwe disease); through an intermediate form (Hand–Schüller–Christian disease) characterized by multifocal, chronic involvement and classically presenting as the triad of diabetes insipidus, proptosis and lytic bone lesions to a solitary or few, indolent chronic lesions of bone or other organs (eosinophilic granuloma). These disorders can present with loosening of teeth and jaw radiolucencies (Figs 1.11.1–1.11.3) and oral ulceration.

## LEUKAEMIA
Leukaemia (Chapter 1.4).

## LIPOMA
Lipoma—benign neoplasms of fatty tissue may produce semi-fluctuant oral swellings (Figs 1.11.4–1.11.6).

## LYMPHOMA
Lymphoma (Chapter 1.4).

## MELANOMA
Melanoma—one of the less common types of skin cancer, but causing the majority of skin cancer-related deaths—is rare in the mouth. Most oral melanomas are thought to arise *de novo*, rarely from oral naevi *Lentigo maligna* (Figs 1.11.7–1.11.9). The most common oral locations for melanoma are the palate and maxillary gingiva. Metastatic melanoma most frequently affects the mandible, tongue and buccal mucosa.

Oral melanoma often is overlooked or clinically misinterpreted as a benign pigmented process until it is well advanced and it frequently presents with metastases in lymph nodes, liver and lungs.

## METASTASES
Metastases to the jaws are usually from carcinomas of the breast or bronchus, thyroid, kidney, liver, oesophagus, colo-rectum, stomach, prostate or uterus (Figs 1.11.10–1.11.14). Metastases are most often seen in the mandible, especially the angle and body. They virtually all present with pain or anaesthesia, expansion of the jaw and/or loosening of the teeth; there may occasionally be external erosion of dental roots.

Intravenous bisphosphonates used in the treatment of metastatic bone disease may predispose to jaw osteochemonecrosis (Chapter 2.8).

**Diagnosis**
Clinical plus imaging and biopsy.

**Management**
Oncological therapy.

## MYXOMA
Myxoma—a neoplasm of primitive connective tissue—mainly affects the heart, but may affect the maxillofacial region (Figs 1.11.15 and 1.11.16).

## NEUROBLASTOMA
Neuroblastoma—one of the most common extracranial solid cancers in childhood and the most common cancer in infancy—arises from neural crest cells mainly in the adrenal glands, neck, chest or spinal cord (Figs 1.11.17 and 1.11.18). Levels of vanillylmandelic acid, or homovanillic acid, are raised in the urine, and meta-iodo-benzyl guanidine scan often defines the lesions.

## NEUROFIBROMA
Neurofibroma (Chapter 1.13).

## NEUROMA
Neuroma, a neoplasm from nerve cells may be seen in the mouth (Figs 1.11.19 and 1.11.20).

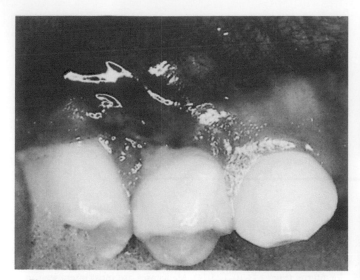

*Figure 1.11.1* Langerhans histiocytosis presenting with ulceration.

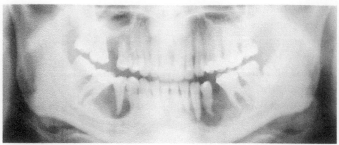

*Figure 1.11.2* Langerhans histiocytosis—osteolytic lesions.

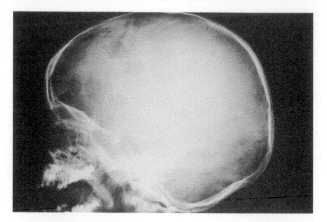

*Figure 1.11.3* Langerhans histiocytosis—osteolytic lesions.

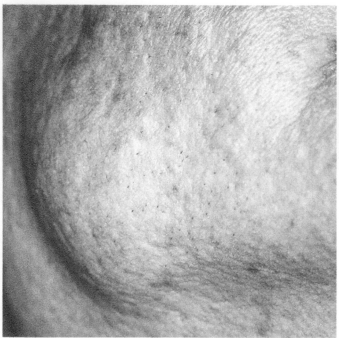

*Figure 1.11.4* Lipoma.

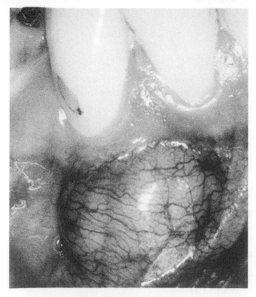

*Figure 1.11.5* Lipoma.

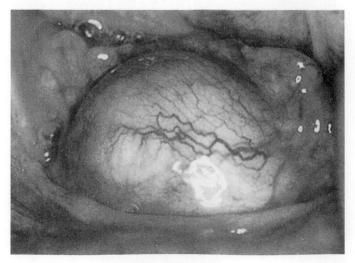

*Figure 1.11.6* Lipoma.

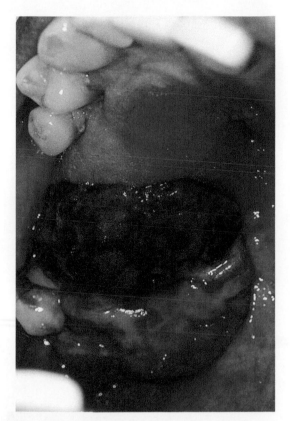

*Figure 1.11.7* Melanoma.

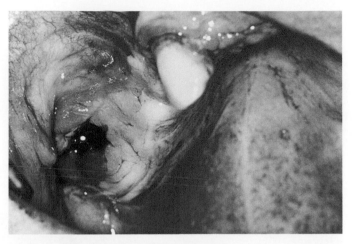

*Figure 1.11.8* Melanoma.

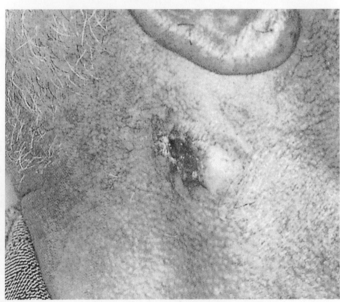

*Figure 1.11.10* Metastasis in lymph node.

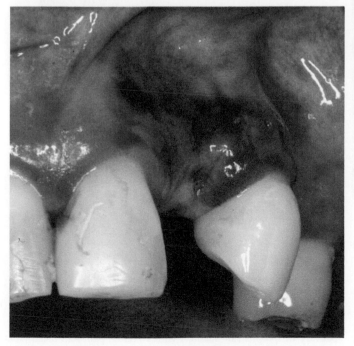

*Figure 1.11.9* Melanoma (lentigo maligna).

## ODONTOGENIC NEOPLASMS

Odontogenic neoplasms affect the jaws (Chapter 2.8).

## ORAL CARCINOMA

Oral carcinoma (Chapter 2.3).

## OSTEOMA

Osteoma—a benign tumour of bone—most commonly affects the skull or facial skeleton (Figs 1.11.21–1.11.23). Large craniofacial osteomas may cause orofacial pain, headache and infection due to obstructed nasofrontal ducts, or ocular signs and symptoms.

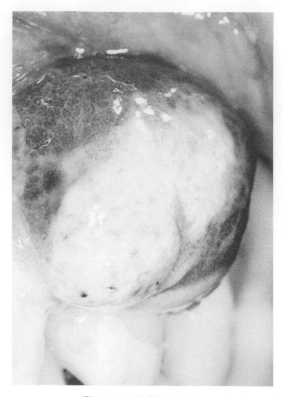

*Figure 1.11.11* Metastasis.

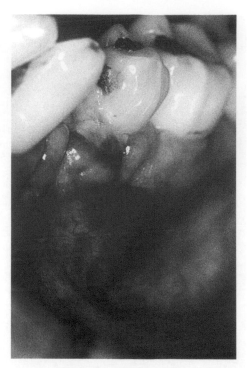

*Figure 1.11.12* Metastasis.

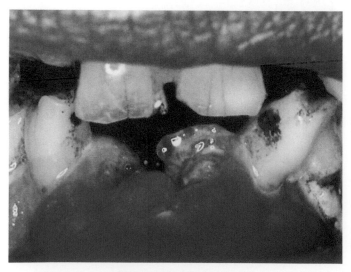

*Figure 1.11.13* Metastasis.

Osteoid osteomas typically affect teenage or young adult males, and can cause intense pain especially pronounced at night, as they secrete pain-inducing prostaglandins.

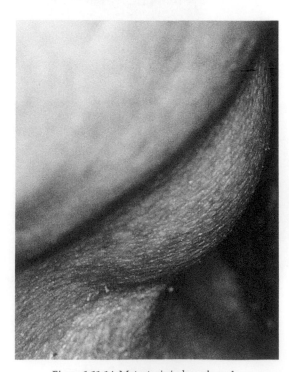

*Figure 1.11.14* Metastasis in lymph node.

## PARANEOPLASTIC SYNDROMES

Paraneoplastic syndromes—paraneoplastic syndromes associated with oral carcinoma are shown in the Box 1.11.1.

## SALIVARY NEOPLASMS

Salivary neoplasms can manifest with swelling, pain and facial palsy (Chapter 2.7).

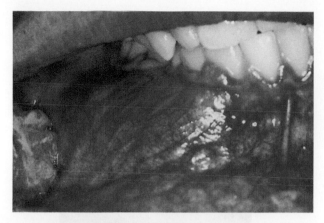

*Figure 1.11.15* Myxoma.

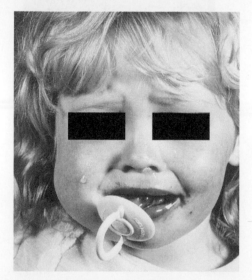

*Figure 1.11.17* Neuroblastoma.

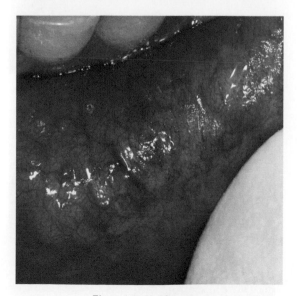

*Figure 1.11.19* Neuroma.

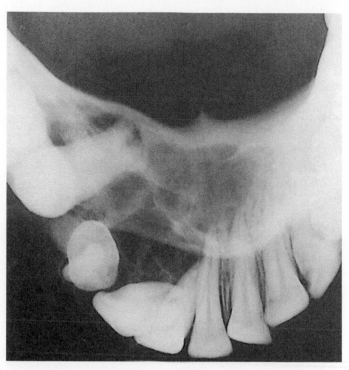

*Figure 1.11.16* Myxoma.

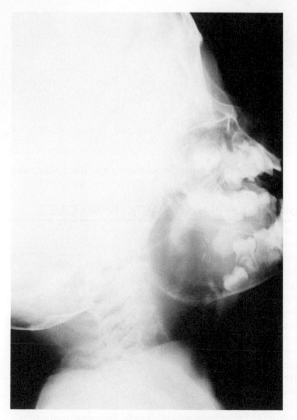

*Figure 1.11.18* Neuroblastoma.

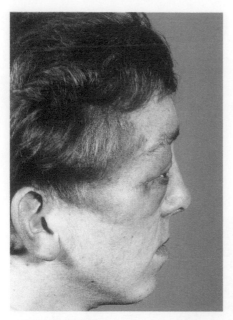

*Figure 1.11.20* Plexiform neurofibroma.

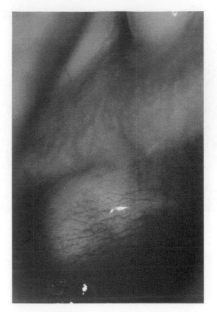

*Figure 1.11.21* Osteoma.

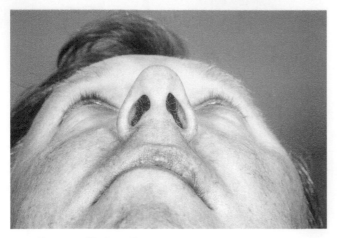

*Figure 1.11.22* Cancellous osteoma and coronoid process.

## Box 1.11.1 PARANEOPLASTIC SYNDROMES

Autoimmune retinal degeneration
Bazex syndrome
Cerebral venous sinus thrombophlebitis
Dermatomyositis
Digital ischaemia
Ectopic production of adrenocorticotrophic hormone
Ectopic production of beta-human chorionic gonadotrophin
Hypercalcaemia, hypercalcaemia–leukocytosis syndrome
Necrotising myopathy
Neutrophilic leukaemoid reaction
Paraneoplastic pemphigus
Pityriasis rotunda
Sweet syndrome
Subacute cerebellar degeneration
Syndrome of inappropriate antidiuretic hormone production
Tripe palm syndrome

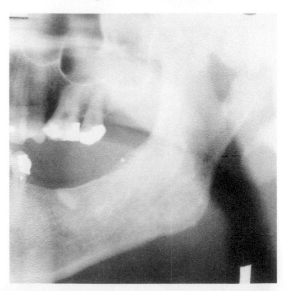

*Figure 1.11.23* Cancellous osteoma and coronoid process.

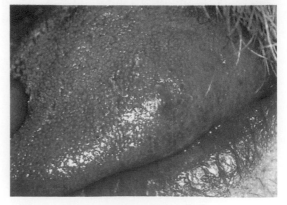

*Figure 1.11.24* Sarcoma—alveolar soft part sarcoma.

## SARCOMAS

Sarcomas are rare malignant neoplasms arising from connective tissue elements. Those that may affect the maxillofacial region include:

- alveolar soft part sarcoma—a slow-growing neoplasm of uncertain origin, that metastasises widely to lungs and brain (Fig. 1.11.24);
- angiosarcoma—an endothelial vascular neoplasm that can affect a variety of sites, is aggressive and tends to recur locally, spread widely, with a high rate of lymph node and systemic metastases (Figs 1.11.25 and 1.11.26); fibrosarcoma—which arises from fibroblasts and tends to recur locally, spread widely, with a high rate of lymph node and systemic metastases (Fig. 1.11.27);
- Kaposi sarcoma may present with red or purple macules or lumps which may ulcerate, most commonly in the maxilla, especially palate or gingivae.
- Osteosarcoma—the most common bone neoplasm and seen mainly in boys around the knee area, or at the ends of long bones or in the jaws (Figs 1.11.28 and 1.11.29); and
- rhabdomyosarcoma—the most common soft tissue sarcoma in children, is thought to arise from skeletal muscle progenitor cells—usually positive for intermediate filaments and other proteins typical of differentiated muscle cells, such as desmin, vimentin, myoglobin, actin and transcription factor myoD. The head and neck is the region most commonly affected but the tumour can arise anywhere except in bone (Figs 1.11.30–1.11.32).

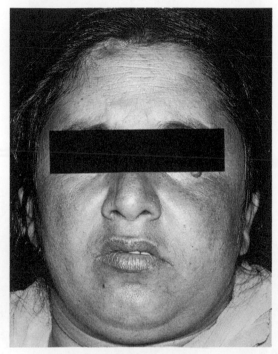

Figure 1.11.25 Sarcoma—angiosarcoma, left maxilla.

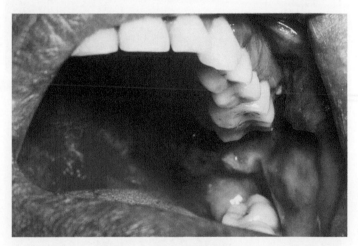

Figure 1.11.26 Sarcoma—angiosarcoma.

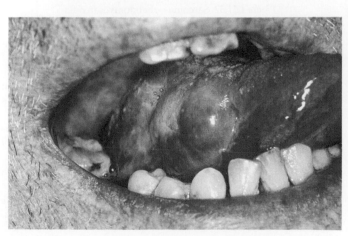

Figure 1.11.27 Sarcoma—fibrosarcoma.

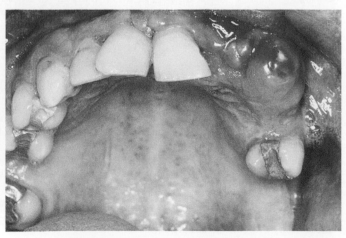

Figure 1.11.28 Sarcoma—osteogenic sarcoma.

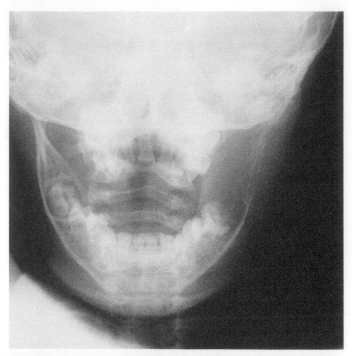

*Figure 1.11.29* Sarcoma—osteogenic sarcoma.

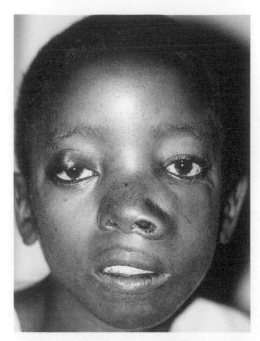

*Figure 1.11.30* Sarcoma—rhabdomyosarcoma.

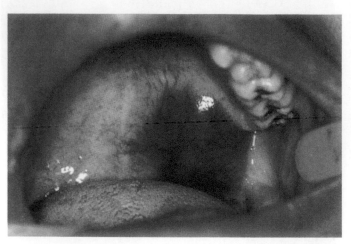

*Figure 1.11.31* Sarcoma—rhabdomyosarcoma.

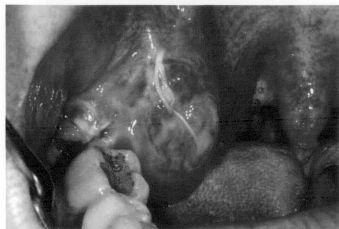

*Figure 1.11.32* Sarcoma—rhabdomyosarcoma.

## FURTHER READING

Al-Hakeem DA, Fedele S, Carlos R, Porter S. Extranodal NK/T-cell lymphoma, nasal type. Oral Oncol 2007; 43: 4–14.

Bagan JV, Scully C. Recent advances in oral oncology 2008; squamous cell carcinoma aetiopathogenesis and experimental studies. Oral Oncol 2009; 45: e45–8.

Capodiferro S, Scully C, Maiorano E, Lo Muzio L, Favia G. Liposarcoma circumscriptum (lipoma-like) of the tongue: report of a case. Oral Dis 2004; 10: 398–400.

Capodiferro S, Scully C, Scivetti M, Lacaita NG, Maiorano E. Nerve sheath myxoma (neurothekeoma) of the tongue: a case report and literature review. J Oral Maxillofac Surg 2006; 64: 705–8.

Chapireau D, Adlam D, Cameron M, Thompson M. Paraneoplastic syndromes in patients with primary oral cancers: a systematic review. Br J Oral Maxillofac Surg 2009. [Epub ahead of print].

Cohan DM, Popat S, Kaplan SE, et al. Oropharyngeal cancer: current understanding and management. Curr Opin Otolaryngol Head Neck Surg 2009; 17: 88–94.

Dios PD, Teijeiro JC, Anguira FB, et al. Synchronous oral leiomyosarcoma and squamous cell carcinoma. Oral Surg Oral Med Oral Pathol 2001; 91: 70–5.

Femiano F, Scully C, Laino G, Battista C. Benign fibrous histiocytoma (BHF) of the cheek: CD 68-KP1 positivity. Oral Oncol 2001; 37: 673–5.

Hirshberg A, Shnaiderman-Shapiro A, Kaplan I, Berger R. Metastatic tumours to the oral cavity—pathogenesis and analysis of 673 cases. Oral Oncol 2008; 44: 743–52.

Leão JC, Caterino-De-Araújo A, Porter SR, Scully C. Human herpesvirus 8 (HHV-8) and the etiopathogenesis of Kaposi's sarcoma. Rev Hosp Clin Fac Med Sao Paulo 2002; 57: 175–86.

Milian MA, Bagan JV, Jimenez Y, et al. Langerhans cell histiocytosis restricted to the oral mucosa. Oral Surg Oral Med Oral Pathol 2001; 91: 76–9.

Patel SG, Prasad ML, Escrig M, et al. Primary mucosal malignant melanoma of the head and neck. Head Neck 2002; 24: 247–57.

Richards A, Costelloe MA, Eveson JW, et al. Oral mucosal non-Hodgkin's lymphoma—a dangerous mimic. Oral Oncol 2000; 36: 556–8.

Scipio JE, Murti PR, Al-Bayaty HF, Matthews R, Scully C. Metastasis of breast carcinoma to mandibular gingiva. Oral Oncol 2001; 37: 393–6.

Scully C, Bagan JV. Recent advances in oral oncology 2008; squamous cell carcinoma imaging, treatment, prognostication and treatment outcomes. Oral Oncol 2009; 45: e25–30.

Scully C, Bagan JV, Hopper C, Epstein JB. Oral cancer: current and future diagnostic techniques. Am J Dent 2008; 21: 199–209.

Scully C, Barrett WA, Gilkes J, Sarner M, Rees M. Oral acanthosis nigricans: the sign of Leser–Trelat syndrome and cholangiocarcinoma. Br J Dermatol 2001; 145: 506–7.

Seoane J, Van der Waal I, Van der Waal RI, et al. Metastatic tumours to the oral cavity: a survival study with a special focus on gingival metastases. J Clin Periodontol 2009; 36: 488–92.

Shen ML, Kang J, Wen YL, et al. Metastatic tumors to the oral and maxillofacial region: a retrospective study of 19 cases in West China and review of the Chinese and English literature. J Oral Maxillofac Surg 2009; 67: 718–37.

Woo VL, Abdelsayed R. Oral manifestations of internal malignancy and paraneoplastic syndromes. Dent Clin North Am 2008; 52: 203–30.

# 1.12 NEPHROLOGICAL DISEASE

- chronic renal failure
- nephrotic syndrome
- oculocerebrorenal syndrome

- renal rickets
- renal transplantation

## CHRONIC RENAL FAILURE

Chronic renal failure (chronic kidney disease) can cause xerostomia, halitosis/taste disturbance, leukoplakia, dental hypoplasia in children, renal osteodystrophy and a bleeding tendency (especially if anticoagulated) (Figs 1.12.1–1.12.3). Furred tongue may be seen in patients on haemodialysis and dental and periodontal health is poor and deteriorates on dialysis. Uraemia and uraemic stomatitis, foetor/halitosis and frosting have been described in end-stage renal disease. Xerostomia can be prominent especially in patients on haemodialysis. Peritoneal dialysis appears to predispose to tuberculous cervical lymphadenitis.

## NEPHROTIC SYNDROME

Nephrotic syndrome—a nonspecific renal disorder in which the kidneys are damaged, causing them to leak large amounts of protein—can manifest with dental hypoplasia.

## OCULOCEREBRORENAL SYNDROME

Oculocerebrorenal syndrome (Lowe syndrome)—caused by an inherited mutation in the *OCRL* gene, mapped to chromosome Xq 26.1—manifests with congenital cataracts, neonatal or infantile hypotonia with subsequent mental impairment and renal tubular dysfunction and may present with multiple unerupted teeth and pericoronal radiolucencies, and extensive calculus deposits.

## RENAL RICKETS

Renal rickets (vitamin D resistant rickets), the result of renal disease, can cause delayed tooth eruption, dental hypoplasia and enlarged pulps (Fig. 1.12.4).

## RENAL TRANSPLANTATION

Renal transplantation necessitates that the patient is T-cell immunosuppressed to prevent graft rejection. Oral complications are mainly those related to the immunosuppression used to prevent graft rejection, and may include infections and neoplasms. An increased susceptibility to lip cancer after transplantation is related to exposure to immunosuppressive agents and UV light. Post-transplantation patients are also prone to lymphoproliferative diseases, Kaposi sarcoma and some carcinomas (Chapter 1.6).

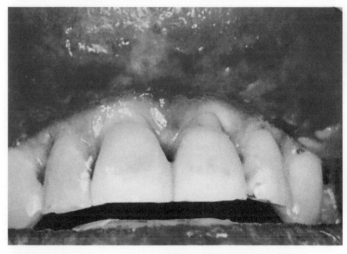

Figure 1.12.2 Chronic kidney disease—ulcers and microbial plaques.

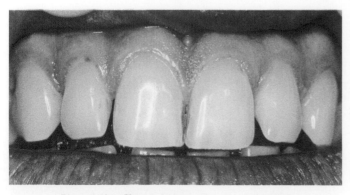

Figure 1.12.1 Chronic kidney disease—oral pallor.

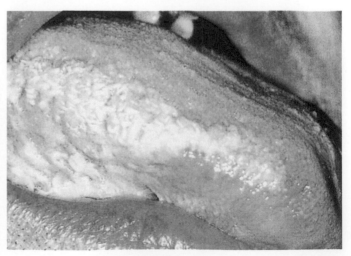

Figure 1.12.3 Chronic kidney disease—uraemic stomatitis.

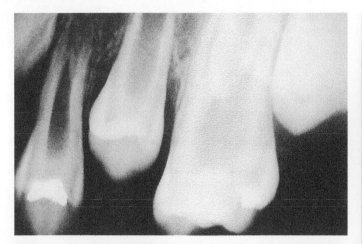

*Figure 1.12.4* Hypophosphataemia showing large pulp chambers and abnormal dentine calcification.

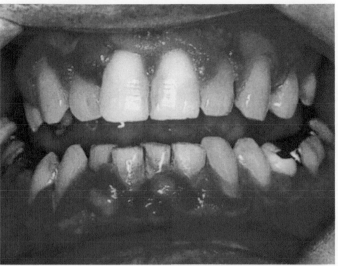

*Figure 1.12.5* Renal transplant showing ciclosporin-induced gingival swelling.

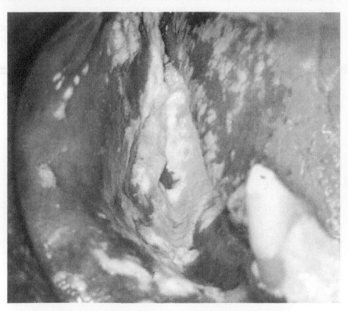

*Figure 1.12.6* Renal transplant showing candidosis.

Drugs used after cardiac transplantation may also produce other maxillofacial adverse side-effects; the most common is gingival swelling caused by ciclosporin or nifedipine (Chapter 1.6) (Figs 1.12.5 and 1.12.6). Sirolimus and tacrolimus may induce mouth ulceration. Chronic periodontitis may be associated with poor prognosis.

## FURTHER READING

Bakathir AA, Margasahayam MV, Al-Ismaily MI. Maxillary hyperplasia and hyperostosis cranialis: a rare manifestation of renal osteodystrophy in a patient with hyperparathyroidism secondary to chronic renal failure. Saudi Med J 2008; 29: 1815–18.

Bayraktar G, Kurtulus I, Kazancioglu R, et al. Oral health and inflammation in patients with end-stage renal failure. Perit Dial Int 2009; 29: 472–9.

Blach A, Franek E, Witula A, et al. The influence of chronic periodontitis on serum TNF-alpha, IL-6 and hs-CRP concentrations, and function of graft and survival of kidney transplant recipients. Clin Transplant 2009; 23: 213–19.

Bots CP, Brand HS, Poorterman JH, et al. Oral and salivary changes in patients with end stage renal disease (ESRD): a two year follow-up study. Br Dent J 2007; 202: E3.

Bots CP, Brand HS, Veerman EC, et al. The management of xerostomia in patients on haemodialysis: comparison of artificial saliva and chewing gum. Palliat Med 2005; 19: 202–7.

Brooks JK, Ahmad R. Oral anomalies associated with the oculocerebrorenal syndrome of Lowe: case report with multiple unerupted teeth and pericoronal radiolucencies. Oral Surg Oral Med Oral Pathol Oral Radiol Endod 2009; 107: e32–5.

Brunello A, Saia G, Bedogni A, Scaglione D, Basso U. Worsening of osteonecrosis of the jaw during treatment with sunitinib in a patient with metastatic renal cell carcinoma. Bone 2009; 44: 173–5.

Cengiz MI, Bagci H, Cengiz S, Yigit S, Cengiz K. Periodontal disease in patients with familial Mediterranean fever: from inflammation to amyloidosis. J Periodontal Res 2009; 44: 354–61.

Cengiz MI, Sümer P, Cengiz S, Yavuz U. The effect of the duration of the dialysis in hemodialysis patients on dental and periodontal findings. Oral Dis 2009; 15: 336–41. [Epub 2009 Mar 23].

Craig RG. Interactions between chronic renal disease and periodontal disease. Oral Dis 2008; 14: 1–7.

Cunha FL, Tagliaferro EP, Pereira AC, Meneghim MC, Hebling E. Oral health of a Brazilian population on renal dialysis. Spec Care Dentist 2007; 27: 227–31.

Davidovich E, Davidovits M, Peretz B, Shapira J, Aframian DJ. The correlation between dental calculus and disturbed mineral metabolism in paediatric patients with chronic kidney disease. Nephrol Dial Transplant 2009; 24: 2439–45.

Dongari-Bagtzoglou A, Dwivedi P, Ioannidou E, et al. Oral Candida infection and colonization in solid organ transplant recipients. Oral Microbiol Immunol 2009; 24: 249–54.

Fisher MA, Taylor GW. A prediction model for chronic kidney disease includes periodontal disease. J Periodontol 2009; 80: 16–23.

Fisher MA, Taylor GW, Papapanou PN, Rahman M, Debanne SM. Clinical and serologic markers of periodontal infection and chronic kidney disease. J Periodontol 2008; 79: 1670–8.

Fitzpatrick JJ, Wilson MH, McArdle NS, Stassen LF. Renal disease and chronic renal failure in dental practice. J Ir Dent Assoc 2008; 54: 215–17.

Fricain JC, Cellerié K, Sibaud V, et al. Oral ulcers in kidney allograft recipients treated with sirolimus. Ann Dermatol Venereol 2008; 135: 737–41.

Garcez J, Limeres Posse J, Carmona IT, Feijoo JF, Diz Dios P. Oral health status of patients with a mild decrease in glomerular filtration rate. Oral Surg Oral Med Oral Pathol Oral Radiol Endod 2009; 107: 224–8.

Gonyea J. Oral health care for patients on dialysis. Nephrol Nurs J 2009; 36: 327–8, 332.

Hajheydari Z, Makhlough A. Cutaneous and mucosal manifestations in patients on maintenance hemodialysis: a study of 101 patients in Sari, Iran. Iran J Kidney Dis 2008; 2: 86–90.

Kshirsagar AV, Craig RG, Moss KL, et al. Periodontal disease adversely affects the survival of patients with end-stage renal disease. Kidney Int 2009; 75: 746–51.

van Leeuwen MT, Grulich AE, McDonald SP, et al. Immunosuppression and other risk factors for lip cancer after kidney transplantation. Cancer Epidemiol Biomarkers Prev 2009; 18: 561–9.

Madore F. Periodontal disease: a modifiable risk factor for cardiovascular disease in ESRD patients? Kidney Int 2009; 75: 672–4.

Masajtis-Zagajewska A, Nowicki M. Influence of dual blockade of the renin-angiotensin system on thirst in hemodialysis patients. Nephron Clin Pract 2009; 112: c242–7. [Epub 2009 Jun 16].

Olczak-Kowalczyk D, Pawłowska J, Cukrowska B, et al. Local presence of cytomegalovirus and Candida species vs oral lesions in liver and kidney transplant recipients. Ann Transplant 2008; 13: 28–33.

Párraga-Linares L, Almendros-Marqués N, Berini-Aytés L, Gay-Escoda C. Effectiveness of substituting cyclosporin A with tacrolimus in reducing gingival overgrowth in renal transplant patients. Med Oral Patol Oral Cir Bucal 2009; 14: e429–33.

Porcu M, Fanton E, Zampieron A. Thirst distress and interdialytic weight gain: a study on a sample of haemodialysis patients. J Ren Care 2007; 33: 179–81.

Proctor R, Kumar N, Stein A, Moles D, Porter S. Oral and dental aspects of chronic renal failure. J Dent Res 2005; 84: 199–208.

Reali L, Zuliani E, Gabutti L, Schönholzer C, Marone C. Poor oral hygiene enhances gingival overgrowth caused by calcineurin inhibitors. J Clin Pharm Ther 2009; 34: 255–60.

Scannapieco FA, Panesar M. Periodontitis and chronic kidney disease. J Periodontol 2008; 79: 1617–19. Erratum in: J Periodontol 2008; 79: 2010.

Shiboski CH, Krishnan S, Besten PD, et al. Gingival enlargement in pediatric organ transplant recipients in relation to tacrolimus-based immunosuppressive regimens. Pediatr Dent 2009; 31: 38–46.

Sung JM, Kuo SC, Guo HR, et al. The role of oral dryness in interdialytic weight gain by diabetic and non-diabetic haemodialysis patients. Nephrol Dial Transplant 2006; 21: 2521–8.

Thorman R, Neovius M, Hylander B. Clinical findings in oral health during progression of chronic kidney disease to end-stage renal disease in a Swedish population. Scand J Urol Nephrol 2009; 43: 154–9.

Ye X, Qian H, Xu P, et al. Nephrotoxicity, neurotoxicity, and mercury exposure among children with and without dental amalgam fillings. Int J Hyg Environ Health 2009; 212: 378–86.

# 1.13 NEUROLOGICAL DISEASE

- abducens (sixth cranial) nerve palsy
- Alzheimer disease
- bulbar palsy
- cerebral palsy (CP)
- cerebrovascular accident
- choreoathetosis
- cranial neuropathies
- Down syndrome
- encephalopathies
- epilepsy
- facial palsy
- Horner syndrome

- hypoglossal nerve palsy
- multiple sclerosis
- neck–tongue syndrome
- neurofibromatosis (NF)
- neurosyphilis
- oculomotor nerve palsy
- Parkinson disease
- Sturge–Weber syndrome
- trigeminal neuralgia
- trigeminal sensory loss
- trochlear nerve palsy
- tuberous sclerosis

## ABDUCENS (SIXTH CRANIAL) NERVE PALSY

Abducens (sixth cranial) nerve palsy is the most common of the isolated ocular motor nerve palsies (Figs 1.13.1 and 1.13.2). A nuclear lesion will cause an ipsilateral gaze palsy and, if the seventh nerve nucleus is also affected, a sixth nerve palsy with ipsilateral facial palsy will result. Raised intracranial pressure can damage the sixth nerve in the subarachnoid space. Petrous or mastoid bone infections, or petrous fractures or nasopharyngeal tumours can result in a sixth nerve palsy with an associated ipsilateral hearing reduction, facial pain and paralysis and photophobia (Gradenigo syndrome). A lesion in the cavernous sinus/superior orbital fissure affecting the sixth nerve may be associated with Horner syndrome or trigeminal involvement.

## ALZHEIMER DISEASE

Alzheimer disease, the most common cause of dementia, is a progressive disease characterized by the development of brain 'plaques' and 'tangles', leading to the death of brain cells. People with Alzheimer disease have no specific maxillofacial manifestations but drooling and, in the absence of good hygiene and diet, caries and inflammatory periodontal disease may manifest.

## BULBAR PALSY

Bulbar palsy is bilateral impairment of the lower cranial nerves—ninth, tenth, eleventh and twelfth, due to a lower motor neurone lesion either at nuclear or fascicular level in the medulla or from bilateral lesions of the lower cranial nerves outside the brainstem. Bulbar palsy may present with palatal palsy and wasting and fasciculation of the tongue, drooling, weakness of the soft palate, absent gag reflex, normal or absent jaw jerk, dysphagia, difficulty in chewing, nasal regurgitation, slurring of speech, choking on liquids and nasal speech.

Pseudobulbar palsy is a clinical syndrome similar to bulbar palsy but the damage affects upper motor neurones.

## CEREBRAL PALSY (CP)

CP is a group of permanent disorders of the development of movement and posture, due to non-progressive disturbances in the developing foetal or infant brain. Characterized by motor disorders, it is often accompanied by disturbances of sensation, perception, communication, cognition and behaviour, by epilepsy and by secondary musculoskeletal problems. Spastic, ataxic and athetoid types of CP are recognized. CP may cause a spastic tongue with dysarthria, drooling, bruxism and attrition, and, if oral hygiene is not maintained, with periodontal disease.

## CEREBROVASCULAR ACCIDENT

Cerebrovascular accident (stroke)—where there is damage in the cerebral cortex or internal capsule to upper motor neurones—may give rise to unilateral facial weakness due to palsy affecting the facial nerve (Fig. 1.13.3) typically with ipsilateral hemiplegia. Strokes may be preceded by lesser forms of damage—transient ischaemic attacks (TIAs) or reversible ischaemic neurological deficits (RINDs). TIAs are typically embolic, and may cause focal cerebral deficits usually lasting less than 60 minutes and recovering fully within 24 hours. RIND is similar but persists for >24 hours.

Medial cerebral artery (MCA) motor stroke is the most common and gives rise to unilateral facial weakness typically with ipsilateral hemiplegia. The upper extremities and face (central facial paresis) are more affected than are the lower extremities. The classic picture is hemiplegia, hemianaesthesia/hyperaesthesia and homonymous hemianopia, with deviation of the head and eyes toward the side of the cerebral lesion. In addition, dominant-hemisphere strokes (usually left) can cause receptive aphasia (inferior division of the MCA supplies Wernicke area) and/or expressive aphasia (superior division of the MCA supplies Broca area). Non-dominant hemisphere strokes can cause defective perception of sensation from one side of the body (amorphosynthesis), hemineglect and visiospatial deficits. Insight and judgment are also affected. There may be a sensory deficit including impaired position sense, tactile localization and two-point discrimination with variable changes in touch, pain and temperature sense.

Anterior cerebral artery (ACA) infarcts if total result in contralateral hemiplegia with severe paralysis of the face, tongue and arm, and marked spastic weakness of the distal lower extremity. ACA strokes are otherwise often well tolerated unless there is infarction of both medial cerebral hemispheres which results in paraplegia, incontinence, abulia (lack of will or initiative) and aphasic symptoms, with frontal lobe personality changes. Complete infarction arising from one ACA distal to the anterior communicating artery results in sensorimotor deficit of the opposite foot and leg, and possibly also the arm, though the face and tongue are spared. Apraxia (loss of the ability to execute or carry out learned purposeful movements), mental and personality changes, primitive

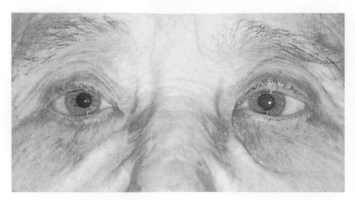

*Figure 1.13.1* Abducens nerve palsy—patient looking ahead.

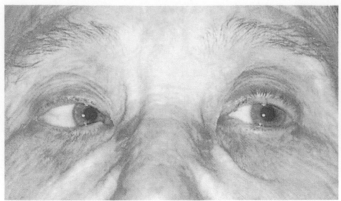

*Figure 1.13.2* Abducens nerve palsy—patient looking to the left, shows that the left nerve is non-functional.

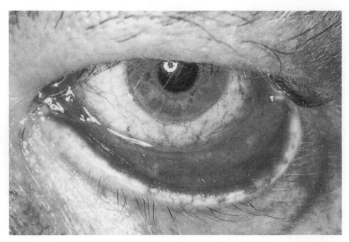

*Figure 1.13.3* Cerebrovascular accident, or stroke showing eyelid palsy.

reflexes, conjugate eye deviation towards the side of the lesion, abulia, and bowel and bladder incontinence are often features.

Posterior cerebral artery (PCA) stroke is often preceded by TIAs causing symptoms mimicking classic migraine attacks. Paraesthesias are common, usually of the face and hands, as are transient spells of hypo- or an-aesthesia. PCA infarction causes contralateral visual field defects of hemianopsia, but often with macular sparing.

Dominant hemisphere PCA lesions usually involve language or memory, dyslexia, colour anomia and alexia (patients who have alexia without agraphia are able to write, speak and spell normally, but cannot read words and sentences or name colours). Non-dominant PCA lesions can cause prosopagnosia (inability to recognise familiar faces).

Although most strokes damage the cerebral cortex, or sometimes the lobes or hemispheres of the brain, some (called *lacunar strokes*) injure deeper structures involved in communication relays between the cortex and brain stem, or relays that help coordinate complex movements. In a lacunar stroke, only very small areas of brain are damaged but their location means they cause significant disability such as from effects on sensation, movement, sight, speech, balance and coordination.

*Sensory strokes* are discussed in Chapter 2.11.

*Ataxic hemiparesis* is most often caused by lesions affecting the internal capsule, corona radiata or pons and causes ataxia and weakness in the arm or leg on one side of the body. The face is rarely affected.

*Dysarthria clumsy-hand syndrome* is caused by a lacunar stroke in the anterior internal capsule and affects the larynx, tongue and other mouth muscles, causing dysarthria and clumsiness of hand movements on one side of the body with difficulty in fine movements (e.g. writing, tying laces or playing musical instruments).

**Clinical features**

Stroke is one of the main causes of facial palsy, when there is often also ipsilateral hemiplegia. There is paralysis mainly of the lower face on the contralateral side to the brain damage, but involuntary movement is preserved; for instance, laughing can still produce facial movement. Stroke-related symptoms depend on the area of brain affected, the extent of damage and the cause, but may include the following:

- Consciousness deficits include sleepiness, stupor, somnolence, lethargy, coma or unconsciousness.
- Hemiplegia (loss of voluntary movement) with paralysis or weakness, or loss of coordination.
- Numbness, paraesthesia or other sensation changes, or in recognising or identifying sensory stimuli (agnosia) resulting in 'neglect' of one side of the body.
- Impaired vision, especially in one eye.
- Language difficulties (aphasia)—slurred, thick, difficult speech or inability to speak—usually the result of a lesion in the left brain, so that most patients are also deprived of the ability to write.
- Difficulty in understanding speech, and with reading or writing.
- Vertigo.
- Swallowing difficulties.
- Personality or emotional changes including depression or apathy.
- Loss of bladder or bowel control.
- Cognitive decline, dementia, easily distracted, impaired judgment, limited attention.

Clinical features of a lacunar stroke can include:

- Weakness or paralysis of face, arm, leg, foot or toes
- Clumsiness of a hand or arm
- Weakness or paralysis of eye muscles
- Sudden numbness
- Difficulty in walking
- Difficulty in speaking.

As a consequence of stroke there may be drooling and plaque retention on the affected side of the mouth, with later gingivitis and halitosis.

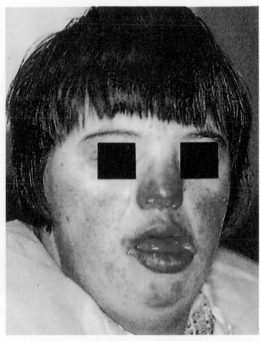

*Figure 1.13.4* Down syndrome facies, showing also cyanosis and tongue posture.

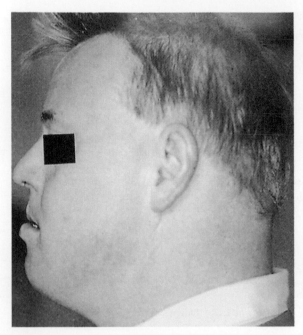

*Figure 1.13.5* Down syndrome showing brachycephaly and maxillary hypoplasia.

Rare consequences of stroke include pseudobulbar or bulbar palsy and impaired vagus nerve function giving rise to impaired unilateral soft palate function. Orolingual angioedema may be a complication of thrombolysis in stroke victims.

### Diagnosis

Diagnosis of stroke is clinical and based on specific neurological, motor and sensory deficits. Tests that may be needed to determine the location and cause of the stroke include:

- CT or MRI of head
- carotid duplex (ultrasound)
- cerebral arteriography
- brainstem evoked response audiometry
- electrocardiogram
- echocardiogram
- clotting and thrombophilia screens.

### Management

All acute stroke patients should be admitted for hospital assessment and care. The airway must be protected and oxygen given. Medical treatment may include:

- anticoagulation
- anti-hypertensive medication
- control of atrial fibrillation
- analgesics.

## CHOREOATHETOSIS

Choreoathetosis—abnormal movements that have a combined choreic and athetoid pattern—can be due to a variety of prenatal and perinatal insults including kernicterus (bilirubin damage to the basal ganglia). It may present with dyskinesia, abnormal jaw and tongue movements with dysarthria, sialorrhoea, possible self-mutilation and green staining of teeth in kernicterus, or hypoplasia of the deciduous dentition in congenital rubella.

## CRANIAL NEUROPATHIES

Cranial neuropathies may be caused by ischaemia in brainstem vascular syndromes or extramedullary vascular disease such as vertebrobasilar dolichoectasia, basilar artery ectasia or aneurysms which may compress multiple cranial nerves—especially third, sixth and fifth. Other causes include internal carotid artery dissection, diabetes, sickle cell disease, Behçet syndrome, multiple sclerosis (MS), connective tissue diseases, granulomatous disorders (e.g. sarcoidosis, Melkersson–Rosenthal syndrome/orofacial granulomatosis/Crohn disease or Wegener granulomatosis) or infections. The latter may be caused by middle ear infections, or by herpesviruses, retroviruses, enteroviruses, *Borrelia burgdorferi* infection (Lyme disease) or leprosy.

Isolated cranial neuropathies can be caused by any of the above, but especially by infections, diabetes or sickle cell disease.

## DOWN SYNDROME

Down syndrome—the most common chromosome anomaly—typically results in a lower than average cognitive ability, and a range of physical anomalies. It can be associated with a range of maxillofacial anomalies including delayed tooth eruption, macroglossia, fissured tongue, cheilitis, maxillary hypoplasia, anterior open bite, hypodontia and periodontal disease (Figs 1.13.4–1.13.15). Early tooth loss is common, not only because some patients have difficulty maintaining oral hygiene, but also because the teeth have short roots and there may be aggressive periodontal destruction.

## ENCEPHALOPATHIES

Encephalopathies may present with tongue dystonia.

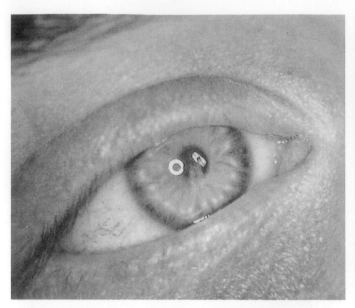

Figure 1.13.6 Down syndrome—Brushfield spots.

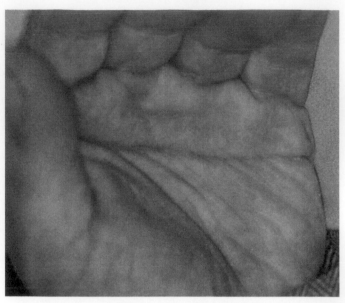

Figure 1.13.7 Down syndrome—palmar (simian) crease.

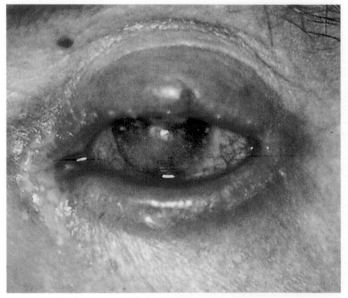

Figure 1.13.8 Down syndrome—blepharitis and visual impairment.

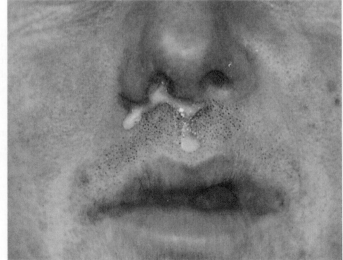

Figure 1.13.9 Down syndrome—nasal discharge from chronic respiratory infection.

## EPILEPSY

Epilepsy—a common chronic neurological disorder characterized by recurrent unprovoked seizures—can result in traumatic injuries to teeth, soft tissues and facial skeleton. Patients may also have the maxillofacial features of any associated disease (e.g. Down syndrome and tuberous sclerosis). Anticonvulsants may precipitate erythema multiforme (Figs 1.13.16–1.13.18). Long-term phenytoin may predispose to gingival swelling and oral ulceration, carbamazepine may lead to dyskinesia of the tongue and clonazepam to xerostomia. Caries appears to be increased.

Birth defects may be found in neonates of women taking anticonvulsants (mainly phenytoin and valproic acid) including deformities of the face and palate, and dental root anomalies (foetal anticonvulsant syndrome). A distinctive facial appearance (broad flat nasal bridge, epicanthic folds and narrow forehead) may be associated with a cluster of major and minor anomalies (spina bifida, cleft lip and/or palate, upper limb abnormalities, lower limb abnormalities, congenital heart disease and kidney defects and central nervous system (CNS) dysfunction). Gingival swelling has been described in some neonates with foetal anticonvulsant syndrome.

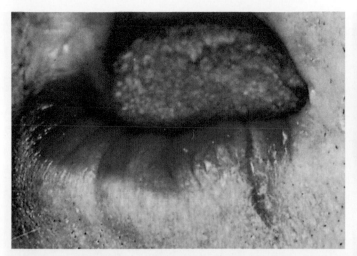

*Figure 1.13.10* Down syndrome—fissured lip.

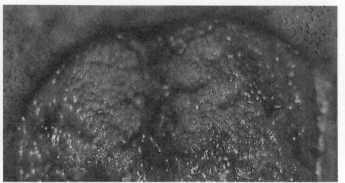

*Figure 1.13.11* Down syndrome—fissured and large tongue.

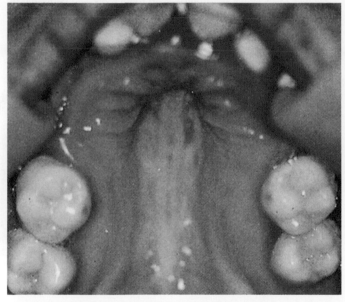

*Figure 1.13.12* Down syndrome—omega palate and hypodontia.

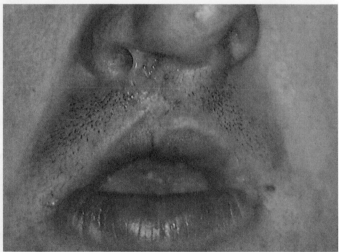

*Figure 1.13.13* Down syndrome; cleft lip (repaired).

## FACIAL PALSY

Facial palsy from any cause may lead to drooling and poor natural cleansing of mouth on same side (Chapter 2.11).

## HORNER SYNDROME

Horner syndrome (Chapter 2.11).

## HYPOGLOSSAL NERVE PALSY

Hypoglossal nerve palsy (Chapter 2.11).

## MULTIPLE SCLEROSIS

MS is the most common disabling neurological condition affecting young adults. Features may include problems with sensation, movement, vision, balance, tremor and mood. Caused by damage to nerve myelin, MS can cause a wide variety of symptoms and may underlie maxillofacial pain, paraesthesia or sensory loss, facial palsy or problems with speech or swallowing. Isolated cranial nerve lesions are rare findings in MS but may affect third, fourth, fifth, sixth, seventh, eighth and twelfth cranial nerves. Hemiaguesia, caused by an ipsilateral MS plaque in the pons, has been reported.

Devic disease, often considered a MS variant, may manifest minor salivary gland inflammation.

## NECK–TONGUE SYNDROME

Neck–tongue syndrome—an unusual disorder of paroxysmal neck pain and tongue paraesthesia, resulting from compression of cervical nerve roots, attributed to damage to lingual afferent fibres travelling in the hypoglossal nerve to the C2 spinal roots. Conservative management is effective in most cases.

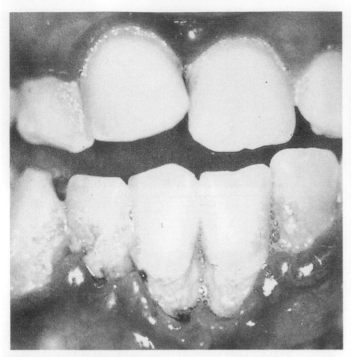

*Figure 1.13.14* Down syndrome—periodontitis.

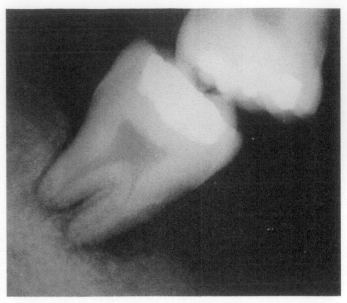

*Figure 1.13.15* Down syndrome—short tooth roots, and periodontitis.

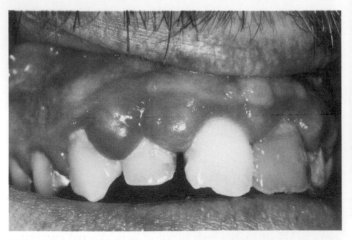

*Figure 1.13.16* Epilepsy—traumatized left maxillary central incisor and gingival swelling.

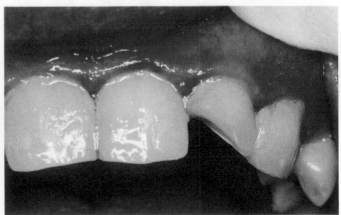

*Figure 1.13.17* Epilepsy—traumatized anterior tooth.

## NEUROFIBROMATOSIS (NF)

NF—a genetic disorder characterized by multiple neuromas. Distinct variants differ from each other genetically, microscopically and clinically. NF-I (related to chromosome 17)—is autosomal dominant and often referred to as von Recklinghausen disease of skin. NF-II (related to chromosome 22) is much less common and largely afflicts the CNS, the hallmark being bilateral acoustic neuromas (vestibular Schwannomas). Neurofibromas and neurilemmomas are the other predominant features of both types. Cutaneous and subcutaneous neurofibromas (Figs 1.13.19 and 1.13.20) may affect any part of the body, including the oral cavity, typically the tongue or palate. Cafe-au-lait hyperpigmented skin patches are seen, especially in the axillary region. Dystrophic kyphoscoliosis is common and there may sometimes be learning impairment and epilepsy, or rarely renal artery stenosis or phaeochromocytoma. One of the most feared complications is development of cancer, mainly neurofibrosarcoma.

Optic nerve or optic chiasmal gliomas may be present. Most patients also have small dome-shaped brown hamartomas (Lisch nodules) on the front of the iris, on slit-lamp examination.

Plexiform neurofibroma may affect the face and erode or invade the adjacent facial skeleton.

## NEUROSYPHILIS

Neurosyphilis—a very rare cause of pain, dysarthria or tongue tremor (Chapter 2.11).

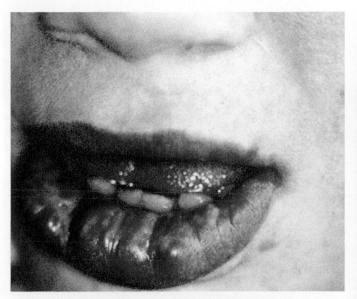

*Figure 1.13.18* Epilepsy showing scarred lip from chronic trauma.

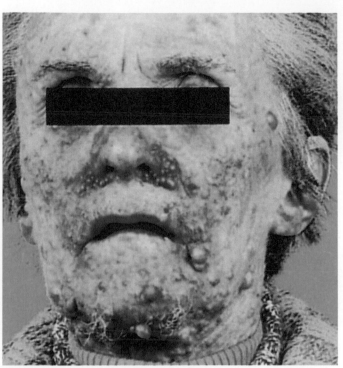

*Figure 1.13.19* Neurofibromatosis.

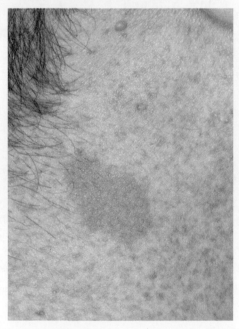

*Figure 1.13.20* Neurofibromatosis—cafe au lait skin plaque.

## OCULOMOTOR NERVE PALSY

Oculomotor nerve palsy may be congenital but is usually a consequence of diabetes, arteriosclerosis, aneurysm of the posterior communicating artery, a space occupying lesion, infection, trauma, MS, HIV/AIDS or cavernous sinus thrombosis. It can result in diplopia, and the affected individual is unable to move the eye normally and, since the nerve also supplies the upper eyelid muscle (levator palpebrae superioris) and the muscles responsible for pupil constriction (termed miosis) and dilation (termed mydriasis), it results in ptosis and miosis.

## PARKINSON DISEASE

Parkinson disease and Parkinsonism, manifest with a resting tremor, stiff muscles, slow movements and difficulty maintaining balance and walking. The face is often expressionless and there is a loss of the blink reflex as a response to gentle tapping of the bridge of the nose. Oculogyric crises may be seen in drug-induced or post-encephalitic disease. There can be hypersalivation from autonomic dysfunction or facial dyskinesias arising from drug therapy (see section 3.5). If severe, these conditions may cause drooling, and tremor of the tongue (serpentine tongue). Taste appreciation may be changed.

## STURGE–WEBER SYNDROME

Sturge–Weber syndrome (Chapter 1.13).

## TRIGEMINAL NEURALGIA

Trigeminal neuralgia often causes severe maxillofacial pain (Chapter 2.11) and may sometimes signify MS, or other serious disease.

## TRIGEMINAL SENSORY LOSS

Trigeminal sensory loss which may be a feature of trauma to the trigeminal nerve or branches, or of malignant or CNS disorders, often presents as 'numb chin syndrome', and may manifest with accidental self-damage (Figs 1.13.21 and 1.13.22) (Chapter 2.11).

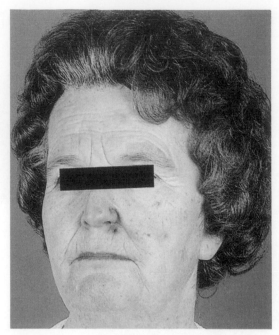

*Figure 1.13.21* Trigeminal sensory loss—nasal trauma.

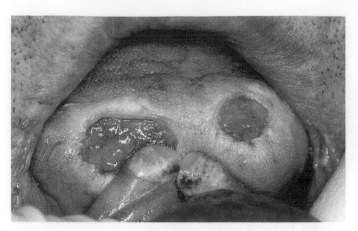

*Figure 1.13.22* Trigeminal sensory loss—trauma in Riley–Day syndrome.

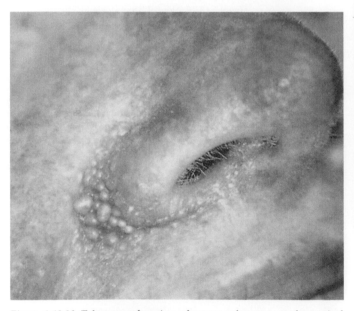

*Figure 1.13.23* Tuberous sclerosis—adenoma sebaceum at the typical location.

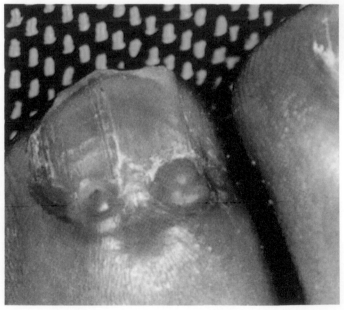

*Figure 1.13.24* Tuberous sclerosis—subungual fibromas.

## TROCHLEAR NERVE PALSY

Trochlear nerve palsy is most commonly caused by head trauma. The trochlear nucleus is unique in that its axons cross the midline before emerging from the brainstem and thus a lesion of the nucleus affects the *contralateral* eye (lesions of all other cranial nuclei affect the *ipsilateral* side). Diabetes, arteriosclerosis, raised intracranial pressure, a space occupying lesion, infection, trauma, MS, HIV/AIDS or cavernous sinus thrombosis may damage the trochlear nerve.

Injury to the nerve causes vertical and torsional diplopia and thus the patient often adopts a posture with the head tilted to one side, chin tucked in.

## TUBEROUS SCLEROSIS

Tuberous sclerosis (epiloia)—a rare genetic condition due to defects in tumour suppressor genes hamartin and tuberin—causes benign tumours in the brain, eyes, heart, kidneys, lungs and skin, and often learning impairment. It may present with adenoma sebaceum, subungual fibromas, 'ash leaf' hypopigmented spots and enamel hypoplasia (Figs 1.13.23–1.13.26), or features of epilepsy.

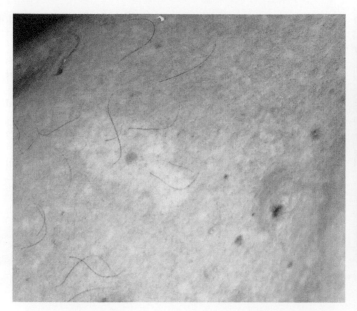

Figure 1.13.25 Tuberous sclerosis—depigmented (ash-leaf) macule.

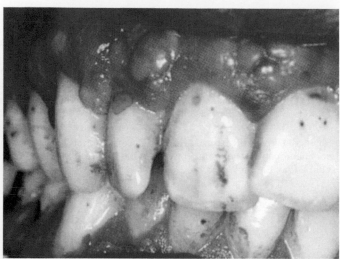

Figure 1.13.26 Tuberous sclerosis—pitting dental hypoplasia and gingival swellings from phenytoin use.

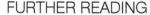

## FURTHER READING

Anjomshoaa I, Cooper ME, Vieira AR. Caries is associated with asthma and epilepsy. Eur J Dent 2009; 3: 297–303.

Arboix A, García-Plata C, García-Eroles L, et al. Clinical study of 99 patients with pure sensory stroke. J Neurol 2005; 252: 156–62.

Arnett PA, Smith MM, Barwick FH, Benedict RH, Ahlstrom BP. Oralmotor slowing in multiple sclerosis: relationship to neuropsychological tasks requiring an oral response. J Int Neuropsychol Soc 2008; 14: 454–62.

Cerero Lapiedra R, Moreno López LA, Esparza Gómez GC. Progressive bulbar palsy: a case report diagnosed by lingual symptoms. J Oral Pathol Med 2002; 31: 277–9.

Chedrawi AK, Fishman MA, Miller G. Neck-tongue syndrome. Pediatr Neurol 2000; 22: 397–9.

Chen WH, Lan MY, Chang YY, et al. Cortical cheiro-oral syndrome: a revisit of clinical significance and pathogenesis. Clin Neurol Neurosurg 2006; 108: 446–50.

Chou KL, Evatt M, Hinson V, Kompoliti K. Sialorrhea in Parkinson's disease: a review. Mov Disord 2007; 22: 2306–13.

Colella G, Giudice A, Siniscalchi G, Falcone U, Guastafierro S. Chin numbness: a symptom that should not be underestimated: a review of 12 cases. Am J Med Sci 2009; 337: 407–10.

Dougherty NJ. A review of cerebral palsy for the oral health professional. Dent Clin North Am 2009; 53: 329–38.

Fatahzadeh M, Glick M. Stroke: epidemiology, classification, risk factors, complications, diagnosis, prevention, and medical and dental management. Oral Surg Oral Med Oral Pathol Oral Radiol Endod 2006; 102: 180–91.

Gallud L, Bagan JV, Cervelló A, et al. Multiple sclerosis as first manifestation in oral and facial area: presentation of four cases. Med Oral Patol Oral Cir Bucal 2006; 11: E141–5.

Igarashi O, Iguchi H, Ogura N, et al. Cheiro-oral-pedal syndrome due to brainstem hemorrhage. Clin Neurol Neurosurg 2006; 108: 507–10. [Epub 2005 Apr 22].

Jamal BT, Herb K. Perioperative management of patients with myasthenia gravis: prevention, recognition, and treatment. Oral Surg Oral Med Oral Pathol Oral Radiol Endod 2009; 107: 612–15.

Javed A, Balabanov R, Arnason BG, et al. Minor salivary gland inflammation in Devic's disease and longitudinally extensive myelitis. Mult Scler 2008; 14: 809–14.

Jeannet PY, Marcoz JP, Kuntzer T, Roulet-Perez E. Isolated facial and bulbar paresis: a persistent manifestation of neonatal myasthenia gravis. Neurology 2008; 70: 237–8.

Kikutani T, Tamura F, Nishiwaki K. Case presentation: dental treatment with PAP for ALS patient. Int J Orofac Myol 2006; 32: 32–5.

Kim DG, Oh SH, Kim HS, et al. Episodic dystonic spasm of the bilateral edge of the tongue during a coma following anoxic encephalopathy. J Clin Neurosci 2009; 16: 1252–3.

Kocer B, Ergan S, Nazliel B. Isolated abducens nerve palsy following mandibular block articaine anesthesia, a first manifestation of multiple sclerosis: a case report. Quintessence Int 2009; 40: 251–6.

McGrath C, McMillan AS, Zhu HW, Li LS. Agreement between patient and proxy assessments of oral health-related quality of life after stroke: an observational longitudinal study. J Oral Rehabil 2009; 36: 264–70. [Epub 2009 Feb 9].

Neves BG, Roza RT, Castro GF. Traumatic lesions from congenital insensitivity to pain with anhidrosis in a pediatric patient: dental management. Dent Traumatol 2009; 25: 545–9.

Oestmann A, Achtnichts L, Kappos L, Gass A, Naegelin Y. "Numb chin syndrome": first presenting syndrome of multiple sclerosis? Dtsch Med Wochenschr 2008; 133: 76–8.

Rodrigues dos Santos MT, Bianccardi M, Celiberti P, de Oliveira Guaré R. Dental caries in cerebral palsied individuals and their caregivers' quality of life. Child Care Health Dev 2009; 35: 475–81.

Rodríguez-Vázquez M, Carrascosa-Romero MC, Pardal-Fernández JM, Iniesta I. Congenital gingival hyperplasia in a neonate with foetal valproate syndrome. Neuropediatrics 2007; 38: 251–2.

Sapir S, Ramig L, Fox C. Speech and swallowing disorders in Parkinson disease. Curr Opin Otolaryngol Head Neck Surg 2008; 16: 205–10.

Scully C, Shotts R. The mouth in neurological disorders. Practitioner 2001; 245: 539–49.

Scully C, Van Bruggen W, Dios PD, Porter SR, Davison M. Down syndrome; lip lesions and *Candida albicans*. Br J Dermatol 2002; 147: 37–40.

Shah M, Deeb J, Fernando M, et al. Abnormality of taste and smell in Parkinson's disease. Parkinsonism Relat Disord 2009; 15: 232–7. [Epub 2008 Jul 7].

Shotts RH, Porter SR, Kumar N, Scully C. Longstanding trigeminal sensory neuropathy of nontraumatic cause. Oral Surg Oral Med Oral Pathol Oral Radiol Endod 1999; 87: 572–6.

Weijnen FG, van der Bilt A, Wokke JH, Wassenberg MW, Oudenaarde I. Oral functions of patients with myasthenia gravis. Ann N Y Acad Sci 1998; 841: 773–6.

Yoshioka I, Shiiba S, Tanaka T, et al. The importance of clinical features and computed tomographic findings in numb chin syndrome: a report of two cases. J Am Dent Assoc 2009; 140: 550–4.

Zakrzewska JM. Classification issues related to neuropathic trigeminal pain. J Orofac Pain 2004; 18: 325–31.

Zakrzewska JM. Facial pain: an update. Curr Opin Support Palliat Care 2009; 3: 125–30.

Zakrzewska JM, Linskey ME. Trigeminal neuralgia. Clin Evid (Online) 2009; pii: 1207.

# 1.14 RESPIRATORY DISEASE

- antral carcinoma
- asthma
- cystic fibrosis (CF)
- lung cancer
- sarcoidosis

- sinusitis
- tonsillitis
- transplantation
- tuberculosis
- Wegener granulomatosis

## ANTRAL CARCINOMA

Antral carcinoma is usually squamous cell carcinoma, seen in older people. The tumour can remain undetected until late. Infiltration of branches of the trigeminal nerve may eventually cause maxillary sensory loss or pain. As the tumour expands the effects of expansion and infiltration of adjacent tissues become apparent as intra-oral alveolar swelling, ulceration of the palate or buccal sulcus; swelling of the cheek; unilateral nasal obstruction often associated with a blood-stained discharge; obstruction of the nasolacrimal duct with epiphora; hypo- or an-aesthesia of the cheek; proptosis and ophthalmoplegia consequent on invasion of the orbit and trismus from infiltration of the muscles of mastication (Figs 1.14.1–1.14.3).

## ASTHMA

Asthma—a predisposition to chronic lung inflammation in which the bronchi are reversibly narrowed—has no specific maxillofacial manifestations but caries, candidosis and angina bullosa haemorrhagica can arise from corticosteroid inhaler use. Caries has arisen as a consequence of sucrose in some medications and, in the past, tetracyclines were often used and caused tooth staining.

## CYSTIC FIBROSIS (CF)

CF or mucoviscidosis—a genetic disease of the exocrine glands secreting mucus, sweat and saliva—can result in sinusitis and antral polyps, bronchiectasis, gastrointestinal, liver and pancreatic disease (and diabetes). It can manifest with salivary gland swelling (especially of the submandibular glands) and dry mouth and sometimes tooth staining from tetracycline use (Figs 1.14.4 and 1.14.5).

## LUNG CANCER

Lung cancer is usually small cell carcinoma, or non-small cell carcinoma, which includes 'squamous' and 'adeno' carcinomas. Lung cancer rarely manifests with oral or cervical, metastases, superior vena cava syndrome, Horner syndrome or palatal pigmentation.

Patients with lung cancer are also more likely to present with second primary tumours in the upper aerodigestive tract—including the mouth.

## SARCOIDOSIS

Sarcoidosis—an uncommon multisystem chronic granulomatous reaction, of unknown aetiology, characterized by non-caseating granulomas—affects especially the lymph nodes and lungs.

### Clinical features

Prevalent particularly in black females, sarcoidosis may present with orofacial lesions that may occasionally precede systemic involvement. Cervical lymphadenopathy may be present. Mucosal nodules, gingival hyperplasia, or labial or salivary gland swellings/masses, or xerostomia are the main features. Heerfordt syndrome (salivary and lacrimal swelling, facial palsy and uveitis) is rare (Figs 1.14.6–1.14.11).

Sarcoidosis has an occasional association with Sjögren syndrome.

### Diagnosis

Diagnosis is by lesional biopsy, chest imaging, gallium scan, raised serum angiotensin converting enzyme and adenosine deaminase, to differentiate from Crohn disease, orofacial granulomatosis, tuberculosis and other conditions such as foreign body reactions or deposits such as amyloid or lymphoma.

Biopsy of minor salivary glands may also reveal granulomas in up to 20% of patients with sarcoidosis, particularly in those with hilar lymphadenopathy.

### Management

Intralesional corticosteroids, systemic steroids and corticosteroid-sparing immunosuppressives are indicated if the lung or eye is involved.

## SINUSITIS

Sinusitis usually follows an upper respiratory tract viral infection. Less commonly it arises after perennial rhinitis, or from odontogenic causes (around 10%)—commonly from dental abscesses, an oroantral fistula, displacement of a tooth or root or foreign body (e.g. endodontic materials, implants, instruments) into the sinus, or sinus perforations during tooth extraction or implant placement. Sinusitis arising from odontogenic infections is typically a mixed aerobic–anaerobic infection, with anaerobes predominant. The most common organisms are anaerobic streptococci, bacteroides, proteus and coliform bacilli. Rare cases of aspergillosis have arisen from endodontic materials entering the sinus.

Sinusitis is also rarely a complication of CF, Kartagener syndrome (immobile cilia and dextrocardia), HIV disease, diabetes and various other immunodeficiencies—when the flora is usually more complex and may contain fungi.

### Clinical features

In bacterial sinusitis, pain is felt over the sinus, especially on moving the head and bending forwards, the cheek may be tender to palpate and the

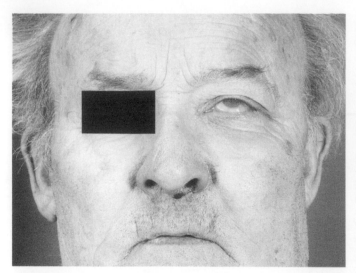

*Figure 1.14.1* Carcinoma of maxillary antrum showing swelling of left cheek and nasal discharge.

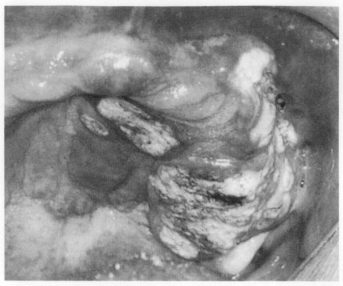

*Figure 1.14.2* Carcinoma of maxillary antrum showing swelling and ulceration of left alveolus and palate.

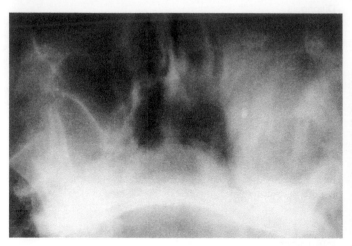

*Figure 1.14.3* Carcinoma of antrum.

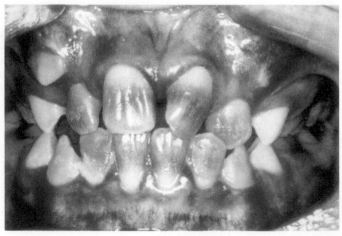

*Figure 1.14.4* Cystic fibrosis—tetracycline stained teeth.

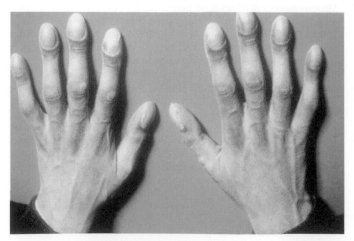

*Figure 1.14.5* Cystic fibrosis—the resulting bronchiectasis is one cause of finger clubbing.

ipsilateral premolars and molars may be tender to percussion. There may be nasal discharge and halitosis.

Ophthalmic symptoms and signs (external ophthalmoplegia, proptosis, visual loss, chemosis and eye lid gangrene), however, are highly suggestive of a mycosis such as zygomycosis, when there may also be nasal discharge/ulceration, infranuclear VI nerve palsy, palatal necrosis, cerebral lobe involvement and hemiparesis. Cavernous sinus thrombosis may follow.

### Diagnosis

A clinical diagnosis can be supported by imaging or endoscopy. Transillumination or occipitomental radiography shows opacities in the affected sinuses (Figs 1.14.12 and 1.14.13). Tilting the head shows if the sinus opacities are fluid.

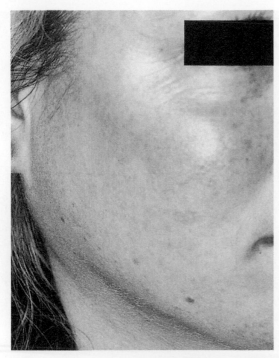

*Figure 1.14.6* Sarcoid causing parotid salivary gland swelling and hypofunction.

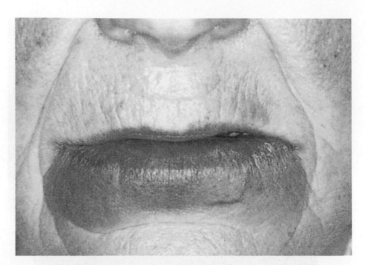

*Figure 1.14.7* Sarcoidosis manifesting as lower lip swelling.

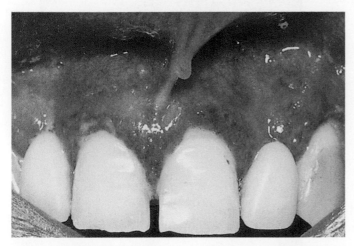

*Figure 1.14.8* Sarcoidosis causing gingival swellings.

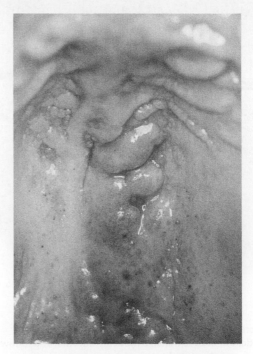

*Figure 1.14.9* Sarcoidosis—palatal lesions.

## Management

Antimicrobials and management of any underlying long-term cause (if possible) are indicated. Any episode of sinusitis not responding to short-term antibacterial therapy, particularly in immunocompromised and diabetic patients, should evoke the diagnosis of zygomycosis.

## TONSILLITIS

Tonsillitis is usually caused by *Streptococcus pyogenes* (Lancefield group A beta haemolytic streptococcus).

### Clinical features

Usually children are affected. An incubation period of 2–4 days is followed by sore throat, dysphagia and fever. The uvula, tonsils and pharynx are diffusely red, with punctate white or yellow tonsillar exudates (Fig. 1.14.14).

Complications, which are rare, can include otitis media, quinsy, sinusitis, rheumatic fever or glomerulonephritis.

### Diagnosis

Clinical plus bacteriological culture and swab.

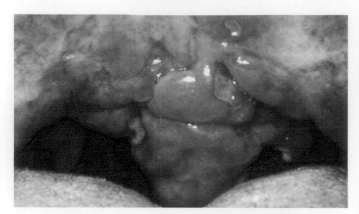

*Figure 1.14.10* Sarcoidosis—oropharyngeal lesions.

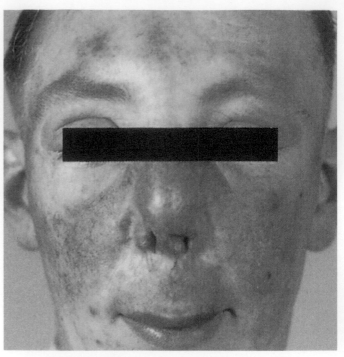

*Figure 1.14.11* Sarcoidosis—lupus pernio.

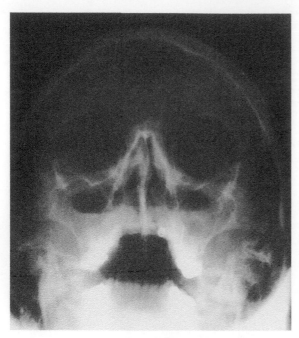

*Figure 1.14.12* Maxillary sinusitis.

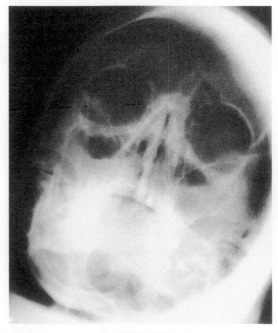

*Figure 1.14.13* Maxillary sinusitis [tilting the head demonstrates that the maxillary radiopacities are liquid (pus)].

## Management

Antibiotics are used to manage the acute infection and follow-up tonsillectomy is sometimes indicated.

## TRANSPLANTATION

Transplantation necessitates that the patient is T-cell immunosuppressed to prevent graft rejection. Oral complications are mainly those related to the immunosuppression used to prevent graft rejection, and may include infections such as candidosis, herpes simplex virus-related ulceration and hairy leukoplakia. An increased susceptibility to lip cancer after transplantation is related to exposure to immunosuppressive agents and UV light. Post-transplantation patients are also prone to lymphoproliferative diseases, Kaposi sarcoma and some carcinomas (Chapter 1.6). Drugs used after lung transplantation may also produce other maxillofacial adverse side-effects; the most common is gingival swelling caused by ciclosporin or nifedipine (Chapter 1.6).

## TUBERCULOSIS

Tuberculosis (Chapter 1.8).

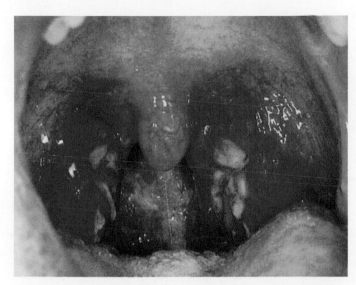

*Figure 1.14.14* Tonsillitis—showing erythematous swollen tonsils and exudates in tonsillar crypts.

## WEGENER GRANULOMATOSIS
Wegener granulomatosis (Chapter 1.1).

## FURTHER READING

Alawi F. Granulomatous diseases of the oral tissues: differential diagnosis and update. Dent Clin North Am 2005; 49: 203–21.

Anjomshoaa I, Cooper ME, Vieira AR. Caries is associated with asthma and epilepsy. Eur J Dent 2009; 3: 297–303.

Anton E. Sarcoidosis presenting as a solitary parotid mass: an uncommon but real diagnostic challenge. Ear Nose Throat J 2007; 86: 188.

Antunes KB, Miranda AM, Carvalho SR, et al. Sarcoidosis presenting as gingival erosion in a patient under long-term clinical control. J Periodontol 2008; 79: 556–61.

Arias-Irimia O, Barona Dorado C, Santos Marino JA, Martínez-Rodriguez N, Martínez-González JM. Meta-analysis of the etiology of odontogenic maxillary sinusitis. Med Oral Patol Oral Cir Bucal 2009; 15: 70–3.

Batal H, Chou LL, Cottrell DA. Sarcoidosis: medical and dental implications. Oral Surg Oral Med Oral Pathol Oral Radiol Endod 1999; 88: 386–90.

Chiapasco M, Felisati G, Maccari A, et al. The management of complications following displacement of oral implants in the paranasal sinuses: a multicenter clinical report and proposed treatment protocols. Int J Oral Maxillofac Surg 2009. [Epub ahead of print].

Hale RG, Tucker DI. Head and neck manifestations of tuberculosis. Oral Maxillofac Surg Clin North Am 2008; 20: 635–42.

Hansen JG, Højbjerg T, Rosborg J. Symptoms and signs in culture-proven acute maxillary sinusitis in a general practice population. APMIS 2009; 117: 724–9.

Hansen SR, Hetta AK, Omdal R. Primary Sjögren's syndrome and sarcoidosis: coexistence more than by chance? Scand J Rheumatol 2008; 37: 485–6.

Kasamatsu A, Kanazawa H, Watanabe T, Matsuzaki O. Oral sarcoidosis: report of a case and review of literature. J Oral Maxillofac Surg 2007; 65: 1256–9.

Kolokotronis AE, Belazi MA, Haidemenos G, Zaraboukas TK, Antoniades DZ. Sarcoidosis: oral and perioral manifestations. Hippokratia 2009; 13: 119–21.

Mehra P, Murad H. Maxillary sinus disease of odontogenic origin. Otolaryngol Clin North Am 2004; 37: 347–64.

Moretti AJ, Fiocchi MF, Flaitz CM. Sarcoidosis affecting the periodontium: a long-term follow-up case. J Periodontol 2007; 78: 2209–15.

Paju S, Scannapieco FA. Oral biofilms, periodontitis, and pulmonary infections. Oral Dis 2007; 13: 508–12.

Rudralingam M, Nolan A, Macleod I, Greenwood M, Heath N. A case of sarcoidosis presenting with diffuse, bilateral swelling of the salivary glands. Dent Update 2007; 34: 439–40, 442.

Scully C, Diz Dios P, Kumar N. Special Care in Dentistry. London: Elsevier, 2007.

Seichter A, Szymański L, Warchoł R. Parotid gland sarcoidosis. Otolaryngol Pol 2007; 61: 491–6.

Suresh L, Radfar L. Oral sarcoidosis: a review of literature. Oral Dis 2005; 11: 138–45.

# 1.15 RHEUMATOLOGICAL AND MUSCULOSKELETAL DISEASE

- cherubism
- cleidocranial dysostosis
- craniofacial dysostosis
- connective tissue diseases
- Ehlers–Danlos syndrome
- Ellis–van Creveld syndrome
- fibrous dysplasia
- lupus erythematosus
- mandibulofacial dysostosis

- myasthenia gravis
- mixed connective tissue disease
- osteogenesis imperfecta
- osteopetrosis
- Paget disease of bone
- reactive arthritis
- rheumatoid arthritis
- scleroderma
- Sjögren syndrome

## CHERUBISM
Cherubism, a rare genetic disorder, causes prominence in the lower face as it may present with bilateral jaw swellings (Fig. 1.15.1).

## CLEIDOCRANIAL DYSOSTOSIS
Cleidocranial dysostosis (dysplasia)—an autosomal dominant condition due to a defect in the *CBFA1* gene—can present with delayed tooth eruption, multiple supernumerary teeth, dentigerous cysts, and short tooth roots, hypoplastic or aplastic clavicles, hyperteleorism, frontal bossing and patent metopic sutures (Figs 1.15.2–1.15.6).

## CRANIOFACIAL DYSOSTOSIS
Craniofacial dysostosis (Crouzon syndrome)—a genetic disorder of the first branchial arch—manifests with cranial synostosis, which usually presents as brachycephaly, and exophthalmos and low set ears. It also manifests with maxillary hypoplasia, and often cleft palate, narrow/high-arched palate, posterior bilateral crossbite and hypodontia.

## CONNECTIVE TISSUE DISEASES
Connective tissue diseases can all cause Sjögren syndrome (SS) and lymph node enlargement.

## EHLERS–DANLOS SYNDROME
Ehlers–Danlos syndrome (cutis hyperelastica)—a group of inherited collagen defects—manifests with disorders affecting skin, muscles, ligaments, blood vessels and visceral organs such as the heart. It may cause temporomandibular joint hypermobility, pulp stones and, rarely periodontitis (Fig. 1.15.7).

## ELLIS–VAN CREVELD SYNDROME
Ellis–van Creveld syndrome (chondroectodermal dysplasia) presents with multiple fraeni, short tooth roots and hypodontia.

## FIBROUS DYSPLASIA
Fibrous dysplasia typically presents as a jaw swelling, usually in the maxilla (Chapter 2.8).

## LUPUS ERYTHEMATOSUS
Lupus erythematosus is a rare autoimmune disease which may manifest with oral white lesions, ulcers or Sjögren syndrome (SS) (Figs 1.15.8–1.15.13). Lupus is usually seen in females in one of two forms:

- Discoid lupus erythematosus (DLE) affects only mucocutaneous tissues: oral lesions are seen in up to 25% of those with cutaneous DLE, mainly in the buccal mucosa, gingiva and lip. Characteristic features include central erythema, white spots or papules, radiating white striae at margins and peripheral telangiectasia. There is a small predisposition to carcinoma.
- Systemic lupus erythematosus (SLE) is a multisystem disorder with autoantibodies directed against nuclei: oral lesions are like those in DLE, but usually more severely ulcerated. SLE may also be associated with SS and, rarely, temporomandibular joint arthritis.

Parvovirus B19 infection has been associated with SLE and a variety of rheumatic manifestations/diseases, including rheumatoid arthritis (RA), and vasculitis.

## MANDIBULOFACIAL DYSOSTOSIS
Mandibulofacial dysostosis (Treacher–Collins syndrome)—a rare genetic disorder characterized by craniofacial deformities such as drooping part of the lateral lower eyelids and coloboma (notch), malformed or absent ears, and downwards slanting eyes—may be associated with mandibular hypoplasia, and often midline clefting defects or cleft palate (Figs 1.5.14 and 1.15.15).

## MYASTHENIA GRAVIS
Myasthenia gravis and other myopathies can cause facial weakness, lingual weakness and dysarthria.

## MIXED CONNECTIVE TISSUE DISEASE
Mixed connective tissue disease (MCTD) may be associated with sensory changes, petechiae, lichenoid mucosal lesions and Sjögren syndrome (Figs 1.15.16 and 1.15.17).

## OSTEOGENESIS IMPERFECTA
Osteogenesis imperfecta (Brittle bone disease, Lobstein syndrome)—a genetic bone disorder caused by mutations in the genes that codify for type I procollagen (i.e. *COL1A1* and *COL1A2*)—is associated with fragile bones and, in some patients, with dentinogenesis imperfecta (Figs 1.15.18, chapter 2.10).

## OSTEOPETROSIS
Osteopetrosis (Albers–Schonberg disease or marble bone disease)—a rare disorder caused by mutations on the *CLCN7* (chloride channel 7)

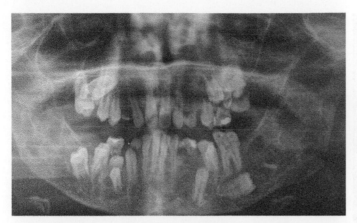

*Figure 1.15.1* Cherubism.

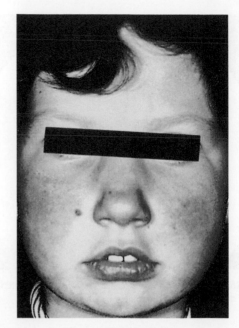

*Figure 1.15.2* Cherubism.

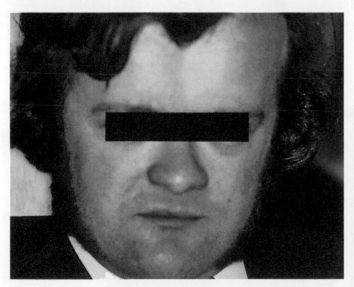

*Figure 1.15.3* Cleidocranial dysplasia showing frontal bossing.

gene, when osteoclasts are defective, in some forms because they lack carbonic acid anhydrase—causes cranial neuropathies, delayed tooth eruption and sometimes osteomyelitis after tooth extractions. Autosomal dominant and recessive forms are recognized.

## PAGET DISEASE OF BONE

Paget disease of bone—a progressive fibro-osseous disease affecting both bone and cementum (osteitis deformans)—is characterized by disorganisation of osteoclast formation. This process is dependent on two cytokines—macrophage colony stimulating factor and receptor activator of NF-kB ligand, and there is a strong genetic component, the genes involved including the sequestosome1 gene (*SQSTM1*).

### Clinical features

Seen mainly in males over 55 years of age, bone remodelling is disrupted, and an anarchic alternation of bone resorption and apposition results in mosaic-like 'reversal lines', often associated with severe bone pain (Figs 1.15.19–1.15.28). In early lesions, bone destruction predomi-

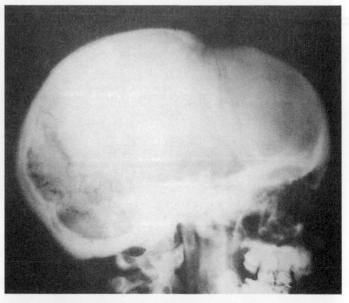

*Figure 1.15.4* Cleidocranial dysplasia showing open sutures and wormian bones.

nates (osteolytic stage) and there is bowing of long bones, especially the tibia and pathological fractures. The increased bone vascularity can lead to high output cardiac failure.

Later, bone apposition increases (osteosclerotic stage) and bones enlarge, with progressive thickening (between these phases is a mixed phase). Paget disease may affect skull, skull base, sphenoid, orbital and frontal bones. The maxilla often enlarges, with widening of the alveolar ridge. Constriction of skull foraminae may cause cranial neuropathies. The dense bone and hypercementosis make tooth extraction difficult, and there is also a liability to haemorrhage and infection.

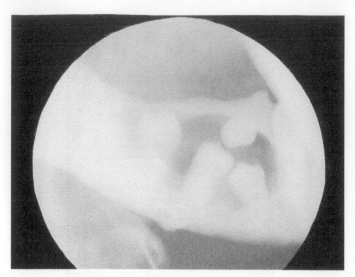

*Figure 1.15.5* Cleidocranial dysplasia showing unerupted, impacted teeth and dentigerous cyst formation.

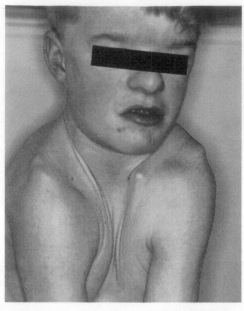

*Figure 1.15.6* Cleidocranial dysplasia clavicular hypoplasia or aplasia allows individuals to approximate their shoulders.

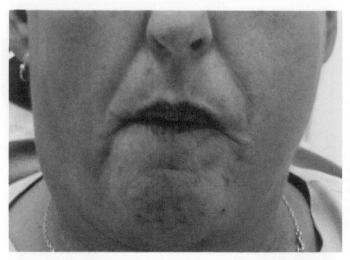

*Figure 1.15.7* Ehlers–Danlos syndrome—temporomandibular joint subluxation.

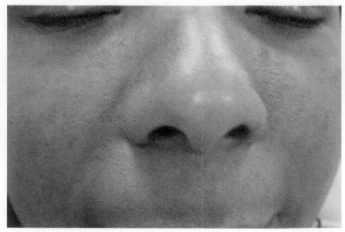

*Figure 1.15.8* Lupus erythematosus—butterfly rash.

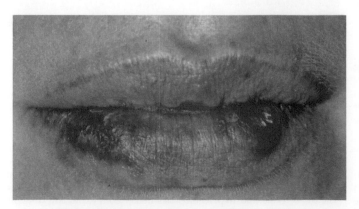

*Figure 1.15.9* Lupus erythematosus affecting the lips.

### Diagnosis

Imaging, biochemistry and histopathology are used. In early lesions, large irregular areas of relative radiolucency (osteoporosis circumscripta) are seen, but later there is increased radiopacity, with appearance of 'cotton wool' pattern. Bone scintiscanning shows localized areas of high uptake. Plasma alkaline phosphatase and urine hydroxyproline levels increase with little or no changes in serum calcium or phosphate levels.

### Management

Bisphosphonates are used but calcitonin may help.

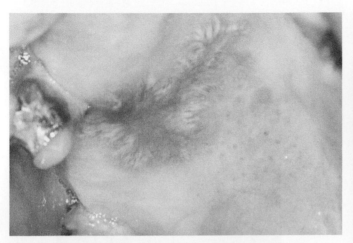

*Figure 1.15.10* Lupus erythematosus lesions may be lichenoid in appearance but often affect the palate.

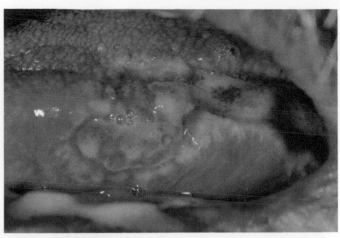

*Figure 1.15.11* Lupus erythematosus lesions resemble lichenoid lesions but with a white brush border to erosions.

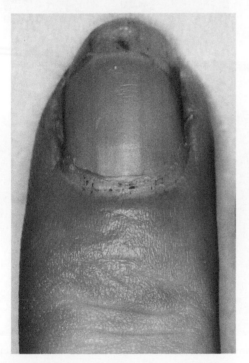

*Figure 1.15.12* Lupus erythematosus nailbed lesions.

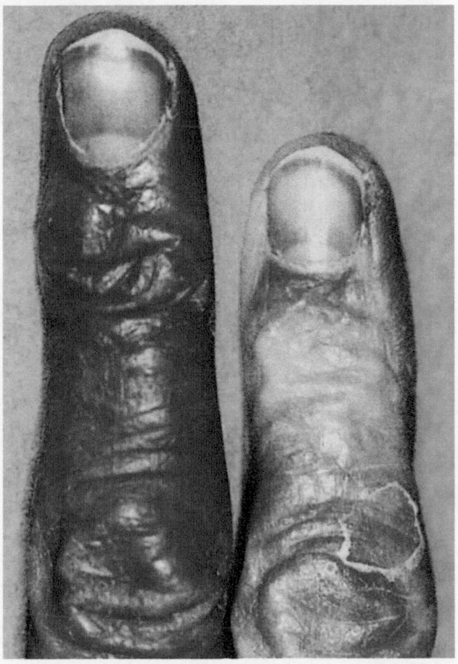

*Figure 1.15.13* Lupus erythematosus—Raynaud phenomenon.

## REACTIVE ARTHRITIS

Reactive arthritis (Reiter syndrome)—a classic triad of arthritis, non-gonococcal urethritis and conjunctivitis—is triggered by enteric or urogenital infections and is associated with human leukocyte antigen (HLA)-B27, although HLA-B27 is not always present in an affected individual, particularly in the presence of HIV. Reactive arthritis may cause oral ulcers or lesions resembling erythema migrans.

## RHEUMATOID ARTHRITIS

RA—a chronic, systemic inflammatory disorder with autoantibodies against immunoglobulins—may affect many tissues and organs, but principally attacks small joints. RA can be associated with SS, and cause temporomandibular arthritis, or drug reactions (e.g. lichenoid). SS is the most common oral association of RA. The temporomandibular joint is commonly affected by arthritis but symptoms are rare: osteoporosis, flattening of the mandibular condyle, marginal irregularities and limited movement with restricted oral opening may be seen. The condyle may necrose in a patient on corticosteroids, leading to a slight anterior open bite, mandibular retrusion and possible obstructive sleep apnoea (Figs 1.15.29–1.15.32).

Oral ulcers may be seen in Felty syndrome because of the neutropenia. Juvenile RA (20% of which is still syndrome, with systemic disease) may interfere with mandibular growth and cause ankylosis.

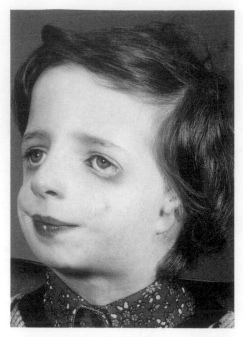

*Figure 1.15.14* Mandibulofacial dysostosis facies and ocular and auricular anomalies.

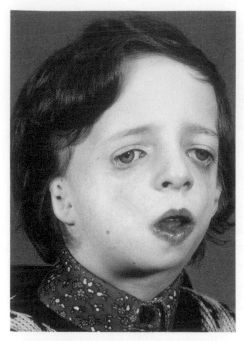

*Figure 1.15.15* Treacher–Collins syndrome.

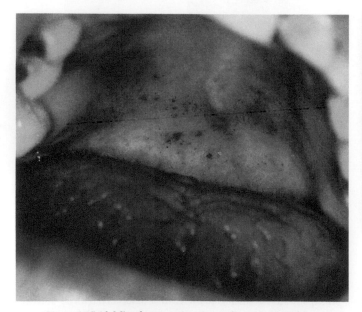

*Figure 1.15.16* Mixed connective tissue disease—petechiae.

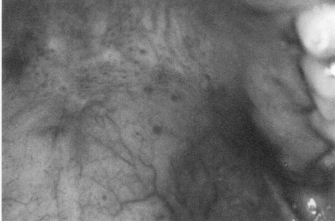

*Figure 1.15.17* Mixed connective tissue disease—palatal lesions.

## SCLERODERMA

Scleroderma (systemic sclerosis)—a chronic autoimmune disease characterized by anti-nuclear, anti-centromere, anti-topoisomerase autoantibodies—can present with vascular alterations and fibrosis.

Scleroderma can present with SS, stiffness of lips, tongue, etc. trismus, telangiectasia, mandibular resorption and periodontal ligament widened on x-ray (Figs 1.15.33–1.15.39). Scleroderma causes skin which becomes tight, waxy and eventually hidebound, and the face smooth with a 'Mona Lisa' appearance and hyperpigmentation.

The lips tighten with radiating furrows—the so-called 'tobacco pouch' mouth—and oral opening is restricted not only by the tight skin but also by pseudoankylosis of the temporomandibular joint. The mandibular condyles, coronoids or zygomatic arches are, rarely, resorbed.

Telangiectasia may appear in the mouth and periorally, especially in the calcinosis Raynaud's, Scleroderma, telangiectasia (CRST) variant or *CREST syndrome*—the association of calcinosis with Raynaud phenomenon, oesophageal dysmobility, scleroderma and telangiectasia. The calcific deposits are most evident in the fingers but there may also be widespread calcification of internal organs.

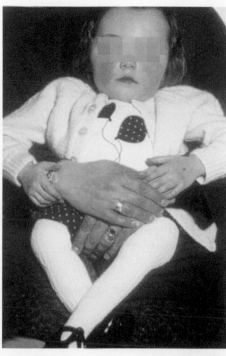

*Figure 1.15.18* Osteogenesis imperfecta—multiple fractures have resulted in substantial deformities.

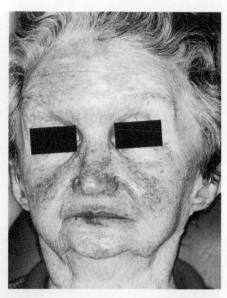

*Figure 1.15.19* Paget disease of bone (osteitis deformans) causing skull swellings.

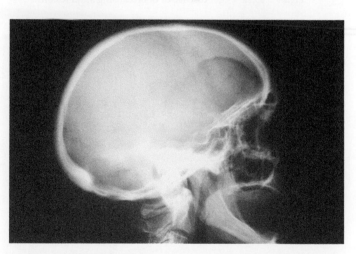

*Figure 1.15.21* Paget disease of bone causing skull radiopacities.

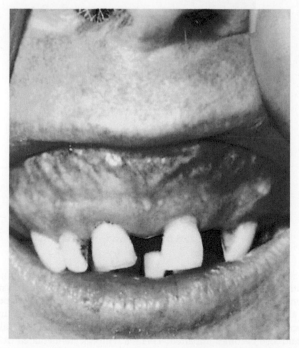

*Figure 1.15.20* Paget disease of bone causing maxillary swelling (leontiasis ossea).

*The limited cutaneous form* affects the skin of the face, hands and arms mainly. Localized scleroderma (Morphoea) presents with lesions typically a perpendicular groove paramedially running from the forehead to the hairline, or on the chin giving a 'coup de sabre' appearance.

*The diffuse cutaneous form* can also affect internal organs, mainly the kidneys, oesophagus, heart and lungs, and can be fatal.

Scleroderma may possibly predispose to oral carcinoma.

## SJÖGREN SYNDROME

SS—the association of dry eyes (keratoconjunctivitis sicca) with dry mouth (xerostomia)—is an autoimmune exocrinopathy which may affect salivary, lacrimal and vaginal glands. It may be found in other family members, is also more common in families that have members

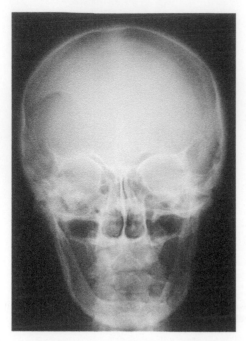

*Figure 1.15.22* Paget disease of bone causing skull lesions.

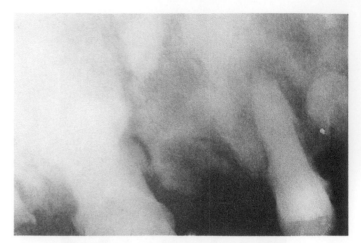

*Figure 1.15.23* Paget disease of bone causing jaw radiopacities with a cotton-wool appearance.

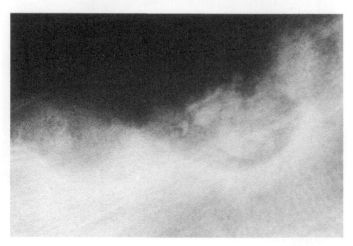

*Figure 1.15.24* Paget disease of bone resulting in osteomyelitis.

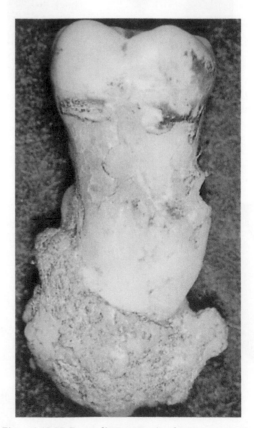

*Figure 1.15.25* Paget disease causing hypercementosis.

with other autoimmune disorders, and may be associated with HLADRB1*15-DRB1*0301 and TAP1-0101 TAP2-0101.

The autoantibodies found in SS are commonly directed against:

- ribonucleoproteins, in SS-1 especially against SS-A (Ro), and in SS-2 against SS-B (La), ds DNA and other extractable nuclear antigens
- IgM [rheumatoid factor (RF)—an IgG antibody against IgM]
- others antigens such as:
  - actin
  - alpha-amylase
  - alpha-fodrin
  - carbonic anhydrase
  - muscarinic M3 receptor
  - salivary duct.

SS pathology appears to start with periductal infiltration of the glands initially mainly by B- but later mainly by T-lymphocytes. The distribution of the membrane pore channel (water channel) protein aquaporin-5 is abnormal in SS, perhaps as a result of paracrine effect of tumour necrosis factor-alpha, and the neurogenic regulation of the salivary gland also becomes impaired. There is lymphocyte-mediated destruction of exocrine glandular acini. Anti-muscarinic 3 receptor antibody plays an important role in cholinergic hyper-responsiveness in SS.

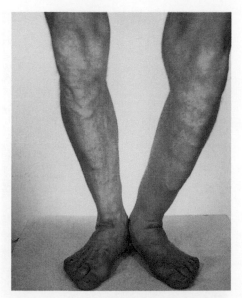

Figure 1.15.26  Paget disease of bone causing tibial bowing.

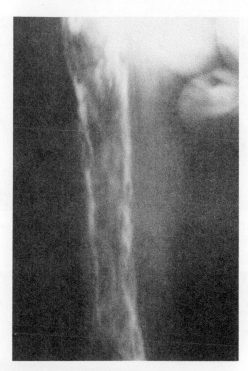

Figure 1.15.27  Paget disease of bone causing lytic lesions.

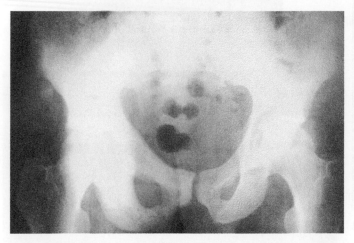

Figure 1.15.28 Paget disease of bone causing ileal and innominate deformities.

Although the salivary acini atrophy, the duct epithelium tends to persist and proliferates sometimes to the extent that the duct lumens may become obliterated, producing islets of epithelium known as 'epimyoepithelial islands'. The fully developed lesion of SS in major glands thus appears as a dense mass of lymphocytes interspersed by islands of epithelium, a pattern termed the 'benign lymphoepithelial lesion'.

Similar syndromes can be produced by viruses [Epstein–Barr virus, hepatitis C, HIV, human T-lymphotropic virus 1 (HTLV-1)]. A Sjögren-like syndrome can also be produced by graft-versus-host-disease (Chapter 1.6).

### Clinical features

Dry eyes and dry mouth if alone are termed primary SS (SS-1) but, if a connective tissue disorder such as RA, SLE, MCTD or scleroderma is present, the condition is termed secondary SS (SS-2). The latter is most common.

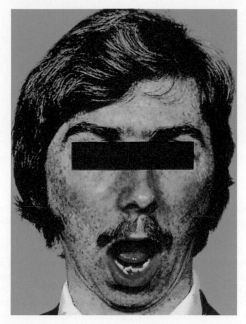

Figure 1.15.29 Rheumatoid arthritis (juvenile rheumatoid arthritis) causing micrognathia.

The clinical spectrum of SS extends from an organ-specific autoimmune process to a systemic disorder. The early manifestations may be non-specific, such as fatigue, arthralgia and Raynaud phenomenon, and it can be 8–10 years from the initial symptoms to full-blown SS.

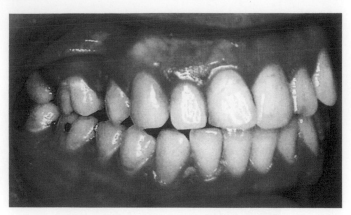

*Figure 1.15.30* Rheumatoid arthritis may lead to condylar necrosis and an anterior open bite.

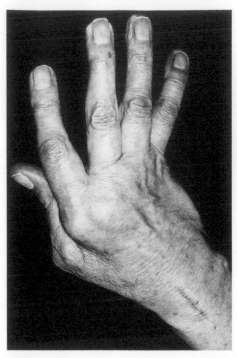

*Figure 1.15.31* Rheumatoid arthritis—typical ulnar deviation of fingers in arthritis mutilans.

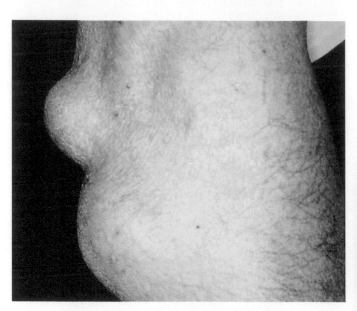

*Figure 1.15.32* Rheumatoid arthritis—rheumatoid nodule in a typical location.

SS presents mainly with eye complaints, including sensations of grittiness, soreness, itching, dryness, blurred vision or light intolerance (Figs 1.15.40–1.15.63). The eyes may be red with infection of the conjunctivae and soft crusts at the angles (keratoconjunctivitis sicca). The lacrimal glands may swell. It is characterized by the occurrence of xerostomia, pharyngolaryngitis sicca, rhinitis sicca, enlarged salivary glands, keratoconjunctivitis sicca, dry skin, decreased sweating, dryness and crusting of the nasal passages, blocking of the Eustachian tubes which can cause deafness, vaginal dryness which can cause dyspareunia, a patchy alopecia, decrease of scalp and body hair, areas of hyperpigmentation and hypopigmentation of the skin, vasculitis, purpura, cataracts and Raynaud syndrome.

- Figure 1.15.63 Sjögren syndrome—rheumatoid arthritis is the most common associated connective tissue disease.Extraoral complications of SS:
- Connective tissue disease in SS-2 usually precedes the onset of dry eyes and dry mouth, and, therefore, patients presenting with dry eyes

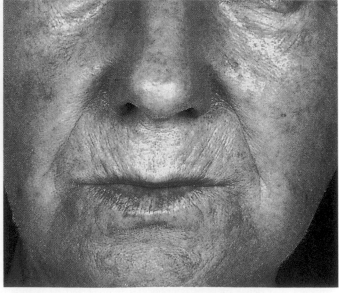

*Figure 1.15.33* Scleroderma—tightened waxy facial skin and lips–tobacco-pouch mouth.

and dry mouth alone probably have SS-1, unless a connective tissue disease manifests within about 1 year. The connective tissue disease in SS-2 is typically longstanding and should be clinically obvious; RA is the most common.

- Extraglandular complaints of SS can include:
  - o Raynaud phenomenon
  - o arthralgia

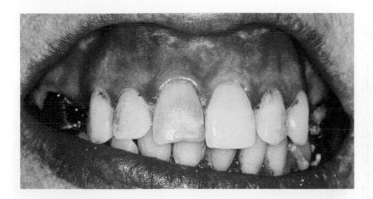

*Figure 1.15.34* Scleroderma—dry mouth from associated Sjögren syndrome.

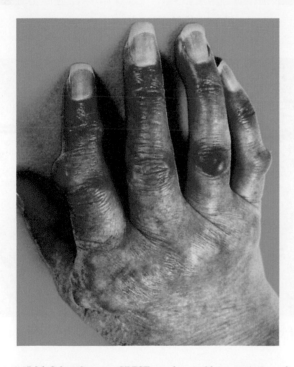

*Figure 1.15.36* Scleroderma—CREST syndrome (the association of calcinosis with Raynaud phenomenon, oesophageal dysmobility, scleroderma and telangiectasia) showing calcinosis and Raynaud phenomenon.

 o myalgia
 o fatigue
 o skin ulceration or rash
 o dyspnoea
 o dry vagina
 o bruising, bleeding and purpura (leukoclastic vasculitis)
 o numbness and other neurological features.
• Associations of SS aside from connective tissue diseases can include:
 o autoimmune (Hashimoto) thyroiditis
 o gastro-oesophageal reflux disease
 o primary biliary cirrhosis
 o B-cell overproduction may eventually lead to lymphoma mostly in primary SS, in mucosal-associated lymphoid tissue (MALT lymphoma) and which may develop into monoclonal gammopathies

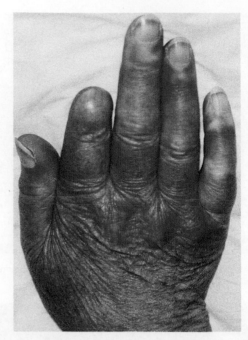

*Figure 1.15.35* Scleroderma—Raynaud syndrome has resulted in digital necrosis.

(such as Waldenstrom macroglobulinaemia). Pseudolymphoma or frank lymphoma should be suspected when there is persistent salivary gland enlargement, lymphadenopathy or lung nodules. Mixed monoclonal cryoglobulins may be found, and when these contain RF cross-reactive for V kappa IIIb related or VH1-related idiotypes, they may be markers for lymphoma.
 o The lungs, brain, nerves, joints, kidneys, thyroid and liver can also be affected in SS.
 o In pregnancy in SS, the autoantibodies may move transplacentally and cause foetal/infant heart block.
• Oral features of SS (often the presenting feature) may include:
 o xerostomia
 o difficulty eating dry foods (the cracker sign)
 o soreness
 o difficulties in controlling dentures in speech and swallowing
 o disturbed taste
 o salivary gland swelling.

Sore and red oral mucosa, and angular stomatitis are usually the result of candidiasis. Dental caries tends to be severe and difficult to control. Ascending (suppurative) sialadenitis is a hazard.

Salivary swelling is occasionally massive and associated with enlarged regional lymph nodes—pseudolymphoma—but B-cell lymphoproliferation may actually become malignant, with a true lymphoma in about 5% of patients with SS. Patients with severe SS are the most likely to develop lymphomas—usually salivary extranodal marginal zone B-cell (MALT) or diffuse large B-cell lymphomas.

**Diagnosis of SS**
Diagnosis is mainly from history and clinical examination. Sialometry is reduced. The Schirmer test measures tear production: a strip of filter paper is held inside the lower eyelid for 5 minutes, when its wetness is

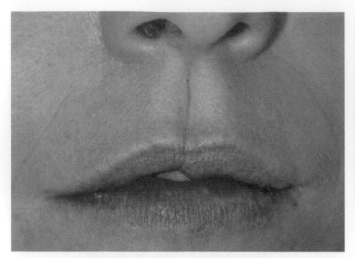

*Figure 1.15.37* Scleroderma—morphoea of philtrum.

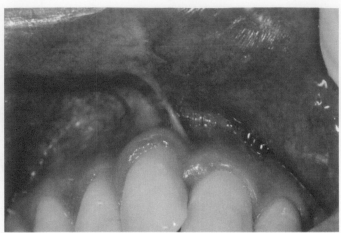

*Figure 1.15.38* Scleroderma—morphoea.

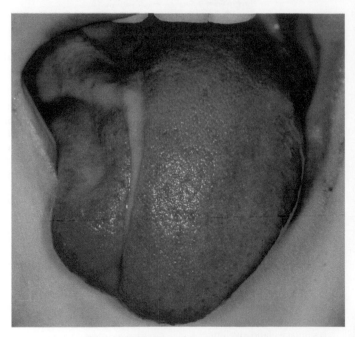

*Figure 1.15.39* Scleroderma—morphoea.

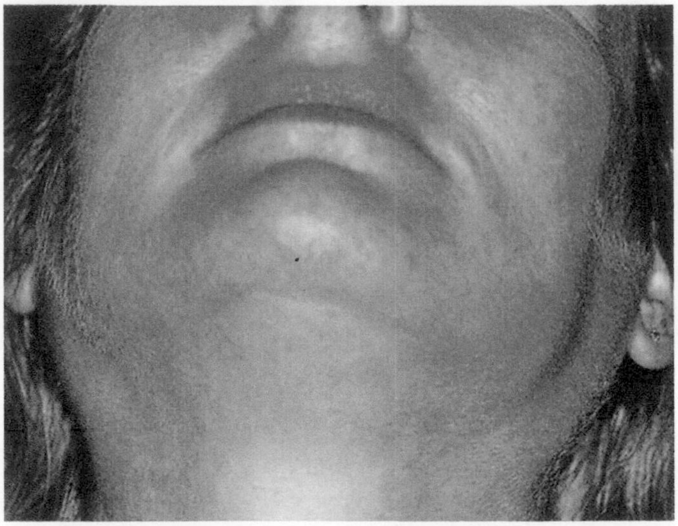

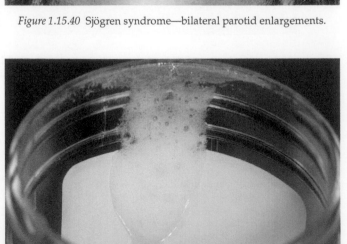

*Figure 1.15.40* Sjögren syndrome—bilateral parotid enlargements.

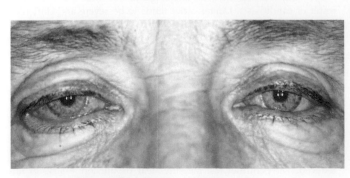

*Figure 1.15.41* Sjögren syndrome—dry eyes.

*Figure 1.15.42* Sjögren syndrome—xerostomia.

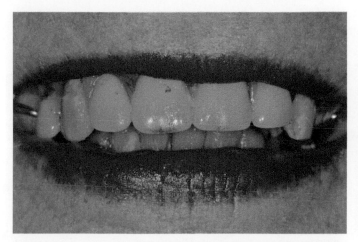

*Figure 1.15.43* Sjögren syndrome—the lipstick sign from lipstick adhering to the dry teeth.

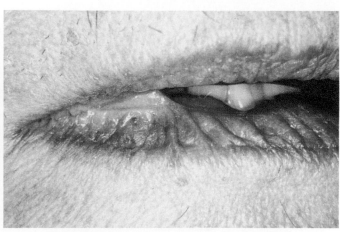

*Figure 1.15.44* Sjögren syndrome—lips adhere if dry.

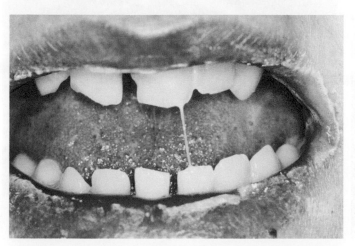

*Figure 1.15.45* Sjögren syndrome—spinbarkheit (threads of saliva).

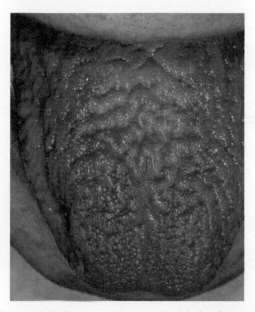

*Figure 1.15.46* Sjögren syndrome—dry lobulated tongue.

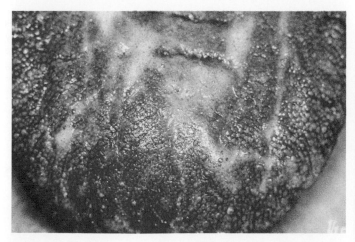

*Figure 1.15.47* Sjögren syndrome—saliva becomes frothy if reduced in amount.

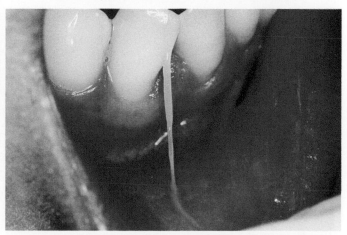

*Figure 1.15.48* Sjögren syndrome—xerostomia.

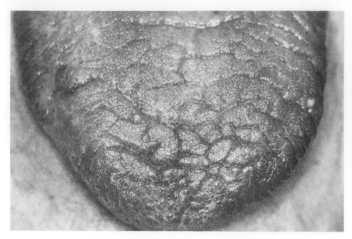

*Figure 1.15.49* Sjögren syndrome—dry fissured tongue.

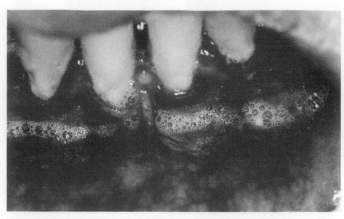

*Figure 1.15.50* Sjögren syndrome—hyposalivation and periodontal disease.

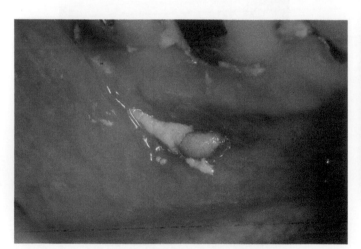

*Figure 1.15.51* Sjögren syndrome—food debris.

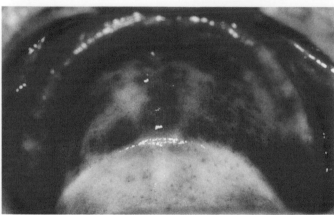

*Figure 1.15.52* Sjögren syndrome—denture-related stomatitis.

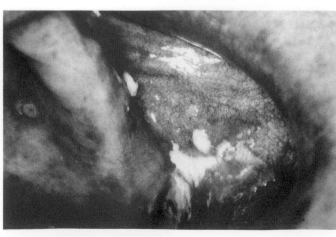

*Figure 1.15.53* Sjögren syndrome—candidosis.

measured with a ruler. Producing <5 mm is usually indicative of SS. Slit lamp examination is done for eye surface dryness.

Helpful investigations can include:

- Serum autoantibodies—particularly RF and antinuclear antibodies known as SS-A (Ro) and SS-B (La), and RF. SS-A is common in many autoimmune diseases (e.g. SLE, SS/SLE overlap syndrome, subacute cutaneous LE, neonatal lupus and primary biliary cirrhosis) including secondary SS. In contrast, anti-La/SS-B is more associated with primary SS.
- Anaemia.
- Raised erythrocyte sedimentation rate or plasma viscosity.
- Labial gland biopsy.
- Salivary studies.

If SS is suspected, specialist referral is warranted since investigations may be needed, and the differential diagnosis may include:

- Viral infections:
  o hepatitis C virus
  o HIV
  o HTLV-1
  o Epstein-Barr virus.

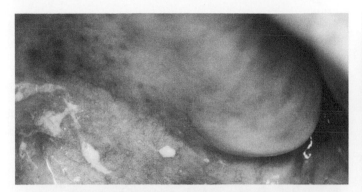

*Figure 1.15.54* Sjögren syndrome—candidosis.

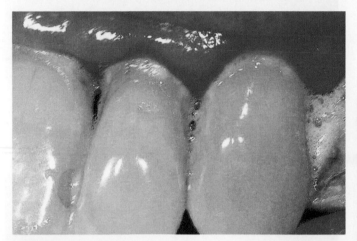

*Figure 1.15.56* Sjögren syndrome—xerostomia and periodontal disease.

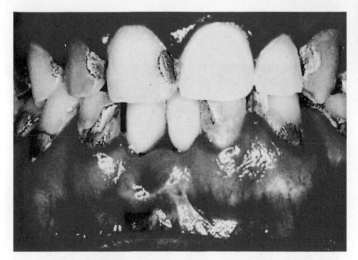

*Figure 1.15.58* Sjögren syndrome—predisposes to caries.

- Sarcoidosis and Heerfordt syndrome.
- Glandular deposits in:
  o haemochromatosis
  o lipoproteinaemias
  o amyloidosis.
- Lymphomas.

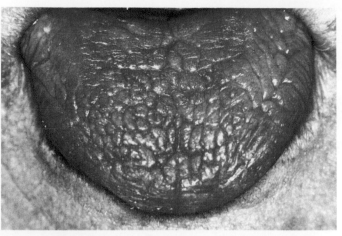

*Figure 1.15.55* Sjögren syndrome—angular stomatitis, dry mouth and fissured tongue

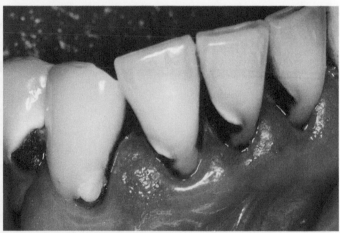

*Figure 1.15.57* Sjögren syndrome—caries.

The diagnosis of SS is mainly on the history, clinical examination and investigation, including:

- ocular symptoms
- oral symptoms
- ocular signs
- autoantibodies
- salivary gland involvement
- histopathology.

The internationally accepted diagnostic criteria for SS are shown in Table 1.15.1.

**Management**

SS remains an incurable condition, since no therapeutic modality has been identified that reliably modifies the course of the disease. Any connective tissue or other disorders should be treated by a physician. Patients with severe extraglandular manifestations are usually treated

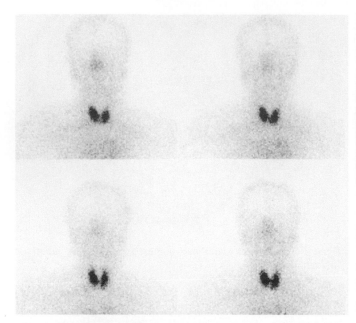

Figure 1.15.59 Sjögren syndrome—salivary scans showing hypofunction.

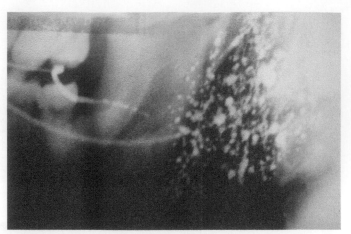

Figure 1.15.60 Sjögren syndrome—sialectasis.

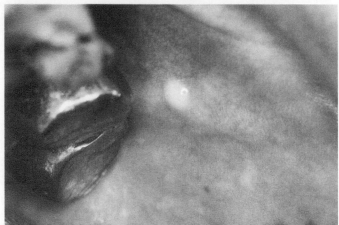

Figure 1.15.62 Sjögren syndrome—pus exuding from Stensen duct in sialadenitis.

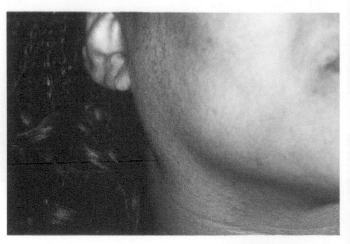

Figure 1.15.61 Sjögren syndrome—parotid sialadenitis.

by a physician with systemic corticosteroids and immunosuppressive drugs such as hydroxychloroquine and occasionally cyclophosphamide. The patient should be followed up regularly, particularly because of the possible complication of lymphoma, which may manifest with:

• firm tender persistent salivary swelling
• lymphadenopathy
• nodular lung lesions
• cough
• dyspnoea
• hepatosplenomegaly.

Other aspects of care are discussed above.

Lymphomas; an oncological opinion is indicated; chemotherapy may be required.

Drugs to control underlying autoimmune disease in SS are experimental only (e.g. ciclosporin and rituximab).

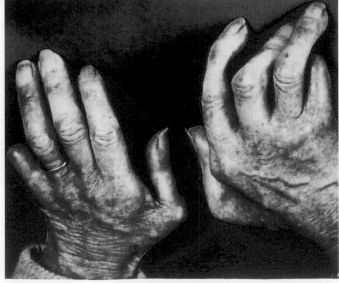

Figure 1.15.63 Sjögren syndrome—rheumatoid arthritis is the most common associated connective tissue disease.

**Table 1.15.1** DIAGNOSTIC CRITERIA (AMERICAN–EUROPEAN) FOR SJÖGREN SYNDROME

| | | |
|---|---|---|
| Ocular symptoms | A positive response to at least one of the following questions: | 1. Have you had daily ocular symptoms or persistent, troublesome dry eyes for more than 3 months? |
| | | 2. Do you have a recurrent sensation of sand or gravel in the eyes? |
| | | 3. Do you use tear substitutes more than three times a day? |
| Oral symptoms | A positive response to at least one of the following questions: | 1. Have you had a daily feeling of dry mouth for more than 3 months? |
| | | 2. Have you had recurrently or persistently swollen salivary glands as an adult? |
| | | 3. Do you frequently drink liquids to aid in swallowing dry food? |
| Ocular signs | That is, objective evidence of ocular involvement defined as a positive result for at least one of the following: | 1. Schirmer I test, performed without anaesthesia (<5mm in 5 minutes) |
| | | 2. Rose Bengal score or other ocular dye score (>4 according to van Bijsterveld scoring system) |
| Histopathology | In minor salivary glands (obtained through normal-appearing mucosa) | Focal lymphocytic sialadenitis evaluated by an expert histopathologist, with a focus score >1, defined as a number of lymphocytic foci (which are adjacent to normal-appearing mucous acini and contain more than 50 lymphocytes) per 4 mm$^2$ of glandular tissue |
| Salivary gland involvement | Objective evidence of salivary gland involvement, defined by a positive result for one of the following: | 1. Unstimulated whole salivary flow </= 1.5 ml in 15 minutes. |
| | | 2. Parotid sialography showing the presence of ductal sialectasis (punctate, cavitatory or destructive pattern) without evidence of obstruction in the major ducts |
| | | 3. Salivary scintigraphy showing delayed uptake, reduced concentration and/or delayed excretion of tracer |
| Autoantibodies | Presence in the serum of the following autoantibodies: | Antibodies to Ro (SS-A) or La (SS-B) antigens, or both |

# FURTHER READING

Aslanidis S, Pyrpasopoulou A, Kontotasios K, Doumas S, Zamboulis C. Parvovirus B19 infection and systemic lupus erythematosus: activation of an aberrant pathway? Eur J Intern Med 2008; 19: 314–18.

D'Cruz DP, Khamashta MA, Hughes GR. Systemic lupus erythematosus. Lancet 2007; 369: 587–96.

Derk CT, Rasheed M, Spiegel JR, Jimenez SA. Increased incidence of carcinoma of the tongue in patients with systemic sclerosis. J Rheumatol 2005; 32: 637–41.

Fischer DJ, Patton LL. Scleroderma: oral manifestations and treatment challenges. Spec Care Dentist 2000; 20: 240–4.

Fox PC. Autoimmune diseases and Sjogren's syndrome: an autoimmune exocrinopathy. Ann NY Acad Sci 2007; 1098: 15–21.

Fox RI. Sjögren's syndrome. Lancet 2005; 366: 321–31.

Georgios K, Helias A, Athanassios K, Eleni M, Konstantinos A. Craniofacial surgical management of a patient with systematic juvenile idiopathic arthritis and Crohn's disease. J Craniofac Surg 2009; 20: 948–50.

Hansen A, Lipsky PE, Dörner T. New concepts in the pathogenesis of Sjögren syndrome: many questions, fewer answers. Curr Opin Rheumatol 2003; 15: 563–70.

López-Labady J, Villarroel-Dorrego M, González N, Pérez R, Mata de Henning M. Oral manifestations of systemic and cutaneous lupus erythematosus in a Venezuelan population. J Oral Pathol Med 2007; 36: 524–7.

Mathews SA, Kurien BT, Scofield RH. Oral manifestations of Sjögren's syndrome. J Dent Res 2008; 87: 308–18.

Mitsias DI, Kapsogeorgou EK, Moutsopoulos HM. Sjögren's syndrome: why autoimmune epithelitis? Oral Dis 2007; 13: 523–32.

Porter S, Scully C. Connective tissue disorders and the mouth. Dent Update 2008; 35: 294–6, 298–300, 302.

Sasaguri K, Ishizaki-Takeuchi R, Kuramae S, et al. The temporomandibular joint in a rheumatoid arthritis patient after orthodontic treatment. Angle Orthod 2009; 79: 804–11.

# 2 COMMON AND IMPORTANT DISORDERS AFFECTING MAXILLOFACIAL REGION: DIFFERENTIAL DIAGNOSIS BY SITE

The history is the most important aspect of diagnosis. The history should include a comprehensive relevant medical, drug, lifestyle habits (tobacco, alcohol, betel, drug use, etc.), travel and social history. The history related to orofacial problems should also include:

- date of onset of symptoms
- swelling details—such as duration and character
- pain details—such as duration, daily timing, character, radiation, aggravating and relieving factors, relationship to meals and associated phenomena
- mouth-opening restriction.

Disorders which affect the oral mucosa may appear to be isolated, but it is important to also consider in the history and examination, the possibility of related systemic disorders or conditions, especially

- blood diseases
- infections
- gastrointestinal disorders
- skin or connective tissue diseases (may also involve genital and/or ocular mucosae)
- drug effects.

## DIAGNOSIS

The teeth, jaws, temporomandibular joints, salivary glands and oral mucosa should be examined. Dental terminology is well described in other texts. Mucocutaneous lesions have a complex terminology as listed below.

Flat lesions

- *Macule*: circumscribed area of altered colour or texture.
- *Petechia*: small haemorrhagic macule (<2 mm).
- *Ecchymosis*: large haemorrhagic macule (>2 mm).

Raised lesions

- *Papule*: elevation <5 mm in diameter.
- *Papilloma*: nipple-like projection, often pedunculated.
- *Plaque*: slightly raised area >5 mm in diameter.
- *Scale*: dry and flat flake of keratin.
- *Stria*: linear elevation.
- *Nodule*: a solid mass in, or under the skin/mucosa, >5 mm in diameter.
- *Tumour*: any tissue enlargement. It is generally avoided as a clinical descriptive term as it is commonly associated with malignancy by patients. The terms 'nodule', 'mass' or even 'swelling' are thus preferable.
- *Haematoma*: an area of extravasated blood inside a tissue.

Fluid-filled lesions

- *Vesicle*: fluid filled elevation <5 mm in diameter.
- *Bulla*: fluid filled elevation >5 mm in diameter.
- *Pustule*: accumulation of pus in the skin/mucosa.

Lesions resulting from tissue loss

- *Atrophy*: thinning of the skin/mucosa and loss of normal markings.
- *Erosion*: partial thickness loss of epidermis/epithelium.
- *Ulcer*: full thickness loss of epidermis/epithelium and dermis/corium.
- *Fissure*: linear slit.
- *Crust (scab)*: dried blood, serum and other exudates covering an ulcerated area. In a moist area this is termed *pseudomembrane*.
- *Scar*: permanent replacement of lost normal tissue by fibrous tissue.

Abnormal passages

- *Fistula*: an abnormal passage between two epithelially lined structures.
- *Sinus*: blind ended track or cavity.

## INVESTIGATIONS

Investigations required should be planned and oriented towards assisting a diagnosis but in relation to mucocutaneous or soft tissue lesions may include:

- Full blood picture
- Haematinics (iron, folate and vitamin B12)
- Plasma viscosity or erythrocyte sedimentation rate or C reactive protein
- Antibodies
  - Autoantibodies
  - Viral antibodies.

Other investigations can include:

- Biopsy
- Ultrasound
- Imaging with radiography or magnetic resonance.

# 2.1 LIPS

- aesthetic conditions
- blisters
- pigmented, red, purple or blue lesions

- soreness, ulceration and pain
- swellings and lumps
- white lesions

---

The lips should be examined in a systematic fashion to ensure that all areas are included. They should first be inspected and examination then is facilitated if the mouth is gently closed and the lips everted.

The lips consist of skin on the external surface and mucous membrane on the inner surface within which are bundles of striated muscle, particularly the *orbicularis oris* muscle. The upper lip includes the *philtrum*, a midline depression, extending from the columella of the nose to the superior edge of the vermilion zone. The *oral commissures* are the angles where the upper and lower lip meet. The epithelium of the lip vermilion is distinctive, with a prominent stratum lucidum and a thin stratum corneum: the dermal papillae are numerous, with a rich capillary supply, which produces the reddish-pink colour of the lips. Melanocytes are abundant in the basal layer of the vermilion of pigmented skin, but are infrequent in white skin. The vermilion zone, the transitional zone between the glabrous skin and the mucous membrane, contains no hair or sweat glands but does contain ectopic sebaceous glands (Fordyce spots)—yellowish pinhead-sized papules particularly seen in the upper lip and at the commissures. They also appear intraorally, mainly in the buccal mucosae. The lips feel slightly nodular because of the contained minor salivary glands, and the labial arteries are readily palpable. The normal labial mucosa appears moist with a fairly prominent vascular arcade and in the lower lip particularly, the many minor salivary glands which are often exuding mucus are visible (Figs 2.1.1–2.1.3) (Figs 2.2.66–2.2.68).

## AESTHETIC CONDITIONS
### Body art
Tattooing of the skin or vermilion and tattooing inside the lip may occasionally be seen. Tattooing of the chin is seen increasingly in Maoris ('Moki'). The vermilion may be tattooed red in some people in Western countries. Tattooing is also seen in some African cultures: a tattooed lower lip in a Sudanese woman, for example, signifies that she is married. The Wodaabe people of Nigeria and Cameroon may tattoo the skin at the angle of the mouth, a practice which has its basis in ritual warding-off of the 'evil eye'. Similar tattoos may be seen on Bedouin women of North Africa.

Maxillofacial piercing may involve a variety of objects and may be seen particularly in persons who have other forms of body art (see also Figs 2.1.4–2.1.7). The placing of jewellery, usually stainless-steel studs, rings or barbells is typically in the lower lip and tongue in some Western cultures but may be seen virtually anywhere on the head and neck. The so-called labrette piercing is usually a central piercing of the lip below the vermilion, carrying a stud or ring. Similar habits have been common for years in certain African cultures and Amazonian cultures, for example, the Suia and Txukahameis tribes of Brazil.

Complications secondary to facial, labial and oral piercings include mainly pain, bleeding, infection, dental fractures and gingival damage. Systemic infections appear to be uncommon.

### Cicatrization
Scarring and sometimes some deformity may follow tissue destruction by, for example, burns, lacerations, gunshot wounds, irradiation, skin diseases such as epidermolysis bullosa or toxic epidermal necrolysis, or infections such as cancrum oris (noma). Some scarring is unavoidable in surgery involving the lips, especially after a very young age. Self-mutilation can result in significant deformity (Fig. 2.1.8).

## Cleft lip and palate (CLP)
### Aetiopathogenesis
Facial clefts are the most common congenital craniofacial abnormalities. The common clefts are cleft lip with or without cleft palate (CL±P), and cleft palate (CP) alone. CLP together are more common than is CL alone.

CL occurs in about 1 per 1000 births: the prevalence being highest in males and in oriental neonates, lower in Caucasian neonates and lowest in neonates of African heritage (approximately 1 per 2500 births) (Fig. 2.1.9).

CP is the fourth most common birth defect—affecting approximately 1 in 700 out of 1000 live births, and is more prevalent in females. There is a familial tendency: when one parent is affected, the risk to a child is about 1 in 10 live births.

The primary palate or premaxilla forms during the 4th–7th weeks of gestation and includes the portion of the alveolar ridge that contains the four maxillary incisors. The secondary palate forms during the 6th–9th weeks of gestation and consists of the remaining hard and all the soft palate. Clefts result from failure of the frontonasal process and/or fusion of the palatal shelves.

More than 400 syndromes may include a facial cleft as one manifestation. Facial clefts are associated with a syndrome in up to 15–60% of cases (and are then termed syndromic clefts). Van der Woude and Waardenberg syndromes are associated with CL, with or without CP. Common syndromes in which CP occurs include Apert, Stickler and Treacher–Collins syndromes. CLP may also be seen in velocardiofacial (Shprintzen), Pierre–Robin and Klippel–Feil syndromes and in various chromosome anomalies (e.g. Down syndrome and Edwards syndrome). A small subgroup of patients have CLP with median facial dysplasia and cerebrofacial malformations, others with laryngotracheal oesophageal clefts (Opitz–Firas or G syndrome) or cranial asymmetry (Opitz or B syndrome).

The cause of non-syndromic CL±P is unclear but there is still a strong genetic component. No single gene defect appears responsible but several loci have been identified in CLP—include transforming growth factor alpha, poliovirus receptor-related 1, retinoic acid receptor alpha, T-box transcription factor-22, glutamic acid decarboxylase, interferon regulatory factor 6, MSX1 (formerly homeobox 7—encodes a member of the muscle segment homeobox gene family) and fibroblast growth factor genes.

CLP is more prevalent in lower socio-economic classes and it is thought that maternal stress, teratogens and various lifestyle factors may increase the risk. Teratogens incriminated include isotretinoin (Accutane)—which also causes birth defects such as brain malformations, learning disability and cardiac problems; thalidomide; anticonvulsants (phenytoin, valproic acid, lamotrigine and carbamazepine) and

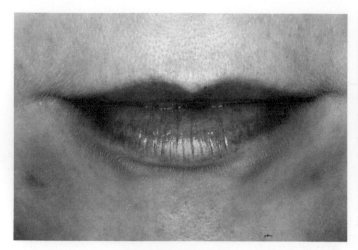

Figure 2.1.1 Normal lips.

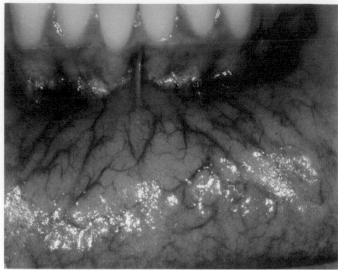

Figure 2.1.2 Normal lower labial mucosa—the minor salivary glands cause the multiple small swellings.

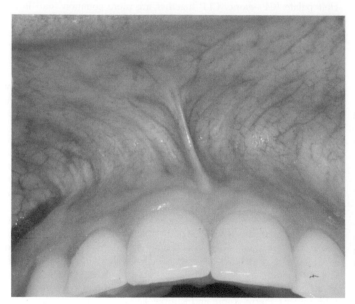

Figure 2.1.3 Normal upper labial mucosa.

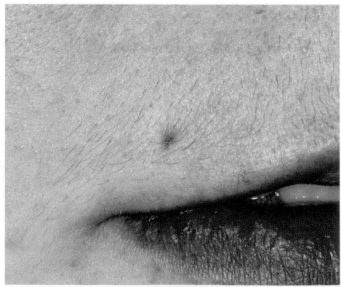

Figure 2.1.4 Labial piercing.

corticosteroids. Potential environmental maternal risk factors include upper respiratory infections, smoking (especially when the mother has glutathione *S*-transferase theta 1-null variants), alcohol use, obesity and diabetes. Paternal smoking has also been implicated as a causal factor. There has been concern about but no real evidence for, aspirin and diazepam as possible causes. Folic acid given peri-conceptually may lower the risk—but the evidence is weak.

'Pierre–Robin' syndrome is the combination of micrognathia, glossoptosis and compromised airway. Features such as CP, or feeding problems are additional. Pierre–Robin sequence (PRS) may occur in isolation or in various genetic syndromes, most commonly Stickler syndrome. Other disorders causing PRS may include velocardiofacial (Shprintzen) syndrome, Treacher–Collins syndrome, trisomy 11q syndrome, trisomy 18 syndrome, deletion 4q syndrome, rheumatoid arthropathy, hypochondroplasia, Möbius syndrome, foetal alcohol syndrome and CHARGE association (a chromosome 8 mutation on

the CHD7 gene manifesting with Coloboma, Heart defects, Atresia of choanae, Retarded growth, Genital defects, Ear anomalies). Stickler syndrome is an autosomal dominant, genetic connective tissue disorder typically associated with mutations in the *COL2A1* gene, characterized by ophthalmological, maxillofacial, auditory and skeletal anomalies. Maxillofacial features include a flat midface with depressed nasal bridge, short nose with anteverted nares and micrognathia. Midline clefting, if present, ranges in severity from a soft palate cleft to PRS. Joint hypermobility leads to osteoarthritis, typically in the 3rd or 4th decade. Sensorineural deafness with high tone loss is typically asymptomatic or mild.

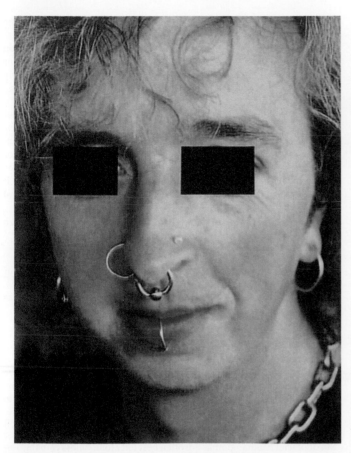

Figure 2.1.5 Body art including a labrette.

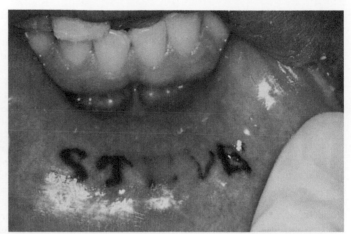

Figure 2.1.6 Body art—a labial tattoo.

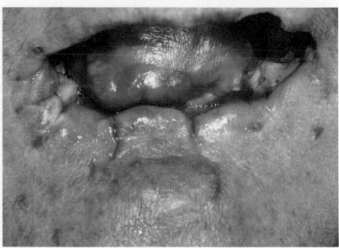

Figure 2.1.8 Lip and tongue scarring and deformity from chronic trauma.

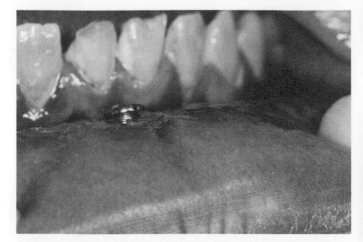

Figure 2.1.7 Body art—lip stud. Gingivitis and chipped mandibular incisors can also be seen.

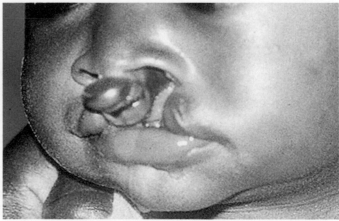

Figure 2.1.9 Cleft lip.

### Clinical features in clefts

Clefts have a major impact on the family from the aesthetic, psychological and functional viewpoints, since the affected neonate is unable to suckle. Clefts are also often accompanied by impaired facial growth, dental anomalies, speech disorders, poor hearing and psychosocial problems.

CP may be incomplete involving only the uvula and the muscular soft palate (velum). A complete CP extends the entire length of the palate.

A high percentage of patients with CP develop otitis media with effusion. Up to 20% have other abnormalities that can affect management: systemic disorders are more frequent in patients with CP than in those with CL alone and include especially skeletal, cardiac, renal and central nervous system defects.

Palatal ulcers seen in neonates with CLP appear to result from trauma from the tongue, and resolve if a palatal plate is fitted. Dental abnormalities include malocclusion (almost 100%), hypodontia (50%), hypoplasia (30%) and supernumerary teeth (20%). Children may have a higher-caries prevalence in both the primary and permanent dentitions, and significantly more gingivitis, especially in the maxillary anterior region. Adult CLP patients may have poorer oral hygiene and more gingivitis. Prevention and continuity of oral health care are essential and a high rate of success can be achieved.

### Diagnosis and management

Healthcare providers that frequently participate in a multidisciplinary CP team include: audiologists, maxillofacial, ear, nose, and throat and plastic surgeons, geneticists, neurosurgeons, nurses, dentists (paediatric dentist/orthodontist/prosthodontist), paediatricians, social workers/psychologists and speech and language pathologists.

*Submucous* CP occurs when the palatal shelves fail to join but the overlying mucous membranes are intact and the muscle attachments of the soft palate are abnormal, causing velopharyngeal insufficiency. It can be recognized by a notched posterior nasal spine, a translucent zone in the midline of the soft palate and a bifid uvula but not all these features are necessarily present, and a bifid uvula may be seen in isolation. About 1 in 1200 births are affected and feeding difficulties, speech defects and middle ear infections may develop in 90% of affected children. Adenoidectomy is contraindicated as it may reveal latent velopharyngeal insufficiency.

### Haemangiomas

Haemangiomas (Chapter 1.1).

Labial haemangiomas, telangiectasia and venous lakes can be aesthetic problems.

Haemangiomas are usually small, deep red or blue-purple, blanch on pressure, are fluctuant to palpation and are level with the mucosa or have a lobulated or raised surface. Haemangiomas (angiomas) are fairly common hamartomas (congenital). They are typically seen in isolation and are of no consequence.

However, a few angiomas may be multiple and/or part of a wider syndrome such as Maffucci or blue rubber bleb naevus syndromes. Large facial haemangiomas, which can involve the lips, may be associated with Sturge–Weber syndrome or Dandy–Walker syndrome, or other posterior cranial fossa malformations. Haemangiomas in some sites may be at risk from trauma or prone to excessive bleeding if damaged (e.g. during tooth extraction). Occasionally, maxillofacial haemangiomas develop phlebolithiasis.

The epithelioid haemangioma (hemangioendothelioma) is a benign vascular anomaly, and has a close relationship with local trauma.

### Clinical features

Haemangiomas are usually symptomless but may cause a lump or coloured area and cosmetic problems if large (Figs 2.1.10–2.1.15). Haemangiomas can also be a problem from bleeding if they lie in areas that may be breached during dental or oral surgical care.

### Diagnosis

Clinical plus aspiration and imaging. Maxillofacial lesions suspected of being haemangiomatous should not be routinely biopsied; aspiration is far safer. Kaposi sarcoma and epithelioid angiomatosis should be excluded. After intravenous administration of contrast medium, enhancement is observed in haemangiomas in areas corresponding to those with high signal on $T_2$-weighted MRI.

### Management

Maxillofacial haemangiomas are often best left alone unless causing aesthetic problems or symptoms. If treatment is required, this is best achieved, if small, with cryosurgery or laser-assisted ablation or, if large, by ligation or angiography-assisted embolization of feeding vessels.

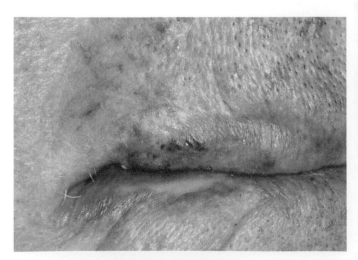

*Figure 2.1.10* Haemangioma.

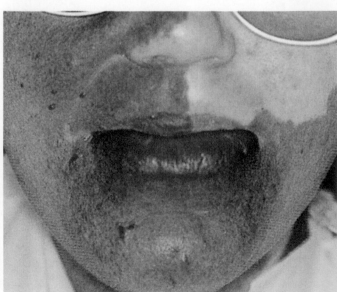

*Figure 2.1.11* Haemangioma in Sturge–Weber syndrome.

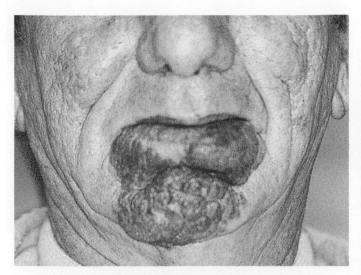

*Figure 2.1.12* Haemangioma.

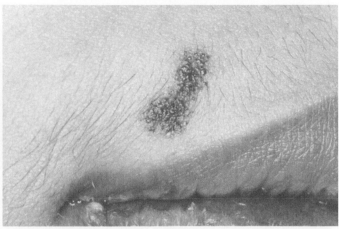

*Figure 2.1.13* Angioma.

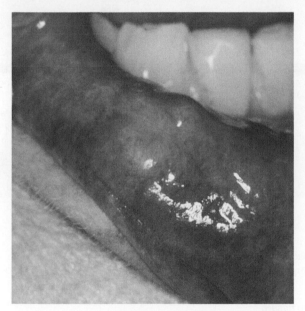

*Figure 2.1.14* Angioma.

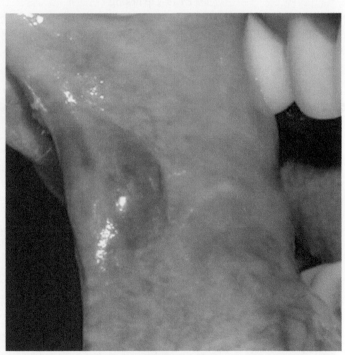

*Figure 2.1.15* Haemangioma.

The treatment of choice for epithelioid hemangioendothelioma because of the unpredictable biological behaviour and recurrence potential is wide local excision.

### Lip-biting

Lip-biting (Morsicatio buccarum).

Lip-biting and lip licking is a common habit, particularly in anxiety states (Figs 2.1.16 and 2.1.17), and may be associated with a few traumatic petechiae. Extreme and fortunately rare cases may result in significant lip destruction, scarring and aesthetic problems—as where there is sensory loss after damage to the trigeminal nerve, and in the rare Riley–Day syndrome, or in psychoses or inborn errors of metabolism such as the Lesch–Nyhan syndrome.

### Lip dimples, pits, fistulas and sinuses

- *Dimples* are common at the commissures.
- *Commissural pits* are distinct definite pits up to 4 mm in diameter and depth, present from infancy, often showing a familial tendency and probably determined by a dominant gene. They are sometimes associated with aural sinuses or pits.
- *Congenital lip pits* or *sinuses* are rare, asymptomatic, small blind fistulae on the vermilion border usually bilateral symmetrical and just to

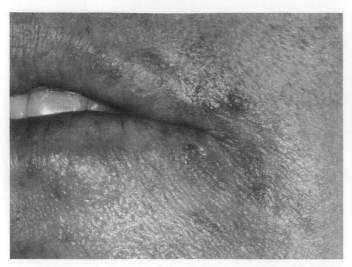

*Figure 2.1.16* Lip licking.

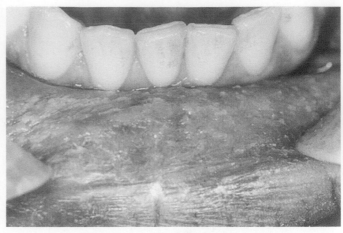

*Figure 2.1.17* Frictional keratosis—lip.

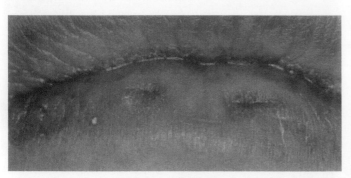

*Figure 2.1.18* Lip pits.

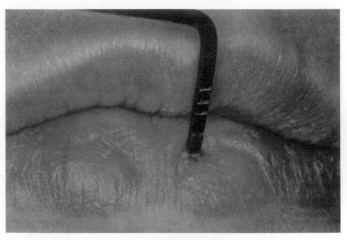

*Figure 2.1.19* Lip pits.

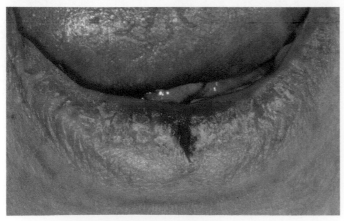

*Figure 2.1.20* Lip fissure.

one side of the midline (Figs 2.1.18 and 2.1.19). Typically seen in females, on the lower lip, and often associated with clefting disorders, they are up to 3–4 mm in diameter, up to 2 cm deep and may communicate with underlying minor salivary glands and exude mucus. The pits are often (67%) associated with CLP (this is the Van der Woude syndrome)—an autosomal dominant syndrome, sometimes seen with syndactyly or talipes equinovarus.

*Diagnosis and management of lip dimples and pits*
Surgical removal may sometimes be indicated for cosmetic purposes.

## Lip fissure
*Aetiopathogenesis*
A fissure may develop in the lip where a patient, typically a child, is mouth-breathing (Figs 2.1.20–2.1.22). Sun, wind, cold weather and smoking are thought to predispose. A hereditary predisposition for weakness in the first branchial arch fusion may exist. Lip fissures are also common in Down syndrome.

Lip fissures are also common when lips swell as, for example, in cheilitis granulomatosa and orofacial granulomatosis/Crohn syndrome (Fig. 2.1.23).

*Clinical features*
Most lip fissures are seen in males, typically median in the lower lip and are chronic, causing discomfort and, from time to time, some bleeding.

*Diagnosis*
Clinical.

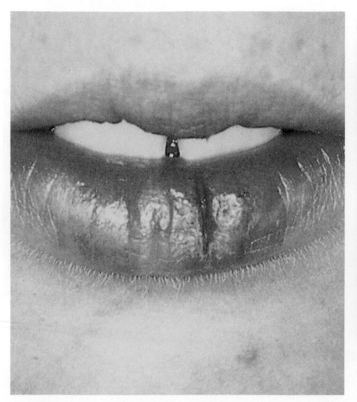

Figure 2.1.21 Lip fissure.

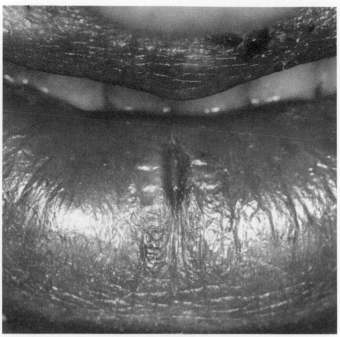

Figure 2.1.22 Lip fissure.

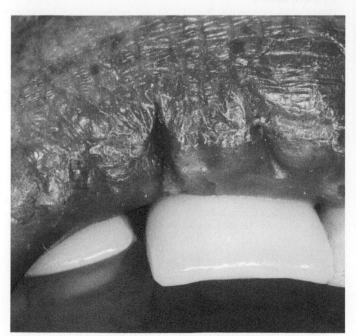

Figure 2.1.23 Lip fissure in Down syndrome.

*Management*
Predisposing factors should be managed if possible. Bland creams may help the lesion heal spontaneously. Applications of 1–2% silver nitrate, 0.5% Balsam of Peru, salicylic acid or antimicrobials may help. If the fissure fails to heal, excision, preferably with a z-plasty or cryosurgery may be needed.

## Sebaceous glands
Sebaceous glands (Fordyce spots; Fordyce granules).

*Aetiopathogenesis*
Sebaceous glands may appear in the mucosa as creamy-yellow dots. They are extremely common: probably 80% of the population has them, but they are rarely evident in infants (though they are present histologically). They may appear in children after the age of 3 years and increase during puberty. They seem to be more obvious in males, in patients with greasy skin and in older people, and may be increased in some rheumatic disorders.

*Clinical features*
Fordyce spots are soft yellowish granules seen mainly in the upper lip, and in the buccal mucosa particularly inside the commissures and sometimes in the retromolar regions or elsewhere (Figs 2.1.24 and 2.1.25) (Figs 2.2.66–2.2.68).

*Diagnosis and management*
Fordyce spots are totally benign, but the occasional patient or physician becomes concerned about them or misdiagnoses them as, for example, thrush, lichen planus or Koplik spots. Biopsy is rarely indicated. Intraoral sebaceous hyperplasia occurs when a lesion, judged to require biopsy has histologic features of one or more well-differentiated sebaceous glands that exhibit no fewer than 15 lobules per gland.

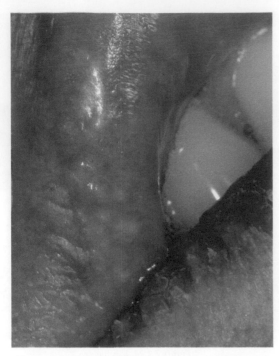

*Figure 2.1.24*  Fordyce spots (ectopic sebaceous glands).

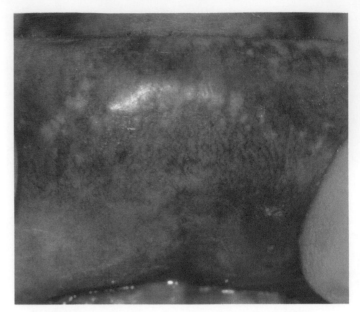

*Figure 2.1.25*  Fordyce spots (ectopic sebaceous glands).

## BLISTERS

Blisters on the lips may have various causes but burns, herpes labialis, allergies, mucoceles, erythema multiforme and autoimmune skin disorders (pemphigus especially) may need to be excluded.

### Bullous disorders

Pemphigoid, pemphigus (Fig. 2.1.26) and erythema multiforme may present with lip blisters (Chapter 1.10).

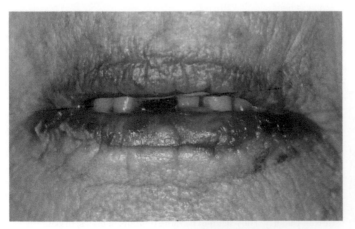

*Figure 2.1.26*  Pemphigus presenting with lip lesions.

### Burns

Burns are most common after the ingestion of hot foods, or exposure to caustic chemicals—including some used in dentistry. Cold injury is uncommon, but follows cryosurgery.

### Herpes labialis

*Aetiopathogenesis*

Herpes simplex virus (HSV), after primary oral or perioral infection (Chapter 1.8), remains latent in the trigeminal ganglion. HSV moves down the trigeminal nerve to produce mucocutaneous lesions if reactivated by factors such as:

- fever
- sunlight
- trauma or
- immunosuppression.

Labial or perioral herpes labialis (cold sores) affect up to 15% of the normal population.

Sebaceous glands with fewer than 15 lobules that form an apparently distinct clinical lesion on the buccal mucosa are considered normal, whereas similar lesions at other intraoral sites are considered ectopic sebaceous glands.

No treatment is indicated, other than reassurance.

### Tattoos

Pigmentation may occur after foreign material (metal or mineral usually) is left in the lip.

### Clinical features

Lesions are seen typically at the mucocutaneous junction, starting as macules which rapidly become papular, vesicular, then pustular over a few days and crust and heal usually without scarring. Any mucocutaneous site can be affected, including the anterior nares (Figs 2.1.27–2.1.47).

Patients with T-cell immune defects in particular are predisposed to recurrent herpes with widespread and persistent lesions. Haemorrhage into lesions produces a deceptive appearance in a leukaemic or other patient with thrombocytopenia.

Impetigo can mimic (or complicate) herpes labialis (Figs 2.1.48 and 2.1.49).

### Diagnosis

Differential diagnosis of herpes labialis is mainly from primary HSV infection (Figs 2.1.32 and 2.1.33), herpes zoster, impetigo or carcinoma (rarely). Diagnosis is largely clinical, though polymerase chain reaction DNA detection, immunodetection, electron microscopy or viral culture is occasionally needed.

### Management

Most patients will have spontaneous remission within 1 week to 10 days but, as the condition is both uncomfortable and unsightly, antiviral treatment is

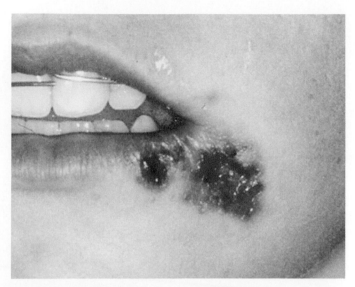

Figure 2.1.27  Herpes simplex virus infection.

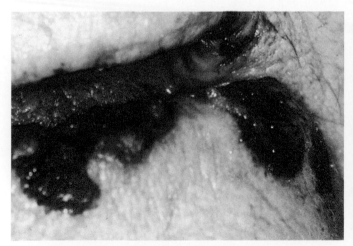

Figure 2.1.28  Herpes simplex virus infection in leukaemia.

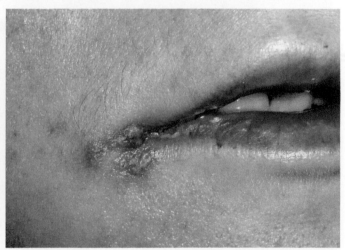

Figure 2.1.29  Herpes simplex virus infection.

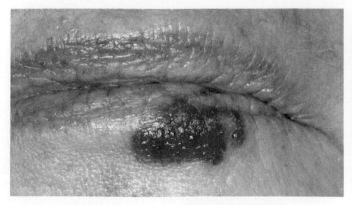

Figure 2.1.30  Herpes simplex virus infection.

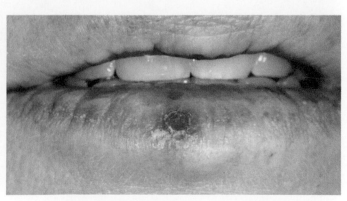

Figure 2.1.31  Herpes simplex virus infection.

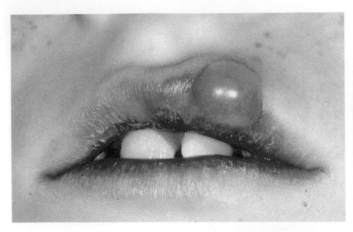

*Figure 2.1.32* Primary herpes simplex virus infection.

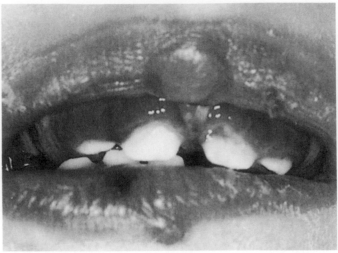

*Figure 2.1.33* Primary herpes simplex virus infection.

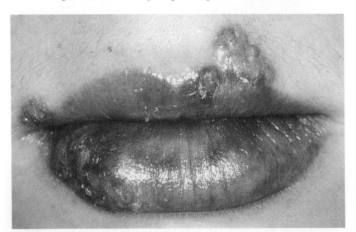

*Figure 2.1.34* Herpes simplex virus infection.

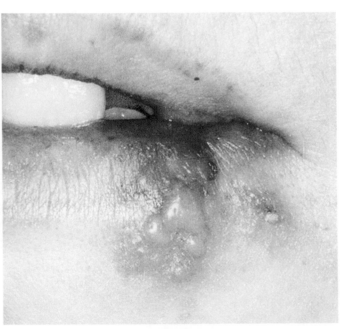

*Figure 2.1.35* Herpes simplex virus infection.

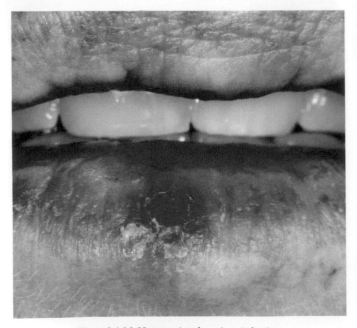

*Figure 2.1.36* Herpes simplex virus infection.

indicated from as early in the disease as possible. Penciclovir 1% cream applied in the prodrome may help abort or control lesions in healthy patients, and appears more effective than aciclovir 5% cream.

Systemic antivirals (aciclovir, valaciclovir and famciclovir) may be needed for more severe cases, especially immunocompromised patients, in whom the lesions may otherwise spread or persist. Antiviral resistance is becoming a significant problem to immunocompromised persons, especially those with severe immune defects: alternative therapies then include foscarnet, *n*-docosanol, idoxuridine or tromantadine hydrochloride.

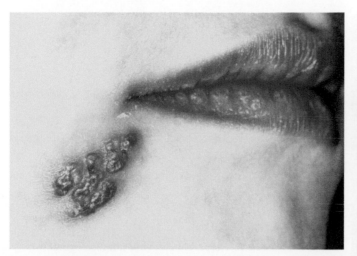

*Figure 2.1.37* Herpes simplex virus infection.

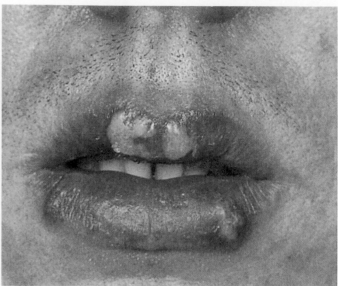

*Figure 2.1.38* Herpes simplex virus infection.

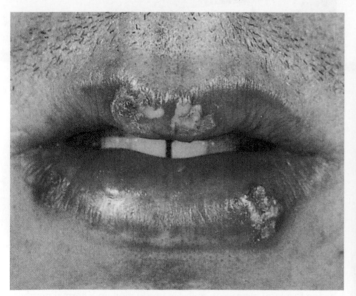

*Figure 2.1.39* Herpes simplex virus infection.

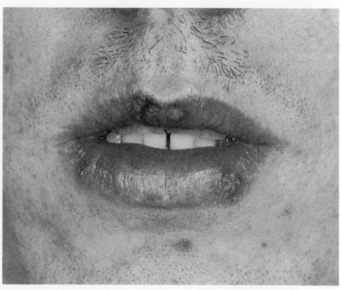

*Figure 2.1.40* Herpes simplex virus infection.

**Mucoceles**

Mucoceles (Chapter 2.7).

Mucoceles are common in the lower labial mucosa (Figs 2.1.50–2.1.53).

## PIGMENTED, RED, PURPLE OR BLUE LESIONS

Lip colour, size and contour vary with skin colour and ethnic origin. Hamangiomas, telangiectases and Kaposi sarcoma may affect the lips. Benign pigmented lesions similar microscopically to racial pigmentation may be seen on the lips. These consist of increased numbers of melanocytes present as single units along the junctional zone without increased melanocyte numbers, clustering or with formation of melanocyte aggregates, similar microscopically to racial pigmentation in the basal epithelial layer often with subepithelial pigment-laden macrophages (melanophages), and they include:

- Melanotic macules consist of increased melanin, without increased numbers of melanocytes.
- Ephelides with sun exposure change in the amount of melanin and consequently colour.
- Melanoacanthomas—rare acquired brown to black usually single benign areas of hyperpigmentation of the mucosa, which can arise suddenly and enlarge, commonly seen on the buccal/commissural

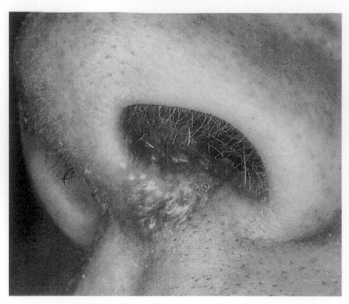

*Figure 2.1.41* Herpes simplex virus infection at anterior nares.

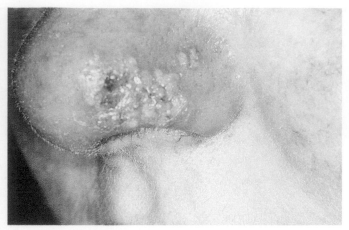

*Figure 2.1.42* Herpes simplex virus infection—nasal.

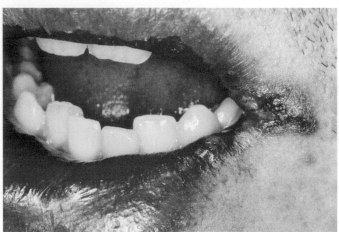

*Figure 2.1.44* Herpes simplex virus infection mimicking angular stomatitis.

### Ephelides

Ephelides (freckles) are circumscribed melanotic macules, typically smaller than 0.5 cm, which appear on sun-exposed areas in childhood, owing to a local increase in melanin production, in a normal number of melanocytes. Ephelides may occasionally involve the lip vermilion (Figs 2.1.54–2.1.56).

### Haemangioma

Haemangioma (angioma).

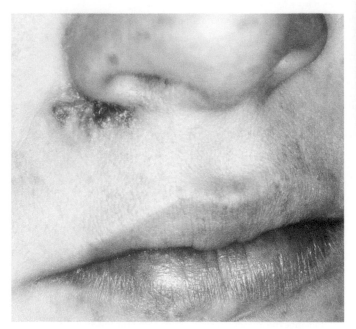

*Figure 2.1.43* Herpes simplex virus infection—perinasally.

### Kaposi sarcoma

Kaposi sarcoma (Chapter 2.4).

### Melanotic macule

*Aetiopathogenesis*

Melanotic macule is an acquired, small, flat, brown to brown-black, asymptomatic, benign lesion, unchanging in character and usually seen

mucosa of women of African heritage. Besides increased melanin in the basal layer they also typically contain dendritic cells with melanin and eosinophils in the upper epithelium. It may be a melanotic macule that appears suddenly as reactive lesions following trauma. Besides increased amount of melanin in the basal layer melanacanthoma also typically shows dendritic cells with melanin and eosinophils in the upper epithelium.

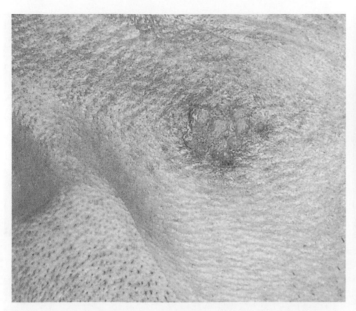

Figure 2.1.45 Herpes simplex virus infection.

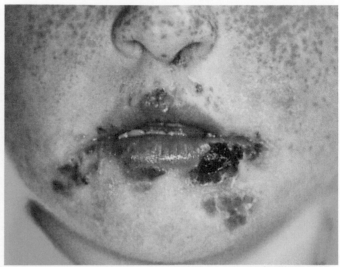

*Figure 2.1.46* Herpes simplex virus infection in a child with T-cell immunodeficiency.

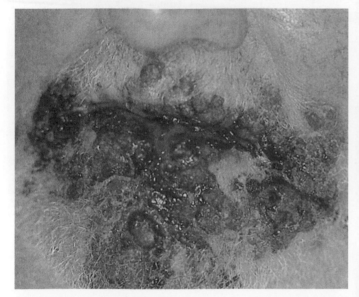

*Figure 2.1.47* Herpes simplex virus infection in an older patient with pneumonia.

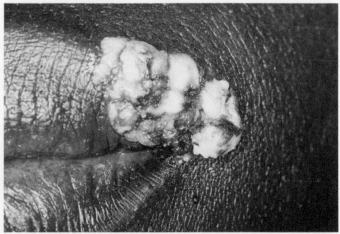

*Figure 2.1.48* Herpes simplex virus infection.

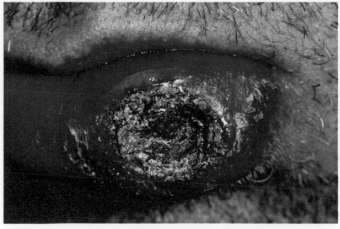

*Figure 2.1.49* Herpes simplex virus infection—with Staphylococcal infection.

in isolation. Labial melanotic macule (on the lip vermilion) is regarded as an entity distinct from intraoral macules (Figs 2.1.57 and 2.1.58).
Melanotic macules may also be seen in:

- Peutz–Jeghers syndrome—circumoral melanosis with intestinal polyposis (below).
- Laugier–Hunziker syndrome—a benign condition of labial, oral, skin and nail hyperpigmentation. Genital involvement is not uncommon.
- HIV infection—most macules are related to primary adrenocortical deficiency or to zidovudine therapy.

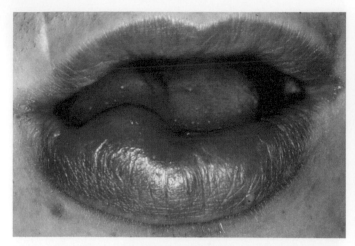

*Figure 2.1.50* Mucocele.

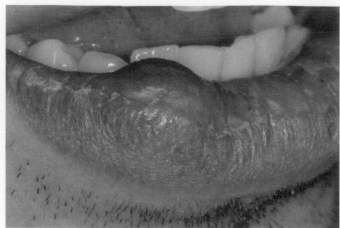

*Figure 2.1.51* Mucocele.

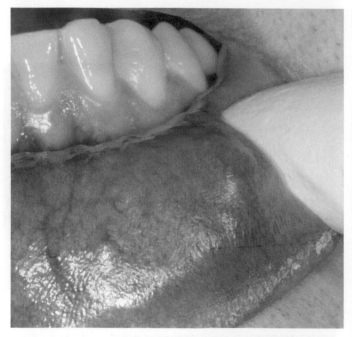

*Figure 2.1.52* Mucocele.

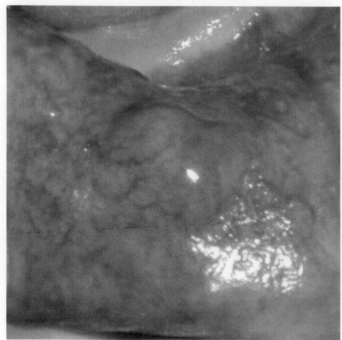

*Figure 2.1.53* Mucocele.

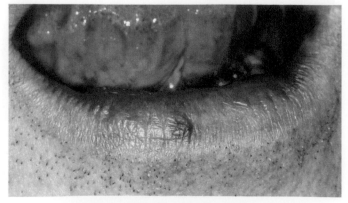

*Figure 2.1.54* Labial melanotic macule.

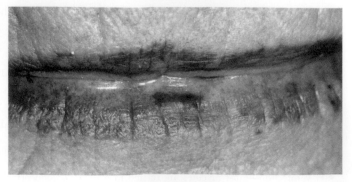

*Figure 2.1.55* Ephelides.

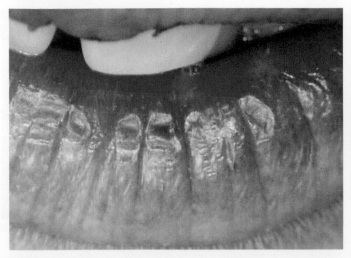

*Figure 2.1.56* Labial melanotic macule.

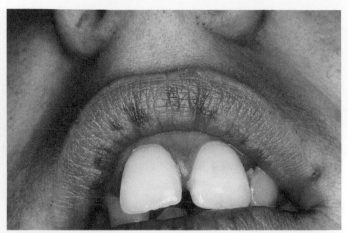

*Figure 2.1.57* Labial melanotic macule.

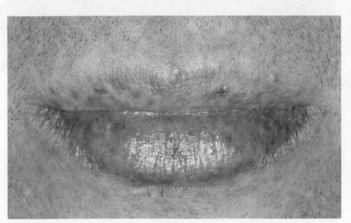

*Figure 2.1.58* Labial melanotic macules.

*Clinical features*
Many macules occur on the vermilion border of the lower lip as solitary lesions (labial melanotic macules). Most melanotic macules are solitary and seen in white adults and their colour ranges from brown to black. The typical macule is a small well-demarcated, uniformly tan to dark brown, round or oval discolouration <7 mm diameter and unchanging in character. Melanotic macules may resemble other lesions such as early melanoma and ephelides, although the latter tend to fade in winter and darken in summer.

*Diagnosis and management*
The melanotic macule has no malignant transformation potential, but an early melanoma could have a similar clinical appearance, so lesions of recent onset, large size, irregular pigmentation, unknown duration or rapidly enlarging should be excised and examined histopathologically. No treatment is required otherwise, except for cosmetic considerations— excision or removal by laser or hidden by lipstick.

**Trauma**
Lip haematomas are common after trauma. Dental local analgesic injections, especially regional blocks, not uncommonly produce a small haematoma which is usually inconsequential unless intramuscular, when it can cause trismus, or is infected, or if the blood tracks extraorally.

Extraoral discolouration and/or swelling may be produced by a haematoma after surgery, especially in the mandibular molar region. Blood may track through fascial planes of the neck to cause extensive bruising, even down to the chest wall and mediastinum. Post-operative oedema is particularly common after poor surgical technique. However, in persons with a bleeding tendency, haematomas can easily arise even with good technique.

Dental local analgesic injections may in contrast produce temporary local pallor because of the contained vasoconstrictor, but this is of no consequence.

**Venous lake**
Venous lake (varix; senile haemangioma).

*Aetiopathogenesis*
Venous dilatation.

*Clinical features*
A solitary bluish-purple soft fluctuant swelling, 2–10 mm in diameter, usually seen on the lower lip vermilion of an elderly person. A venous lake may be only a trivial cosmetic problem or it can bleed severely after trauma.

*Diagnosis*
Clinical; the lesion also empties on prolonged pressure.

*Management*
Venous lake can be left alone or excised, or treated with cryotherapy, electrocautery, infrared coagulation or argon laser.

## SORENESS, ULCERATION AND PAIN
**Burns**
Burns due to thermal, chemical or electrical insults are uncommon, but may be iatrogenic (e.g. trauma to an anaesthetized lower lip) (Figs 2.1.59 and 2.1.60). Burns present as blisters followed by localized areas of superficial ulceration that usually heal within 7–10 days. Some patients with burning mouth syndrome complain of a sensation of burning in the lips, and some drugs such as angiotensin converting enzyme inhibitors (ACEIs) cause 'scalded lip syndrome'.

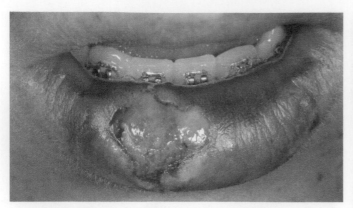

*Figure 2.1.59* Labial ulceration from trauma.

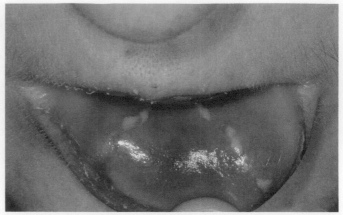

*Figure 2.1.60* Labial ulceration from trauma in a seizure.

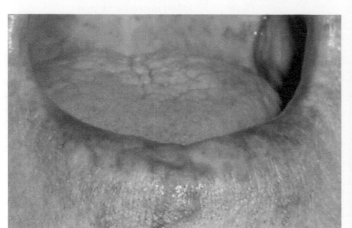

*Figure 2.1.61* Actinic stomatitis (cheilitis).

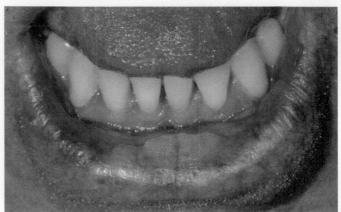

*Figure 2.1.62* Actinic stomatitis.

## Cheilitis

Cheilitis (inflammation of the lips) can present with blistering and/or swelling, and can have many causes. It usually arises as a primary disorder of the lip vermilion as a contact reaction to cosmetics, lip salves, dentifrices, mouthwashes, dental materials or even some food and drink but there are other causes.

## Actinic cheilitis

Actinic cheilitis (actinic keratosis of lip, solar keratosis, solar cheilosis) due to acute sunburn is common, and clinically resembles 'chapping'.

### Aetiopathogenesis

Sunlight can damage the lips and skin, particularly the vermilion of the lower lip. Mainly seen in Caucasians in the tropics less in people with coloured skins, sun damage is most common in:

- hot, dry regions
- outdoor workers
- fair-skinned people.

Particularly at risk are individuals whose lifestyles include much time spent outdoors, especially farmers, sailors, windsurfers, skiers, mountaineers, golfers, etc. Other forms of radiation that can cause similar changes include arc-welding.

### Clinical features

- Acute cheilitis due to acute sunburn is common, and clinically resembles 'chapping'.
- Attacks of herpes simplex may also be induced by sunlight.
- Actinic cheilitis is a chronic premalignant keratosis of the lip caused by long exposure to solar irradiation. Most actinic cheilitis is, therefore, seen:
  o on the lower lip, with sparing of the oral commissures
  o in fair-skinned men
  o in the fourth to eight decades of life
  o particularly in those who have had prolonged exposure to sunlight.

Actinic cheilitis is a chronic condition which may evolve into squamous cell carcinoma of the lip. In the early stages of actinic cheilitis there may be redness and oedema, but later the lip becomes dry and scaly and wrinkled with grey to white changes in pigmentation. Lesions may appear as a smooth or scaly, friable patch or can involve the entire lip. At times, the border between the vermilion and the skin or mucosa becomes indistinct. At times, vesicles may appear which rupture to form superficial erosions. Vertical fissuring and crusting may be seen (Figs 2.1.61 and 2.1.62), particularly in cold weather, although sometimes the condition improves during the winter months. Later, the epithelium becomes palpably thickened with small greyish white plaques.

Eventually, warty nodules may form and, eventually, one or more may undergo malignant change.

The possibility of malignant change must always be considered when there are suspect features such as:

• ulceration
• a red and white blotchy appearance with an indistinct vermilion border
• generalized atrophy with focal areas of whitish thickening
• persistent flaking and crusting.

Cancer in actinic cheilitis is more aggressive than some others; approximately 10% of carcinomas whose origin is in the lip metastasize.

### Diagnosis

A careful history and a biopsy are often indicated. The need for early detection of actinic changes and preventive management is important in actinic cheilitis since squamous cell carcinoma must be excluded whenever an erosion or ulcer is present.

It must be remembered that actinic cheilitis rarely may be an early manifestation of a genetic susceptibility to light damage as in xeroderma pigmentosum or part of the syndrome of actinic prurigo. Lupus erythematosus and lichen planus must also be considered in the differential diagnosis.

### Management

*Prevention* is advised, especially in high risk individuals. Particular care is needed in patients with photosensitivity disorders such as xeroderma pigmentosum, and in those whose exposure to ultraviolet (UV) light, especially UVB is high, such as mountaineers and skiers. Sun avoidance or the use of UV barriers (sunscreens) or even in extreme instances a shield, are advised.

*Management of established actinic cheilitis* is required both to relieve symptoms and to try to prevent development of squamous cell carcinoma. This is best achieved by the removal of the premalignant epithelium by:

*Topical chemoexfoliants* including 5-fluorouracil, tretinoin or trichloroacetic acid.

*Surgery.* Cryosurgery is effective in the majority of instances but for refractory or widespread disease, laser or surgical excision with advancement of a mucosal flap (vermilionectomy) (*lip shave*) or electrodesiccation, or curettage may be required.

*Laser ablation.* Carbon dioxide laser vaporization of the vermilion is simple, easy-to-use and offers excellent results with no post-operative paraesthesiae or significant scarring.

*Vermilionectomy.* The vermilion border is excised with a scalpel and the wound closed by advancing the labial mucosa to the skin. This can be combined with wedge resection if cancer has developed. Postoperative complications are generally more than with laser ablation and include paraesthesiae, lip pruritus and labial scar tension.

Following management, prevention of recurrence by the regular use of a UVA and UVB protective sunscreen is advisable. Contact cheilitis may occasionally be induced by lipsticks or lip salves via contact allergy, or by the photosensitizing action of certain ingredients.

## Angular cheilitis

*Angular cheilitis* (angular stomatitis, cheilosis, perleche).

Angular cheilitis is inflammation at the commissures of the lips.

### Aetiopathogenesis

A number of factors (infective, mechanical, nutritional or immunological) may be implicated alone or in combination. Angular cheilitis is most often chronic, seen in older patients, and due to infective and/or mechanical causes. Denture-related stomatitis may predispose to angular stomatitis. Although *Candida albicans* is the prevalent organism, *Staphylococcus aureus* and other micro-organisms may sometimes be isolated.

Diabetes mellitus, malignancy, HIV-infection and anaemia can increase the probability of angular cheilitis. Rarely, angular stomatitis is a manifestation of iron deficiency, or of vitamin deficiency—when there may also be glossitis and mouth ulcers, or of an immune defect (Figs 2.1.63–2.1.74). Cheilitis is common in Down syndrome, the large tongue and the constant dribbling possibly being contributory factors, along with immune deficiency. Swollen lips in Crohn disease, or orofacial granulomatosis also predispose to fissures and angular cheilitis. Angular cheilitis associated with candidosis may also be a manifestation of an underlying immunological deficiency such as diabetes or HIV disease.

The recurrent trauma of dental flossing, and hypersalivation are rare causes of angular cheilitis.

### Clinical features

Angular cheilitis is bilateral and most commonly presents as roughly triangular areas of erythema and oedema at both commissures. Atrophy,

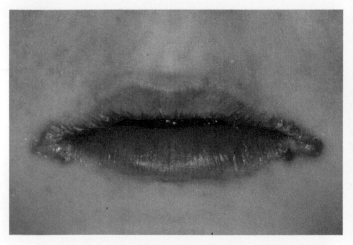

*Figure 2.1.63* Angular stomatitis in orofacial granulomatosis.

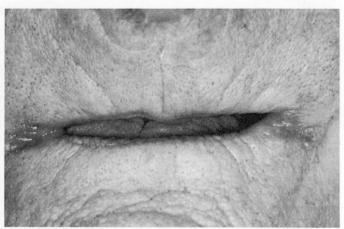

*Figure 2.1.64* Angular stomatitis in vitamin B12 deficiency.

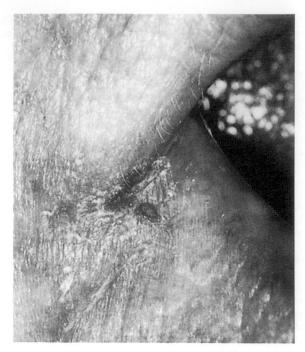

Figure 2.1.65 Angular stomatitis.

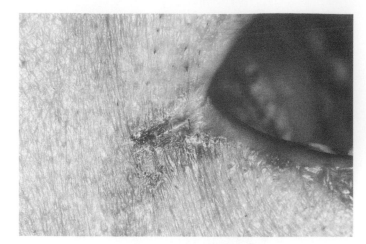

Figure 2.1.66 Angular stomatitis.

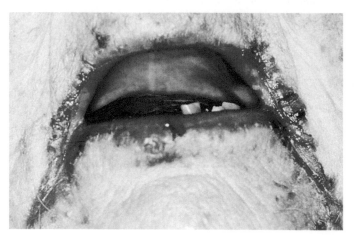

Figure 2.1.67 Angular stomatitis.

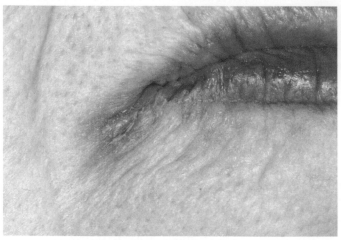

Figure 2.1.68 Angular stomatitis.

erythema, ulceration, crusting and scaling may be seen. Recurrent exudation and crusting are frequent. An eczematous dermatitis may extend some distance onto the cheek or chin as an infective eczematoid reaction or as a reaction to topical medicaments. In long-standing lesions, suppuration and granulation tissue may develop. Lesions occasionally extend beyond the vermilion border onto the skin in the form of linear furrows or fissures radiating from the angle of the mouth (rhagades) mainly in the more severe forms, especially in denture wearers.

Unilateral lesions are uncommon, usually induced by trauma and are short-lived.

*Diagnosis*
Diagnosis is usually by clinical examination alone. Inspection may reveal palatal erythema caused by associated denture-related stomatitis,

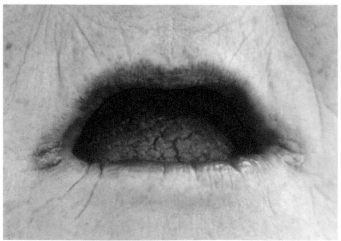

Figure 2.1.69 Angular stomatitis.

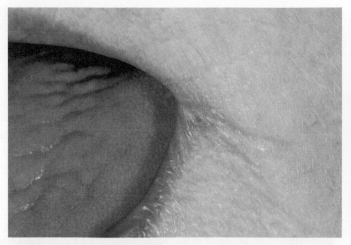

*Figure 2.1.70* Angular stomatitis.

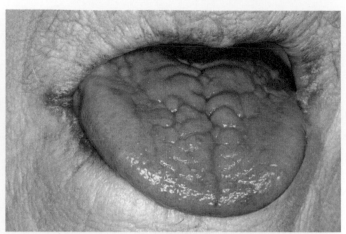

*Figure 2.1.71* Angular stomatitis.

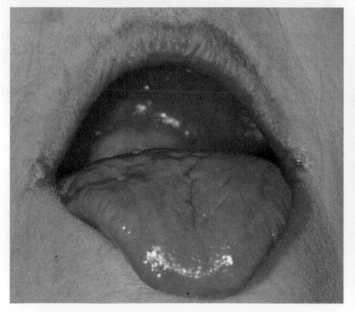

*Figure 2.1.72* Angular stomatitis in iron deficiency.

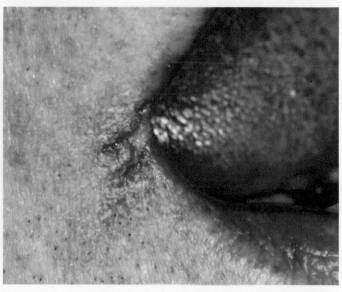

*Figure 2.1.73* Angular stomatitis.

usually due to candidosis. An underlying nutritional deficiency may be revealed by a depapillated tongue in iron deficiency, a depapillated glossy red tongue in folate deficiency or a reddish-purple depapillated tongue in vitamin B deficiency.

Angular cheilitis accompanied by alopecia, diarrhoea and non-specific oral ulcerations, most commonly of the tongue and buccal mucosa, suggests a zinc deficiency.

### Management

Mechanical predisposing factors should be corrected. A change in dentures may be necessary; new prostheses which restore facial contour may help. Underlying systemic disease must be sought and treated, and a course of oral iron and vitamin B supplements may be helpful in indolent cases.

If infection is the cause of angular cheilitis, treatment will only be effective if the underlying disease process is also treated. Mixed infections of Candida and Staphylococcus respond best to topical miconazole, and Staphylococcus infection alone clears with topical antibiotics such as fucidin. Denture-related stomatitis should be treated with both an anti-fungal application to the fitting surface of the denture together with nystatin or amphotericin tables or lozenges.

The skin lesions should be swabbed. Miconazole may be preferable treatment for candidosis (cream applied locally, together with the oral gel) as it has some Gram-positive bacteriostatic action but there is a high relapse rate unless treatment is prolonged. Miconazole is absorbed systemically and may occasionally potentiate the action of warfarin, phenytoin and the sulphonylureas. Polyenes such as nystatin or amphotericin (as cream or ointment) should, therefore, be tried first in patients taking these drugs. Staphylococcal infection can be treated with fusidic acid ointment or cream at least four times daily.

Recurrence of angular cheilitis must be prevented by eliminating organisms from their reservoir. Dentures harbour Candida and require

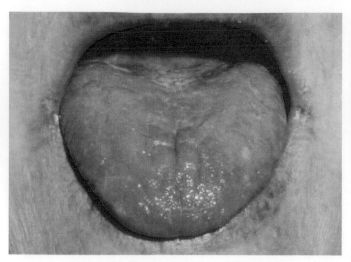

*Figure 2.1.74* Angular stomatitis in candidosis.

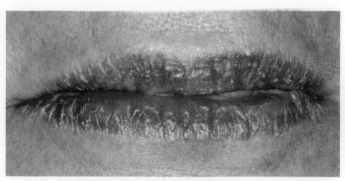

*Figure 2.1.75* Chapped lips.

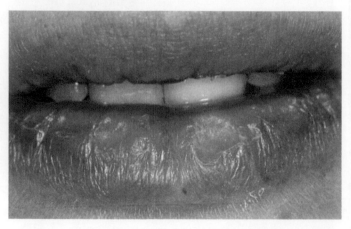

*Figure 2.1.76* Chapped lips.

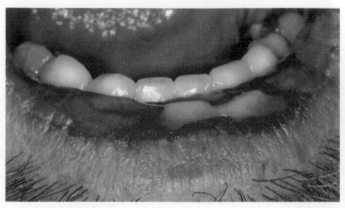

*Figure 2.1.77* Cheilitis—contact reaction to medicament.

proper disinfection. Dentures should be kept out of the mouth during sleep and stored in a candidacidal solution such as hypochlorite.

In rare intractable cases, surgery or occasionally collagen injections may be useful to try and restore normal commissural anatomy.

### Chapping of the lips

*Aetiopathogenesis*

Chapping is a lip reaction with scaling in response to adverse environmental conditions, usually exposure to freezing cold or hot, dry winds.

*Clinical features*

The lips become sore, cracked and scaly and the affected subject tends to lick the lips, or to pick or chew at the scales, which may aggravate the condition (Figs 2.1.75 and 2.1.76).

*Diagnosis*

Clinical.

*Management*

Application of an emollient such as petrolatum (petroleum jelly), avoidance of the causative environmental conditions and additional factitious damage usually suffice.

### Contact cheilitis

*Aetiopathogenesis*

Contact or allergic cheilitis is an inflammatory reaction of the lips provoked by the irritant or allergic sensitizing action of chemical agents, sometimes also with a phototoxic effect. Both type I and type IV hypersensitivity reactions may be responsible.

Many substances have been incriminated but most cases are caused by:

- lipsticks
- lip salves
- tartar-control toothpastes
- mouthwashes
- dental materials
- foods and flavourings
- cane reed instruments.

*Clinical features*

There may be labial erythema, oedema, vesicles, weeping, crusts, scales or fissures (Fig. 2.1.77).

*Diagnosis*

If an allergic reaction is suspected, skin patch tests using the appropriate concentrations of the substances concerned may be helpful.

*Management*

If the offending substance is identified and avoided, the inflammation will subside spontaneously. If needed, topical corticosteroids will both give symptomatic relief and calm inflammation. Mid-potency corticosteroids such as fludrocortisone, especially in ointment bases, are usually effective but should be restricted to short-term use since their long-term use can produce atrophy.

Cheilitis can arise as a result of drug allergy or as a pharmacological effect. Erythema multiforme, which is commonly caused by drugs, can produce haemorrhagic crusting of the lips.

## Exfoliative cheilitis

Exfoliative cheilitis (factitious cheilitis, le tic de lèvres).

*Aetiopathogenesis*

Exfoliative cheilitis is a chronic superficial inflammatory disorder characterized by hyperkeratosis and desquamation of the vermilion, with persistent scaling. Most cases occur in girls or young women, the majority of whom seem to have a personality disorder and indeed, a psychogenic

cause was proposed by the French, designating this 'le tic des levres' to indicate manipulation as being the basis. There appears to be no association with dermatological or systemic disease, though some cases are infected with Candida species and rare cases are seen in HIV disease.

In some cases the condition appears to start with chapping or with atopic eczema, and then develops into a habit tic. A preoccupation with the lips is prevalent in some individuals and many cases are thought to be factitious, caused by repeated self-induced trauma such as repetitive biting, picking, lip sucking, chewing or other manipulation of the lips. Exacerbations have been associated with stress and some have been shown to regress with psychotherapy and antianxiolytic or antidepressant treatment.

*Clinical features*

Exfoliative cheilitis often starts in the centre of the lower lip and spreads to involve the whole of the lower or of both lips. The patient may complain of irritation or burning and can be observed frequently biting or sucking the lips. Persistent scaling of the vermilion is seen (Figs 2.1.78–2.1.81) and may have a somewhat cyclical nature. The lips can be

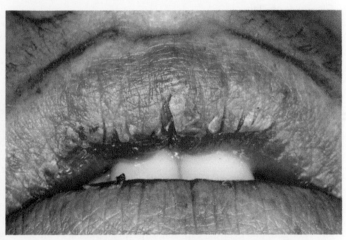

Figure 2.1.79  Exfoliative cheilitis.

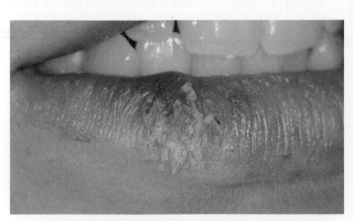

Figure 2.1.78  Exfoliative cheilitis.

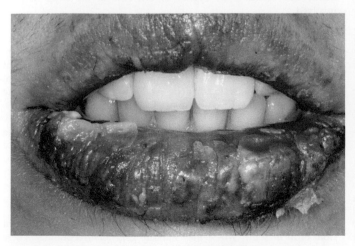

Figure 2.1.80  Exfoliative cheilitis.

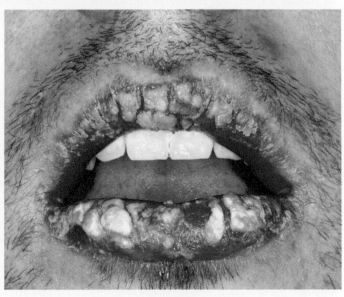

Figure 2.1.81  Exfoliative cheilitis.

covered with a shaggy yellowish coating. Lip scaling and crusting is more or less confined to the vermilion border, persisting in varying severity for months or years.

### Diagnosis

Similar superficial scaling may be present in actinic cheilitis, contact cheilitis, glandular cheilitis, lupus erythematosus, Candida infections and HIV infection. Biopsy is sometimes indicated.

### Management

Some cases resolve spontaneously or with improved oral hygiene. Reassurance and topical corticosteroids may be helpful in others but often exfoliative cheilitis is refractory to treatment, even including topical fluorinated corticosteroids. Indeed, the peeling in some cases is accentuated by topical medications.

When a factitial cause is suspected, a psychiatric consultation and care may be beneficial; some require psychotherapy, antidepressants or tranquillizers.

## Glandular cheilitis

Glandular cheilitis (cheilitis glandularis) is a rare, chronic inflammatory disorder of minor salivary glands in which there is mucus hypersecretion.

### Aetiopathogenesis

Cheilitis glandularis is an idiopathic condition which, in a few cases, has apparently been familial. It was originally thought that cheilitis glandularis was due to inflammation of enlarged heterotopic salivary glands, but the glands often appear normal in size, depth and histology. It is possible that the excessive salivary secretion from minor salivary glands in this condition might be an unusual clinical response to irritation of the lip from some other cause such as actinic damage, repeated licking, etc.

### Clinical features

Glandular cheilitis usually affects the lower lip. The lip appears swollen, enlarged, and everted, exposing superficial puncta of the salivary ducts along the mucosal vermilion border. The puncta may be macular or papular in appearance and may be topped with red, white or black dots and release thick sticky mucus that forms a crust on the lip surface as it dries.

The everted lip mucosa develops metaplasia and squamous cell carcinoma can arise (in some series in 20–30% of cases).

Three types of cheilitis glandularis are recognized:

1. The simple type (puente) consists of multiple asymptomatic papular lesions containing dilated minor salivary gland ducts.
2. The superficial suppurative type (Baelz) may present with superficial erosions, crust formation and induration, possibly representing secondary bacterial infection, followed by inflammation and enlargement of the lip.
3. The deep suppurative type (Volkman) includes abscess and fistulous tract formation. The lip is considerably and permanently enlarged, with episodes of pain, tenderness and increased swelling.

### Diagnosis

Biopsy is indicated. Histological findings range from no change to hypertrophy and hyperplasia of the minor salivary glands. In the milder forms there is often some fibrosis surrounding the salivary glands, and in the more severe forms there may be a dense, chronic, inflammatory infiltrate, but only rarely is there genuine salivary gland hyperplasia or ductal ectasia.

### Management

A wide range of modalities including cryosurgery have been used with limited success. Conservative approaches include systemic antibiotics, corticosteroids, antihistamines, lip balms and sunscreens. In advanced disease, surgery is the management of choice because of the risk of malignancy. If the lips are grossly enlarged, excision of an elongated ellipse of tissue may be required, and in other cases shave vermilionectomy may be all that is necessary.

## Granulomatous cheilitis

Granulomatous cheilitis (cheilitis granulomatosa).

### Aetiopathogenesis

Granulomatous cheilitis is an uncommon chronic swelling of the lip due to granulomatous inflammation from a range of aetiologies.

The cause of cheilitis granulomatosa is unknown, but there may be:

- a genetic predisposition
- Melkersson–Rosenthal syndrome (MRS)—the term used when there is cheilitis with facial palsy and plicated tongue. Melkersson described recurrent facial palsy in association with labial oedema and Rosenthal added plicated tongue to the syndrome. MRS is characterized by a triad, typically with an onset in childhood or youth, of recurrent facial paralysis (in 30% of cases), chronic oedema of face and lips, and fissured tongue (lingua plicata). It may have autosomal dominant inheritance with variable expressivity, there is a chronic granulomatous aetiopathogenesis and there is a suggestion of a responsible gene mapping to chromosome 9p11.
- Miescher cheilitis—the term used when the granulomatous changes are confined to the lip and is generally regarded as a monosymptomatic form of the MRS although the possibility remains that these may be two separate diseases.
- Crohn disease—regional ileitis may follow some years later.
- Orofacial granulomatosis.

### Clinical features

The onset is usually in young adult life and has no gender or racial predilection. Labial swelling occurs in about 75% and facial swelling in 50% of patients. The earliest manifestation is sudden diffuse or occasionally nodular swellings of the lip or face, involving in decreasing order of frequency, the upper lip, the lower lip and one or both cheeks. Less commonly the forehead, the eyelids or one side of the scalp may be involved.

Cheilitis granulomatosa is episodic with non-tender swelling and enlargement of one or both lips. The upper lip is involved slightly more often than the lower lip and may feel soft, firm or nodular on palpation. The normal lip architecture is eventually altered by the presence of lymphoedema and non-caseating granulomas in the lamina propria. Lingual, palatal, gingival and buccal involvement also may occur. At the first episode the oedema typically subsides completely in hours or days, but after recurrent attacks the swelling may persist, and slowly increases in degree (Figs 2.1.82–2.1.86). The swelling eventually becomes permanent. Recurrences can range from days to years; however, once chronicity is established, the enlarged lip appears cracked and fissured with reddish-brown discolouration and scaling. The fissured lip becomes painful. It eventually acquires the consistency of firm rubber. After some years, the swelling may very slowly regress.

There may be splitting of the lips and angular stomatitis.

A fissured or plicated tongue is seen in 20–40% of cases. It is present from birth in some, which may indicate genetic susceptibility. There may be loss of sense of taste and decreased salivary gland secretion.

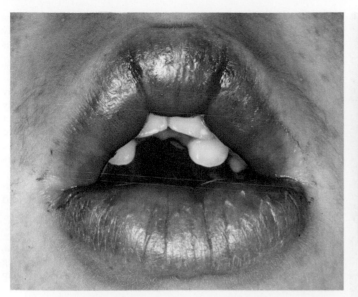

Figure 2.1.82 Cheilitis granulomatosa in orofacial granulomatosis.

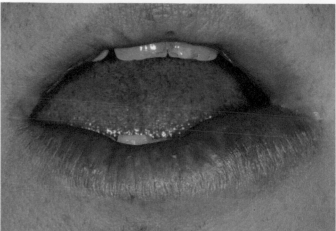

Figure 2.1.83 Cheilitis granulomatosa.

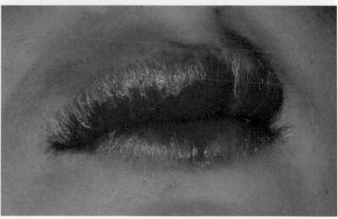

Figure 2.1.85 Cheilitis granulomatosa.

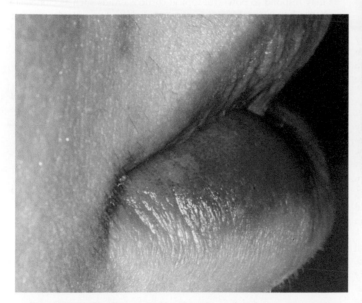

Figure 2.1.84 Cheilitis granulomatosa in orofacial granulomatosis.

Facial palsy of the lower motor-neurone type occurs in some 30% of cases. It may precede the attacks of oedema by months or years, but more commonly develops later. Though intermittent at first, the palsy may become permanent. It may be unilateral or bilateral, and partial or complete. Other cranial nerves (the olfactory, auditory, glossopharyngeal and hypoglossal) may occasionally be affected. Involvement of the central nervous system has also been reported, but the significance of the resulting symptoms is easily overlooked as they are very variable, sometimes simulating multiple sclerosis but often with a poorly defined association of psychotic and neurological features. Autonomic disturbances may occur.

### Diagnosis

The many causes of oedema of the lips make the diagnosis one based on exclusion, on clinical signs and on histological examination. The essential feature is the chronic non-tender swelling of lip or face. In the early attacks clinical differentiation from angioedema may be impossible in the absence of either plicated tongue or facial palsy but persistence of the swelling between attacks should suggest the diagnosis.

In the established cases, other causes of macrocheilia must be excluded. Ascher syndrome associated with blepharochalasia is likely to cause confusion—though the swelling of the lip is caused by redundant salivary tissue and is present from childhood. Lymphoma and amyloid disease are rare differential diagnoses.

Biopsy of the swollen lip or facial tissues is indicated but, during the early stages, shows only lymphoedema and perivascular lymphocytic infiltration. However, although the histological changes are not always conspicuous or specific in many cases of long duration, the infiltrate becomes more dense and pleomorphic and small focal granulomas are formed, indistinguishable from Crohn disease or sarcoidosis. In some cases, small granulomas occur in the lymphatic walls. Similar changes may be present in cervical lymph nodes.

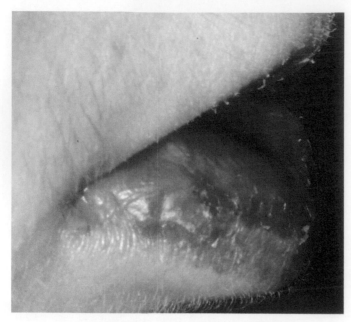

*Figure 2.1.86* Cheilitis granulomatosa.

Investigation of the gastrointestinal tract (endoscopy, radiography and biopsy) is mandatory to exclude Crohn disease. Investigations such as chest radiography, serum ACE and a gallium scan may be required to exclude sarcoidosis. Patch tests may be indicated to exclude reactions to various foodstuffs or additives.

### Management

MRS seems to respond well to corticosteroid treatment and occasionally systemic sulphasalazine or other antimicrobials (metronidazole, minocycline and rothixromycin), or other agents (clofazimine, ketotifen, infliximab or thalidomide) are required.

Surgery and irradiation have little place. Surgery alone is relatively unsuccessful and the best results are from reduction cheiloplasty with intralesional triamcinolone and systemic tetracycline. Corticosteroid injections must be given periodically after surgery or there may be an exaggerated recurrence.

Sarcoidosis—asymptomatic swelling of the parotid glands or cervical nodes, and less frequently the lips, may accompany systemic sarcoid. Superficial or deep seated red submucosal nodules may develop intraorally and on the lips. Non-tender, well circumscribed, brownish-red or violaceous nodules with superficial ulceration have also been reported on the lips in patients with sarcoidosis. The oral and lip lesions may occasionally precede systemic involvement. Biopsy of the minor salivary glands will reveal non-caseating granulomas in up to 20% of patients, even without lip involvement, particularly in those with hilar lymphadenopathy.

### Plasma cell cheilitis

Plasma cell cheilitis (plasma cell orificial mucositis).

### Aetiopathogenesis

Plasma cell cheilitis is a rare inflammatory disorder of the lips with a characteristic band-like infiltrate of plasma cells in the upper lamina propria/dermis. Plasma cell cheilitis is the counterpart of Zoon plasma cell balanitis and similar conditions (under a wide variety of names) can affect not only the penis, but also the vulva, buccal mucosa, palate, gingiva, tongue, epiglottis and larynx. The cause is unknown, presumably immunological. Precipitants may include a range of substances such as additives to cosmetics or dentifrices.

### Clinical features

Plasma cell cheilitis is a benign disorder that is not associated with any known dermatosis, but affects the lips and other mucosae close to body orifices—plasma cell orificial mucositis. It presents usually on the lower lip in an elderly person as glistening red circumscribed flat or raised patches. The lip may be thick and fissured with ulceration and may be accompanied by tenderness and sensitivity to certain foods. It also may involve the oral mucosa.

A similar lesion which tends to form a tumourous mass with a hyperkeratotic surface reportedly after trauma and needs to be differentiated from extramedullary plasmacytoma has been called *plasma-acanthoma*.

### Diagnosis

The possibility of a plasma cell dyscrasia and an underlying myeloma, and extramedullary plasmacytoma should be excluded. Underlying provocative factors should be identified: patch testing can be helpful in eliminating contact hypersensitivity factors.

### Management

Underlying provocative factors should be eliminated. Plasma cell cheilitis may respond to powerful topical corticosteroids such as clobetasol, or to the intralesional injection of triamcinolone. Interestingly, systemic corticosteroids are of variable benefit. The effectiveness of corticosteroid-sparing immunosuppressives is unclear.

### Nutritional cheilitis

Severe nutritional deficiency, especially pellagra, can cause the vermilion zone to become shiny and cracked, sometimes with eroded areas. Milder degrees of deficiency cause angular cheilitis. Oral ulcers and glossitis may also be present.

### Traumatic cheilitis

Trauma from habits such as lip-licking, use of various musical instruments and in some occupations may cause cheilitis.

## SWELLINGS AND LUMPS

Lip swelling may be caused by oedema (allergic, inflammatory or traumatic), deposits (e.g. amyloidosis) or neoplasms.

### Allergic angioedema

#### Aetiopathogenesis

Lip, facial and/or oral swelling may be a feature of hereditary angioedema (Chapter 2.1) and of allergic angioedema—a type 1 response mediated by leukotrienes and vasoactive amines released from mast cells and basophils in an IgE-mediated response to an allergen. Allergic angioedema may be induced by allergens such as:

- Foods; especially beef, pork or lamb. Reactions appear due to IgE antibodies to galactose-alpha-1,3-galactose (alpha-gal), a carbohydrate commonly expressed on non-primate mammalian proteins
- Food additives such as benzoic and sorbic acids
- Drugs
  - Antibiotics
  - Antihypertensives

o Captopril
o Doxorubicin
o Nonsteroidal anti-inflammatory drugs
o Opiates
o Sedatives
● Other allergens
o Vaccines.

Angioedema may be induced by a range of drugs, especially ACEIs, due to a rise in levels of bradykinins and/or altered levels or function of C1 esterase inhibitor. People of African heritage may be at particular risk. Defective degradation of vasoactive peptide substrates of ACE, such as bradykinin or substance P, may contribute via non-ACE pathways to the pathogenesis of ACEI-associated angioedema. Bradykinin and des-arginine 9-bradykinin, two powerful vasodilatory and pro-inflammatory peptides and substance P, substrates of ACE, increase vascular permeability and cause tissue oedema. The amino-terminal degradation of these peptides, by aminopeptidase P and dipeptidyl peptidase IV, may be impaired in people with ACEI-associated angioedema.

Orolingual angioedema is also a potentially life-threatening complication of alteplase (plasminogen activator) treatment in stroke patients, especially in those using ACEI.

*Clinical features*
Angioedema presents with the sudden onset of painless, circumscribed, non-pitting swelling of the face (around the eyes, chin and lips), tongue, feet, genitalia and trunk, which persists from a few hours to 2–3 days. Involvement of the upper airways can result in rapidly fatal respiratory obstruction and the risk of asphyxiation, unless appropriate interventions are taken.

*Diagnosis*
Clinical; from the rapid development of oedematous swelling, especially when there is a prior history. Angioedema is characterized by the transient nature of the swelling and the lack of scaling. Orolingual haematoma as a differential diagnosis can be excluded by CT scan.

*Management*
Mild angioedema—antihistamines or a sympathomimetic agent such as ephedrine.

Severe angioedema—intramuscular adrenaline (epinephrine) is the first line agent. Systemic corticosteroids or antihistamines are of lesser importance.

## Deposits
Amyloidosis and other deposits are rare causes of lip swelling.

## Haematoma
Haematoma (Chapter 2.2).

## Inflammatory causes
Labial swelling may be seen in infections such as odontogenic or cutaneous infections, or inflammatory conditions such as Crohn disease, orofacial granulomatosis or sarcoidosis.

## Neoplastic
Squamous cell carcinoma is the most common malignancy to affect the lip. It is seen particularly in older males but the male:female differential is declining.

*Aetiopathogenesis*
Lip cancer:

● involves the sun-exposed lower lip, more than the upper lip and may follow actinic cheilitis
● is seen more in outdoor workers and rural populations than in office workers or urban populations
● is seen more in fair-skinned than dark-skinned people.

Actinic radiation thus is a main risk factor but other factors may include low socio-economic class, tobacco smoking, syphilis, poor dentition, infection with HSV or human papillomaviruses (HPV) and immune suppression; for example, lip cancer is increased in immunosuppressed renal transplant recipients.

Genetic risk factors include xeroderma pigmentosum, recessive dystrophic epidermolysis bullosa, oculocutaneous albinism, discoid lupus erythematosus and cheilitis glandularis.

*Clinical features*
Lip carcinoma affects the lower lip in 90% and typically presents with thickening, induration, crusting or ulceration, usually at the vermilion border of the lower lip just to one side of midline. A lip carcinoma can, however, present in many ways (Figs 2.1.87–2.1.95), including as a:

● nodule
● ulcer
● red plaque
● white plaque
● fissure.

Metastasis is primarily to submental and submandibular lymph nodes.

*Diagnosis*
Lip carcinoma must be differentiated from herpes labialis, keratoacanthoma, basal cell carcinoma and chronic infections such as deep mycoses.

Biopsy is invariably indicated. It is also crucial to determine whether cervical lymph nodes are involved, or if there are other primary neoplasms in the upper aerodigestive tract, or metastases elsewhere.

*Management*
Carcinoma of the lip is readily treated by surgery and/or irradiation. Patients with carcinoma of the lip tend to present early and the prognosis is usually good, with 5-year survival rates ranging from 70% to 90%.

## Other neoplasms
Lymphomas, salivary gland neoplasms, Kaposi sarcoma and other neoplasms are uncommon causes of lip swelling.

## Pyogenic granulomas
Pyogenic granulomas (Fig. 2.1.96) (Chapter 2.3).

## Silicone granulomas
Facial cosmetic procedures may include injection of dimethicone—the liquid form of silicone (dimethylpolysiloxane)—or other fillers for soft tissue augmentation. This material can induce a granulomatous inflammatory response. The diagnosis of the granulomatous foreign-body reactions may be challenging because of their microscopic resemblance to liposarcoma. Topical imiquimod has been successfully used to treat this.

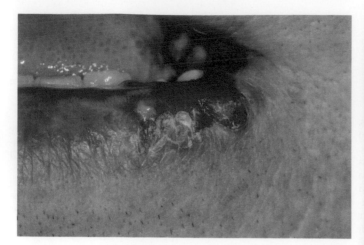

*Figure 2.1.87* Carcinoma of the lip.

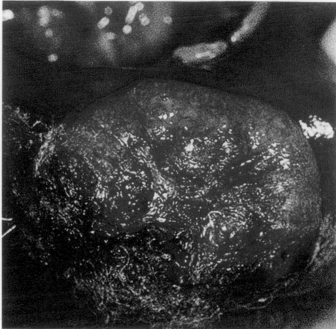

*Figure 2.1.88* Carcinoma of the lip.

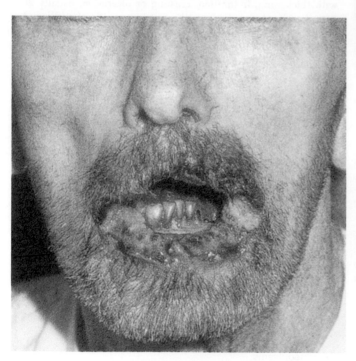

*Figure 2.1.89* Carcinoma of the lip.

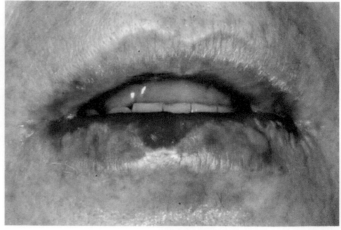

*Figure 2.1.90* Carcinoma of the lip.

### Traumatic

Trauma is a common cause of lip swelling. Child abuse (or other non-accidental injury) may need to be excluded: bruised and swollen lips, lacerated fraenum and even subluxed teeth or fractured jaws can be features.

### Warts

HPV can be responsible for warts on the lips (Figs 2.1.97–2.1.100).

## WHITE LESIONS

### Actinic cheilitis

Actinic cheilitis (page 194).

### Candidosis

Candidosis (Chapter 1.8).

### Carcinoma

Carcinoma (Chapter 2.3).

### Leukoplakia

Leukoplakia (Figs 2.1.101–2.1.104) (Chapter 2.2).

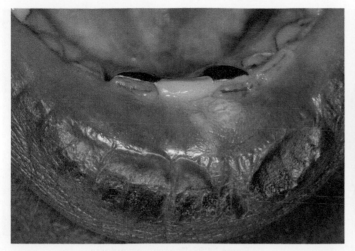

*Figure 2.1.91* Carcinoma of the lip.

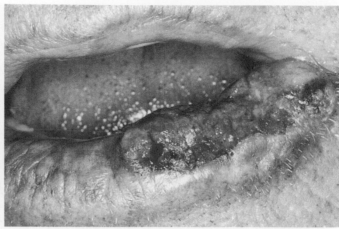

*Figure 2.1.92* Carcinoma of the lip.

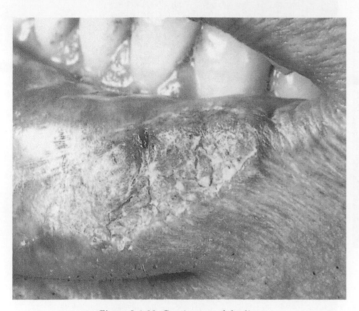

*Figure 2.1.93* Carcinoma of the lip.

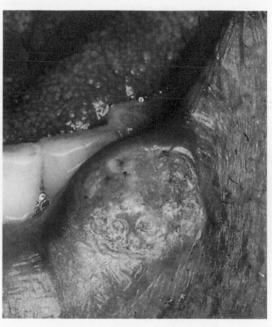

*Figure 2.1.94* Carcinoma of the lip.

### Lichen planus
Lichen planus (Figs 2.1.105–2.1.107) (Chapter 1.10).

### Venous lake
Venous lake (Fig. 2.1.108).

Seen mainly on the lower lip in older people, this is similar to an angioma.

### Vitiligo
Vitiligo is typically autoimmune and may occasionally affect the lips (Figs 2.1.109 and 2.1.110). Melanocytes, pigment epithelium of retina and choroid all derive developmentally from the neural crest, and share the susceptibility to damage in vitiligo, a common acquired disorder. Vitiligo is characterized by well-marginated milky white spots on the skin resulting from loss of melanocytes and is associated with the risk of ocular abnormalities and some autoimmune disorders and retinal pigmentary anomalies in the absence of ophthalmologic complaints may be detected in some patients. Autoimmune diseases like thyroid diseases, Addison disease, pernicious anaemia and insulin-dependent diabetes mellitus may be seen and auto antibodies against other organs may be detected in the absence of clinical evidence of the diseases. Premature greying of the hair and alopecia areata are important cutaneous associations in some patients.

The commonest modality of treatment is systemic or topical psoralen and UVA (PUVA) therapy, which consists of use of psoralen compounds followed by exposure to UV radiation in the 320–400 nm range (UVA).

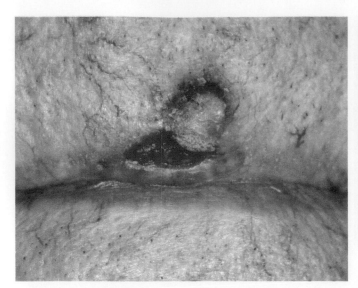

Figure 2.1.95 Carcinoma of the lip.

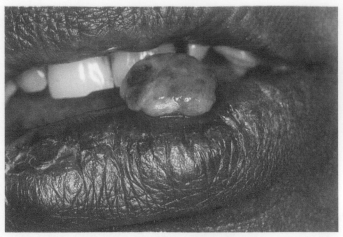

Figure 2.1.96 Pyogenic granuloma.

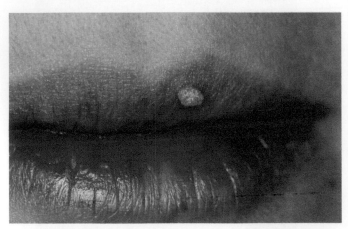

Figure 2.1.97 Human papillomavirus infection—verruca vulgaris.

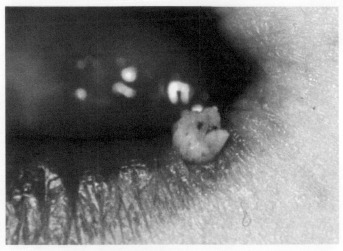

Figure 2.1.98 Human papillomavirus infection—wart.

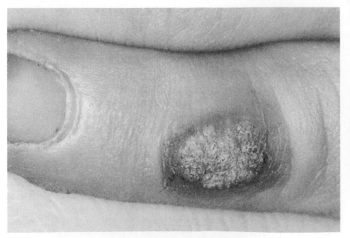

Figure 2.1.99 Human papillomavirus infection—wart.

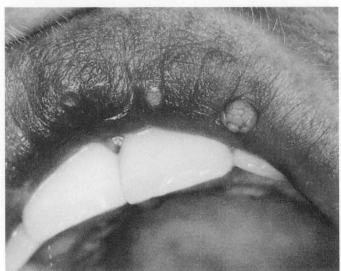

Figure 2.1.100 Human papillomavirus infection—wart.

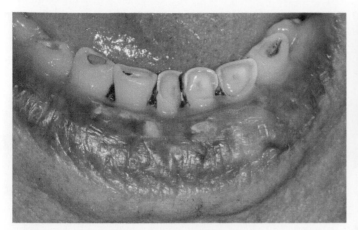

Figure 2.1.101  Leukoplakia.

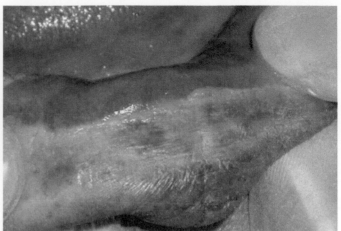

Figure 2.1.102  Leukoplakia.

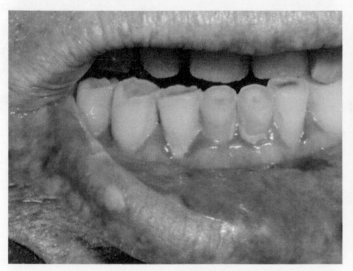

Figure 2.1.103  Leukoplakia.

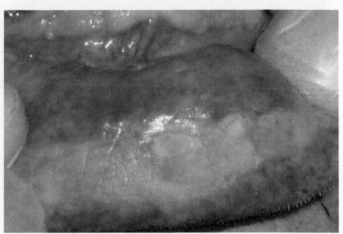

Figure 2.1.104  Leukoplakia.

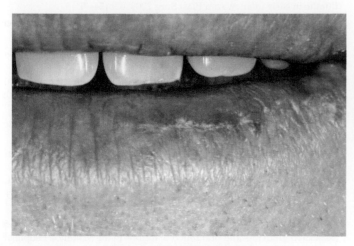

Figure 2.1.105  Lichen planus.

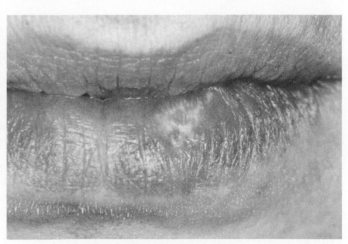

Figure 2.1.106  Lichen planus.

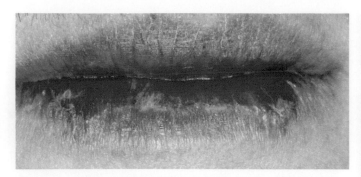

*Figure 2.1.107* Lichen planus.

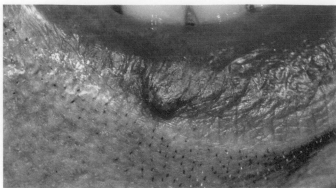

*Figure 2.1.108* Venous lake.

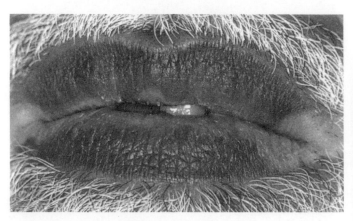

*Figure 2.1.109* Vitiligo.

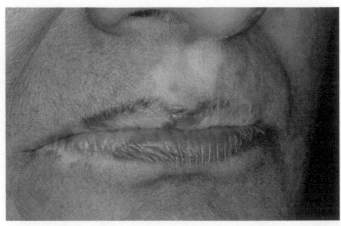

*Figure 2.1.110* Vitiligo.

Corticosteroids are also used in the management of vitiligo. Multiple surgical modalities are also available for selected patients.

**White sponge naevus**
White sponge naevus (Chapter 1.10).

## FURTHER READING

Ah-Weng A, Natarajan S, Velangi S, Langtry JA. Venous lakes of the vermillion lip treated by infrared coagulation. Br J Oral Maxillofac Surg 2004; 42: 251–3.

Andrade ES, Sobral AP, Laureano Filho JR, Santos ME, Camargo IB. Cheilitis glandularis and actinic cheilitis: differential diagnoses—report of three unusual cases. Dermatol Online J 2009; 15: 5.

Antunes LA, Kuchler EC, de Andrade Risso P, Maia LC. Oral chemical burns caused by self-medication in a child: case report. J Burn Care Res 2009; 30: 740–3.

Arduino PG, Porter SR. Oral and perioral herpes simplex virus type 1 (HSV-1) infection: review of its management. Oral Dis 2006; 12: 254–70.

Arduino PG, Porter SR. Herpes simplex virus type 1 infection: overview on relevant clinico-pathological features. J Oral Pathol Med 2008; 37: 107–21.

Ayangco L, Rogers 3rd RS. Oral manifestations of erythema multiforme. Dermatol Clin 2003; 21: 195–205.

Bukar A, Danfillo IS, Adeleke OA, Ogunbodede EO. Traditional oral health practices among Kanuri women of Borno State, Nigeria. Odontostomatol Trop 2004; 27: 25–31.

Chen WL, Zhang B, Li JS, et al. Liquid nitrogen cryotherapy of lip mucosa hemangiomas under inhalation general anesthesia with sevoflurane in early infancy. Ann Plast Surg 2009; 62: 154–7.

Combes J, Mellor TK. Treatment of chronic lip fissures with carbon dioxide laser. Br J Oral Maxillofac Surg 2009; 47: 102–5.

Comi AM. Pathophysiology of Sturge–Weber syndrome. J Child Neurol 2003; 18: 509–16.

Crinzi RA, Palm NV, Mostofi R, Indresano AT. Management of a dental infection in a patient with Sturge–Weber disease. J Am Dent Assoc 1980; 101: 798–800.

Dahan D, Fenichel GM, El-Said R. Neurocutaneous syndromes. Adolesc Med 2002; 13: 495–509.

De Moor RJ, De Witte AM, Delmé KI, et al. Dental and oral complications of lip and tongue piercings. Br Dent J 2005; 199: 506–9.

Dibart S, De Feo P, Surabian G, et al. Oral piercing and gingival recession: review of the literature and a case report. Quintessence Int 2002; 33: 110–12.

Fabian FM, Mumghamba EG. Tooth and lip mutilation practices and associated tooth loss and oral mucosal lesions in the Makonde People of southeast Tanzania. East Afr Med J 2007; 84: 183–7.

Farrier JN, Perkins CS. Plasma cell cheilitis. Br J Oral Maxillofac Surg 2008; 46: 679–80.

Glass LF, Maize JC. Morsicatio buccarum et labiorum (excessive cheek and lip biting). Am J Dermatopathol 1991; 13: 271–4.

Hodgson TA, Malik F, Hegarty AM, Porter SR. Topical tacrolimus: a novel therapeutic intervention for recalcitrant labial pemphigus vulgaris. Eur J Dermatol 2003; 13: 142–4.

Kaugars GE, Heise AP, Riley WT, Abbey LM, Svirsky JA. Oral melanotic macules. A review of 353 cases. Oral Surg Oral Med Oral Pathol 1993; 76: 59–61.

Kaugars GE, Pillion T, Svirsky JA, et al. Actinic cheilitis: a review of 152 cases. Oral Surg Oral Med Oral Pathol Oral Radiol Endod 1999; 88: 181–6.

Kuo HW, Yang CH. Venous lake of the lip treated with a sclerosing agent: report of two cases. Dermatol Surg 2003; 29: 425–8.

Leão JC, Ferreira AM, Martins S, et al. Cheilitis glandularis: an unusual presentation in a patient with HIV infection. Oral Surg Oral Med Oral Pathol Oral Radiol Endod 2003; 95: 142–4.

Levin L, Zadik Y, Becker T. Oral and dental complications of intra-oral piercing. Dent Traumatol 2005; 21: 341–3.

Levine N. White lesions on the lip. Geriatrics 2001; 56: 16.

López-Pintor R, Hernández G, de Arriba L, de Andrés A. Comparison of oral lesion prevalence in renal transplant patients under immunosuppressive therapy and healthy controls. Oral Dis 2009; Jul 27. [Epub ahead of print].

Martins WD, Westphalen FH, Westphalen VP. Microstomia caused by swallowing of caustic soda: report of a case. J Contemp Dent Pract 2003; 4: 91–9.

Martis J, Bhat R, Nandakishore B, Shetty JN. A clinical study of vitiligo. Indian J Dermatol Venereol Leprol 2002; 68: 92–3.

Olivier JH. Fordyce granules on the prolabial and oral mucous membranes of a selected population. SADJ 2006; 61: 072–4.

Ophaswongse S, Maibach HI. Allergic contact cheilitis. Contact Dermatitis 1995; 33: 365–70.

Ozgür F, Tunçbilek G. Bilateral congenital pits of the upper lip. Ann Plast Surg 2000; 45: 658–61.

Petruzzi M, De Benedittis M, Pastore L, et al. Isolated lichen planus of the lip. Int J Immunopathol Pharmacol 2007; 20: 631–5.

Porter SR, Scully C, Kainth B, Ward-Booth P. Multiple salivary mucoceles in a young boy. Int J Paediatr Dent 1998; 8: 149–51.

Rocha N, Mota F, Horta M, et al. Plasma cell cheilitis. J Eur Acad Dermatol Venereol 2004; 18: 96–8.

Rogers 3rd RS, Bekic M. Diseases of the lips. Semin Cutan Med Surg 1997; 16: 328–36.

Scully C. A review of common mucocutaneous disorders affecting the mouth and lips. Ann Acad Med Singapore 1999; 28: 704–7.

Scully C, van Bruggen W, Diz Dios P, et al. Down syndrome: lip lesions (angular stomatitis and fissures) and Candida albicans. Br J Dermatol 2002; 147: 37–40.

Scully C, Eisen D, Rogers R, Porter SR, Bagan J. Dermatology of the Lips. Oxford: Isis Medical Media, 2000: 1–180.

Scully C, el-Kabir M, Samaranayake LP. Candida and oral candidosis: a review. Crit Rev Oral Biol Med 1994; 5: 125–57.

Shulman JD, Lewis DL, Carpenter WM. The prevalence of chapped lips during an army hot weather exercise. Mil Med 1997; 162: 817–19.

Sun ZJ, Zhang L, Zhang WF, et al. Epithelioid hemangioendothelioma of the oral cavity. Oral Dis 2007; 13: 244–50.

Taniguchi S, Kono T. Exfoliative cheilitis: a case report and review of the literature. Dermatology 1998; 196: 253–5.

Thomas-Sohl KA, Vaslow DF, Maria BL. Sturge–Weber syndrome: a review. Pediatr Neurol 2004; 30: 303–10.

Van Doorne L, De Maeseneer M, Stricker C, Vanrensbergen R, Stricker M. Diagnosis and treatment of vascular lesions of the lip. Br J Oral Maxillofac Surg 2002; 40: 497–503.

Venning VA, Frith PA, Bron AJ, Millard PR, Wojnarowska F. Mucosal involvement in bullous and cicatricial pemphigoid. A clinical and immunopathological study. Br J Dermatol 1988; 118: 7–15.

van der Waal RI, Schulten EA, van der Meij EH, et al. Cheilitis granulomatosa: overview of 13 patients with long-term follow-up—results of management. Int J Dermatol 2002; 41: 225–9.

Yu TC, Kelly SC, Weinberg JM, Scheinfeld NS. Isolated lichen planus of the lower lip. Cutis 2003; 71: 210–12.

Zadik Y. Iatrogenic lip and facial burns caused by an overheated surgical instrument. J Calif Dent Assoc 2008; 36: 689–91.

# 2.2 ORAL MUCOSA

- aesthetic conditions
- blisters
- pigmented, red, purple or blue lesions
- soreness, ulceration and pain
- swellings and lumps
- white lesions

Complete visualization with a good source of light is essential for examination of the oral mucosa, which is most readily inspected if the mouth is held half-open. All mucosal surfaces should be examined, starting away from the location of any known lesions. If the patient wears any removable prostheses these must be removed in the first instance, although it may be necessary later to replace the prostheses to assess fit, function and relationship to any lesion. The labial mucosa, buccal mucosa, floor of mouth and ventrum of tongue, dorsal surface of the tongue, hard and soft palates, gingivae and teeth should be examined in sequence (Figs 2.2.1–2.2.4).

The intraoral mucosa is divided into masticatory, lining and specialized types. *Masticatory mucosa* (hard palate, gingiva) is adapted to the forces of pressure and friction and is keratinized. *Lining mucosa* (buccal, labial and alveolar mucosa, floor of mouth, ventral surface of tongue, soft palate, lips) is non-keratinized.

The vascular pattern and minor salivary glands so prominent in the labial mucosa are not obvious in the buccal mucosa but Fordyce spots may be conspicuous, particularly near the commissures and retromolar regions in adults.

Place the surface of a dental mirror against the buccal (cheek) mucosa; the mirror should lift off easily but, if it adheres to the mucosa, then xerostomia is present.

## AESTHETIC CONDITIONS

### Body art

Body piercing is a cause of some concern since bleeding or oedema can occasionally be pronounced, widespread and a hazard to the airway. Thereafter, the permanent jewellery is placed and worn constantly, to avoid the perforation closing over spontaneously. Speech can be impaired and the teeth and gingiva may be damaged by the jewellery. Pyogenic granulomas can occasionally arise about the jewellery.

## BLISTERS

Blisters on the oral mucosa may have various causes but burns, mucoceles, erythema multiforme, epidermolysis bullosa, angina bullosa haemorrhagica and autoimmune skin disorders (pemphigoid and pemphigus especially) may need to be excluded.

## PIGMENTED, RED, PURPLE OR BLUE LESIONS

### Addison disease

Addison disease (Chapter 1.2).

### Betel nut effects

Betel use, typically in a quid with tobacco, not only causes discolouration of the oral mucosa and teeth (Fig. 2.2.5), but can also predispose to potentially malignant disorders such as oral submucous fibrosis (OSMF)

and leukoplakia, and also to oral carcinoma. Betel users are also predisposed to a number of systemic problems, including:

- Cancer and potentially malignant conditions
  - OSMF
  - oral cancer
  - oesophageal cancer
  - pancreatic cancer
  - hepatocellular cancer
- Cardiovascular and diabetes
  - hypertension
  - metabolic syndrome
- Adverse birth outcomes
  - lower male to female sex ratio
  - lower birth weight
  - reduced birth length
- Others
  - liver cirrhosis
  - chronic kidney disease
  - contact dermatitis
  - periodontitis
  - urinary calculi (related to use of calcium hydroxide 'chuna' in the betel quid).

### Candidosis

Some forms of candidosis such as erythematous candidosis (EC) (Figs 2.2.6 and 2.2.7) produce red mucosal lesions. Dental appliance wearing, smoking, dry mouth, antibiotics or corticosteroids (Chapter 1.6) as well as systemic immunodeficiencies can predispose to EC which may particularly be seen in the palate or on the tongue as red, depapillated areas on the dorsum (Fig. 2.2.8). Lesions are often asymptomatic but a moderate growth of Candida can be demonstrated on culture from the lesions. EC may be seen in smokers, diabetics and others who are immunocompromised, and is the commonest maxillofacial manifestation of HIV disease. Treatment is with antiseptics such as chlorhexidine and topical antifungal drugs, along with treatment of the underlying disorder such as HIV or diabetes mellitus. Smoking cessation should also be encouraged.

### Drug-induced hyperpigmentation

Superficial (extrinsic) mucosal staining may be caused particularly by chlorhexidine, betel and tobacco use and also iron, bismuth subsalicylate, some antimicrobial agents and various other substances.

Facial and/or oral intrinsic hyperpigmentation may be caused in particular by drugs (see Section 3.5), such as:

- adrenocorticotrophic hormone
- antimalarials
- busulphan
- chemicals (various)
- clofazimine
- contraceptive pill
- ketoconazole

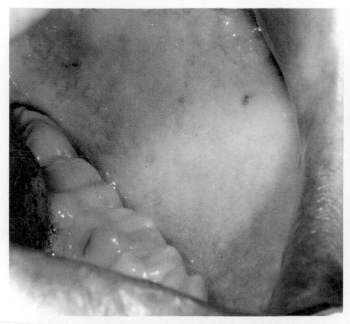

*Figure 2.2.1* Normal buccal mucosa.

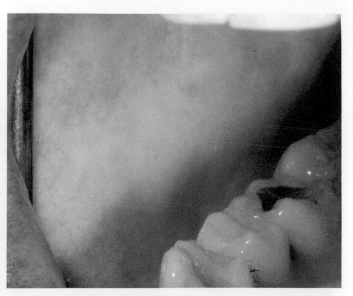

*Figure 2.2.2* Normal buccal mucosa.

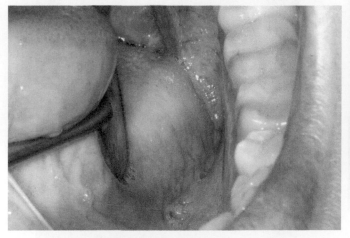

*Figure 2.2.3* Normal floor of mouth.

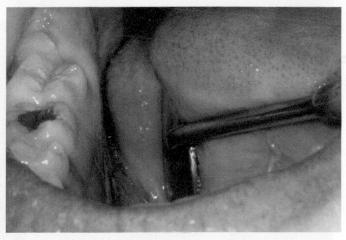

*Figure 2.2.4* Normal floor of mouth.

- minocycline
- phenothiazines
- phenytoin
- zidovudine.

Various chemicals which may produce hyperpigmentation and a photosensitive dermatitis include furocumarine, bergamot oil and eugenol—which may be found in perfumes, sprays, creams, mouthwashes and breath fresheners.

Chloasma (perioral hyperpigmentation) may arise during pregnancy or in patients using the oral contraceptive or various other products (see Section 3.5 and Chapter 1.2). It may rarely be a feature of healthy individuals not receiving medication.

Bismuth and lead caused a line at the gingival margin where sulphides deposited in areas of poor oral hygiene. Arsenic binds to keratins and chronic intoxication leads to mucositis, pigmentation and facial oedema. Arsenic poisoning causes 'rain-drop' hyperpigmentation of the skin with hyperkeratosis of the palms and soles and white transverse striae on the nails (Mees' lines). Arsenic poisoning is now rare and usually follows the ingestion of pesticides containing arsenates.

Minocycline is taken up by bone which it can stain black, and this may show through the mucosa. There have been occasional reports of mucosal hyperpigmentation unrelated to bone involvement (e.g. on the tongue).

### Erythroplasia

Erythroplasia (erythroplakia) is the oral lesion with the most severe epithelial dysplasia and greatest predilection to develop to carcinoma: it contains areas of dysplasia, carcinoma in situ or invasive carcinoma in virtually every instance.

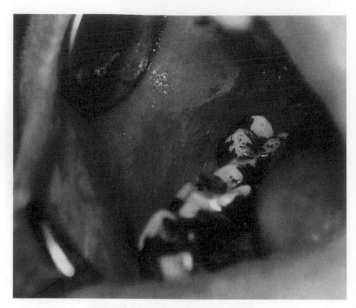

*Figure 2.2.5* Drug staining—betel use.

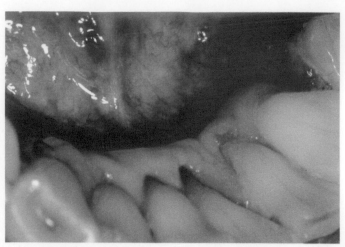

*Figure 2.2.6* Candidosis beneath a lower denture.

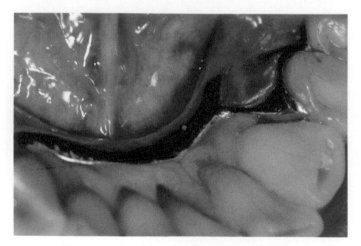

*Figure 2.2.7* Candidosis—patient from Figure 2.2.6.

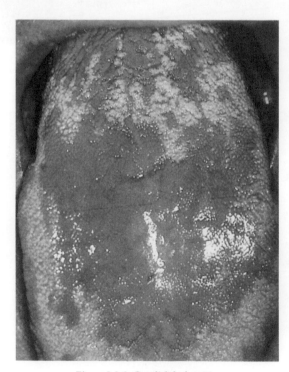

*Figure 2.2.8* Candidal glossitis.

*Aetiopathogenesis*
Tobacco and alcohol use are often implicated.

*Clinical features*
Erythroplastic lesions are well-defined velvety red plaques. Some erythroplakias are associated with white patches, and are then termed speckled leukoplakia. Erythroplasia is seen mainly in older males, usually in the buccal mucosa (Fig. 2.2.9) or palate.

*Diagnosis*
Similar clinical appearances can be seen in inflammatory and atrophic lesions (e.g. in deficiency anaemias, geographic tongue and lichen planus). A biopsy should be undertaken to confirm the diagnosis and histopathologically detect epithelial dysplasia or carcinoma.

*Management*
Any possible causal factor such as tobacco use should be stopped. The lesion should be removed, though there is no reliable evidence for the efficacy of this approach. It is likely that similar disease will develop at the same, or another, oral mucosal site at some time following removal of the original lesion.

There is also no hard evidence as to the ideal frequency of follow-up, but it has been suggested that patients with mucosal potentially malignant disorders be clinically re-examined:

- within 1 month
- at 3 months

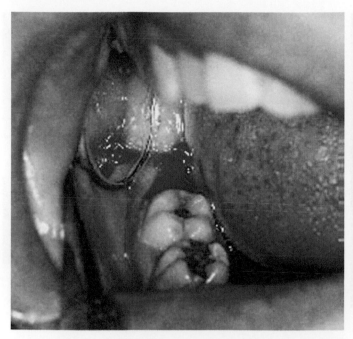

*Figure 2.2.9* Erythroplasia (erythroplakia).

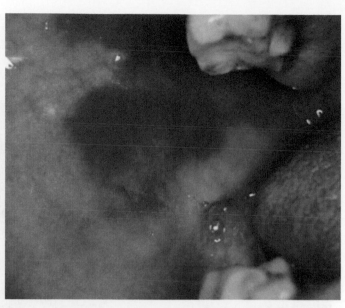

*Figure 2.2.10* Trauma from local anaesthetic injection—causing haematoma.

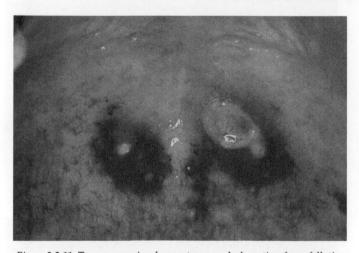

*Figure 2.2.11* Trauma causing haematoma and ulceration from fellatio.

- at 6 months
- at 12 months
- at least annually thereafter.

### Haematomas
Haematomas (Figs 2.2.10–2.2.12) (Chapter 1.4).

### Haemangioma
Haemangioma (Figs 2.2.13 and 2.2.14) (Chapter 2.1).

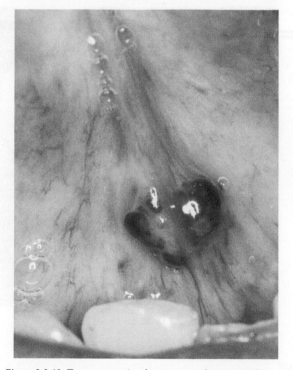

*Figure 2.2.12* Trauma causing haematoma from cunnilingus.

### Melanoacanthoma
Melanoacanthoma (Fig. 2.2.15) (Chapter 2.1).

### Melanotic macules
Melanotic macules (Figs 2.2.16 and 2.2.17) (Chapter 2.1).

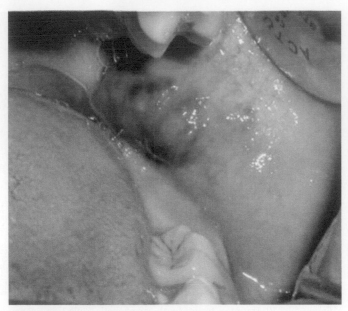

*Figure 2.2.13* Haemangioma.

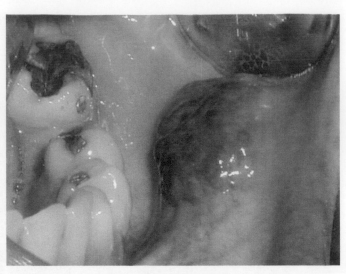

*Figure 2.2.14* Haemangioma.

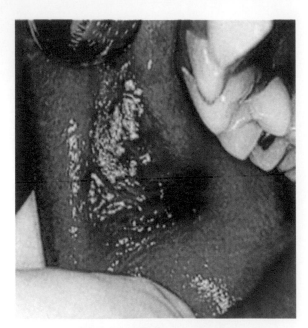

*Figure 2.2.15* Melanoacanthoma.

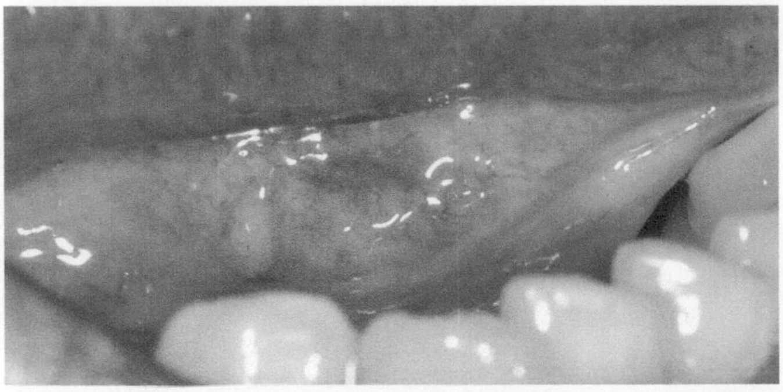

*Figure 2.2.16* Melanotic macule.

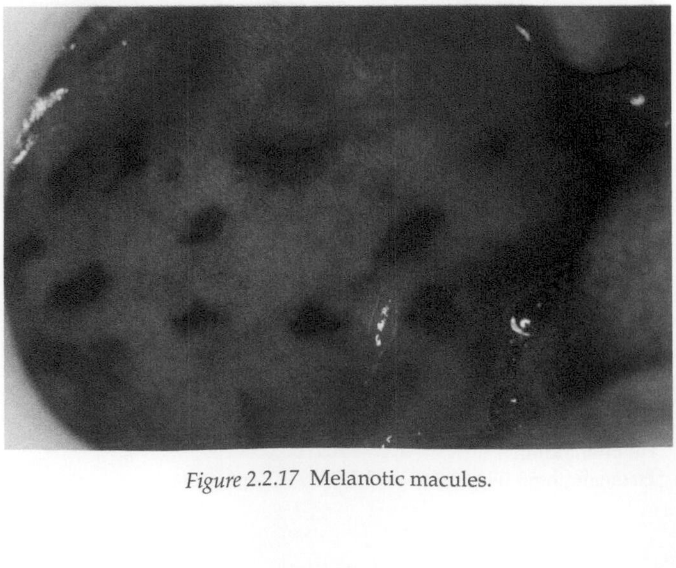

## Naevi

*Aetiopathogenesis*

Congenital. Approximately half of the naevi are histologically of the intradermal (intramucosal) type; one-third are blue naevi, many others are compound naevi and some are junctional naevi.

*Clinical features*

Most intraoral melanotic naevi are benign, circumscribed, small, greyish or brownish macules seen on the hard palate or in the buccal mucosa (Fig. 2.2.18).

*Figure 2.2.17* Melanotic macules.

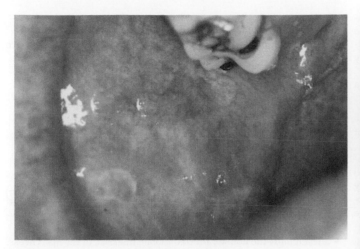

*Figure 2.2.18* Naevi.

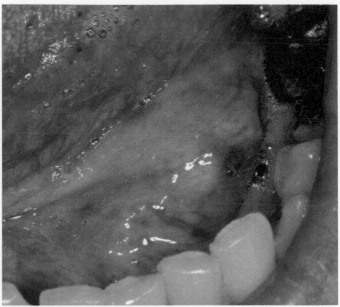

*Figure 2.2.19* Amalgam tattoo.

The most common are intramucosal naevi, seen typically in the palate or buccal mucosa as brown macules or papules. Less common are oral melanotic macules, intramucosal naevus and compound, junctional and blue naevi and naevi of Ota.

Naevi of Ota are seen mainly in young female Japanese, affect the first or second divisions of the trigeminal nerve with pigmentation of the choroid and iris (oculodermal melanocytosis).

*Diagnosis*
Clinical plus biopsy.

*Management*
Excision or observation. Few pigmented naevi progress to melanoma.

**Pigmentary incontinence**
Pigmentary incontinence may rarely be seen in lichen planus and can persist after the lichen planus has resolved.

**Tattoos**
*Aetiopathogenesis*
Dental amalgam can be incorporated into the tissues accidentally during conservative dentistry procedures and is a common cause of acquired oral hyperpigmentation. Other foreign bodies may result from facial trauma and may even enter the maxillary antrum. In soft tissues they can lead to hyperpigmented lesions: for example, palatal pigmentation from graphite (a pencil lead) is occasionally seen.

*Clinical features*
Amalgam tattoo usually appears as a bluish-black macule in the gingiva or vestibule, especially in the mandible in the premolar–molar region (Fig. 2.2.19). If used as a retrograde root-filling material as it was in the past, amalgam may cause discolouration high on the alveolar mucosa towards the vestibule.

*Diagnosis*
Clinical plus imaging—but not all amalgam tattoos show on radiography.

*Management*
Excision if the diagnosis is uncertain.

# SORENESS, ULCERATION AND PAIN
**Allergic reactions**
Latex, and other rubber products, such as dental dam, eugenol and other essential oils, various dentifrices, mouthwashes and cosmetics occasionally induce allergic reactions in the oral mucosa (see also Chapter 1.6). Drugs rarely may induce a fixed drug eruption.

Orofacial granulomatosis may have a background in hypersensitivity to components of some food and drinks (Chapters 1.3 and 2.1).

**Aphthae**
Aphthae [recurrent aphthae, recurrent aphthous stomatitis (RAS)].

*Aetiopathogenesis*
The aetiology of RAS is not entirely clear, and, therefore, they are termed 'idiopathic'. There is no evidence that RAS is a classical autoimmune disease, since there is no association with systemic autoimmune disorders, none of the common autoantibodies are found, and RAS may resolve spontaneously with increasing age.

Despite many studies trying to identify a causal micro-organism, RAS does not at present appear to be infectious, contagious or sexually transmitted. However, cross-reacting antigens between the oral mucosa and micro-organisms may be involved. Reactions to heat shock proteins (HSP) is one possibility. Patients with RAS have circulating lymphocytes reactive with peptide 91–105 of HSP 65-60.

It seems likely that a minor degree of immunological dysregulation underlies aphthae. Immune mechanisms that appear to play a role in people with a genetic predisposition to oral ulceration include:

- T-helper cells (gamma-delta cells), which predominate in the early RAS lesions, along with some natural killer (NK) cells.
- Cytotoxic cells then appear in the lesions and there is evidence for an antibody-dependent cellular cytotoxicity reaction.
- Mononuclear cells, T-cells, neutrophils and NK cells may, therefore, be involved.

RAS may not be a single condition but rather may be the manifestation of a group of disorders of quite different aetiology. There are also patients who suffer from aphthous-like ulcers (ALU) in systemic disorders such as HIV infection, Behçet syndrome and auto-inflammatory syndromes.

A number of predisposing factors can be identified—but in only a minority of patients with RAS.

- There is a genetic predisposition to RAS, as shown by a positive family history in about one-third of patients and an increased frequency of human leukocyte antigen (HLA) types (HLA-A2, A11, B12 and DR2).
- In up to 20% of patients; deficiencies of iron, folic acid (folate) or vitamin B (haematinics) may be found. Iron deficiency is usually due to chronic haemorrhage (e.g. from the gastrointestinal or genitourinary tract). Folic acid deficiencies may be dietary, or related to malabsorption or drugs (alcohol, anticonvulsants, carbamazepine and some cytotoxic drugs). Vitamin $B_{12}$ deficiency can arise particularly in vegans, in pernicious anaemia, after gastrectomy, and in ileal disease (e.g. Crohn's disease). Imerslund–Grasbeck syndrome is a rare autosomal recessive familial syndrome caused by selective malabsorption of vitamin $B_{12}$ resulting in megaloblastic anaemia (juvenile pernicious anaemia). Histamine $H_2$ receptor antagonists (cimetidine, ranitidine and omeprazole) can also impede vitamin $B_{12}$ absorption.
- In about 3% of patients with RAS, coeliac disease (gluten-sensitive enteropathy)—an allergic reaction to gluten in wheat—is seen.
- Cessation of smoking may precipitate or exacerbate RAS in some cases, but the reason is unclear.
- Psychological stress may underlie some cases of RAS and ulcers appear to exacerbate during school or university examination times.
- Trauma from biting the mucosa or from dental appliances (e.g. orthodontic) may lead to some aphthae.
- Endocrine factors are relevant in a small number of women where RAS are related to the fall in progestogen level in the luteal phase of the menstrual cycle, or to the contraceptive pill, and then RAS may regress temporarily in pregnancy.
- Allergies to food occasionally underlie RAS, and there is a high incidence of atopy.
- Sodium lauryl sulphate (SLS), a detergent in some oral healthcare products, may produce oral ulceration, in a small number of individuals.

### Clinical features

Patients with classical RAS have no clinically detectable systemic symptoms or signs. If ulceration affects the genitals or other mucosae, or there are other features (e.g. fevers), the diagnosis cannot be of RAS alone—rather of ALU.

There are three main clinical types of RAS, though any significance of these distinctions is unclear (they could be three distinct disorders):

- minor aphthous ulcers (MiAUs) (80% of all RAS)
- major aphthous ulcers (MjAUs)
- herpetiform ulcers (HU).

MiAU (Mikulicz ulcer):

- occur mainly in the 10–40 year age group
- consist of small round or ovoid ulcers 2–4 mm in diameter (Figs 2.2.20–2.2.24), in groups of only a few ulcers (1–6) at a time, with initially yellowish floors surrounded by an erythematous halo and some oedema but the floors assume a greyish hue as healing and epithelialization proceeds
- affect mainly the non-keratinized mobile mucosae of the lips, cheeks, floor of the mouth, sulci or ventrum of the tongue

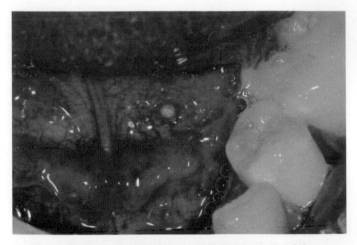

*Figure 2.2.21* Recurrent aphthous stomatitis—minor aphthae.

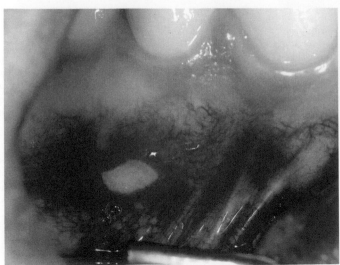

*Figure 2.2.22* Recurrent aphthous stomatitis—minor aphthae.

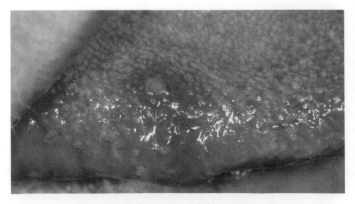

*Figure 2.2.20* Recurrent aphthous stomatitis.

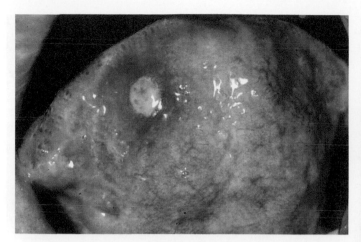

Figure 2.2.23 Recurrent aphthous stomatitis—minor aphthae.

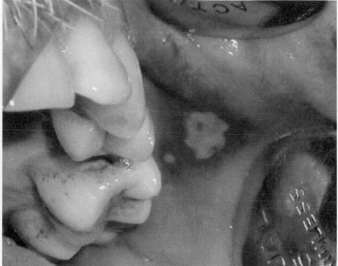

Figure 2.2.24 Recurrent aphthous stomatitis—minor aphthae.

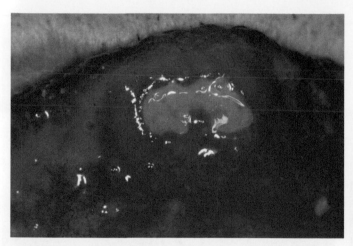

Figure 2.2.25 Recurrent aphthous stomatitis—major aphthae.

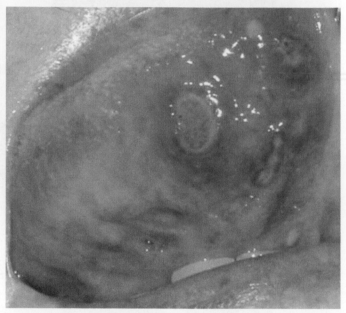

Figure 2.2.26 Recurrent aphthous stomatitis—major aphthae.

- often causes minimal symptoms
- heal in 7–10 days
- leave little or no evidence of scarring
- recur at intervals of 1–4 months.

MjAU (Sutton ulcers or periadenitis mucosa necrotica recurrens):

- are round or ovoid occur in groups of only a few ulcers (1–6) at one time but reach a large size, usually about 1 cm in diameter or even larger
- are found on any area of the oral mucosa, including the keratinized dorsum of the tongue or palate (Figs 2.2.25–2.2.28)
- heal slowly over 10–40 days
- recur extremely frequently
- may heal with scarring
- occasionally are found with a raised erythrocyte sedimentation rate or plasma viscosity.

HU (Cooke aphthae):

- are found in a slightly older age group than the other RAS
- are found mainly in females

- begin with vesiculation which passes rapidly into multiple minute pinhead-sized discrete ulcers (Figs 2.2.29 and 2.2.30) which increase in size and coalesce to leave large, round, ragged ulcers
- involve any oral site, including the keratinized mucosa
- heal in 10 days or longer
- are often extremely painful
- recur so frequently that ulceration may be virtually continuous.

*Diagnosis*
Diagnosis of RAS must be based on the history and clinical features, since no specific tests are available. ALU may be seen in:

- Immune deficiencies such as HIV, cyclical neutropenia and other immune defects.

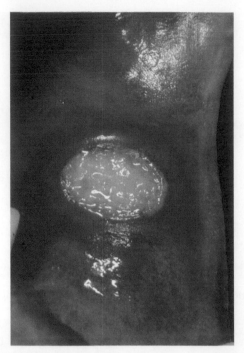

*Figure 2.2.27* Recurrent aphthous stomatitis—major aphthae.

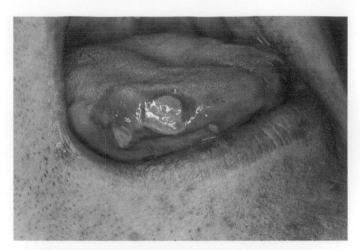

*Figure 2.2.28* Recurrent aphthous stomatitis—major aphthae.

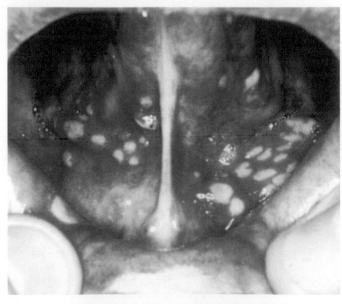

*Figure 2.2.29* Recurrent aphthous stomatitis—herpetiform ulcers.

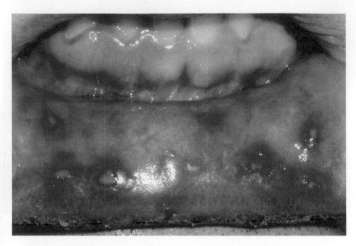

*Figure 2.2.30* Recurrent aphthous stomatitis—herpetiform ulcers.

- Drug use, especially non-steroidal anti-inflammatory drugs and nicorandil.
- Behçet syndrome, where mouth ulcers are seen along with ulcers of the genitals.
- Auto-inflammatory syndromes, for example, periodic fever, aphthous stomatitis, pharyngitis and cervical adenitis syndrome in children, which resolves spontaneously and rarely has long-term sequelae. Corticosteroids are highly effective symptomatically; tonsillectomy and cimetidine treatment have been effective in a few patients.

- Sweet syndrome, in which mouth ulcers are found with conjunctivitis, episcleritis and inflamed tender skin papules or nodules.

Biopsy of RAS is rarely indicated, and is only usually needed where a different diagnosis is suspected but, in order to exclude the systemic disorders discussed above, it is often useful to undertake investigations on:

- blood
  - erythrocyte sedimentation rate (or plasma viscosity)
  - a full blood picture
  - haemoglobin
  - white cell count and differential
  - red cell indices
  - red cell folate assay.
- serum
  - ferritin levels (or other iron studies)
  - vitamin B$_{12}$ measurements
  - transglutaminase assays (positive in coeliac disease).

*Management*
Disorders where ALU are also seen should be excluded.

- Predisposing factors should be corrected:
  - ○ ensure patients avoid trauma, avoid hard or sharp foods (e.g. toast, potato crisps) and brush their teeth atraumatically (e.g. by using a small-headed, soft toothbrush)
  - ○ if SLS is implicated, this should be avoided
  - ○ any iron or vitamin deficiency should be corrected, once the cause of that deficiency has been established
  - ○ if there is an obvious relationship to certain foods, these should be excluded from the diet; patch-testing to reveal allergies may be indicated
  - ○ the occasional patient who relates ulcers to the menstrual cycle or to an oral contraceptive may benefit from suppression of ovulation with a progestogen, or a change in the oral contraceptive
  - ○ causal drugs should be excluded.
- Relief of pain and reduction of ulcer duration.
- Topical corticosteroids can often control RAS. The major concern of adrenal suppression with long-term and/or repeated application has rarely been addressed, although the preparations noted below appear not to cause this problem:
  - ○ topical hydrocortisone hemisuccinate pellets
  - ○ topical triamcinolone acetonide in carboxymethyl cellulose paste
  - ○ stronger topical corticosteroids (e.g. betametasone sodium phosphate).
- Topical tetracycline (e.g. doxycycline) as a mouth rinse may provide relief and reduce ulcer duration, but tetracyclines should be avoided in children under 12 years old who might ingest them and develop tooth staining.
- Good oral hygiene should be maintained; chlorhexidine or triclosan mouthwashes may help.
- Anti-inflammatory agents; there is a spectrum of topical agents such as benzydamine and amlexanox that may help in the management of RAS.
- If RAS fails to respond to these measures, systemic immunomodulators may be required, under specialist supervision. These include:
  - ○ corticosteroids systemically (e.g. prednisolone)
  - ○ colchicine
  - ○ thalidomide.

## Carcinoma
Carcinoma (Chapter 2.3).

## Coxsackie virus infections
Coxsackie virus infections (Chapter 1.8).

## Crohn disease
Crohn disease (Chapter 1.3).

## Drug-induced or chemical mucositis and ulceration
A range of drugs may produce mucositis and/or oral ulceration (see Section 3.5) but the most consistent association is with caustic or cytotoxic chemotherapeutic agents (Fig. 2.2.31). Chemical burns from the mistaken ingestion of acids can cause severe erosions. Chemicals such as acids (chromic, trichloracetic, phosphoric) used during dental procedures can cause ulcers. Self-curing resins, especially epoxy resins for oral use may also produce mucosal erosions, as may various mouthwashes. Rubber-based or silicone-based impression materials occasionally

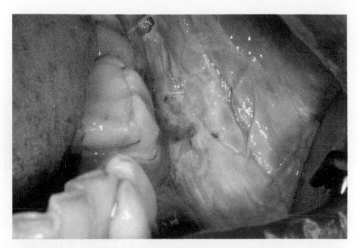

*Figure 2.2.31* Burn—trichlorophenol burn.

produce an erosive reaction. Lesions of erythema multiforme, of toxic epidermal necrolysis, or lesions resembling lichen planus, lupus erythematosus, leukoplakia, pemphigoid or pemphigus may be drug-induced.

## Eosinophilic ulcer
Eosinophilic ulcer (traumatic eosinophilic granuloma; traumatic ulcerative granulomatous disease).

*Aetiopathogenesis*
Eosinophilic ulcer may be traumatic in aetiology; histology shows extensive eosinophilic cell infiltration, throughout the submucosa, histologically similar to CD30+ lymphoproliferative disorders. The peripheral blood eosinophil count is normal.

*Clinical features*
Eosinophilic ulcer is a rare self-limiting single ulcer that often appears on the tongue.

*Diagnosis and management*
Clinical features and biopsy are indicated if the ulcer persists. Conservative excision or incisional biopsy usually effect resolution.

## Erythema multiforme
Erythema multiforme (Figs 2.2.32 and 2.2.33) (Chapter 1.10).

## Graft-versus-host disease
Graft-versus-host disease (Fig. 2.2.34) (Chapter 1.6).

## Herpesvirus infections
Herpesvirus infections (Fig. 2.2.35) (Chapter 1.8).

## Ionizing radiation-induced epithelial changes
Ionizing radiation-induced epithelial changes (Chapter 1.6).

## Lichen planus
Lichen planus (Fig. 2.2.36) (Chapter 1.10).

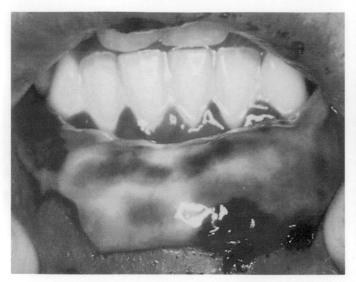

Figure 2.2.32 Erythema multiforme.

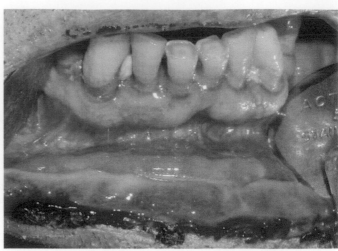

Figure 2.2.33 Erythema multiforme.

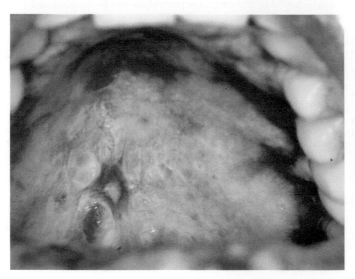

Figure 2.2.34 Mucositis in graft-versus-host-disease.

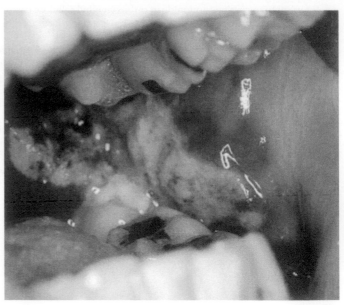

Figure 2.2.35 HIV disease—necrotising stomatitis associated with herpes simplex virus.

**Mycoses**

Mycoses (Chapter 1.8).

**Neutrophil defects**

Neutrophil defects (Fig. 2.2.37) (Chapter 1.4).

**Pemphigoid**

Pemphigoid (Figs 2.2.38 and 2.2.39) (Chapter 1.10).

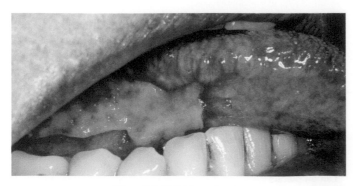

Figure 2.2.36 Lichen planus.

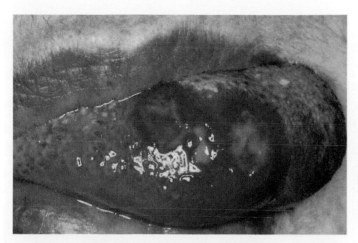

*Figure 2.2.37* Neutropenia—ulceration.

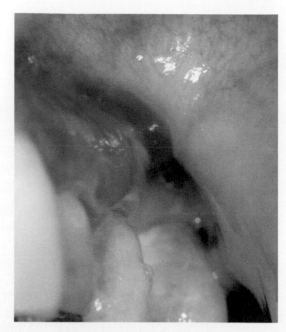

*Figure 2.2.38* Pemphigoid vesiculation.

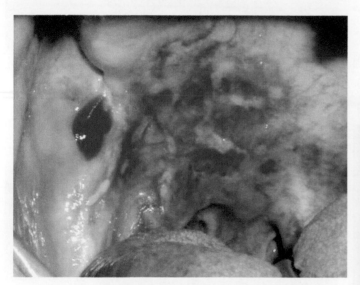

*Figure 2.2.39* Pemphigoid erosions.

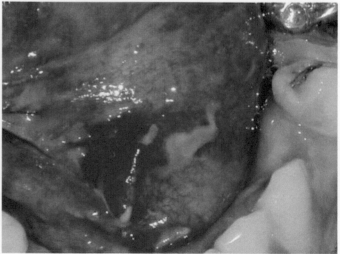

*Figure 2.2.40* Pemphigus erosions.

## Pemphigus
Pemphigus (Figs 2.2.40 and 2.2.41) (Chapter 1.10).

## Syphilis
Syphilis (Fig. 2.2.42) (Chapter 1.8).

## Traumatic ulcers
Trauma may result in haematoma or ulcer formation, commonly seen as a consequence of chronic trauma such as from a sharp tooth cusp or by accidental biting, hard foods, appliances such as dentures or orthodontic appliances, or following dental treatment, non-accidental injury or even orogenital sexual habits (Figs 2.2.43–2.2.50). Chronic self-induced traumatic ulcers may be seen in self-mutilation in a disturbed patient or in learning impairment.

Neonates occasionally develop a palatal ulcer (Bednar ulcer) which it is thought may be caused by trauma from the examining finger of the paediatrician. The lingual fraenum can be traumatized by repeated rubbing over the lower incisor teeth in children with recurrent bouts of coughing as in whooping cough, termed Riga–Fedes disease. A similar lesion can be seen in cunnilingus tongue.

## Tuberculosis
Tuberculosis (Chapter 1.8).

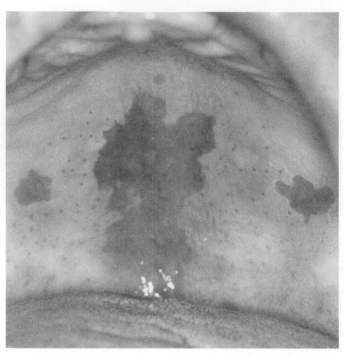

*Figure 2.2.41* Pemphigus—early erosions in paraneoplastic pemphigus.

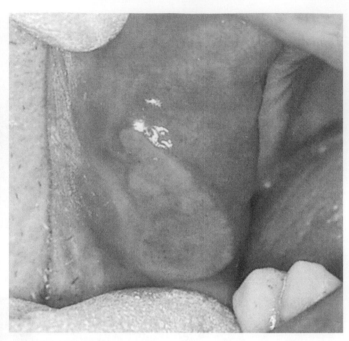

*Figure 2.2.42* Syphilis—ulceration of primary chancre (Hunterian ulcer).

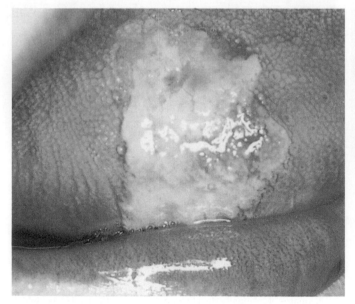

*Figure 2.2.43* Traumatic ulceration.

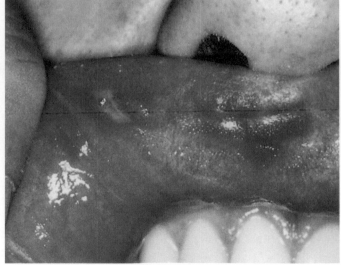

*Figure 2.2.44* Traumatic ulceration—non-accidental.

# SWELLINGS AND LUMPS
## Carcinoma
Carcinoma (Figs 2.2.51–2.2.53) (Chapter 2.3).

## Crohn disease
Crohn disease (Figs 2.2.54 and 2.2.55) (Chapter 1.3).

## Denture-induced hyperplasia
Denture-induced hyperplasia (epulis fissuratum).

*Aetiopathogenesis*
A denture margin (flange) may cause ulceration of the vestibule, and the chronic irritation may produce hyperplasia.

*Clinical features*
The denture often fits neatly into the groove between the hyperplastic leaves of tissue (Figs 2.2.56 and 2.2.57).

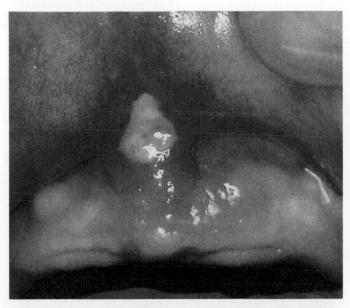

*Figure 2.2.45* Traumatic ulceration of fraenum in non-accidental injury.

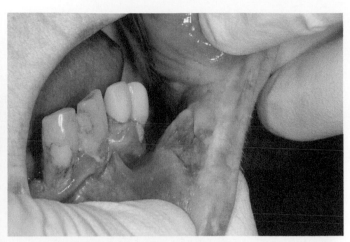

*Figure 2.2.46* Traumatic ulceration—self-harm in learning impairment.

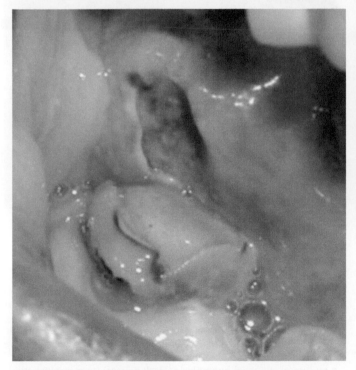

*Figure 2.2.47* Traumatic ulceration from the lower molar tooth.

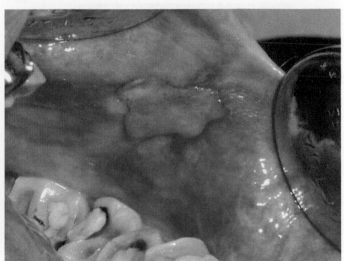

*Figure 2.2.48* Traumatic ulceration.

*Diagnosis*
Clinical.

*Management*
This condition is quite benign but, very occasionally, hyperplasia results from a lesion proliferating beneath and impinging on a denture flange. Excision is the usual treatment.

**Fibrous lump**
Fibrous lump (fibroepithelial polyp).

*Aetiopathogenesis*
Fibrous lumps may be related to irritation, but this is not always evident. They are totally benign.

*Clinical features*
The lesion may present as a lump (Figs 2.2.58 and 2.2.59) or a so-called 'leaf fibroma', although it is not actually a true fibroma.

*Diagnosis*
Biopsy is prudent.

*Management*
Excision.

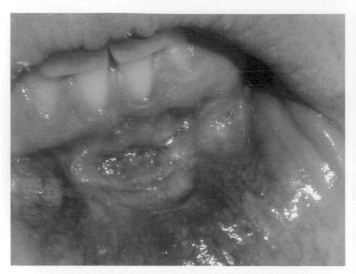

*Figure 2.2.49* Traumatic ulceration—deliberate self-harm.

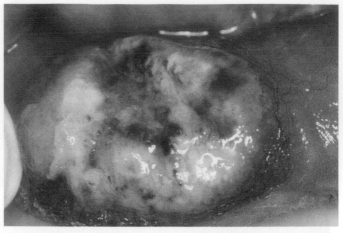

*Figure 2.2.50* Traumatic ulceration—biting of an anaesthetized lip.

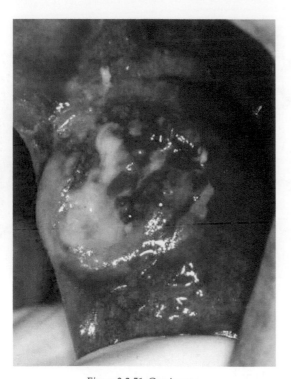

*Figure 2.2.51* Carcinoma.

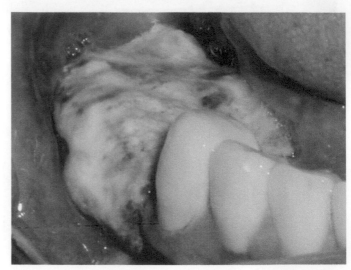

*Figure 2.2.52* Carcinoma.

## Haemangioma

Haemangioma (Chapter 2.1).

## Human papillomavirus (HPV) infections

*Aetiopathogenesis*
There are over 100 HPVs described.

*Clinical features*
HPV can cause oral or perioral

- verruca vulgaris (common wart)—typically on the lip
- papilloma—most common on the palate or gingiva. The cauliflower-like appearance is obvious but indistinguishable from a wart (Fig. 2.2.60)
- condyloma acuminatum (genital wart)—mainly in the anterior mouth. The lesions are increasingly common, especially in sexually active patients and as a complication of HIV disease
- multifocal epithelial hyperplasia (Heck disease), seen in some ethnic groups such as south American natives, associated with HPV-13 and HPV-32, appears as multiple papules mainly on the lateral tongue, lower lip and occlusal line—sites typically traumatized. It usually resolves spontaneously after puberty.

HPV-16 and other types have also been implicated in oropharyngeal carcinoma.

*Diagnosis*
Clinical and biopsy.

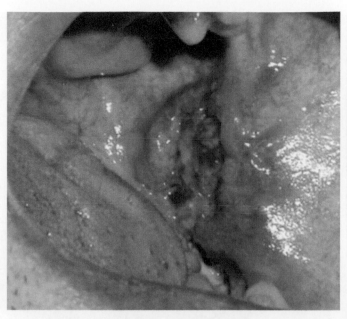

*Figure 2.2.53* Carcinoma.

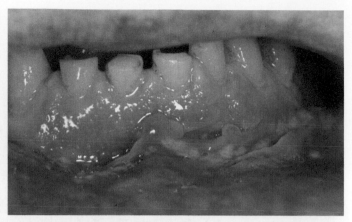

*Figure 2.2.54* Crohn disease—mucosal tags and gingival granulomas.

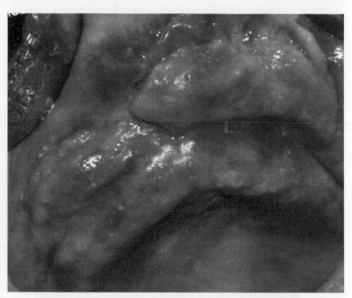

*Figure 2.2.56* Fibroma—denture-related fibroma.

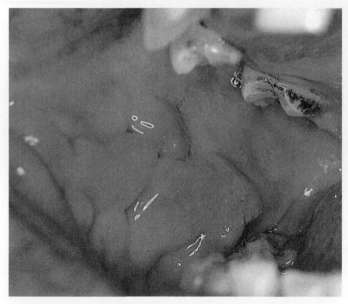

*Figure 2.2.55* Crohn disease—mucosal cobblestoning.

### Mucocoele
Mucocoele (Chapter 2.7).

### Pyogenic granuloma
Pyogenic granuloma (Figs 2.1.96 and 2.2.61) (Figs 2.3.57 and 2.3.58) (Chapter 2.5).

*Management*
Excision or podophyllin. The efficacy of newer agents such as imiquimod in the treatment of oral lesions is not known.

### Surgical emphysema
*Aetiopathogenesis*
Dental instrumentation using air-turbine handpieces or air syringes occasionally introduces air into the tissues.

*Clinical features*
Surgical emphysema is recognized by acute swelling, crackling on palpation.

### Lymphangioma
Lymphangioma (Chapter 2.1).

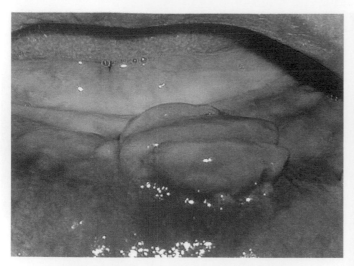

*Figure 2.2.57* Fibroma—denture-related fibroma.

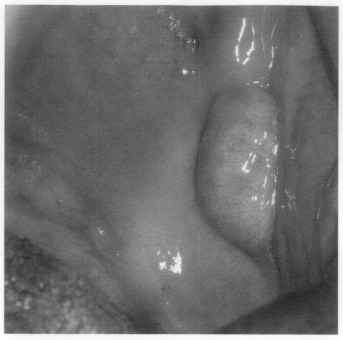

*Figure 2.2.58* Fibrous lump.

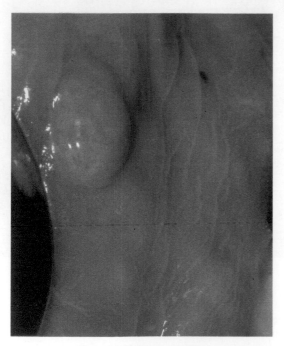

*Figure 2.2.59* Fibrous lump.

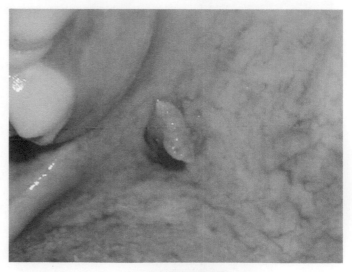

*Figure 2.2.60* Papilloma.

*Diagnosis*
Clinical.

*Management*
Early recognition is essential to prevent such life-threatening rare complications as airway obstruction, deep neck infection or mediastinitis.

# WHITE LESIONS
## Burns
Burns (Figs 2.2.62 and 2.2.63) (Chapter 1.6).

## Candidosis
Candidosis (candidiasis, acute pseudomembranous candidosis, moniliasis, thrush).

*Aetiopathogenesis*
Candida species are common oral commensals, and orogenital and anogenital transmission is possible. Candida can proliferate if the local ecology changes or if immune defences fall. Apart from neonates, who have no immunity to Candida species, candidosis indicates an immunocompromised patient, or a local disturbance in oral flora (such as that caused by xerostomia, radiotherapy, antibiotic treatment or corticosteroids).

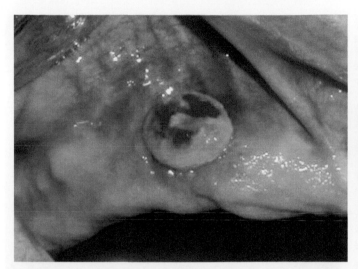

*Figure 2.2.61* Pyogenic granuloma.

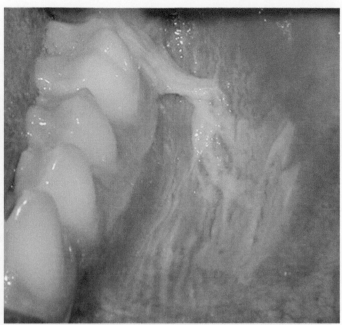

*Figure 2.2.62* Drug burn from topical application of aspirin.

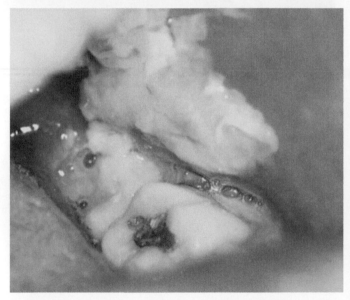

*Figure 2.2.63* Drug burn from topical application of analgesic to reduce toothache.

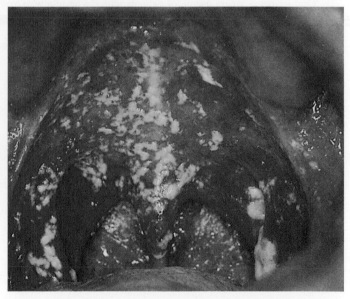

*Figure 2.2.64* Candidosis—acute pseudomembranous.

Candidosis can, for example, be an early feature of HIV or related disease, or leukaemia. *Candida albicans* is the most common and virulent species but *C. tropicalis, C. parapsilosis, C. guilliermondii, C. krusei* and *C. dubliniensis* may also be implicated—especially in immunocompromised persons. In severely immunocompromised patients, there may also be other fungal infections, such as Aspergillus, Mucor or Trichosporon species.

*Clinical features*
Acute pseudomembranous candidosis (thrush) appears as white flecks or plaques, which are easily removed with gauze to leave an erythematous base, typically seen in the palate or upper buccal vestibule posteriorly (Fig. 2.2.64).

*Diagnosis*
Diagnosis is clinical but can, if necessary, be supported by:

- identification of blastospores and pseudohyphae in stained lesional smears
- culture, usually on Sabouraud or dextrose Sabouraud medium.

However, investigations can be complicated by the facts that:

- up to about 50% of the population are carriers
- any attempt at quantitation of Candida is affected by time of sampling and the way in which the specimen is handled.

Other investigations may include:

- Appropriate assessment of immune function—indicated mainly in HIV disease or chronic mucocutaneous candidosis.
- Tests of thyroid, parathyroid and adrenocortical function—since some endocrine disorders may be associated with chronic mucocutaneous candidosis.
- Haemoglobin, white blood cell counts, corrected whole blood folate, vitamin $B_{12}$ and serum ferritin—since oral candidosis is occasionally associated with nutritional deficiencies or blood dyscrasias.

### Management

Few patients have spontaneous remission unless the condition is solely related to, for example, the use of an antimicrobial, or a topical corticosteroid, and thus, in other cases, treatment is often indicated. Often, attention to the underlying cause will avoid the need for prolonged or repeated courses of antifungal treatment. Intermittent or prolonged topical antifungal treatment may be necessary where the underlying cause is unavoidable or incurable.

Treatment includes the following:

- Avoid or reduce smoking.
- Treat any local predisposing cause such as xerostomia.
- Improve oral hygiene; chlorhexidine has some anti-candidal activity.
- Antifungals:
  - Topical antifungal agents are useful for most lesions restricted to the oral cavity and are available as suspensions, tablets and creams. Oral suspensions are useful for patients with dry mouth who may have difficulty in dissolving tablets. Available preparations include: nystatin, amphotericin, miconazole or fluconazole.
  - Systemic antifungals are increasingly used, especially fluconazole, but may interact with anti-HIV and other medications.

### Candidal leukoplakia

*Aetiopathogenesis*
Smoking, HIV infection or deficiencies of haematinics may underlie chronic candidosis.

*Clinical features*
Chronic hyperplastic candidosis, or candidal leukoplakia, is a firm white adherent plaque, usually seen inside the commissures (Fig. 2.2.65), or on the tongue. Candidal leukoplakia may also be a speckled red and white lesion. These leukoplakias are suggested to have a higher malignant potential than many forms.

*Diagnosis*
Diagnosis is clinical but supported by biopsy and can, if necessary, also be supported by:

- identification of blastospores and pseudohyphae in stained smears from a lesion
- culture, usually on Sabouraud or dextrose Sabouraud medium
- histology stained by periodic acid Schiff.

Other investigations:

- Tests of immune function are indicated mainly in HIV disease or chronic mucocutaneous candidosis.
- Tests of thyroid, parathyroid and adrenocortical function are warranted in selected individuals.
- Estimates of haemoglobin, white blood cell counts, corrected whole blood folate, vitamin $B_{12}$ and serum ferritin may occasionally be relevant.

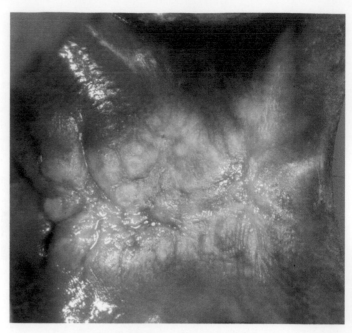

*Figure 2.2.65* Candidal leukoplakia.

### Management

Candidal leukoplakia warrants excision, as the lesion may also contain areas of epithelial dysplasia. There remains little evidence that topical or antifungal therapy will be of benefit. All affected patients, however, should be advised to reduce any tobacco usage.

### Multifocal chronic candidosis

Multifocal chronic candidosis may occur in the palate in apposition to the tongue lesion—the 'kissing lesions'. Multifocal chronic candidosis may appear as red, white or mixed lesions and is usually seen in smokers.

### Carcinoma

Carcinoma (Chapter 2.3).

### Fordyce spots

Fordyce spots (Figs 2.2.66–2.2.68) (Chapter 2.1).

### Grafts

Skin graft of a defect following excision of a carcinoma remains paler than the mucosa, becomes wrinkled and white and may grow hairs. Mucosal grafts from the palate for periodontal treatment are less white than skin grafts.

### Keratosis

*Aetiopathogenesis*
Repeated friction can result in keratosis, and this is typically seen on edentulous ridges (benign alveolar ridge keratosis), or surrounding

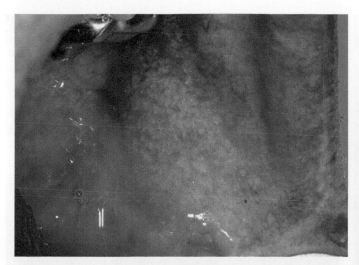

*Figure 2.2.66* Fordyce spots.

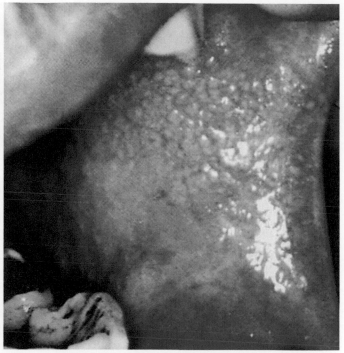

*Figure 2.2.67* Fordyce spots.

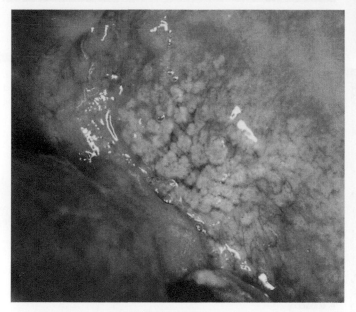

*Figure 2.2.68* Fordyce spots.

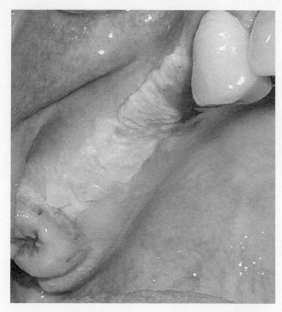

*Figure 2.2.69* Keratosis—benign alveolar ridge keratosis.

chronic traumatic ulcers. Smoking and tobacco-related habits are the other most common identifiable causes of keratoses (hyperkeratosis). Sanguinaria may also cause a white lesion.

*Clinical features*
Most keratoses are flat and smooth-surfaced (homogeneous) white lesions, and benign (Figs 2.2.69 and 2.2.70).

*Diagnosis*
Although dysplasia is unlikely in most cases of keratosis, biopsy is often indicated to determine the precise histopathology and exclude dysplasia.

*Management*
Patients should be encouraged to reduce or cease any tobacco habit.

Excision and regular clinical and/or histopathological review are recommended—despite the lack of evidence for such a regimen.

**Leukoedema**
*Aetiopathogenesis*
Leukoedema is not a mucosal disease but a normal variant.

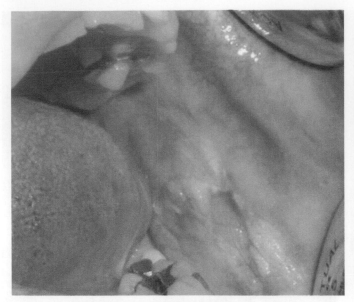

*Figure 2.2.70* Leukoplakia—frictional keratosis.

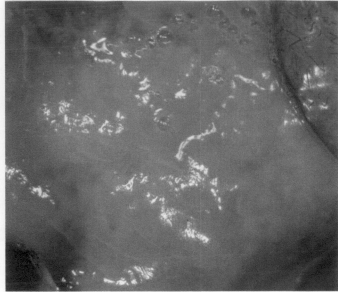

*Figure 2.2.71* Leukoedema.

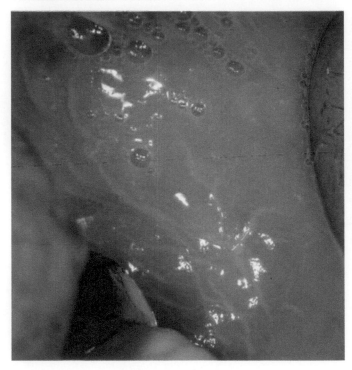

*Figure 2.2.72* Leukoedema.

*Clinical features*
Leukoedema is the description of very faint whitish lines in some normal buccal mucosae, seen very often in coloured races (Figs 2.2.71 and 2.2.72).

*Diagnosis*
The whitish lines disappear if the mucosa is stretched—a diagnostic test. The lines disappear if the mucosa is stretched when the cheek is pushed in from outside. Confusion with lichen planus should thereby be avoided.

*Management*
Reassurance only.

## Leukoplakia

Oral leukoplakia as defined by WHO is 'a predominantly white lesion of the oral mucosa that cannot be characterized as any other definable lesion'.

*Aetiopathogenesis*
Leukoplakia may be idiopathic but, in some, predisposing factors are habits such as the use of:

• tobacco
• alcohol
• betel: the betel leaf contains allylbenzene compounds such as chavibetol, chavicol, estragole, eugenol and methyl eugenol, and may be included in the betel quid (paan), along with betel nut (*Areca catechu*) and often various spices, tobacco and/or slaked lime.
• sanguinarine (pseudochelerythrine)—a quaternary benzophenanthridine alkaloid extracted from plants including bloodroot (*Sanguinaria canadensis*), Mexican prickly poppy *Argemone mexicana*, *Chelidonium majus* and *Macleaya cordata*—and was used in some oral healthcare products. It is a potent suppressor of NF-κB activation and induces a rapid apoptotic response by glutathione-depletion.

Some white lesions have a microbial pathogenesis, such as:

• Chronic candidal infection—common in speckled leukoplakias. *C. albicans* can cause or colonize other keratoses, particularly in smokers, and is especially likely to form speckled leukoplakias at commissures. They may be dysplastic and have higher malignant potential than some other keratoses. Candidal leukoplakias may respond to antifungals and stopping smoking.

- HPV—proliferative verrucous leukoplakia is a diffuse white and/or papillary lesion seen in elderly patients, often associated with, HPV and which has an inexorably slow progression to verrucous or squamous cell carcinoma, over one or two decades. Polymorphisms at XRCC1, one of the DNA repair loci, may modulate the risk of tobacco-related leukoplakia and cancer in HPV-infected individuals.
- Tertiary syphilis—the malignant potential of syphilitic leukoplakia is suggested to be high.
- Epstein–Barr virus is associated with oral *hairy* leukoplakia, which is quite different from other leukoplakias and not usually grouped with them. This condition appears to be benign and self-limiting and is seen in the immunocompromised and as a complication of HIV infection. It usually has a corrugated surface and affects the margins of the tongue almost exclusively.

### Clinical features

Leukoplakias vary in size: some are small and focal, others more wide-spread—occasionally involving very large areas of the oral mucosa—and in other patients several discrete separate areas of leukoplakia can be seen. Leukoplakia has a wide range of clinical presentations, from homogeneous white plaques, which can be faintly white or very thick and opaque, to nodular white lesions, or lesions admixed with red lesions (Figs 2.2.73–2.2.81).

The malignant potential depends on the appearance, histopathology (i.e. degree of dysplasia), some aetiological factors and perhaps the site of the lesion.

Verrucous or nodular keratoses have a higher malignant potential than that of homogeneous keratoses. A variant termed proliferative verrucous leukoplakia is seen especially in the buccal mucosa in older women and about one-half eventually develop carcinoma.

Keratosis on the ventrum of the tongue and floor of the mouth has a higher malignant potential than similar lesions elsewhere. Seen especially in middle-aged or older women, the sublingual keratosis is usually bilateral.

The surface may have a so-called 'ebbing tide' appearance, resembling the appearance of sand on the beach as the tide ebbs, and the lesion may be a mixture of white and red lesions: a speckled leukoplakia.

Speckled leukoplakias have the highest malignant potential of the leukoplakia, and these may have a candidal association, and are typically located at the commissures or on the tongue dorsum.

### Appearance

- Homogeneous leukoplakias: the most common type, are uniformly white plaques—common in the buccal (cheek) mucosa and usually of low malignant potential. Sometimes lesions are widespread, suggesting there are widespread molecular changes in the mucosa.
- Non-homogeneous or heterogeneous leukoplakias: nodular, verrucous and speckled leukoplakias which consists of white patches or nodules in a red, often eroded, area of mucosa have a high risk of malignant transformation and therefore are far more serious.

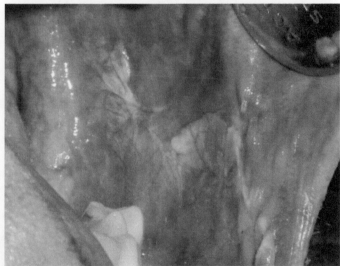

*Figure 2.2.74* Leukoplakia.

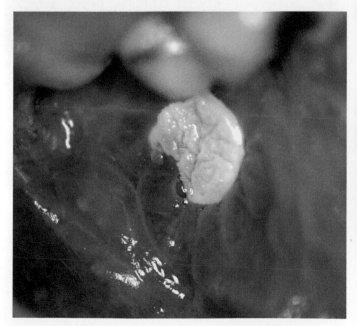

*Figure 2.2.73* Leukoplakia—homogeneous leukoplakia.

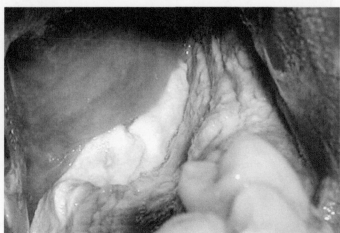

*Figure 2.2.75* Leukoplakia—verrucous leukoplakia.

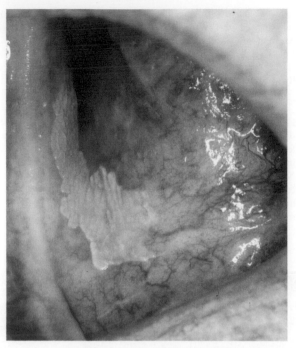

Figure 2.2.76 Leukoplakia—in floor of mouth (sublingual keratosis).

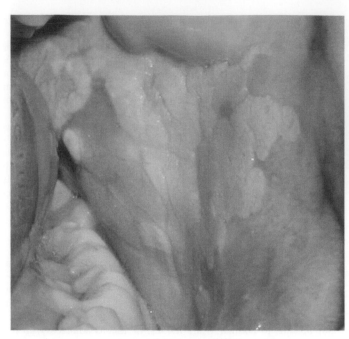

Figure 2.2.77 Leukoplakia.

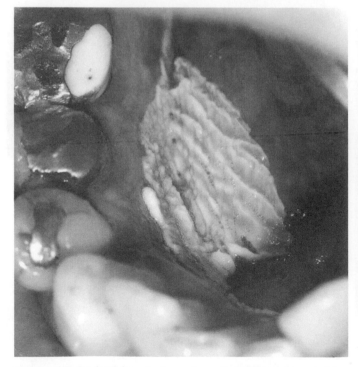

Figure 2.2.78 Leukoplakia—in floor of mouth (sublingual keratosis)—ebbing tide appearance.

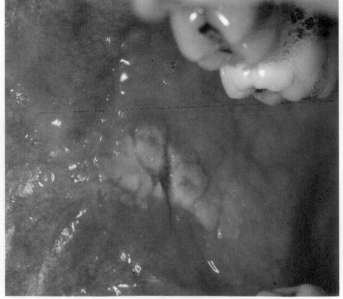

Figure 2.2.79 Leukoplakia—from tobacco chewing.

## Site

High-risk sites for malignant transformation include the soft palate complex and ventrolateral tongue and floor of the mouth (where sublingual keratosis has a particularly high risk of malignant change). Sublingual keratosis is more common in women than men, has a typical 'ebbing-tide' appearance clinically and has a high malignant potential.

## Diagnosis

There are no clinical signs or symptoms which reliably predict whether a leukoplakia will undergo malignant change, and thus there must be

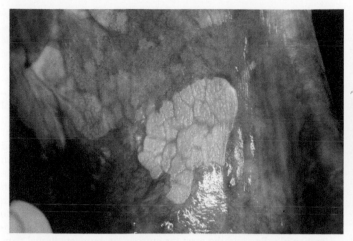

*Figure 2.2.80* Leukoplakia—homogeneous leukoplakia.

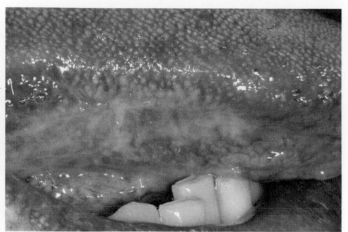

*Figure 2.2.81* Leukoplakia—in floor of mouth (sublingual keratosis).

use of microscopy to detect dysplasia. Biopsy is generally indicated and is certainly mandatory for those leukoplakias which are:

- in patients with previous or concurrent head and neck cancer
- non-homogeneous, that is:
  - ○ have red areas
  - ○ are verrucous
  - ○ are indurated
- in a high-risk site such as the floor of the mouth or the tongue
- focal
- with symptoms
- without obvious aetiological factors.

Overall,

- 2–5% of all leukoplakias become malignant in 10 years
- 5–20% of leukoplakias are dysplastic
- 10–35% of leukoplakias showing dysplasia proceed to carcinoma in 10 years.

It is not at present possible to reliably predict which lesions will progress to carcinoma. Over the last few years, much effort has gone into identifying the genetic changes that underlie progression to oral carcinoma. Currently, the most predictive markers of transformation to carcinoma are:

- Histology—dysplasia
- Cancer history
- Chromosomal polysomy (ploidy)
- Chromosomal loss of heterozygosity (LOH) at 3p or 9p
- p53 protein expression.

Ploidy may become useful in this respect, but at the present time remains controversial. Staining with tolonium chloride (toluidine blue) can delineate areas of severe oral epithelial dysplasia or frank carcinoma and thus may be an aid to determining a site of biopsy.

*Management*
Leukoplakia can be totally benign or sometimes can be precancerous or a marker for cancer elsewhere in the upper aerodigestive tract. The prevalence of malignant transformation in leukoplakias ranges from 2% to 35% over 10 years and is highest in lesions with severe dysplasia.

While the potentially malignant nature of leukoplakias is often stressed, several studies have shown that dysplastic lesions can sometimes regress spontaneously or if risk factors are removed, with rates ranging from 9% to 60%. However, although some patients have spontaneous remission of leukoplakia, the lesion may be potentially malignant and thus both behaviour (lifestyle) modification and active treatment of the lesion are indicated.

- Patient information is an important aspect in management.
- Removal of known risk factors (tobacco, alcohol and trauma) is a mandatory first step. Up to 60% of leukoplakias regress or totally disappear if tobacco use is stopped. Leukoplakias induced by smokeless tobacco may resolve if the habit is stopped. Success is difficult to achieve: in one series of 145 patients operated on for oral leukoplakias, only 20 gave up smoking and only 5 stopped drinking alcohol.
- The patient should be re-examined 3 months after instituting this.
- If the lesion persists, it should be removed if possible and is the treatment of choice. However, many patients with leukoplakias belong to lower socio-economic groups and do not always accept or understand the need to re-attend. Therefore, many suggest removing the lesion at an earlier stage.

Medical therapies

- Up to 30% of leukoplakias can markedly improve or even resolve when aetiological factors are removed and medical therapies (anti-inflammatory and antimycotic agents) used. Some candidal leukoplakias respond at least partially to antifungal drugs (smoking should also be stopped) and dysplasia may regress.
- Topical anticancer drugs or retinoids can cause regression and are generally well tolerated and effective, but their efficacy is only temporary, and perhaps their best indication is when the location or extent of the lesion render surgical removal difficult. Topical treatment of leukoplakia with podophyllin solution or bleomycin has induced some regression or even total resolution of dysplasia and clinical lesions, and lesions recur more slowly than after surgery. The efficacy of photo dynamic therapy, in which a light-sensitizing dye is given to the patients, and laser shone on the lesion to activate the dye and cause necrosis of the pathological tissue, still remains to be fully determined.
- Since leukoplakias are only *potentially* cancerous, it is generally accepted that radiotherapy or systemic chemotherapy are inappropriate treatments.

Surgery

- Surgery is an obvious option for the management of leukoplakia, certainly for patients with high predisposition to malignant transformation, such as leukoplakias that are:
  - speckled
  - verrucous
  - from high-risk sites, including the floor of the mouth/ventrum of the tongue, or soft palate/fauces
  - in a patient with previous cancer in the upper aerodigestive tract
  - dysplastic
  - polysomic (aneuploidy or tetraploidy)
  - tested positive for genetic markers such as mutated tumour suppressor factor p53, or LOH on chromosomes 3p or 9p.

- 'Watchful waiting' and excision only when signs of cancerization creates a dilemma since even excised leukoplakias which show only dysplasia on prior biopsy may still contain carcinomatous foci. In one series of removed leukoplakias, 5–10% of lesions were found to be malignant on removal, although they had been judged both clinically to be benign and on preoperative biopsy were negative for severe dysplasia or malignancy. Even when surgical specimens of excised leukoplakias showed only orthokeratosis, or parakeratosis with epithelial hyperplasia (no dysplasia) and minimal inflammation, some 5% of such patients subsequently developed oral squamous cell carcinoma.
- Resection with a scalpel or laser is probably the most effective and safe means of removing pathologic tissue since—unlike the case with cryosurgery, coagulation or laser vaporization—a specimen for pathologic evaluation (of histology and margins) is produced, and the pain and postoperative scarring are less with these techniques than with coagulation. Finally, laser excision (usually with the carbon dioxide laser) seems to have advantage over the use of a scalpel, as intraoperative bleeding and the need for mucosal or dermoepidermal flaps are reduced.
- Follow-up; patients should be regularly checked at 3, 6 and 12 months, and then annually for any:
  - size change
  - appearance of red lesions
  - ulceration
  - recurrences
  - new lesions.

### Lichen planus

Lichen planus (Figs 2.2.82 and 2.2.83) (Chapter 1.10).

### Linea alba

Linea alba (occlusal line) is a simple line of frictional keratosis seen usually bilaterally in the buccal mucosae (occasionally along the margin of the tongue), horizontally aligned with the occlusal surfaces of the teeth, sometimes with small vertical lines coincident with the interdental areas (Figs 2.2.84–2.2.87).

This is more obvious in patients with parafunctional habits such as jaw clenching or tooth-grinding, and in those with temporomandibular pain-dysfunction syndrome.

No treatment is required, although if lesions extend beyond sites of likely trauma it may be advantageous to confirm the diagnosis histopathologically.

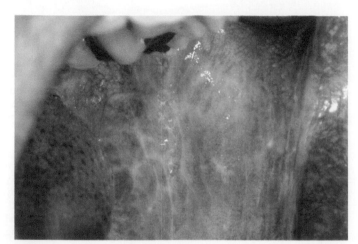

Figure 2.2.82 Lichen planus.

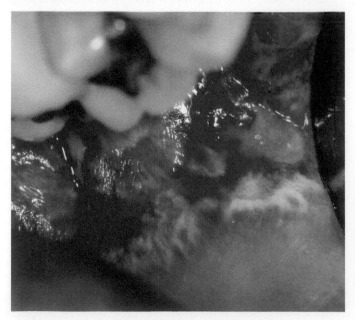

Figure 2.2.83 Lichen planus.

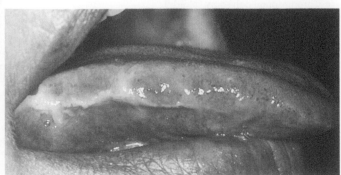

Figure 2.2.84 Linea alba.

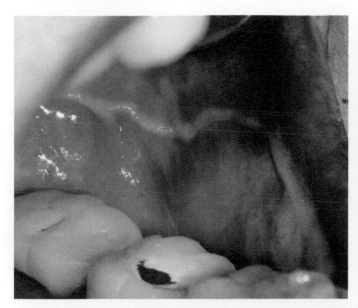

*Figure 2.2.85* Linea alba.

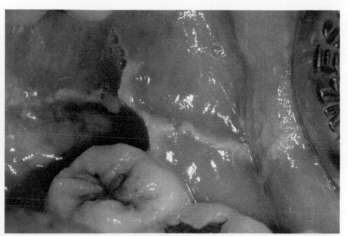

*Figure 2.2.86* Linea alba.

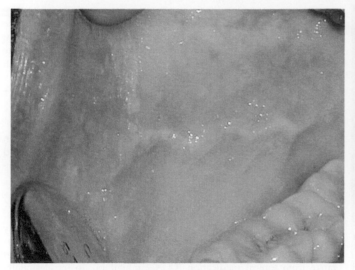

*Figure 2.2.87* Linea alba.

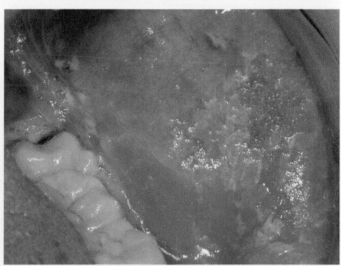

*Figure 2.2.88* Morsicatio buccarum.

### Measles
Measles (rubeola) (Chapter 1.8).

### Morsicatio buccarum
Morsicatio buccarum (cheek biting).

*Aetiopathogenesis*
Cheek biting is especially seen in anxious patients, and those with other psychologically related disorders, for example, temporomandibular pain-dysfunction syndrome. Rarely, severe self-mutilation is seen in;

- psychiatric disorders
- learning impairment
- rare syndromes such as Lesch–Nyhan syndrome or those with insensitivity to pain [e.g. familial dysautonomia (Riley–Day syndrome)].

*Clinical features*
Abrasion of superficial epithelium leaves whitish fragments on a reddish background (Figs 2.2.88–2.2.90). Lesions are invariably restricted to lower labial mucosa and/or buccal mucosa near occlusal line on one or both sides.

*Diagnosis*
This is a clinical diagnosis but, if lesions extend beyond sites of likely trauma, it may be advantageous to establish the histopathological diagnosis.

Differentiate from other causes of white lesions—particularly white sponge naevus.

*Management*
Stop the habit if possible.

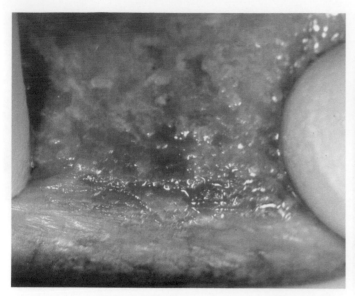

*Figure 2.2.89* Morsicatio buccarum.

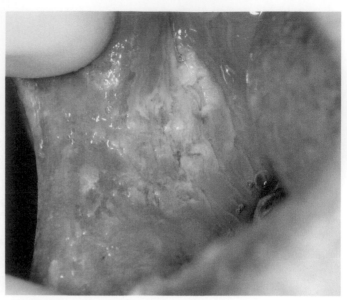

*Figure 2.2.90* Morsicatio buccarum.

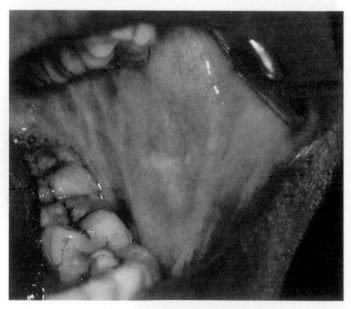

*Figure 2.2.91* Oral submucous fibrosis—showing vertical bands in buccal mucosa.

## Oral submucous fibrosis

### Aetiopathogenesis

OSMF is a chronic disorder seen only in persons who use betel (*A. catechu*) nuts, pan masala or gutkha. The lesions of OSMF appear to be due to nut constituents such as copper, alkaloids, tannin and catechin which act by increasing collagen cross-linking or other effects. There may be some genetic predisposition.

### Clinical features

OSMF can affect the oral and sometimes pharyngeal mucosa, and develops insidiously, often initially presenting with oral dysaesthesia and a non-specific vesicular stomatitis. Later symmetrical fibrosis of the cheeks, lips, tongue or palate develops, and may be noted as vertical bands running through the mucosa. This can become so severe that the affected site becomes white and firm, with severely restricted mouth opening (Fig. 2.2.91).

There is epithelial atrophy and carcinoma may eventually develop—possibly in up to 8%.

### Diagnosis

OSMF is usually easily diagnosed clinically, since it is extremely rare in people not of Asian extraction. There is a history of betel chewing and no history of other injury or surgery. Diagnosis can be confirmed if necessary by biopsy, and haematology often reveals coexistent anaemia.

### Management

Management is first to stop areca nut use. Asymptomatic cases should be observed only. Symptomatic cases with restricted opening may respond to physiotherapy to stretch the restrictive bands but there is as yet no other reliably effective therapy for OSMF. Medical therapies range from topical medication (COX-2 inhibitors); to intralesionally injected medicaments such as corticosteroids, collagenase or hyaluronidase; to systemic medication with lycopene or pentoxifylline. Surgical therapies range from laser release of the bands to excision of the 'scarred' tissue and split skin, radial forearm or other flap procedures.

## White sponge naevus

White sponge naevus (Chapter 1.10).

## FURTHER READING

Abdollahi M, Radfar M. A review of drug-induced oral reactions. J Contemp Dent Pract 2003; 4: 10–31.

Arduino PG, Surace A, Carbone M, et al. Outcome of oral dysplasia: a retrospective hospital-based study of 207 patients with a long follow-up. J Oral Pathol Med 2009; 38: 540–4.

Bagan JV, Jimenez Y, Sanchis JM, et al. Proliferative verrucous leukoplakia: unusual locations of oral squamous cell carcinomas, and field cancerization as shown by the appearance of multiple OSCCs. Oral Oncol 2004; 40: 440–3.

Blomgren J, Berggren U, Jontell M. Fluconazole versus nystatin in the treatment of oral candidosis. Acta Odontol Scand 1998; 56: 202–5.

Burge S, Kuffer R, Scully C, Porter SR. Recurrent aphthous stomatitis. Oral Dis 2006; 12: 1–21.

Chawla O, Burke GA, MacBean AD. The eosinophilic ulcer revisited. Dent Update 2007; 34: 56–7.

Cox S, Zoellner H. Physiotherapeutic treatment improves oral opening in oral submucous fibrosis. J Oral Pathol 2009; 38: 220–6.

Craig RM Jr, Vickers VA, Correll RW. Erythroplastic lesion on the mandibular marginal gingiva. J Am Dent Assoc 1989; 119: 543–4.

De Moor RJ, De Witte AM, Delmé KI, et al. Dental and oral complications of lip and tongue piercings. Br Dent J 2005; 199: 506–9.

Diz Dios P, Scully C. Adverse effects of antiretroviral therapy: focus on orofacial effects. Expert Opin Drug Saf 2002; 1: 307–17.

Eisen D. Disorders of pigmentation in the oral cavity. Clin Dermatol 2000; 18: 579–87.

Ellepola AN, Samaranayake LP. Oral candidal infections and antimycotics. Crit Rev Oral Biol Med 2000; 11: 172–98.

Fedorowicz Z, Chan Shih-Yen E, Dorri M, et al. Interventions for the management of oral submucous fibrosis. Cochrane Database Syst Rev 2008; (4): CD007156.

Femiano F, Gombos F, Scully C. Recurrent aphthous stomatitis unresponsive to topical corticosteroids: a study of the comparative therapeutic effects of systemic prednisone and systemic sulodexide. Int J Dermatol 2003; 42: 394–7.

Glass LF, Maize JC. Morsicatio buccarum et labiorum (excessive cheek and lip biting). Am J Dermatopathol 1991; 13: 271–4.

Hashem FK, Al Khayal Z. Oral burn contractures in children. Ann Plast Surg 2003; 51: 468–71.

Holmstrup P, Axéll T. Classification and clinical manifestations of oral yeast infections. Acta Odontol Scand 1990; 48: 57–9.

Jaber MA, Porter SR, Speight P, et al. Oral epithelial dysplasia: clinical characteristics of western European residents. Oral Oncol 2003; 39: 589–96.

Jiang X, Hu J. Drug treatment of oral submucous fibrosis: a review of the literature. J Oral Maxillofac Surg 2009; 67: 1510–15.

Jurge S, Kuffer R, Scully C, Porter SR. Recurrent aphthous stomatitis. Oral Dis 2006; 12: 1–21.

Karki AJ, Stokes MM, Fraser JS, Adlam DM. Surgical emphysema following a restorative procedure: a case report. Dent Update 2006; 33: 171–2, 174.

Katz J, Guelmann M, Stavropolous F, Heft M. Gingival and other oral manifestations in measles virus infection. J Clin Periodontol 2003; 30: 665–8.

Kaugars GE, Heise AP, Riley WT, Abbey LM, Svirsky JA. Oral melanotic macules. A review of 353 cases. Oral Surg Oral Med Oral Pathol 1993; 76: 59–61.

Kissel SO, Hanratty JJ. Periodontal treatment of an amalgam tattoo. Compend Contin Educ Dent 2002; 23: 930–2, 934, 936.

Lenane P, Powell FC. Oral pigmentation. J Eur Acad Dermatol Venereol 2000; 14: 448–65.

Lodi G, Sardella A, Bez C, Demarosi F, Carrassi A. Interventions for treating oral leukoplakia. Cochrane Database Syst Rev 2001; (4): CD001829.

Lodi G, Scully C, Carrozzo M, et al. Current controversies in oral lichen planus: report of an international consensus meeting. Part 1. Viral infections and etiopathogenesis. Oral Surg Oral Med Oral Pathol Oral Radiol Endod 2005; 100: 40–51.

Lodi G, Scully C, Carrozzo M, et al. Current controversies in oral lichen planus: report of an international consensus meeting. Part 2. Clinical management and malignant transformation. Oral Surg Oral Med Oral Pathol Oral Radiol Endod 2005; 100: 164–78.

Martelli H Jr, Pereira SM, Rocha TM, et al. White sponge nevus: report of a three-generation family. Oral Surg Oral Med Oral Pathol Oral Radiol Endod 2007; 103: 43–7.

McCullough MJ, Abdel-Hafeth S, Scully C. Recurrent aphthous stomatitis (RAS) revisited; clinical features, associations, and new association with infant feeding patterns? J Oral Pathol Med 2007; 36: 615–20.

Meleti M, Vescovi P, Mooi WJ, van der Waal I. Pigmented lesions of the oral mucosa and perioral tissues: a flow-chart for the diagnosis and some recommendations for the management. Oral Surg Oral Med Oral Pathol Oral Radiol Endod 2008; 105: 606–16.

Majumder M, Indra D, Roy PD, et al. Variant haplotypes at XRCC1 and risk of oral leukoplakia in HPV non-infected samples. J Oral Pathol 2009; 38: 174–80.

Owens BM, Johnson WW, Schuman NJ. Oral amalgam pigmentations (tattoos): a retrospective study. Quintessence Int 1992; 23: 805–10.

Ozcelik O, Haytac MC, Akkaya M. Iatrogenic trauma to oral tissues. J Periodontol 2005; 76: 1793–7.

Pandya S, Chaudhary AK, Singh M, Mehrotra R. Correlation of histopathological diagnosis with habits and clinical findings in oral submucous fibrosis. Head Neck Oncol 2009; 1: 10.

Petti S. Pooled estimate of world leukoplakia prevalence: a systematic review. Oral Oncol 2003; 39: 770–80.

Porter SR, Hegarty A, Kaliakatsou F, Hodgson TA, Scully C. Recurrent aphthous stomatitis. Clin Dermatol 2000; 18: 569–78.

Porter SR, Scully C. Aphthous ulcers: (recurrent). Clin Evid 2006; 16: 539–40.

Praetorius F. HPV-associated diseases of oral mucosa. Clin Dermatol 1997; 15: 399–413.

Reibel J. Prognosis of oral pre-malignant lesions: significance of clinical, histopathological, and molecular biological characteristics. Crit Rev Oral Biol Med 2003; 14: 47–62.

Reichart PA, Nguyen XH. Betel quid chewing, oral cancer and other oral mucosal diseases in Vietnam: a review. J Oral Pathol Med 2008; 37: 511–14.

Reichart PA, Phillipsen HP. Betel chewer's mucosa—a review. J Oral Pathol Med 1998; 27: 239–42.

Reichart PA, Samaranayake LP, Philipsen HP. Pathology and clinical correlates in oral candidiasis and its variants: a review. Oral Dis 2000; 6: 85–91.

Reichart PA. Oral manifestations in HIV infection: fungal and bacterial infections, Kaposi's sarcoma. Med Microbiol Immunol (Berl) 2003; 192: 165–9.

Scully C, Bagan JV. Adverse drug reactions in the orofacial region. Crit Rev Oral Biol Med 2004; 15: 221–39.

Scully C, Carrozzo M. Oral mucosal disease: lichen planus. Br J Oral Maxillofac Surg 2008; 46: 15–21.

Scully C, el-Kabir M, Samaranayake LP. Candida and oral candidosis: a review. Crit Rev Oral Biol Med 1994; 5: 125–57.

Scully C, Gorsky M, Lozada-Nur F. The diagnosis and management of recurrent aphthous stomatitis–a consensus approach. J Am Dent Assoc 2003; 134: 200–7.

Scully C, Hodgson T. Recurrent oral ulceration: aphthous-like ulcers in periodic syndromes. Oral Surg Oral Med Oral Pathol Oral Radiol Endod 2008; 106: 845–52.

Scully C, Porter S. ABC of oral health. Swellings and red, white, and pigmented lesions. BMJ 2000; 321: 225–8.

Scully C, Porter S. Orofacial disease: update for the dental clinical team: 2. Ulcers, erosions and other causes of sore mouth. Part I. Dent Update 1998; 25: 478–84.

Scully C, Porter S. Orofacial disease: update for the dental clinical team: 5. Lumps and swellings. Dent Update 1999; 26: 214–17.

Scully C, Porter S. Orofacial disease: update for the dental clinical team: 3. White lesions. Dent Update 1999; 26: 123–9.

Scully C, Porter S. Orofacial disease: update for the dental clinical team: 4. Red, brown, black and bluish lesions. Dent Update 1999; 26: 169–73.

Scully C, Porter SR. Oral mucosal diseases: recurrent aphthous stomatitis. Br J Oral Maxillofac Surg 2008; 46: 198–206.

Scully C, Sudbo J, Speight PM. Progress in determining the malignant potential of oral lesions. J Oral Pathol Med 2003; 32: 251–6.

Scully C. Oral precancer: preventive and medical approaches to management. Eur J Cancer B Oral Oncol 1995; 31B: 16–26.

Scully C, Eisen D, Rogers R, Porter SR, Bagan J. Dermatology of the Lips. Oxford: Isis Medical Media, 2008: 1–180.

Scully C, Porter SR. Oral mucosal disease: recurrent aphthous stomatitis. Br J Oral Maxillofac Surg 2008; 46: 198–206.

Scully C. Aphthous ulceration. N Engl J Med 2006; 355: 41–8.

Segura S, Pujol RM. Eosinophilic ulcer of the oral mucosa: a distinct entity or a non-specific reactive pattern? Oral Dis 2008; 14: 287–95.

Seward GR. Amalgam tattoo. Br Dent J 1998; 184: 470–1.

Solomon LW. Chronic ulcerative stomatitis. Oral Dis 2008; 14: 383–9.

Syrjanen S, Puranen M. Human papillomavirus infections in children: the potential role of maternal transmission. Crit Rev Oral Biol Med 2000; 11: 259–74.

Syrjanen S. Human papillomavirus infections and oral tumors. Med Microbiol Immunol (Berl) 2003; 192: 123–8.

Taybos G. Oral changes associated with tobacco use. Am J Med Sci 2003; 326: 179–82.

Telang GH, Ditre CM. Blue gingiva, an unusual oral pigmentation resulting from gingival tattoo. J Am Acad Dermatol 1994; 30: 125–6.

Tilakaratne WM, Klinikowski MF, Saku T, Peters TJ, Warnakulasuriya S. Oral submucous fibrosis: review on aetiology and pathogenesis. Oral Oncol 2006; 42: 561–8.

Treister NS, Magalnick D, Woo SB. Oral mucosal pigmentation secondary to minocycline therapy: report of two cases and a review of the literature. Oral Surg Oral Med Oral Pathol Oral Radiol Endod 2004; 97: 718–25.

van der Waal I. The diagnosis and treatment of precancerous lesions. FDI World 1995; 4: 6–9.

Wakefield Y, Pemberton MN. Oro-facial thermal injury caused by food heated in a microwave oven. Dent Update 2009; 36: 26–7.

Warnakulasuriya S, Reibel J, Bouquot J, Dabelsteen E. Oral epithelial dysplasia classification systems: predictive value, utility, weaknesses and scope for improvement. J Oral Pathol Med 2008; 37: 127–33.

# 2.3 TONGUE

- aesthetic conditions
- congenital conditions
- pigmented, red, purple or blue lesions
- soreness, ulceration and pain
- swellings and lumps
- white lesions

---

The specialized mucosa on the dorsum of the tongue, adapted for taste and mastication, is keratinized.

The posterior third of the tongue, difficult to visualize, contains the *lingual tonsils*—round or oval prominences of lymphoid tissue with intervening lingual crypts lined by non-keratinized epithelium, lying between the epiglottis posteriorly and the circumvallate papillae anteriorly. It is usually divided in the midline by a ligament. The lingual tonsils are part of *Waldeyer oropharyngeal ring* of lymphoid tissue.

The posterior third of the tongue is embryologically and anatomically distinct from the anterior two-thirds (the oral tongue) and the two parts are joined at a V-shaped groove, the *sulcus terminalis*. The anterior (oral) tongue bears a number of different papillae.

*Circumvallate papillae*, each surrounded by a deep groove into which open ducts of the serous minor salivary glands are 8–12 large papillae, adjacent and anterior to the sulcus terminalis. The lateral walls of these papillae contain taste buds.

*Foliate papillae*: 4–11 parallel ridges alternating with deep grooves in the mucosa—lie on the lateral margins posteriorly and also have taste buds.

*Filiform papillae* which form an abrasive surface to control the food bolus as it is pressed against the palate cover the entire surface of the anterior two-thirds of the tongue dorsum.

*Fungiform papillae* are fewer, mushroom-shaped, red structures covered by non-keratinized epithelium and with taste buds on their surface are scattered between the filiform papillae, mainly anteriorly.

The tongue dorsum is best inspected by protrusion, when it can be held with gauze. A healthy child's tongue is rarely coated but a mild coating is not uncommon in healthy adults. The posterior aspect of the floor of the mouth is the most difficult area to examine well and one where lesions are most likely to be missed. The floor of mouth and tongue ventrum is best examined by asking the patient to push the tongue first into the palate then into each cheek in turn. This raises for inspection the floor of the mouth, an area where tumours may start (the 'coffin' or 'graveyard' area of the mouth) (Figs 2.3.1–2.3.5). During this part of the examination the quantity and consistency of saliva should be assessed. Examine for the normal pooling of saliva in the floor of the mouth.

The voluntary tongue movements and sense of taste should be formally tested. Abnormalities of tongue movement (neurological or muscular disease) may be obvious from dysarthria or involuntary movements and any fibrillation or wasting noted.

Taste sensation can be tested with salt, sweet, sour, bitter and *unami* by applying solutions of salt, sugar, vinegar (acetic acid), 5% citric acid and glutamate to the tongue on a cotton swab or cotton bud.

A range of local and systemic disorders can affect the tongue; this chapter highlights only those that are seen particularly or exclusively in that location.

## AESTHETIC CONDITIONS
### Body art
The practice of tongue piercing is a cause of some concern since bleeding or oedema can occasionally be pronounced, widespread and a hazard to the airway. Thereafter, the permanent jewellery is placed and worn constantly, to avoid the perforation closing over spontaneously (Fig. 2.3.6). Speech can be impaired and the teeth and gingiva may be damaged by the jewellery. Tongue piercing provides a potential reservoir for periodontopathogenic bacteria.

Tongue splitting is another form of body art.

## CONGENITAL CONDITIONS
### Ankyloglossia
Ankyloglossia (tongue-tie).

*Aetiopathogenesis*
Ankyloglossia, or tongue-tie, is usually a congenital anomaly: there may be a family history of ankyloglossia, and sometimes deviation of the epiglottis or larynx. The association of ankyloglossia with cleft palate is inherited as a semi-dominant disorder related to chromosome Xq21: the T-box transcription factor gene *TBX22* is mutated.

In some other patients, maternal cocaine use has been implicated.

*Clinical features*
Ankyloglossia is caused by a tight lingual fraenum and, therefore, the tongue cannot be fully protruded (Fig. 2.3.7). A similar effect can be seen after surgery or burns, if there is scarring in the area.

There is no evidence that ankyloglossia interferes seriously with speech but it can result in difficulty in using the tongue to cleanse food away from the teeth and vestibules.

The opposite effect is seen in Ehlers–Danlos syndrome, where there is a genetic connective tissue abnormality resulting in joint hypermobility and the tongue can be protruded far enough to touch the tip of the nose (Gorlin sign).

*Diagnosis*
Clinical.

*Management*
If necessary, fraenectomy will relieve ankyloglossia.

### Erythema migrans
Erythema migrans (geographic tongue, benign migratory glossitis or migratory stomatitis).

*Aetiopathogenesis*
Erythema migrans is a very common and benign inflammatory condition of the tongue, quite distinct from the cutaneous disorder of the same name. In oral erythema migrans the filiform papillae desquamate in irregular demarcated areas.

The aetiology is unknown, but many patients with erythema migrans have a positive family history and many patients with a fissured tongue (scrotal tongue) also have lingual erythema migrans. There are reports of associations with human leukocyte antigen (HLA)-B15 and DR7, but HLA findings have been equivocal.

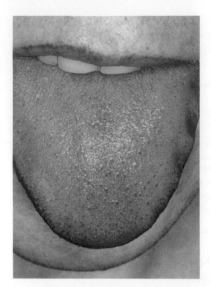

*Figure 2.3.1* Normal tongue.

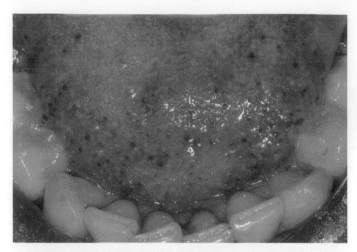

*Figure 2.3.2* Normal tongue showing racial pigmentation.

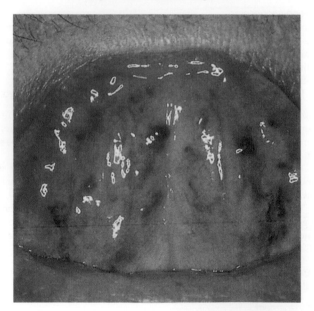

*Figure 2.3.3* Normal tongue with varices—ventrum.

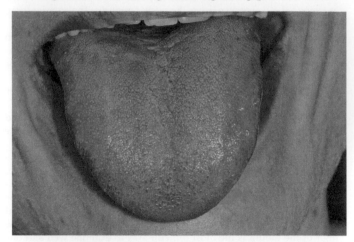

*Figure 2.3.4* Normal tongue—dorsum.

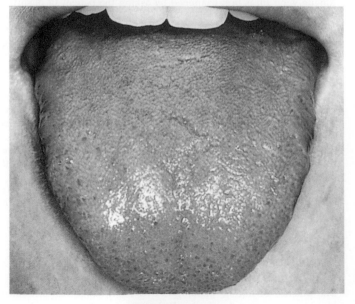

*Figure 2.3.5* Normal tongue—dorsum.

Clinically and histologically similar oral lesions may be seen in Reiter syndrome, generalized pustular psoriasis and acrodermatitis continua of Hallopeau.

Some patients with lingual erythema migrans have atopic allergies such as hay fever and a few relate the oral lesions to a particular food, for example, cheese, or to stress.

Purported associations with diabetes may be coincidental.

### Clinical features

Erythema migrans may be asymptomatic or may cause soreness, especially on eating spicy or acidic foods. Erythema migrans is characterized by map-like red areas with increased thickness of intervening filiform papillae. Alternatively, there are rounded, sometimes scalloped, reddish areas with a white margin. These patterns change from day to day and even within a few hours. Rarely, other sites, such as the labial or palatal mucosa, are also affected (Figs 2.3.8–2.3.16). There are no known complications.

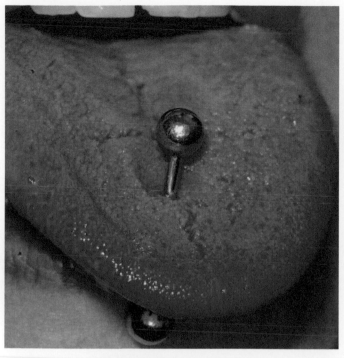

*Figure 2.3.6* Body art—tongue stud.

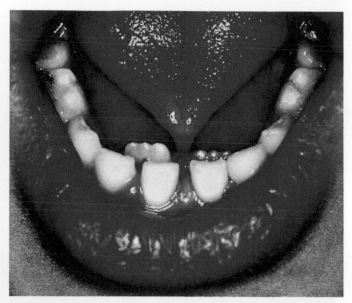

*Figure 2.3.7* Ankyloglossia.

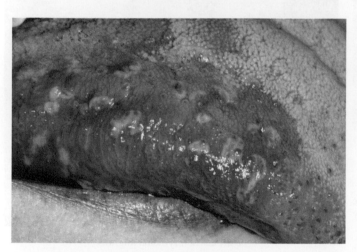

*Figure 2.3.8* Erythema migrans.

There are rare examples where the lesion is persistent and unchanging (erythema migrans perstans is the rather inappropriate term used).

*Diagnosis*
Clinical examination usually suffices to differentiate erythema migrans from deficiency glossitis, lichen planus (LP), candidosis, psoriasis or rarely, larva migrans.

*Management*
Benzydamine hydrochloride spray or mouthwash may provide symptomatic relief. Retinoids and tetracyclines have been advocated by some

and topical corticosteroids may be symptomatically helpful—but there is no effective treatment.

**Fissured tongue**
Fissured tongue (scrotal or plicated tongue).

*Aetiopathogenesis*
Fissured tongue is a common developmental anomaly affecting up to 15% of the population. Fissured tongue has no known associations with systemic disease, but it may be commonly seen in:

• Down syndrome
• Melkersson–Rosenthal syndrome.

*Clinical features*
Fissured tongue gives rise to fissures that radiate from the centre of the dorsum to the lateral borders (Figs 2.3.17 and 2.3.18). Tongue protrusion may make the fissures more obvious. It may only first be noticed after puberty. In about 20% of cases there may also be erythema migrans.

*Diagnosis*
The diagnosis is usually clear-cut from clinical features. The lobulated tongue of xerostomia (e.g. as in Sjögren syndrome) must be differentiated (Fig. 2.3.19) (Chapter 1.15).

*Management*
Reassure: the condition is of no serious consequence.

**Lingual thyroid**
*Aetiopathogenesis*
The thyroid arises embryonically from an invagination of lingual mucosa and remnant may remain within the posterior tongue. Some 10% of cadaver tongues contain thyroid tissue, although clinical presentation is much less common.

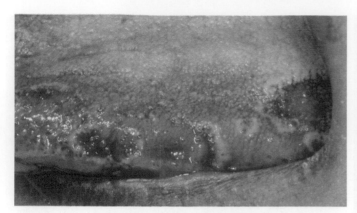

*Figure 2.3.9* Erythema migrans.

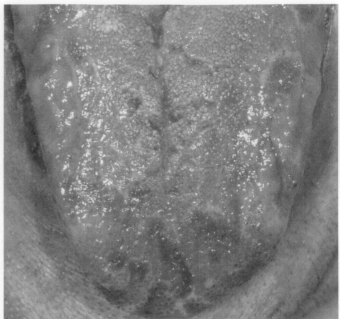

*Figure 2.3.10* Erythema migrans.

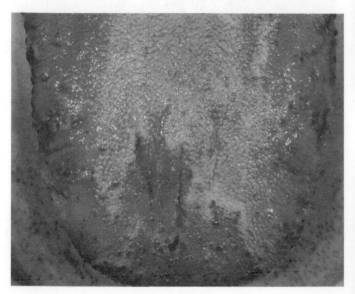

*Figure 2.3.11* Erythema migrans.

*Clinical features*
Midline asymptomatic smooth-surfaced lumps in the posterior tongue occasionally prove to be due to a lingual thyroid. Complications may include hypothyroidism in up to 20%, dysplasia, dysarthria or dyspnoea.

*Diagnosis and management*
The neck should be examined and MRI and $^{99m}$Tc pertechnetate radionuclide scan performed to ensure there is a normal thyroid gland in the neck, before such a lump is excised, since in about 75% of cases no thyroid tissue is present in the neck.

### Lymphangioma
*Aetiopathogenesis*
Lymphangioma is a hamartoma containing lymph.

*Clinical features*
The surface may have a typical 'frogspawn' appearance. Lymphangioma is uncommon in the mouth, usually solitary and seen mainly in the anterior tongue (Fig. 2.3.20) or lip.

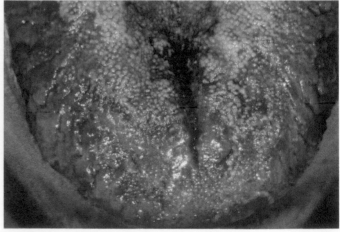

*Figure 2.3.12* Erythema migrans.

Patients with lymphatic malformations of the tongue base often have extensive disease and risk of serious complications and death.

*Diagnosis*
Clinical, but contrast-enhanced $T_1$-weighted MRI can be used to differentiate between lymphangiomas and deep haemangiomas.

*Management*
Small lymphangiomas need no treatment. Larger lesions may require excision, although cryotherapy, laser therapy and sclerotherapy can be useful and radiofrequency ablation has been reported. Embolization may also be possible.

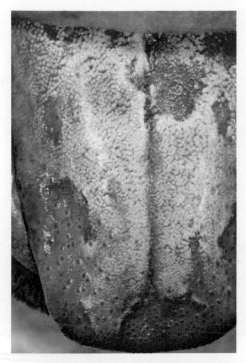

*Figure 2.3.13* Erythema migrans.

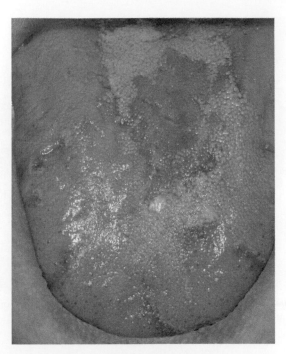

*Figure 2.3.14* Erythema migrans.

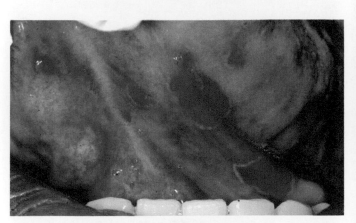

*Figure 2.3.15* Erythema migrans.

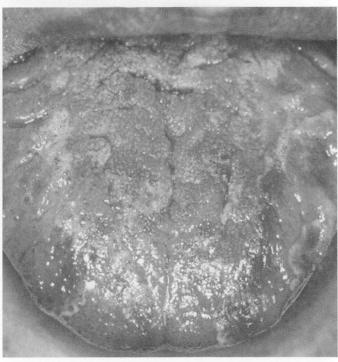

*Figure 2.3.16* Erythema migrans.

# PIGMENTED, RED, PURPLE OR BLUE LESIONS

## Angina bullosa haemorrhagica

Angina bullosa haemorrhagica (Chapter 2.4).

## Black hairy tongue

### Aetiopathogenesis

Superficial transient brown discolouration of the dorsum of the tongue and sometimes other soft tissues may be caused by cigarette smoking, tobacco or betel chewing, some drugs (such as iron salts), some foods and beverages (such as coffee, tea and liquorice) and chlorhexidine.

Black hairy tongue is more common in people with hyposalivation, where the diet is soft, where antimicrobials are used, and where oral hygiene is wanting and appears to be caused by the accumulation of epithelial squames and the proliferation of chromogenic micro-organisms.

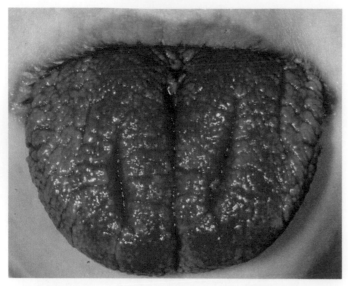

*Figure 2.3.17* Fissured (scrotal tongue) and angular stomatitis in orofacial granulomatosis.

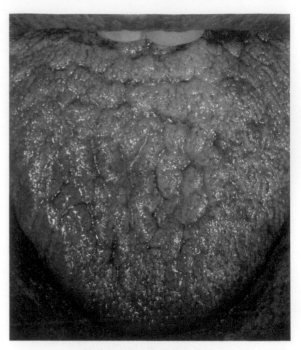

*Figure 2.3.18* Fissured tongue.

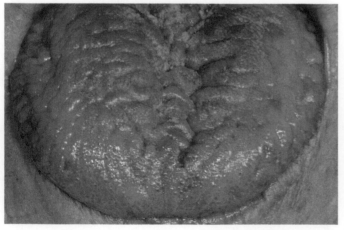

*Figure 2.3.19* Fissured tongue in Sjögren syndrome.

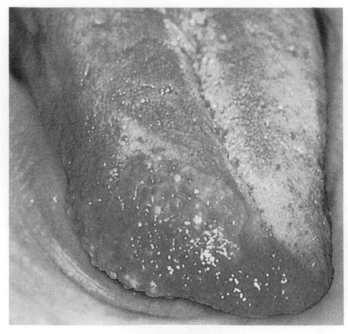

*Figure 2.3.20* Lymphangioma.

*Clinical features*
Black hairy tongue (Figs 2.3.21 and 2.3.22) affects the posterior dorsum of the tongue; there is often a triangular area of discolouration pointing anteriorly. The filiform papillae are excessively long and stained and black or brown.

*Diagnosis*
Clinical.

*Management*
Such discolouration, although not uncommon, is usually of obvious aetiology, is easily removed and is of little consequence. Patients with black hairy tongue may find the condition improves by eating pineapple or sucking a peach stone, increasing their oral hygiene, scraping the tongue with a tongue-scraper, or brushing the tongue with a hard toothbrush, using sodium bicarbonate mouthwashes.

**Haematoma**
Haematoma (Chapter 2.1).

**Haemangioma**
Haemangioma (Figs 2.3.23–2.3.26).

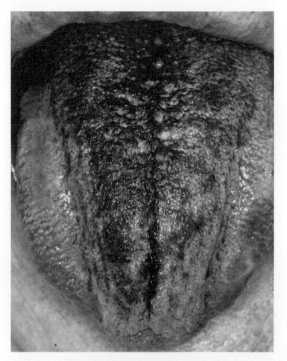

*Figure 2.3.21* Black hairy tongue.

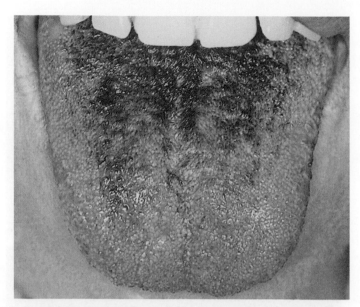

*Figure 2.3.22* Black hairy tongue.

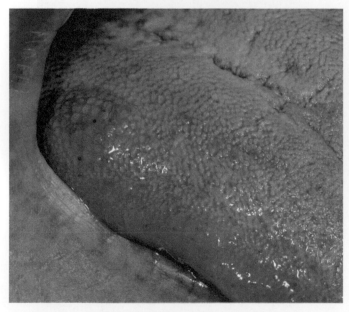

*Figure 2.3.23* Angioma (haemangioma).

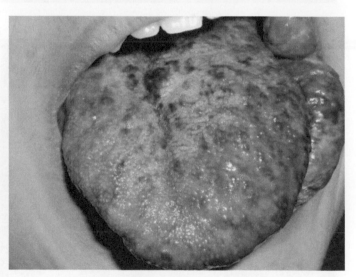

*Figure 2.3.24* Angioma (haemangioma).

## Kaposi sarcoma

Kaposi sarcoma (Chapter 1.7).

## Median rhomboid glossitis

Median rhomboid glossitis (central papillary atrophy).

*Aetiopathogenesis*

Median rhomboid glossitis was originally thought to be caused by persistence of the tuberculum impar, but it is rarely seen in children. It is now known to be associated with candidosis. Smoking, denture wearing and, occasionally, immune defects (including HIV) and diabetes predispose.

*Clinical features*

Median rhomboid glossitis is typically a symptomless, red or mixed red and white, depapillated, rhomboidal area in the midline of the dorsum of the tongue, just anterior to the sulcus terminalis and of somewhat rhomboidal shape (Figs 2.3.27–2.3.29). Occasionally, there is a nodular component.

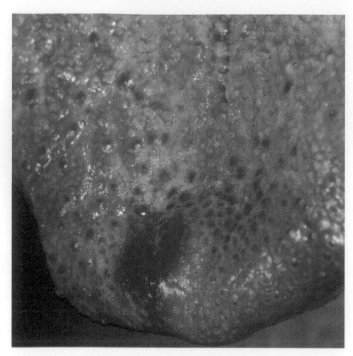

*Figure 2.3.25* Angioma (haemangioma).

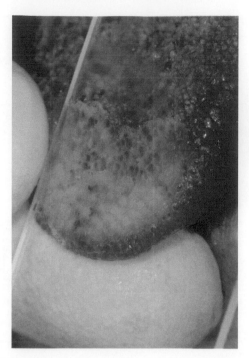

*Figure 2.3.26* Angioma (haemangioma) showing effect of pressure.

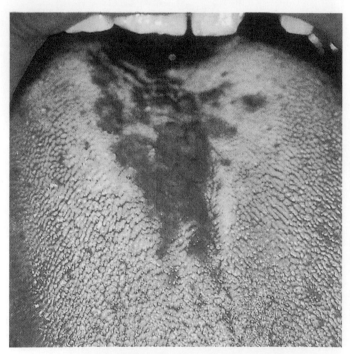

*Figure 2.3.27* Candidal median rhomboid glossitis.

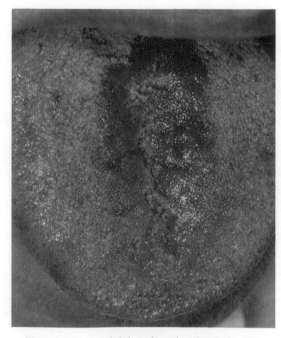

*Figure 2.3.28* Candidal median rhomboid glossitis.

There may also sometimes be a coexistent erythematous candidosis 'kissing' lesion in the palate—which some have termed 'chronic oral multifocal candidosis'.

*Diagnosis*

Median rhomboid glossitis is usually diagnosed on clinical grounds, although biopsy may be indicated, since some lesions are nodular and may clinically simulate a neoplasm. Histology shows irregular candida-induced pseudoepitheliomatous epithelial hyperplasia that may resemble a carcinoma histopathologically but it is not a malignant condition. Oral carcinoma is rare at this site—but not unknown.

In view of the possible association with immunodeficiency and chronic mucocutaneous candidosis (Chapter 1.7), assessment of the full blood cell count and appropriate physician referral may be warranted in some cases.

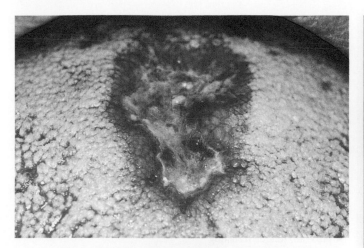

Figure 2.3.29  Candidal median rhomboid glossitis.

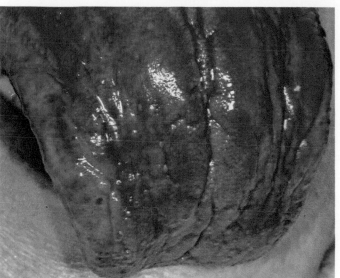

Figure 2.3.30  Glossitis.

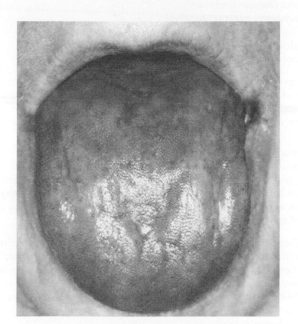

Figure 2.3.31  Glossitis in iron deficiency.

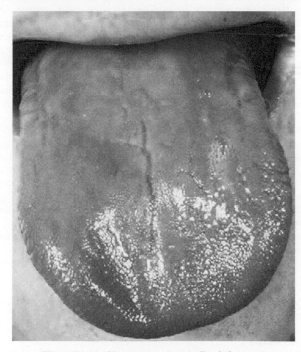

Figure 2.3.32  Glossitis in vitamin B$_{12}$ deficiency.

*Management*
Median rhomboid glossitis may respond to smoking cessation and to the use of antifungals.

**Racial**
Racial (Fig. 2.5.53) (Chapter 2.5).

# SORENESS, ULCERATION AND PAIN
## Atrophic glossitis
Atrophic glossitis (lingual papillary atrophy) is usually due to haematinic deficiency (Fig. 2.3.30–2.3.33), but atrophy may also be seen after repeated ulceration, burns or irradiation.

**Burning tongue**
Burning tongue [glosspyrosis; burning mouth syndrome (BMS); stomatodynia].

*Aetiopathogenesis*
The International Association for the Study of Pain have defined BMS as 'a distinctive nosological entity characterized by unremitting oral burning or similar pain in the absence of detectable mucosal changes' while the International Headache Society defines it as 'an intraoral burning sensation for which no medical or dental cause can be found'.

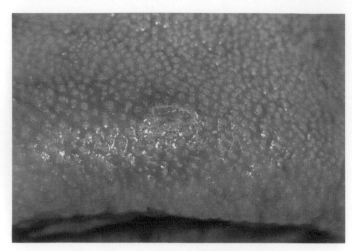

*Figure 2.3.33* Glossitis in vitamin B$_{12}$ deficiency.

A burning sensation in the mouth, especially the tongue, may also be caused by vitamin or iron deficiency, diabetes mellitus, long-standing xerostomia, drugs such as angiotensin converting enzyme (ACE) inhibitors or protease inhibitors, or lesions such as erythema migrans. Patients with BMS have none of the aforementioned features, although they may complain of symptoms of xerostomia (in the absence of relevant signs).

A psychogenic cause, such as anxiety, depression or cancerophobia, can be identified in about 20% of cases. The BMS may seem to have a precipitant such as a dental intervention or respiratory tract infection, but these are unlikely to be of aetiological relevance.

It has been suggested recently that BMS is a disorder of reduced pain threshold and that patients are 'super-tasters'—with a raised sensitivity to taste. Hypotheses include that BMS is due to a neuropathy, with:

- neurological transduction interruption induced by salivary compositional alterations, or
- changes in the nigrostriatal dopaminergic system which causes trigeminal excitability or
- loss of central inhibition from taste damage in the chorda tympani and/or glossopharyngeal nerve or
- a sympathetic activity-mediated disorder affecting the trigeminal induced by trauma or varicella zoster virus infection.

A unilateral burning sensation may be neurological in origin, often due to a brainstem lesion.

### Clinical features

BMS most frequently affects the tongue, but it can also affect the palate or, less commonly, the lips or lower alveolus. The complaint is bilateral and:

- variably
  - burning
  - scalded
  - tingling
- persistent but does not disturb sleep
- prolonged > 4 months
- unlikely to spontaneously remit until after several years
- not worsened by eating: rather it is tends to be relieved by eating and drinking
- reduced by alcohol.

There are often also multiple oral and/or other psychogenic-related complaints, such as:

- dry mouth
- dysgeusia
- thirst
- headaches
- chronic back pain
- irritable bowel syndrome
- dysmenorrhoea.

### Diagnosis

Oral examination is important to exclude organic causes of similar discomfort, such as:

- allergies
- bruxism/tongue thrusting
- candidosis
- dermatoses such as LP, dry mouth and drugs such as ACE inhibitors and protease inhibitors
- erythema migrans (geographic tongue)
- fissured tongue
- glossitis such as caused by haematinic deficiency
- hormonal problems such as diabetes and hypothyroidism.

Investigations indicated may include psychological screening using, for example, the hospital anxiety and depression scale, sialometry and haematological/serological assessment for anaemia, haematinic deficiency, diabetes and hypothyroidism, and possible causes of xerostomia.

### Management

About 50% of patients with BMS remit spontaneously within 6 or 7 years, but few have spontaneous remission in the short term, and thus treatment is usually indicated. Patients should avoid anything that aggravates symptoms, such as sparkling wines, citrus drinks and spices.

- Patient information is crucial in management, providing positive reinforcement of the likelihood that the symptoms are not a reflection of significant oral or systemic disease, and that in many instances resolve spontaneously.
- Some patients respond to topical benzydamine rinse or spray; topical capsaicin cream; a clonazepam tablet sucked locally; or alpha-lipoic acid—systemically.

Cognitive behavioural therapy or a specialist referral may be indicated.
Antidepressants and anxiolytics may be of some benefit, but should only be prescribed if there is evidence of a proven underlying affective disorder. Possible therapies include:

- amitriptyline
- clonazepam
- dosulepin
- doxepin
- fluoxetine
- nortriptyline
- trazodone.

Gabapentin, or lafutidine (an H2 receptor antagonist) may also be of benefit.

Active dental or oral surgical treatment, or attempts at 'hormone replacement', in the absence of any specific indication, should be avoided.

## Candidosis
Candidosis (Chapter 1.8).

## Acute atrophic candidosis
Acute atrophic candidosis (antibiotic sore tongue).

Broad spectrum antimicrobials such as tetracycline or ampicillin, and corticosteroids, predispose to an acute atrophic candidosis that causes soreness or a burning sensation, especially of the tongue.

## Erythematous candidosis
This is akin to median rhomboid glossitis.

## Deficiency glossitis
Deficiency glossitis page 247.

## Erythema migrans
Erythema migrans page 239.

## Foliate papillitis
*Aetiopathogenesis*
The foliate papillae are normally of variable size and shape and they occasionally swell if irritated mechanically or if there is an upper respiratory infection.

*Clinical features*
The foliate papillae, found on the lateral border of the tongue, at the junction of the anterior two-thirds with the posterior third, may cause discomfort and be swollen and/or erythematous (Fig. 2.3.34).

Inflammation of the lingual tonsils may also give rise to concern as it may present with pain and dysphagia.

*Diagnosis*
Clinical.

*Management*
Located at a site of high predilection for lingual cancer, enlarged foliate papillae may give rise to anxiety about cancer. Reassurance is indicated.

## Trauma
Lingual soreness can arise from the patient pressing or moving the tongue consciously or subconsciously on the teeth (Figs 2.3.35–2.3.37).

## Ulceration
Ulceration (Chapter 2.2).

Lingual ulceration can arise from local causes such as trauma, burns or mucositis, from aphthae, drugs, neoplasms or systemic disease (haematological, infectious, gastrointestinal, mucocutaneous) (Figs 2.3.38–2.3.46).

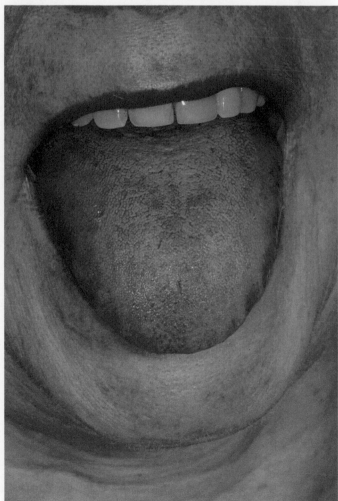

*Figure 2.3.35* Trauma—causing crenation.

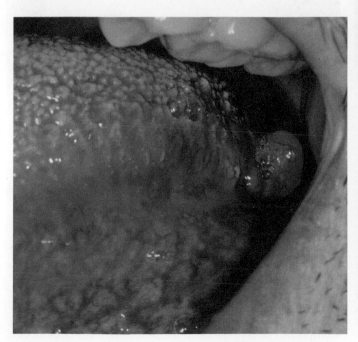

*Figure 2.3.34* Foliate papillitis.

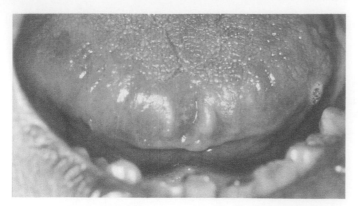

*Figure 2.3.36*  Trauma—tooth indents on tongue.

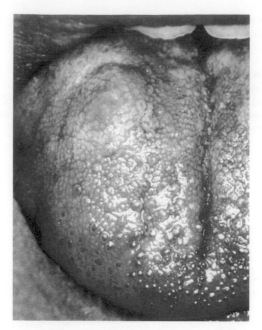

*Figure 2.3.37*  Trauma—haematoma.

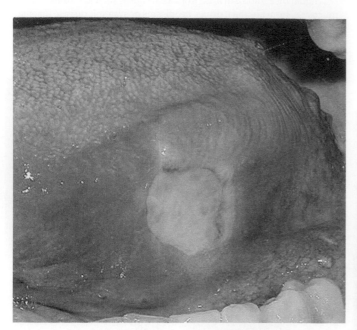

*Figure 2.3.38*  Traumatic ulceration.

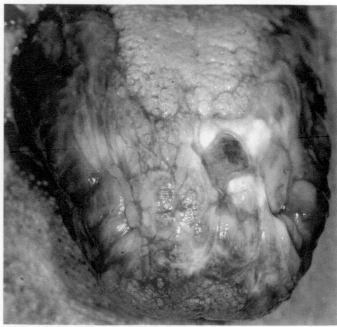

*Figure 2.3.39*  Lichen planus.

# SWELLINGS AND LUMPS

### Angiomas

Angiomas (Chapter 2.1).

### Deposits

Amyloidosis is a rare cause of lingual swelling.

### Neoplasms

Oral squamous cell carcinoma (OSCC) is the most common oral cancer and amongst the 10 most common cancers worldwide. It appears most commonly on the tongue. The number of new mouth (oral) and oropharyngeal cancers are estimated to be 300,000 cases worldwide, amounting to around 3% of total cancers.

Cancers of the oral cavity are classified according to site by the International Classification of Diseases (ICD):

- lip (ICD-10, C00),
- tongue (ICD-10, C01, C02),
- gum (ICD-10, C03),
- floor of the mouth (ICD-10, C04),
- unspecified parts of the mouth (ICD-10, C06), tonsil (ICD-10, C09), oropharynx (ICD-10, C10) and other ill-defined sites (ICD-10, C14).

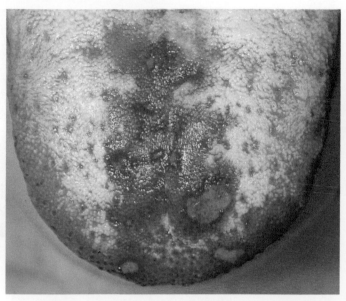

Figure 2.3.40 Herpetic ulceration (herpes simplex virus).

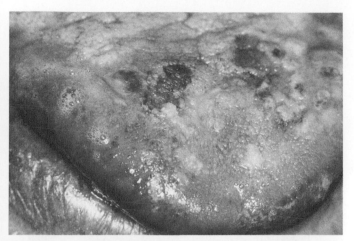

Figure 2.3.41 Herpetic ulceration (herpes simplex virus) in HIV disease.

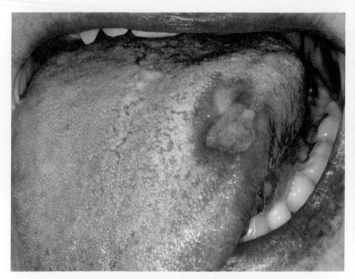

Figure 2.3.42 Drug-induced ulceration.

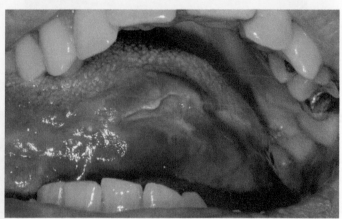

Figure 2.3.43 Drug-induced ulceration (phenytoin).

Other malignant oral neoplasms include:

- Epithelial malignancies other than squamous carcinomas:
  ○ arising from a surface (e.g. melanoma)
  ○ maxillary antral carcinoma (or other neoplasms)
  ○ glandular (e.g. salivary gland)
  ○ intrabony epithelial (e.g. odontogenic).
- Secondary carcinomas:
  ○ within a lymph node (e.g. metastasis from the mouth)
  ○ within bone (e.g. metastasis from lung, breast, kidney, stomach, liver cancer).
- Sarcomas:
  ○ in muscle (e.g. rhabdomyosarcoma)
  ○ in bone (e.g. osteosarcoma)

○ in connective tissue (e.g. sarcoma)
○ from blood vessels (e.g. Kaposi sarcoma).
- Lymphoreticular neoplasms:
  ○ lymphomas.

*Aetiopathogenesis*

OSCC arises as a consequence of multiple molecular events causing genetic damage affecting many chromosomes and genes, which leads to DNA changes and eventually to one of the main features that appears to precede the onset of malignancy—epithelial dysplasia.

Predisposing factors (risk factors) for OSCC include especially:

- age
- a number of lifestyle factors
  ○ tobacco use
  ○ alcohol use
  ○ betel quid use (some 22% of the world's population use betel)
  ○ ethnic minority groups
  ○ lower socio-economic groups.
- Micro-organisms such as Candida, syphilis and human papilloma-viruses (HPV) have been detected in some OSCC where they may play a role. HPV-16 is particularly implicated in oropharyngeal cancer.

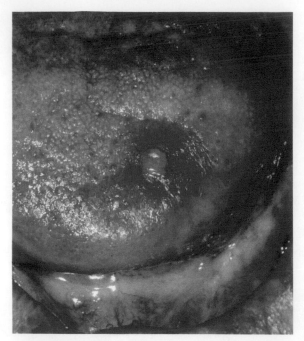

Figure 2.3.44  Drug-induced ulceration (alendronate).

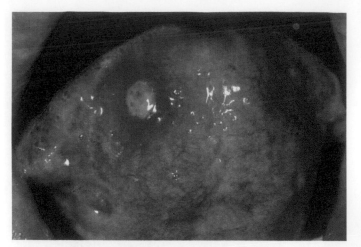

Figure 2.3.45  Recurrent aphthous stomatitis.

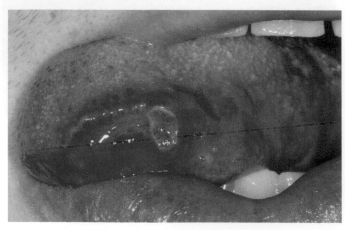

Figure 2.3.46  Recurrent aphthous stomatitis.

- There is concern that cannabis use may predispose to OSCC.
- Diets rich in fresh fruits and vegetables and in vitamin A may have a protective effect.

Potentially malignant (precancerous) lesions which can progress to OSCC include, especially:

- Erythroplasia (erythroplakia): the most likely lesion to progress to severe dysplasia or carcinoma.
- Leukoplakia (Chapter 2.2):
  o proliferative verrucous leukoplakia
  o sublingual leukoplakia
  o candidal leukoplakia
  o syphilitic leukoplakia.

Potentially malignant (precancerous) conditions include:

- actinic cheilitis
- lichenoid lesions; cases of dysplasia with a lichenoid appearance (lichenoid dysplasia)
- discoid lupus erythematosus
- submucous fibrosis
- previous oral malignancy
- immunosuppression
- Fanconi anaemia
- syphilitic glossitis
- dyskeratosis congenita
- Paterson–Brown–Kelly syndrome (sideropenic dysphagia; Plummer–Vinson syndrome)
- scleroderma
- diabetes.

*Clinical features*

OSCC is seen predominantly in older people, but intraoral cancer is increasing, especially in younger adults. OSCC is seen predominantly in males, but the male/female differential is decreasing. There is marked inter-country variation in both the incidence of and mortality from oral cancer. In addition, there is also growing evidence of intra-country and ethnic differences in incidence and mortality, especially recorded in the United Kingdom and United States.

OSCC may present clinically as a (Figs 2.3.47–2.3.55):

- Granular ulcer with fissuring or raised rolled everted (exophytic) margins.
- Red lesion (erythroplasia).
- White lesion.
- Mixed white and red lesion.
- Lump, sometimes with abnormal supplying blood vessels.
- Lump/ulcer which is indurated (i.e. a firm infiltration beneath the mucosa).
- Non-healing extraction socket.
- Lesion fixed to deeper tissues or to overlying skin or mucosa.
- Some 25% of OSCC in the developed world affects the tongue, the common intraoral site.

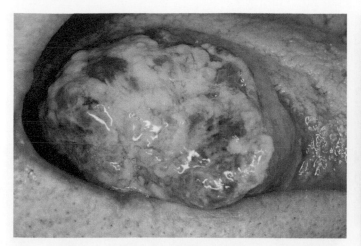

*Figure 2.3.47* Carcinoma.

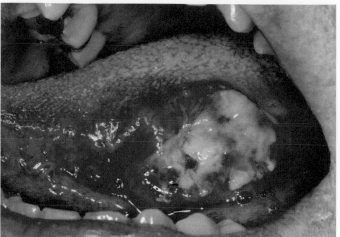

*Figure 2.3.48* Carcinoma.

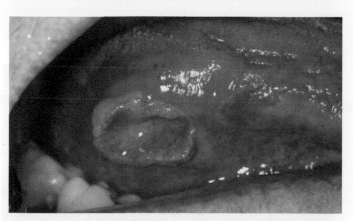

*Figure 2.3.49* Carcinoma.

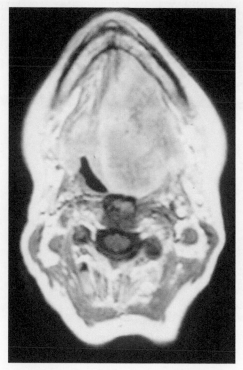

*Figure 2.3.50* Carcinoma (MRI scan).

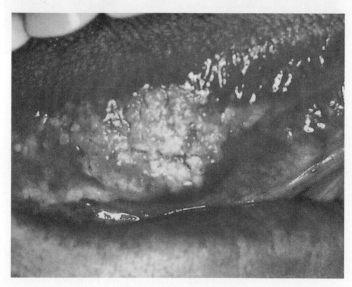

*Figure 2.3.51* Carcinoma.

- The majority of OSCC involve the lateral border of the tongue and/or the floor of the mouth, but the very invasive nature of these tumours makes difficult the precise definition of the site of origin. Nevertheless, most arise from the lower part of the mouth raising questions as to why this site appears predisposed to tumour development. Perhaps carcinogens pool in saliva in this so-called 'graveyard' or 'coffin' area?
- In the developing world, where OSCC arises mainly from betel use, OSCC is most common in the buccal mucosa.
- Most intraoral tumours are larger than 2 cm in diameter at presentation.
- Carcinomas in the anterior mouth are usually detected at an earlier stage than are carcinomas in the posterior oral cavity.

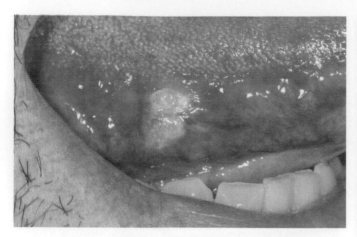

*Figure 2.3.52* Carcinoma.

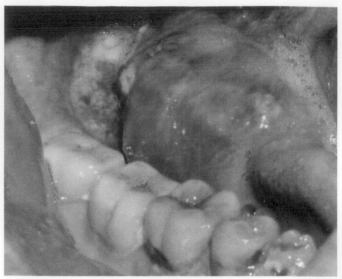

*Figure 2.3.53* Carcinoma.

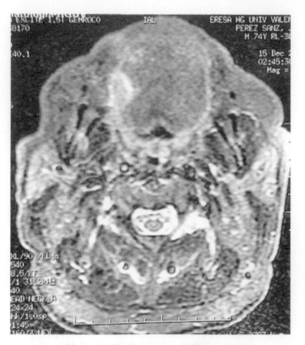

*Figure 2.3.54* Carcinoma (MRI scan).

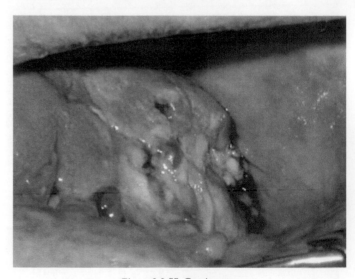

*Figure 2.3.55* Carcinoma.

- Lymph node enlargement, especially if there is hardness in a lymph node or fixation. Enlarged cervical nodes in a patient with oral carcinoma may be caused by infection, reactive hyperplasia secondary to the tumour or metastatic disease. Occasionally, a 'positive' lymph node is detected in the absence of any obvious primary tumour.
- Second primary tumours (SPTs) in the aerodigestive tract may be seen in those with OSCC.

*Diagnosis*

- Clinicians should be aware that single ulcers, lumps, red patches or white patches, particularly if any of these are persisting for more than 3 weeks, may be manifestations of frank malignancy. There should be a high index of suspicion, especially of a solitary lesion present for over 3 weeks: biopsy is invariably indicated.
- The whole oral mucosa should be examined as there may be widespread dysplastic mucosa ('field change') or even a SPT, and the cervical lymph nodes must be examined. Frank tumours should be inspected and palpated to determine the extent of spread.
- Examination under general anaesthetic may be indicated especially for patients with:
  ○ tumours in the posterior tongue
  ○ tumours where the margins cannot be readily defined
  ○ an enlarged cervical node but no visible primary neoplasm. Blind biopsy of the tonsil or fossa of Rosenmuller may then be indicated. Positron emission tomography (PET) may also be helpful to identify latent primary neoplasms

○ any suggestion of a SPT; these patients may then need panendoscopy of larynx, pharynx and oesophagus
- OSCC should be staged according to the TNM (tumour, node, metastases) classification of the International Union against Cancer—according to tumour size, nodal metastases and distant metastases—since this classification relates well to overall survival rate (i.e. the earlier the tumour, the better the prognosis and the less complicated is the treatment).

When deciding which investigations to undertake, three principles are crucial to:

- Confirm the diagnosis histopathologically, and determine if there is malignant disease elsewhere, whether there are:
  ○ Bone, muscles or cervical lymph nodes involved.
  ○ Other primary tumours (typically in the upper aerodigestive tract—mouth, nares, pharynx, larynx, oesophagus). There is controversy as to the need for endoscopy in all cases to detect such tumours.
  ○ Metastases, which initially are to regional lymph nodes and later to liver, bone and brain. Imaging may detect abnormalities that escape clinical examination.
- Ensure that the patient is as prepared as possible for the major surgery required, particularly in terms of their understanding and consent, general anaesthesia, potential blood loss and ability to metabolize drugs.
- Address any potential dental or oral problems preoperatively, to avoid later complications such as osteoradionecrosis.

These three principles almost invariably indicate the following investigations:

- Lesional biopsy.
- Biopsy or fine needle aspiration of equivocal neck lymph nodes.
- Jaw radiography (often rotating pantomography), though this is inadequate to exclude bone invasion.
- Chest radiography or CT. This is important as a preanaesthetic check, especially in patients with known pulmonary or airways disease, and to demonstrate SPTs or metastases to lungs or hilar lymph nodes, ribs or vertebrae.
- MRI or CT of the primary site, of the head and neck, and suspected sites of distant metastases, and MRI scans of the neck to delineate the extent of cervical node metastases. Some units routinely examine the chest and abdomen. Diffusion-weighted imaging and the apparent diffusion coefficient can help in the differential diagnosis of carcinomas from lymphomas, and may also help differentiate benign from malignant tumours. MRI is particularly useful to determine:
  ○ tumour spread
  ○ bone involvement
  ○ nodal metastases.
- PET (now routine in some units) or single photon emission computed tomography.
- Electrocardiography.
- Blood tests:
  ○ full blood picture and haemoglobin
  ○ blood for grouping and cross-matching
  ○ urea and electrolytes
  ○ liver function tests.

In selected cases other investigations which may be indicated include:

- bronchoscopy, if chest radiography reveals any lesions
- endoscopy of the upper aerodigestive tract, especially if there is a history of tobacco use
- gastroscopy, if a per-endoscopic gastrostomy is to be used for feeding

- liver ultrasound, if there is hepatomegaly or abnormal liver function
- Doppler duplex flow studies, in planning radial free forearm flaps
- angiography, in planning lower limb free flaps.

*Management*
Cancer treatment and planning decisions are based on

- tumour size, nodal status and metastases
- wishes of the patient
- social circumstances
- co-existent medical conditions.

Cancer treatment and planning involves a multidisciplinary team that includes a range of specialties: surgeons, pathologists, anaesthetists, oncologists, nursing staff, dental staff, nutritionists, speech and physiotherapists, maxillofacial prosthodontists, social workers and others.

**Treatment modalities**

- OSCC is now treated largely by surgery and/or radiotherapy to control the primary tumour and metastases in the draining cervical lymph nodes.
- Intraoral cancers < 4 cm in diameter may be treated equally effectively by surgery or radiotherapy.
  ○ T1 tumours are generally managed surgically.
  ○ T2 tumours are also generally managed surgically.
  ○ T3 tumours are generally treated by surgery followed by radiotherapy if there is extracapsular spread or multiple lymph node involvement.
  ○ T4 tumours may be treated with chemo-radiotherapy using docetaxel (T), cisplatin (P) and 5-fluorouracil (F) (TPF).
  ○ Targeted therapy is increasingly used.

**Other neoplasms**
Other neoplasms (Chapter 1.11).

**Fibrous lumps**
Fibrous lumps (Fig. 2.3.56).

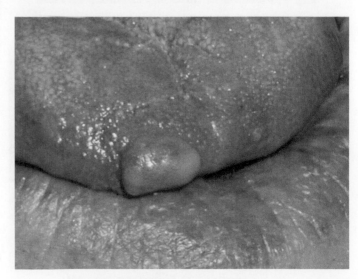

*Figure 2.3.56* Fibrous lump.

### Oedema

Oedema from trauma, infection or allergy may cause swelling.

### Pyogenic granulomas

Pyogenic granulomas (Figs 2.3.57 and 2.3.58) (Chapter 2.5).

### Warty lesions

Warty lesions (Figs 2.3.59–2.3.61) (Chapter 1.8).

## WHITE LESIONS

### Candidosis

Candidosis (thrush, candidosis, acute pseudomembranous candidosis, moniliasis) (Fig. 2.3.62A and B).

### Furred tongue

*Aetiopathogenesis*

Coating of the tongue is quite commonly seen in healthy adults, particularly in edentulous patients, those who are on a soft, non-abrasive diet, those with poor oral hygiene or those who are fasting. The coating in these instances appears to be of epithelial, food and microbial debris which collects since it is not mechanically removed. Indeed, the tongue is the main reservoir of some micro-organisms such as *Candida albicans* and some streptococci. The tongue may be coated with off-white debris in many illnesses, particularly

- febrile diseases
- xerostomia
- ill patients, especially those with poor oral hygiene or who are dehydrated.

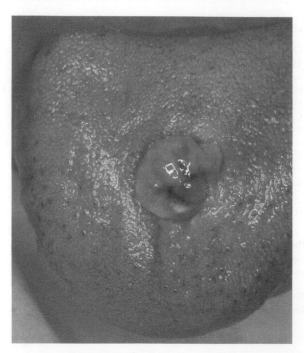

*Figure 2.3.57* Pyogenic granulomas.

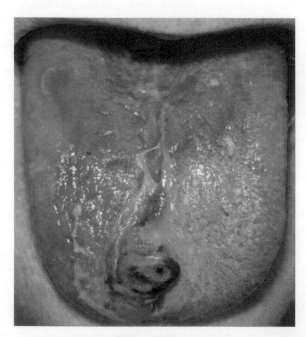

*Figure 2.3.58* Pyogenic granulomas.

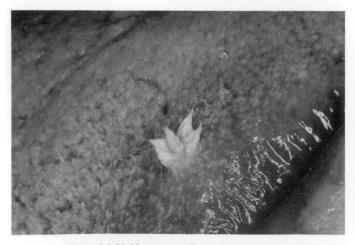

*Figure 2.3.59* Human papillomavirus infection.

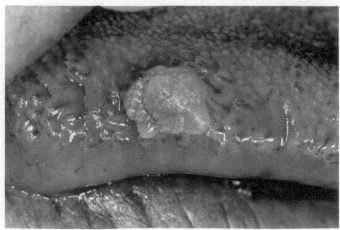

*Figure 2.3.60* Human papillomavirus infection.

*Clinical features*
Furring of the tongue dorsum only.

*Diagnosis*
The history is important to exclude a congenital or hereditary cause of an adherent white lesion. The clinical appearances may strongly suggest the diagnosis but investigations are often required if the white lesion does not scrape away from the mucosa with a gauze. Biopsy is then often indicated.

*Management*
Treatment is of the underlying cause.

## Hairy leukoplakia
*Aetiopathogenesis*
Hairy leukoplakia is a common, corrugated (or 'hairy') white lesion usually seen on the tongue mainly in HIV/AIDS and other immuno-compromising states. Hairy leukoplakia is caused by Epstein–Barr virus (EBV) and has no known malignant potential.

*Clinical features*
Hairy leukoplakia is:

• a white lesion that is not removed by wiping with a gauze
• seen mainly on the lateral margins of the tongue (Fig. 2.3.63)
• not known to be premalignant
• a predictor of poor prognosis in HIV disease
• sometimes associated with lymphoma elsewhere.

*Diagnosis*
Diagnosis is largely clinical, supported by immunohistochemical confirmation of the presence of intra-epithelial EBV within the lesional tissue, and HIV testing.

*Management*
Treatment is not required, since the lesion is almost always asymptomatic and has no malignant potential. Of note, however, the condition often resolves with aciclovir or valaciclovir or other agents active against EBV, or with restoration of immune function in HIV disease following use of antiretroviral agents.

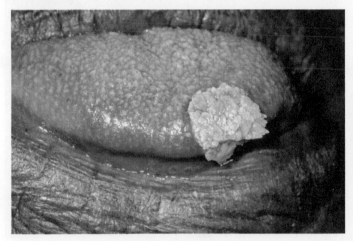

*Figure 2.3.61* Human papillomavirus infection—genital wart (condyloma acuminatum).

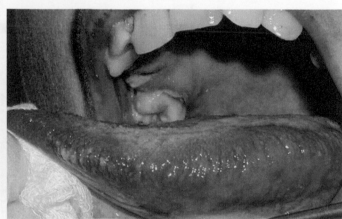

*Figure 2.3.63* Hairy leukoplakia.

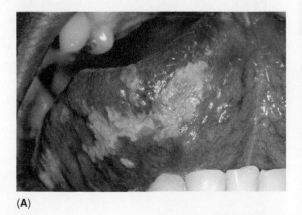

**(A)**

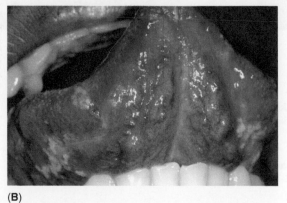

**(B)**

*Figure 2.3.62* (**A**) Candidosis in HIV disease. (**B**) Candidosis in HIV disease after wiping with gauze.

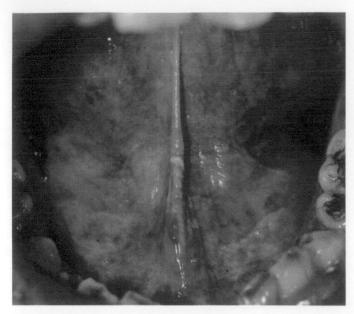

Figure 2.3.64 Leukoplakia.

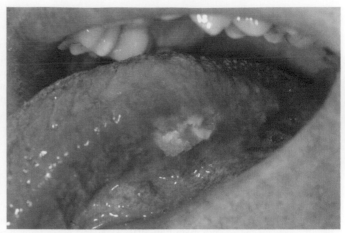

Figure 2.3.65 Leukoplakia—verrucous leukoplakia.

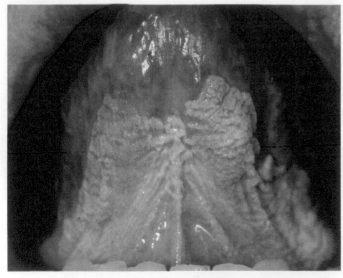

Figure 2.3.66 Leukoplakia—sublingual keratosis.

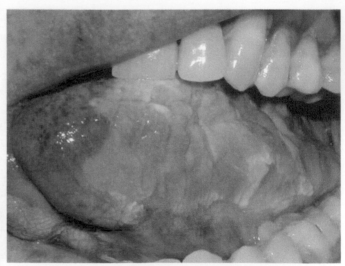

Figure 2.3.67 Leukoplakia.

**Leukoplakia**
Leukoplakia (Figs 2.3.64–2.3.68).

**Lichen planus**
LP (Figs 2.3.69–2.3.75).

**Trauma**
Trauma (Fig. 2.3.76).

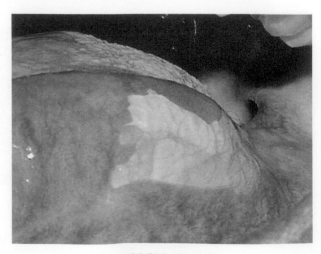

Figure 2.3.68 Leukoplakia.

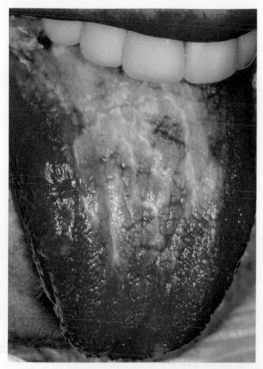

*Figure 2.3.69* Lichen planus.

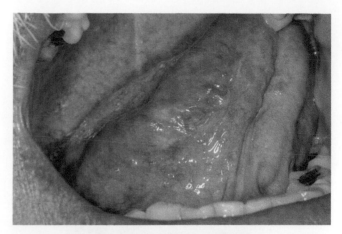

*Figure 2.3.70* Lichen planus.

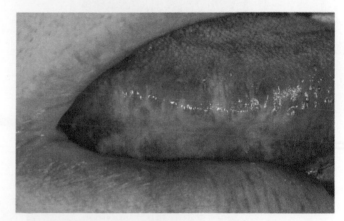

*Figure 2.3.72* Lichen planus.

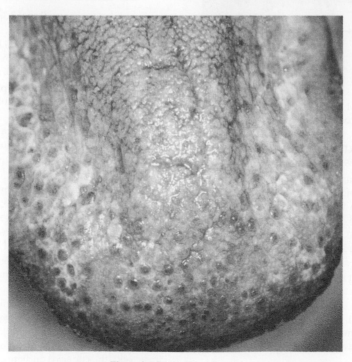

*Figure 2.3.71* Lichen planus.

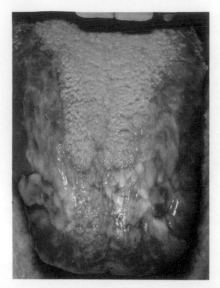

*Figure 2.3.73* Lichen planus.

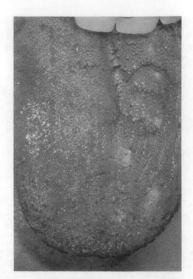

*Figure 2.3.74* Lichen planus.

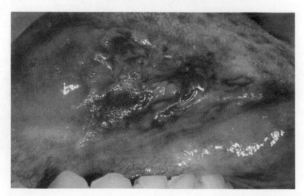

*Figure 2.3.75* Lichen planus—malignant transformation.

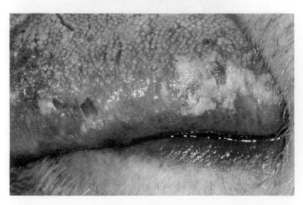

*Figure 2.3.76* Trauma.

## FURTHER READING

Arduino PG, Surace A, Carbone M, et al. Outcome of oral dysplasia: a retrospective hospital-based study of 207 patients with a long follow-up. J Oral Pathol Med 2009; 38: 540–4.

Azizkhan RG, Rutter MJ, Cotton RT, et al. Lymphatic malformations of the tongue base. J Pediatr Surg 2006; 41: 1279–84.

Bagan J, Jimenez Y, Gómez D, et al. Collagen telopeptide (serum CTX) and its relationship with the size and number of lesions in osteonecrosis of the jaws in cancer patients on intravenous bisphosphonates. Oral Oncol 2008; 44: 1088–9. [Epub 2008 Apr 8].

Bagan JV, Jimenez Y, Murillo J, et al. Lack of association between proliferative verrucous leukoplakia and human papillomavirus infection. J Oral Maxillofac Surg 2007; 65: 46–9.

Bagan JV, Jimenez Y, Sanchis JM, et al. Proliferative verrucous leukoplakia; high incidence of gingival squamous cell carcinoma. J Oral Pathol Med 2003; 32: 379–82.

Bagan JV, Murillo J, Poveda R, et al. Proliferative verrucous leukoplakia (PVL); unusual locations of oral squamous cell carcinomas (OSCC), and field cancerization as shown by the appearance of multiple OSCCs. Oral Oncol 2004; 40: 440–3.

Campisi G, Panzarella V, Giuliani M, et al. Human papilloma virus: its identikit and controversial role in oral oncogenesis, premalignant and malignant lesions. Int J Oncol 2007; 30: 813–23.

Cavalcanti DR, da Silveira FR. Alpha lipoic acid in burning mouth syndrome – a randomized double-blind placebo-controlled trial. J Oral Pathol Med 2009; 38: 254–61.

Colella G, Cappabianca S, Giudice A, Scully C. Liver ultrasound in oral squamous cell carcinoma. Oral Biosci Med 2004; 1: 55–60.

Di Felice R, Lombardi T. Foliate papillitis occurring in a child: a case report. Ann Dent 1993; 52: 17–18.

Esmeili T, Lozada-Nur F, Epstein J. Common benign oral soft tissue masses. Dent Clin North Am 2005; 49: 223–40.

Femiano F, Gombos F, Scully C. Oral proliferative verrucous leukoplakia; open trial of surgery compared with combined therapy using surgery and methisoprinol. Int J Oral Maxillofac Surg 2001; 30: 318–22.

Femiano F, Gombos F, Scully C. Burning mouth syndrome (BMS): double blind controlled study of alpha-lipoic acid (thioctic acid) therapy. J Oral Pathol Med 2002; 31: 267–9.

Femiano F, Gombos F, Scully C. Burning mouth syndrome (BMS); the efficacy of lipoic acid on subgroups. J Eur Assoc Dermatol Venereol 2004; 18: 676–8.

Femiano F, Gombos F, Scully C, Busciolano M, De Luca P. Burning mouth syndrome (BMS); controlled open trial of the efficacy of alpha-lipoic acid (thioctic acid) on symptomatology. Oral Dis 2000; 6: 274–7.

Femiano F, Gombos F, Scully C. Burning mouth syndrome (BMS): open trial of psychotherapy alone, medication with alpha-lipoic acid (thioctic acid) and combination therapy. Med Oral Patol Oral Cir Bucal 2004; 9: 8–13.

Femiano F, Gombos F, Scully C, et al. Oral leukoplakia; open trial of topical therapy with calcipotriol compared with tretinoin. Int J Oral Maxillofac Surg 2001; 30: 402–6.

Firoozmand LM, Paschotto DR, Almeida JD. Oral piercing complications among teenage students. Oral Health Prev Dent 2009; 7: 77–81.

Frezzini C, Leao JC, Porter S. Current trends of HIV disease of the mouth. J Oral Pathol Med 2005; 34: 513–31.

Gandolfo S, Pentenero M, Broccoletti R, et al. Toluidine blue uptake in potentially malignant oral lesions in vivo: clinical and histological assessment. Oral Oncol 2006; 42: 89–95.

Genden EM, Ferlito A, Bradley PJ, Rinaldo A, Scully C. Neck disease and distant metastases. Oral Oncol 2003; 39: 207–12.

Graells J, Ojeda RM, Muniesa C, Gonzalez J, Saavedra J. Glossitis with linear lesions: an early sign of vitamin B12 deficiency. J Am Acad Dermatol 2009; 60: 498–500.

Horn C, Thaker HM, Tampakopoulou DA, et al. Tongue lesions in the pediatric population. Otolaryngol Head Neck Surg 2001; 124: 164–9.

Jaber MA, Porter SR, Bain L, Scully C. Lack of association between hepatitis C virus and oral epithelial dysplasia in British patients. Int J Oral Maxillofac Surg 2003; 32: 181–3.

Jaber MA, Porter SR, Speight P, Eveson JW, Scully C. Oral epithelial dysplasia: clinical characteristics of western European residents. Oral Oncol 2003; 39: 589–96.

Lai YT, Chen HS, Chang YL. Lingual thyroid. Otolaryngol Head Neck Surg 2009; 140: 944–5.

Maeda M, Maier SE. Usefulness of diffusion-weighted imaging and the apparent diffusion coefficient in the assessment of head and neck tumors. J Neuroradiol 2008; 35: 71–8. [Epub 2008 Mar 5].

Marino R, Capaccio P, Pignataro L, Spadari F. Burning mouth syndrome: the role of contact hypersensitivity. Oral Dis 2009; 15: 255–8.

Martinez EM, Bagan JV, Jimenez Y, Scully C. Evaluation of dental health and the need for dental treatment prior to radiotherapy in 83 patients with head and neck cancer. Oral Biosci Med 2004; 1: 181–5.

Miloğlu O, Göregen M, Akgül HM, Acemoğlu H. The prevalence and risk factors associated with benign migratory glossitis lesions in 7619 Turkish dental outpatients. Oral Surg Oral Med Oral Pathol Oral Radiol Endod 2009; 107: e29–33.

Mra Z, Chien J. Kaposi's sarcoma of the tongue. Otolaryngol Head Neck Surg 2000; 123(1 Pt 1): 151.

Navone R, Pentenero M, Rostan I, et al. Oral potentially malignant lesions: first level micro-histological diagnosis from tissue fragments sampled in liquid-based diagnostic cytology. J Oral Pathol Med 2008; 37: 358–63; Feb 19. [Epub ahead of print].

Pass B, Brown RS, Childers EL. Geographic tongue: literature review and case reports. Dent Today 2005; 24: 54, 56–7.

Patel NJ, Sciubba J. Oral lesions in young children. Pediatr Clin North Am 2003; 50: 469–86.

Pentenero M, Carrozzo M, Pagano M, et al. Oral mucosal dysplastic lesions and early squamous cell carcinomas: underdiagnosis from incisional biopsy. Oral Dis 2003; 9: 68–72.

Petti S, Scully C. Oral cancer: the association between nation-based alcohol-drinking profiles and oral cancer mortality. Oral Oncol 2005; 41: 828–34.

Petti S, Scully C. Association between different alcoholic beverages and leukoplakia among non- to moderate- drinking adults: a matched case-control study. Eur J Cancer 2006; 42: 521–7.

Pierro VS, Maia LC, Primo LG, Soares FD. Case report: the importance of oral manifestations in diagnosing iron deficiency in childhood. Eur J Paediatr Dent 2004; 5: 115–18.

Poate TWJ, Buchanan JAG, Hodgson TA, et al. An audit of the efficacy of the oral brush biopsy technique in a specialist oral medicine unit. Oral Oncol 2004; 40: 829–34.

Popovtzer A, Shpitzer T, Bahar G, et al. Squamous cell carcinoma of the oral tongue in young patients. Laryngoscope 2004; 114: 915–17.

Powell FC. Glossodynia and other disorders of the tongue. Dermatol Clin 1987; 5: 687–93.

Rapidis A, Gullane P, Langdon J, et al. Major advances in the knowledge and understanding of the epidemiology, aetiopathogenesis, diagnosis, management and prognosis of oral cancer. Oral Oncol 2009; 45: 299–300.

Reichart PA, Samaranayake LP, Philipsen HP. Pathology and clinical correlates in oral candidiasis and its variants: a review. Oral Dis 2000; 6: 85–91.

Reis-Filho JS, Souto-Moura C, Lopes JM. Classic Kaposi's sarcoma of the tongue: case report with emphasis on the differential diagnosis. J Oral Maxillofac Surg 2002; 60: 951–4.

Sarti GM, Haddy RI, Schaffer D, Kihm J. Black hairy tongue. Am Fam Physician 1990; 41: 1751–5.

Scully C. Oral squamous cell carcinoma; from an hypothesis about a virus, to concern about possible sexual transmission. Oral Oncol 2002; 38: 227–34.

Scully C, Bagan JV. Oral squamous cell carcinoma; overview of current understanding of aetiopathogenesis, and clinical implications. Oral Dis 2009; 15: 388–99; April 2. [Epub ahead of print].

Scully C, Bagan JV, Hopper C, Epstein JB. Oral cancer; current and future diagnostic techniques. Am J Dent 2008; 21: 199–209.

Scully C, Bedi R. Ethnicity and oral cancer. Lancet Oncol 2000; 1: 37–42.

Scully C, Chen M. Tongue piercing (oral body art). Br J Oral Maxillofac Surg 1994; 32: 37–8.

Scully C, Field JK, Tanzawa H. Genetic aberrations in oral or head and neck squamous cell carcinoma (SCCHN): 1. Carcinogen metabolism, DNA repair and cell cycle control. Oral Oncol 2000; 36: 256–63.

Scully C, Field JK, Tanzawa H. Genetic aberrations in oral or head and neck squamous cell carcinoma (SCCHN): 2. Chromosomal aberrations. Oral Oncol 2000; 36: 311–27.

Scully C, Field JK, Tanzawa H. Genetic aberrations in oral or head and neck squamous cell carcinoma (SCCHN): 3. Clinico-pathological applications. Oral Oncol 2000; 36: 404–13.

Scully C, el-Kabir M, Samaranayake LP. Candida and oral candidosis: a review. Crit Rev Oral Biol Med 1994; 5: 125–57.

Scully C, Sudbo J, Speight PM. Progress in determining the malignant potential of oral lesions. J Oral Pathol Med 2003; 32: 251–6.

Shotts R, Scully C. How to identify and deal with tongue problems. Pulse 2002; 62: 73–6.

Suter VG, Bornstein MM. Ankyloglossia: facts and myths in diagnosis and treatment. J Periodontol 2009; 80: 1204–19.

Terai H, Shimahara M. Atrophic tongue associated with Candida. J Oral Pathol Med 2005; 34: 397–400.

Toida M, Kato K, Makita H, et al. Palliative effect of lafutidine on oral burning sensation. Oral Pathol 2009; 38: 262–8.

Van Borsel J, Cornelis C. Tongue piercing and speech. J Otolaryngol Head Neck Surg 2009; 38: 11–15.

Warnakulasuriya S, Sutherland G, Scully C. Tobacco, oral cancer, and treatment of dependence. Oral Oncol 2005; 41: 244–60.

Ziebolz D, Hornecker E, Mausberg R. Microbiological findings at tongue piercing sites—implications to oral health. Int J Dent Hyg 2009; 7: 256–62.

# 2.4 PALATE AND FAUCES

- aesthetics
- blisters
- red, purple or blue lesions
- soreness, ulceration and pain
- swellings and lumps
- white lesions

The palate and fauces consist of a hard anterior and soft posterior palate, the tonsillar area and pillars of the fauces, and the oropharynx. The mucosa of the hard palate is firmly bound down as a mucoperiosteum (similar to the gingivae) and with no obvious vascular arcades. Rugae are present anteriorly on either side of the incisive papilla that overlies the incisive foramen.

The soft palate and fauces may show a faint vascular arcade. In the soft palate, just posterior to the junction with the hard palate, is a conglomeration of minor salivary glands, a region which is often also yellowish (Figs 2.4.1 and 2.4.2).

The palate should be inspected and movements examined when the patient says 'Aah'. Using a mirror, this also permits inspection of the posterior tongue, tonsils, oropharynx and can even offer a glimpse of the larynx. Glossopharyngeal palsy may lead to uvula deviation to the contralateral side.

Surprisingly few conditions are found in the palate; this chapter highlights those that are seen particularly or exclusively there.

Cleft palate is a dramatic lesion with multiple implications. Torus palatinus is a common central developmental abnormality. Other lumps are most commonly caused by unerupted teeth. Acquired lumps are often dental abscesses, but fibrous lumps, human papillomavirus-associated warts, neoplasms, particularly salivary, Kaposi sarcoma (KS) and lymphomas must be excluded.

Mucosal lesions are also uncommon in the palate. Ulceration is uncommon, except in burns, trauma, localized oral purpura, pemphigus and lupus erythematosus. Erythematous candidosis may affect the palate—denture-related stomatitis is a common form. Pigmented lesions in the palate are usually naevi but KS has and melanoma have a predilection for this site also. White lesions may be seen in the palate, especially in smoker's keratosis, leukoplakia and candidosis and, on the palatal gingivae, lichen planus.

## AESTHETICS

### Bifid uvula (cleft uvula)

Bifid or cleft uvula (Fig. 2.4.3) is a fairly common minor manifestation of a submucous cleft palate but is of little other consequence.

### Cleft lip and palate

*Aetiopathogenesis*

Cleft lip and palate has a familial tendency; when one parent is affected, the risk to a child is about 1 in 10 live births.

*Clinical features*

The cleft is on the left in over 60% of patients, although the cleft may be bilateral (Fig. 2.4.4). Cleft lip and palate are, in about 20% of cases, associated with anomalies of head and neck, extremities, genitalia or heart. Morphoea may have a similar appearance (Fig. 2.4.5).

*Diagnosis*

Diagnosis is clinical but imaging and other studies are indicated.

*Management*

Management is with long-term multidisciplinary care, involving oral and maxillofacial surgeons, orthodontists, prosthodontists and speech therapists.

### Velopharyngeal dysfunction (VPD)

Causes of VPD and hypernasality range from structural to neuromuscular causes and include:

- cleft palate
- submucous cleft palate—often defined by a bifid or double uvula, muscular diastasis of the soft palate and notching of the posterior border of the hard palate—but may be occult. These patients may be especially predisposed to VPD if the local anatomy changes, such as post-adenoidectomy
- Down syndrome
- Kabuki syndrome—cleft palate, cardiac abnormalities (typically aortic coarctation), muscular hypotonia and characteristic facial features
- velocardiofacial syndrome
- neurofibromatosis
- myotonic dystrophy
- muscular dystrophy.

VPD may be acquired after stroke or head injury, and in multiple sclerosis, amyotrophic lateral sclerosis or Parkinson disease.

VPD significantly impacts speech intelligibility. Diagnosis is from the history and physical examination, speech assessment, and nasendoscopy and radiographic multiplanar videofluoroscopy. Treatment consists of prosthetic management or surgery, supplemented with speech therapy.

## BLISTERS

Palatal blisters may be caused most commonly, by burns or by mucoceles, by localized oral purpura, or occasionally by bullous disorders such as pemphigoid.

## RED, PURPLE OR BLUE LESIONS

### Candidosis; chronic atrophic

Candidosis; chronic atrophic (denture-related stomatitis) (Chapter 1.8).

*Aetiopathogenesis*

Chronic atrophic candidosis is common beneath complete upper dentures, especially in older people.

- Factors that are usually *not* significant include:
  - Allergy to the dental material (if it were, denture-related stomatitis would affect mucosae other than just that beneath the appliance)
  - Trauma; the condition is more common beneath maxillary dentures than mandibular dentures, yet trauma is more common under the latter
  - Pharmacological agents
  - Smoking.

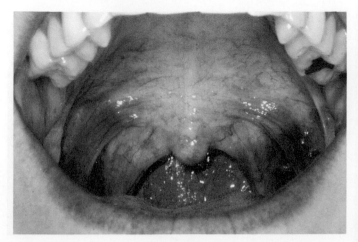

*Figure 2.4.1* Normal palate.

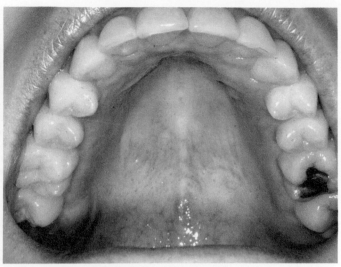

*Figure 2.4.2* Normal palate.

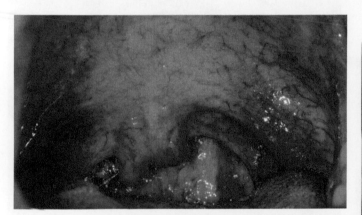

*Figure 2.4.3* Bifid uvula.

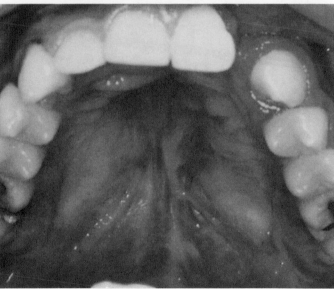

*Figure 2.4.4* Cleft palate (repaired).

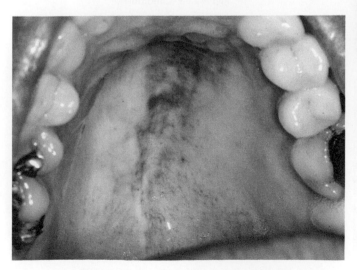

*Figure 2.4.5* Morphoea affecting the palate.

- Dental appliance wearing (mainly maxillary dentures), especially when worn throughout the night, or with a dry mouth, is the major predisposing factor. Dentures can produce a number of ecological changes, including accumulation of microbial plaque (bacteria and/ or yeasts) on and in the fitting surface of the denture and the underlying mucosa. This plaque undergoes sequential development, and is colonized by *yeasts* such as *Candida*, which are isolated in up to 90% of persons with denture-related stomatitis. It may be that the decreased salivary flow and a low pH under the denture probably will result in a high *Candida* enzymatic activity, which can cause mucosal inflammation.

When *Candida* species are involved in denture-related stomatitis, the more common terms '*Candida*-associated denture stomatitis', 'denture-induced candidosis' or 'chronic atrophic candidosis' are used. The most frequently isolated organism is *Candida albicans*; however, even 66% of denture wearers have such yeasts but no stomatitis and it is not clear why only some denture-wearers develop denture-related stomatitis. *Candida*, however, is not the only micro-organism associated with denture-related stomatitis; occasionally other factors such as bacterial infection, high carbohydrate diet or mechanical irritation are at play—and there might be immune factors. Most patients appear otherwise healthy and have no serious cell-mediated immune defects, though they may sometimes be deficient in migration-inhibition factor and may have overactive suppressor T-cells, or other T-lymphocyte or phagocyte defects. Diabetes and HIV are very rare underlying factors.

*Clinical features*

Denture-related stomatitis although formerly termed denture sore mouth, is usually asymptomatic unless complicated by thrush (Figs 2.4.5–2.4.10) or angular stomatitis.

It manifests as chronic erythema and oedema of the mucosa that contacts the fitting surface of the denture, usually a complete upper denture

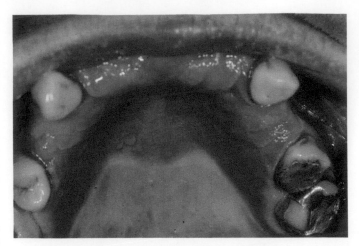

*Figure 2.4.7* Denture-related stomatitis.

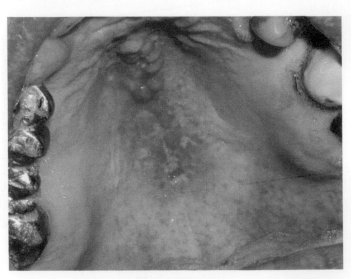

*Figure 2.4.9* Candidosis.

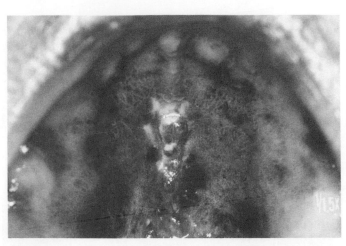

*Figure 2.4.6* Candidosis.

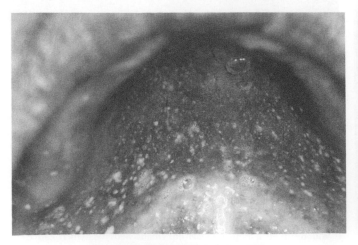

*Figure 2.4.8* Denture-related stomatitis.

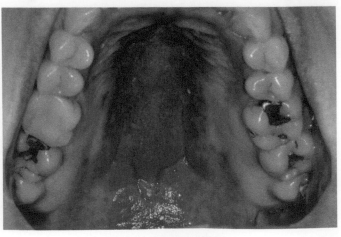

*Figure 2.4.10* Candidosis.

(the denture-bearing area); the mucosa beneath lower dentures is rarely involved.

Newton described three types increasing in severity:

- Type 1—a localized simple inflammation or a pinpoint hyperaemia.
- Type 2—an erythematous or generalized simple type presenting as more diffuse erythema involving a part of, or the entire, denture-covered mucosa.
- Type 3—a granular type (inflammatory papillary hyperplasia) commonly involving the central part of the hard palate and the alveolar ridge (Figs 2.4.11 and 2.4.12).

*Diagnosis*
This is a clinical diagnosis and there is very rarely any need for haematological, serological or urinary investigations for any underlying immune defect such as diabetes mellitus or HIV disease, unless of course the denture-related stomatitis is accompanied by other fungal disease (e.g. angular stomatitis) or oral/systemic features of immunosuppression. Mycological investigation of denture-associated stomatitis is rarely warranted.

*Management*
Any underlying systemic disease should be treated where possible. The denture plaque and fitting surface are infested with *Candida* and other organisms, so these should be cleaned and disinfected. Chlorhexidine gluconate or alkaline peroxide, alkaline hypochlorite, acid, yeast lytic enzyme, proteolytic enzyme or other disinfectant is suitable. Hypochlorite is also an effective anti-candidal, but can turn chrome cobalt dentures black. Dentures should be left out of the mouth during sleep, and stored in an antiseptic denture cleanser. Denture soak solutions containing benzoic acid completely eradicate *C. albicans* from the denture surface as they are taken up into the acrylic resin and eliminate the organism from the internal surface of the prosthesis. A protease-containing denture soak (alcalase protease) is also an effective way of removing denture plaque, especially when combined with brushing.

- The mucosal infection is eradicated by brushing the palate and using antifungals for 4 weeks. Effective agents include nystatin pastilles or suspension, amphotericin lozenges or miconazole gel or fluconazole suspension or tablets, administered concurrently with an oral antiseptic such as chlorhexidine, which has antifungal activity. Miconazole lacquer, or antifungals such as fluconazole in tissue conditioners applied to the denture fitting surface are also effective.
- Studies of sensitivity to antifungal agents have shown that isolates from different strains are sensitive to amphotericin and nystatin, but less sensitive to miconazole. Fluconazole is as effective as newer agents such as itraconazole. The cyclodextrin solution of itraconazole and capsule preparations of itraconazole are equally effective adjuncts in the treatment but, because of adverse effects, capsules are preferred.

**Drug pigmentation**
Drug pigmentation (Fig. 2.4.13) (Chapter 1.6).

**Erythroplasia**
Erythroplasia (Figs 2.4.14 and 2.4.15) (Chapter 2.2).

**Haemangioma**
Haemangioma (Fig. 2.4.16) (Chapter 2.1).

**Haematoma**
Haematoma (Chapter 2.1).

**Kaposi sarcoma**
KS (Chapter 1.7).

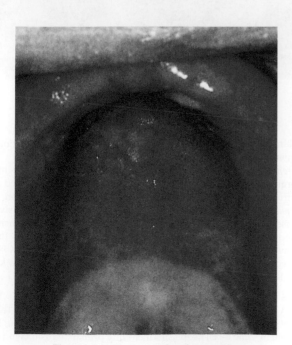

*Figure 2.4.11* Denture-related stomatitis.

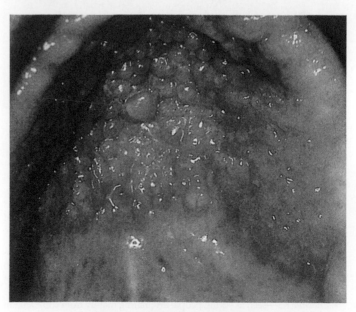

*Figure 2.4.12* Papillary hyperplasia.

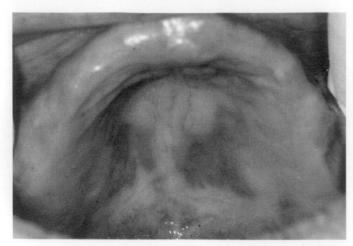

*Figure 2.4.13* Mepacrine palatal pigmentation.

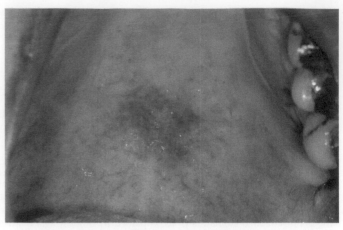

*Figure 2.4.14* Erythroplasia.

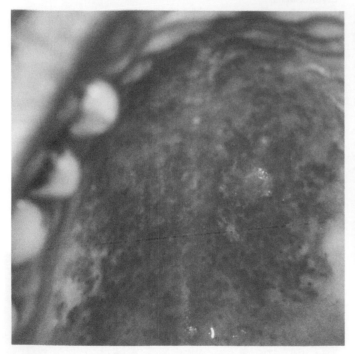

*Figure 2.4.15* Erythroplasia.

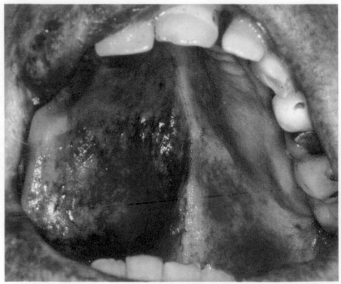

*Figure 2.4.16* Angioma.

### Aetiopathogenesis

KS is a malignant neoplasm of endothelial cells caused by Kaposi sarcoma herpesvirus (KSHV) infection. KS is a multifocal tumour characterized by deregulated angiogenesis, proliferation of spindle cells and extravasation of inflammatory cells and erythrocytes. There is a range of varieties of KS which include:

- *Classic KS*—the original type of KS described, a relatively indolent disease affecting older men of Eastern European or Mediterranean basin descent, where there are higher rates of KSHV than the remainder of Europe.
- *Endemic KS*—seen in young people originating mainly from sub-Saharan countries in Africa, and a more aggressive disease which infiltrates the skin extensively, especially on the lower limbs. The populations frequently have greater than 50% rate of KSHV infection.
- *Transplant related KS*—became recognized when an KSHV-infected organ was transplanted into a person not previously exposed to the virus or when the recipient already harboured KSHV infection.
- *Epidemic KS*—first recognized during the 1980s as an aggressive disease in patients with AIDS. KSHV is usually sexually transmitted and KS is over 300 times more common in AIDS patients than in renal transplant recipients. In 1994, a virus isolated from a KS lesion revealed it to be the eighth human herpesvirus (HHV-8)—now known as KSHV.

KS arises from endothelial cells and the causative agent is KSHV (HHV-8)—which may be acquired sexually and non-sexually (e.g. via saliva). KSHV is responsible for all types of KS and, in addition, is also present in some B-cell neoplasms including primary effusion lymphoma and multicentric Castleman disease. Infection is thought to be life-long so that persons infected with KSHV may develop KS years later if they develop AIDS or become otherwise immunocompromised.

KSHV encodes genes that stimulate cellular, and counter the host immune response. KSHV is a unique virus that incorporates into its genome, cellular genes that cause tumours ('molecular piracy'); these genes may help cells proliferate and migrate, and avoid apoptosis, and KSHV evades the immune system. Infection of endothelial cells, leads to rapid suppression of Toll-like receptor-4 (TLR4) expression, a mechanism of immune escape as TLR4 mediates innate immunity against KSHV. HIV-infected individuals carrying a mutant TLR4 allele appear more likely to develop Castleman disease. Activation of the interleukin-6 receptor signalling pathway and constitutive signalling of viral G protein-coupled receptor play an important role in the activation, proliferation and transformation of KSHV-infected endothelial cells.

KS is generally not considered a true sarcoma but rather a cancer of lymphatic endothelium which forms vascular channels that fill with blood cells, giving the tumour its characteristic bruise-like appearance. Endothelial cells harbour the KSHV genome, and are thought to be the precursors of the KS spindle cells which become the predominant cell type in plaque- and nodular-stage KS lesions. KS lesions contain KSHV proteins (latency-associated nuclear antigen) uniformly detectable in KS cancer cells.

### Clinical features

KS lesions are initially red, purple or brown macules later becoming nodules that may be red, purple, brown or black, typically found on the skin, but spread elsewhere is common, especially to the respiratory tract, gastrointestinal tract and the mouth. Usually oral lesions are part of more widespread disease but, in AIDS, KS typically involves the palate or gingivae (Fig. 2.4.17).

### Diagnosis

Diagnosis is confirmed by biopsy. Blood tests to detect antibodies against KSHV have been developed and can be used to determine if a patient is at risk for transmitting infection to his or her sexual partner, or if an organ is infected prior to transplantation. Unfortunately, there is little screening for persons at risk for becoming infected with KSHV, such as transplant patients.

Epithelioid angiomatosis, haemangiomas, lymphomas and purpura may need to be differentiated.

### Management

Management is treatment of the underlying predisposing condition if possible. In 40% or more of patients with AIDS-associated KS, the Kaposi lesions will shrink with highly active antiretroviral therapy. KS lesions of HIV disease may partially or completely resolve with ART, although local inflammation about existing sites of KS can transiently increase in the immune reconstitution syndrome (Chapter 1.7).

Local therapies for oral KS using radiotherapy and/or chemotherapy are now rarely employed. Patients with a few local lesions can be treated with local measures such as radiation therapy but surgery is generally not recommended as KS can appear in wound edges. More widespread disease, or disease affecting internal organs, is generally treated with systemic therapy with alpha interferon, vinca alkaloids systemically or intralesionally, liposomal anthracyclines or paclitaxel.

### Localized oral purpura

Localized oral purpura (Angina bullosa haemorrhagica).

### Aetiopathogenesis

Localized oral purpura is a fairly common condition that mimics pemphigoid. Seen mainly in older patients or sometimes after use of corticosteroid inhalers, in most instances it is idiopathic.

### Clinical features

Patients present with blood blisters, typically on the soft palate, often after eating (Figs 2.4.18–2.4.20). There is subepithelial vesiculation and an ulcer which has been described as a 'sunburst ulcer' results.

### Diagnosis

This condition must be differentiated from pemphigoid, and acquired epidermolysis bullosa in particular. Biopsy may be indicated.

### Management

If a corticosteroid inhaler is used—optimize the inhaler technique and instruct patient to gargle with water after inhaler use. Otherwise, reassurance is all that can be offered.

### Naevi

Naevi (Figs 2.4.21 and 2.4.22) (Chapter 2.2).

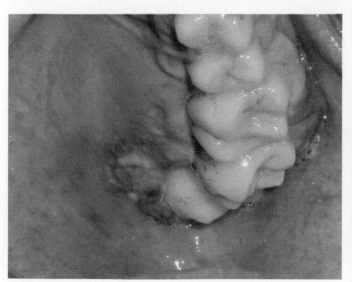

*Figure 2.4.17* Kaposi sarcoma.

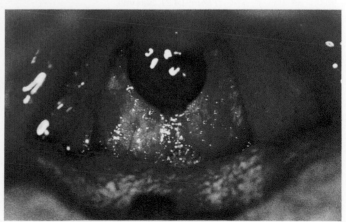

*Figure 2.4.18* Angina bullosa haemorrhagica.

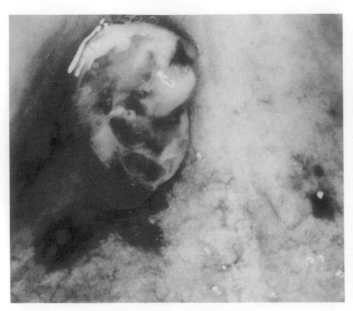

*Figure 2.4.19* Angina bullosa haemorrhagica.

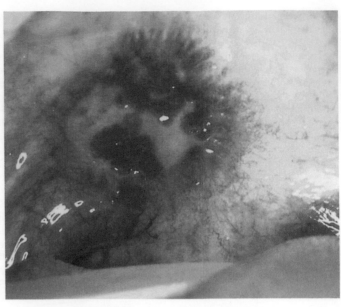

*Figure 2.4.20* Angina bullosa haemorrhagica.

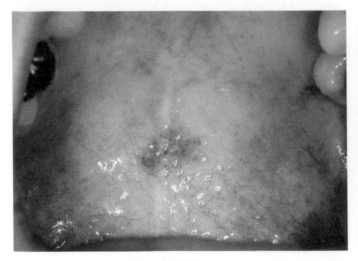

*Figure 2.4.21* Naevus.

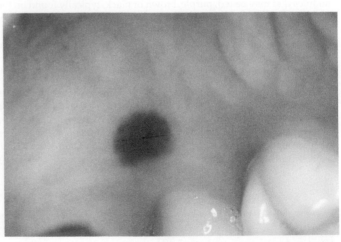

*Figure 2.4.22* Naevus.

**Melanoma**

Melanoma (Fig. 2.4.23) (Chapter 2.2).

**Racial**

Racial (Fig. 2.4.24) (Chapter 2.2).

**Tattoos**

Tattoos (Chapter 2.1).

# SORENESS, ULCERATION AND PAIN

Palatal ulceration can arise from local causes such as trauma, burns or mucositis, from aphthae, drugs, neoplasms or systemic disease (haematological, infectious, gastrointestinal, mucocutaneous) (Figs 2.4.25–2.4.32). Aphthae occasionally affect the palate—mainly the soft palate/fauces. Most common causes in the hard palate are burns, trauma, herpetic recurrences and pemphigoid.

### Necrotizing sialometaplasia (NSM)

*Aetiopathogenesis*

NSM is an uncommon, benign, self-limited inflammatory lesion of both major and minor salivary glands, commonly associated with tissue ischaemia. It is seen predominantly in young adult males—most of whom smoke tobacco—and in palatal minor salivary glands. An occasional association with bulimia has been reported. Diagnosis is from histology showing foci of eosinophilic granulocytes with lobular infarction or necrosis, bland-appearing nuclear morphology of squamous

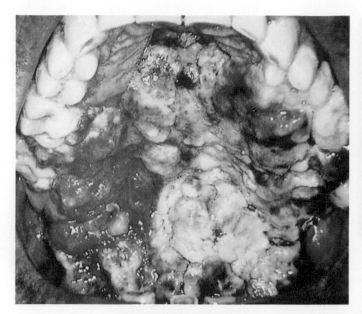

*Figure 2.4.23* Melanoma.

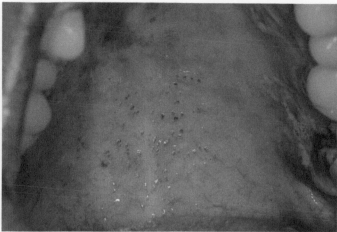

*Figure 2.4.24* Racial pigmentation.

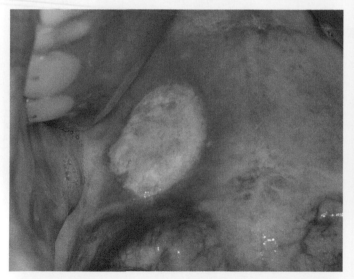

*Figure 2.4.25* Aphthous-like ulceration.

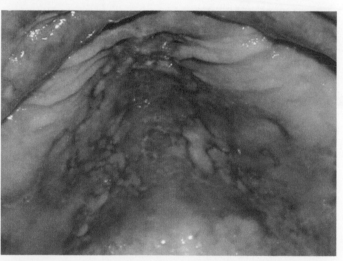

*Figure 2.4.26* Pemphigoid.

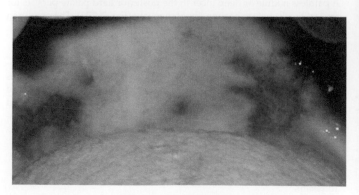

*Figure 2.4.27* Pemphigus.

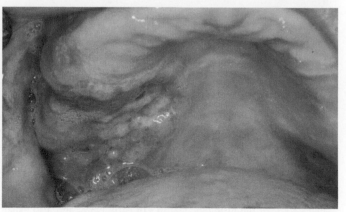

*Figure 2.4.28* Carcinoma.

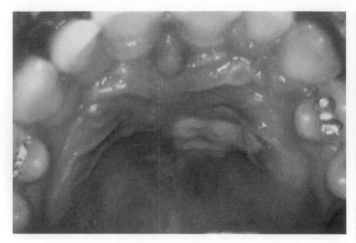

Figure 2.4.29 Burn.

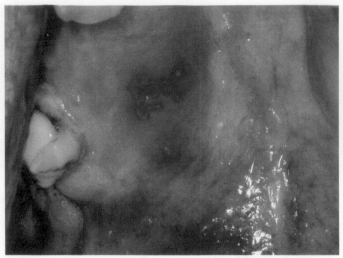

Figure 2.4.30 Herpes simplex virus infection.

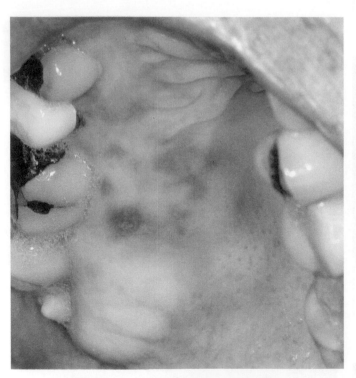

Figure 2.4.31 Herpes simplex virus infection.

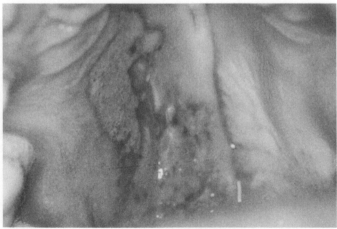

Figure 2.4.32 Herpes simplex virus infection.

*Clinical features*

A painless nodule or deep ulcer in the posterior hard palate persists for several weeks before healing spontaneously (Fig. 2.4.33). The condition occasionally arises in the tongue, lip or elsewhere.

*Diagnosis and management*

This benign self-limiting condition must be differentiated from malignancy. Biopsy reveals necrosis and pseudoepitheliomatous changes probably resulting from squamous metaplasia following infarction of minor salivary glands. NSM can also be seen in some carcinomas and other neoplasms. Identification of myoepithelial cells and CK7 expression may help to distinguish NSM from its mimics. The lesion resolves spontaneously.

**Tonsillitis**

Tonsillitis (Chapter 1.15).

cells, and simultaneous metaplasia of ducts and mucous acini, supplemented with focal to absent immunoreactivity for p53, low immunoreactivity for MIB1 (Ki-67), CK7 expression, and the presence of 4A4/p63- and calponin-positive myoepithelial cells.

*Subacute necrotizing sialadenitis* is an uncommon inflammatory condition that shows acinar necrosis surrounded by a dense polymorphous inflammatory infiltrate with focal exuberant tissue eosinophilia and shares some of the histologic features of early NSM, and also usually affects palatal minor salivary glands.

# SWELLINGS AND LUMPS
## Fibrous lumps
Fibrous lumps (Figs 2.4.34–2.4.36) (Chapter 2.2).

## Neoplasms
Neoplasms (Chapter 1.11).

Minor salivary gland neoplasms, lymphomas and KS are amongst the most common neoplasms seen in the palate but carcinomas arising from the oral epithelium or maxillary antrum may be seen (Figs 2.4.37–2.4.41).

## Papillary hyperplasia
### Aetiopathogenesis
Papillary hyperplasia of the palate is a benign condition of unknown aetiology, but it is often more obvious where a denture is worn and where there is denture-related stomatitis. However, papillary hyperplasia can also appear in the absence of dentures.

### Clinical features
Papillary lesions in the palatal vault (Figs 2.4.42 and 2.4.43).

### Diagnosis
Clinical. Papillomatous lesions in the vault of the palate may occasionally result from obstructed ducts of minor salivary glands or sarcoidosis which should be excluded.

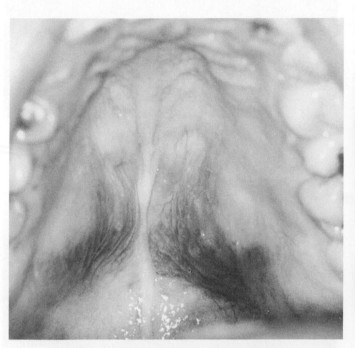

*Figure 2.4.33* Necrotizing sialometaplasia.

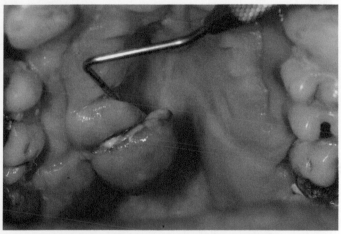

*Figure 2.4.34* Fibrous—denture granulomas.

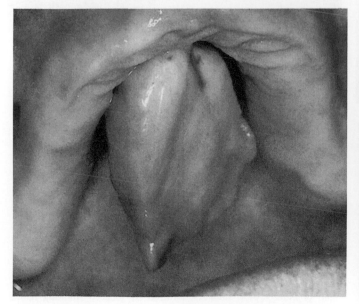

*Figure 2.4.35* Fibrous lump.

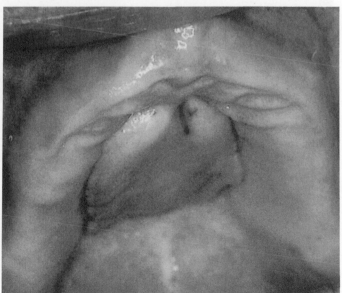

*Figure 2.4.36* Fibrous lump.

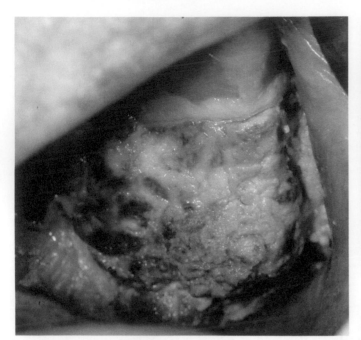

Figure 2.4.37 Carcinoma.

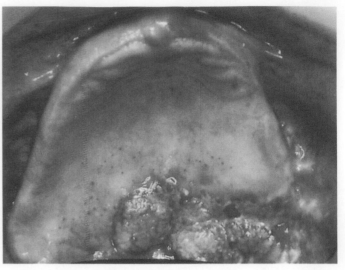

Figure 2.4.38 Carcinoma.

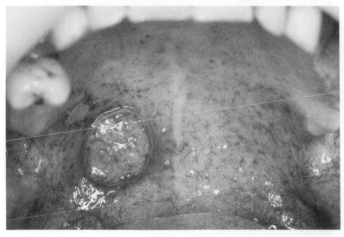

Figure 2.4.39 Carcinoma.

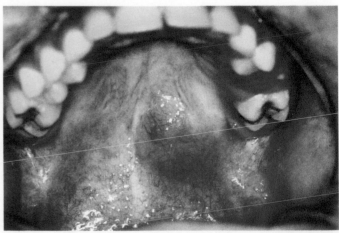

Figure 2.4.40 Salivary gland neoplasm.

*Management*
Reassurance.

**Torus palatinus**
Torus palatinus (Fig. 2.4.44) (Chapter 2.8).

**Warty lesions**
Warty lesions (Figs 2.4.45–2.4.47) (Chapter 1.8).

# WHITE LESIONS
**Candidosis**
Candidosis (Figs 2.4.48–2.4.52) (Chapter 1.8).

**Carcinoma**
Carcinoma (Fig. 2.4.53) (Chapter 2.3).

**Keratosis**
Keratosis (stomatitis nicotina; Smoker's palate).

*Aetiopathogenesis*
Stomatitis nicotina is a fairly common lesion, seen typically in middle-aged or elderly pipe smokers, induced by tobacco smoking habits. Reverse smoking is also a potent cause.

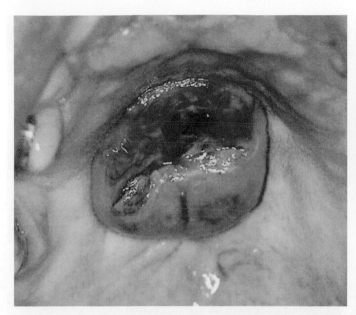

Figure 2.4.41 Salivary gland neoplasm.

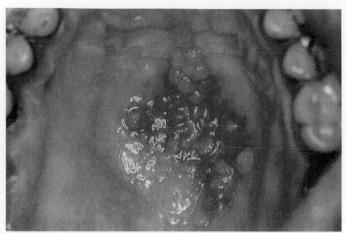

Figure 2.4.42 Papillary hyperplasia.

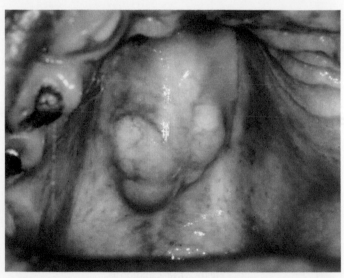

Figure 2.4.44 Torus palatinus.

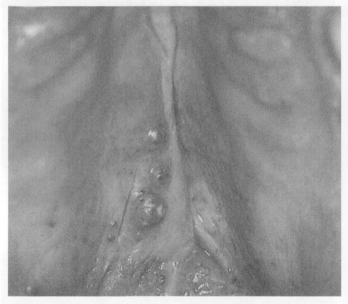

Figure 2.4.43 Papillary hyperplasia.

*Clinical features*

The palate is diffusely white but the orifices of the minor salivary glands are obvious as red spots (Figs 2.4.54–2.4.58). If a denture is worn, the mucosa is protected from the tobacco smoke by the denture and appears normal in contrast to the non-denture bearing area.

*Diagnosis*

Clinical.

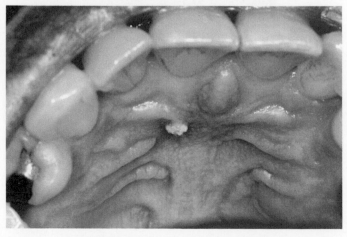

Figure 2.4.45 Human papillomavirus infection.

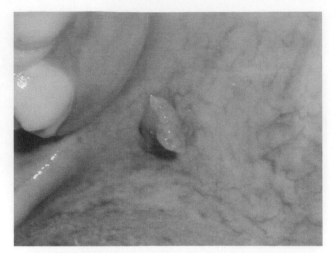

*Figure 2.4.46* Human papillomavirus infection.

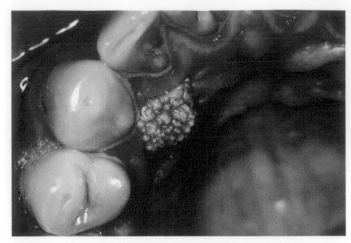

*Figure 2.4.47* Human papillomavirus infection.

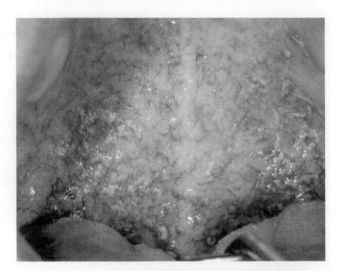

*Figure 2.4.48* Candidosis.

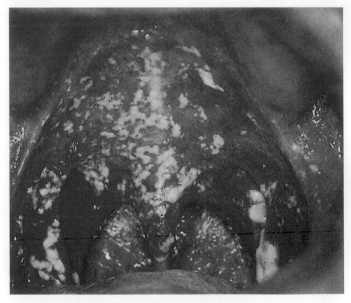

*Figure 2.4.49* Candidosis.

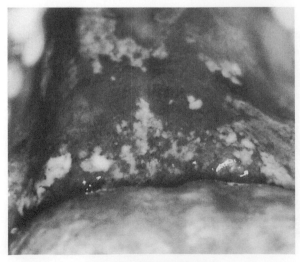

*Figure 2.4.50* Candidosis.

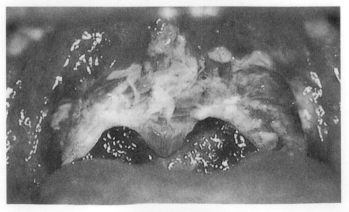

*Figure 2.4.51* Candidosis.

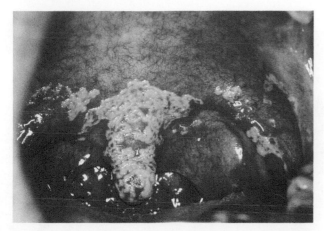

Figure 2.4.52 Candidosis.

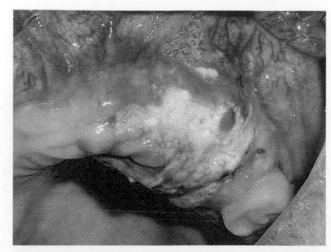

Figure 2.4.53 Carcinoma.

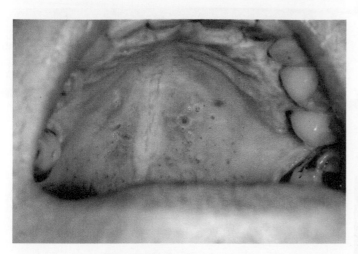

Figure 2.4.54 Smokers keratosis.

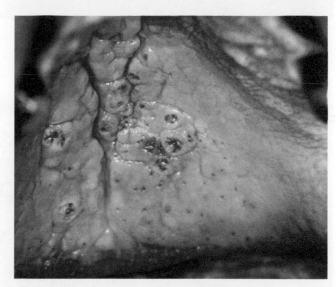

Figure 2.4.55 Keratosis—stomatitis nicotina.

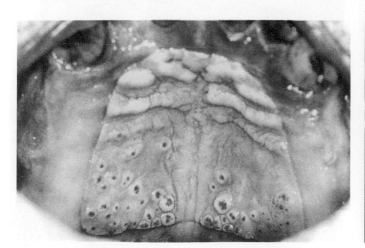

Figure 2.4.56 Keratosis—stomatitis nicotina.

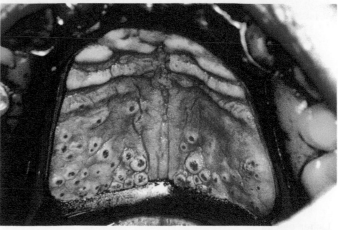

Figure 2.4.57 Keratosis—stomatitis nicotina (same patient as Fig. 2.4.56).

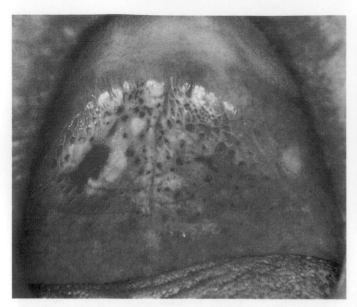

*Figure 2.4.58* Keratosis—stomatitis nicotina.

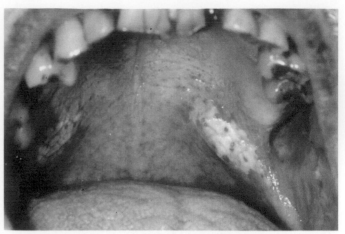

*Figure 2.4.59* Leukoplakia—tobacco-related keratosis.

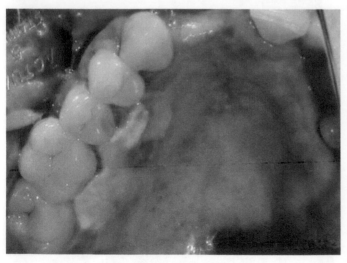

*Figure 2.4.60* Leukoplakia.

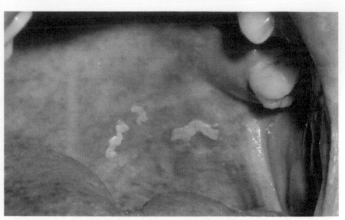

*Figure 2.4.61* Leukoplakia.

*Management*

Smoker's keratosis is usually a benign lesion that regresses if tobacco smoking is stopped.

**Leukoplakia**

Leukoplakia (Figs 2.4.59–2.4.63) (Chapter 2.2).

**Lichen planus**

Lichen planus (Figs 2.4.64–2.4.66) (Chapter 1.10).

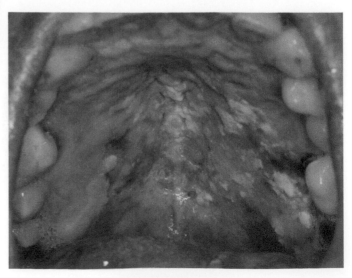

*Figure 2.4.62* Leukoplakia—tobacco related.

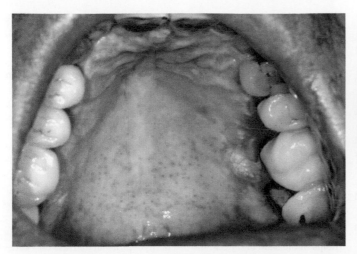

*Figure 2.4.63* Leukoplakia and lichen planus.

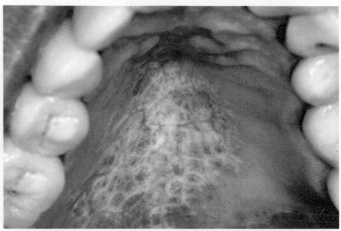

*Figure 2.4.64* Lichen planus.

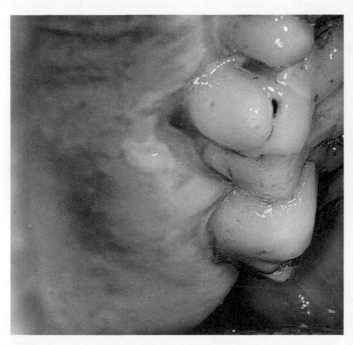

*Figure 2.4.65* Lichen planus.

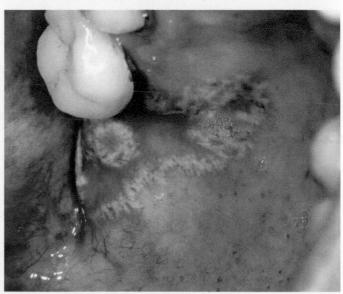

*Figure 2.4.66* Lichen planus.

**Lupus erythematosus**

Lupus erythematosus (Chapter 1.15).

**Oral submucous fibrosis**

Oral submucous fibrosis (Fig. 2.4.67) (Chapter 2.2).

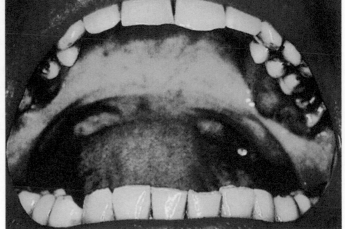

*Figure 2.4.67* Oral submucous fibrosis.

# FURTHER READING

Arduino PG, Carrozzo M, Pentenero M, Bertolusso G, Gandolfo S. Non-neoplastic salivary gland diseases. Minerva Stomatol 2006; 55: 249–70.

Biesbrock AR, Aguirre A. Multiple focal pigmented lesions in the maxillary tuberosity and hard palate: a unique display of intraoral junctional nevi. J Periodontol 1992; 63: 718–21.

Carlson DL. Necrotizing sialometaplasia: a practical approach to the diagnosis. Arch Pathol Lab Med 2009; 133: 692–8.

Cohan DM, Popat S, Kaplan SE, et al. Oropharyngeal cancer: current understanding and management Curr Opin Otolaryngol Head Neck Surg 2009; 17: 88–94.

Dominguez-Malagon H, Mosqueda-Taylor A, Cano-Valdez AM. Necrotizing sialometaplasia of the palate associated with angiocentric T-cell lymphoma. Ann Diagn Pathol 2009; 13: 60–4.

Eppley BL, van Aalst JA, Robey A, Havlik RJ, Sadove AM. The spectrum of orofacial clefting. Plast Reconstr Surg 2005; 115: 101e–14e.

Flint SR. Necrotizing sialometaplasia: an important diagnosis—review of the literature and spectrum of clinical presentation. J Ir Dent Assoc 2005; 51: 26–8.

Frezzini C, Leao JC, Porter S. Current trends of HIV disease of the mouth. J Oral Pathol Med 2005; 34: 513–31.

Jainkittivong A, Aneksuk V, Langlais RP. Oral mucosal conditions in elderly dental patients. Oral Dis 2002; 8: 218–23.

Jugessur A, Farlie PG, Kilpatrick N. The genetics of isolated orofacial clefts: from genotypes to subphenotypes. Oral Dis 2009; 15: 437–53.

Komínek P, Blasch P. Necrotizing sialometaplasia: a potential diagnostic pitfall. Ear Nose Throat J 2006; 85: 604–5.

Lager I, Altini M, Coleman H, Ali H. Oral Kaposi's sarcoma: a clinicopathologic study from South Africa. Oral Surg Oral Med Oral Pathol Oral Radiol Endod 2003; 96: 701–10.

Lausten LL, Ferguson BL, Barker BF, Cobb CM. Oral Kaposi sarcoma associated with severe alveolar bone loss: case report and review of the literature. J Periodontol 2003; 74: 1668–75.

Leao JC, Porter S, Scully C. Human herpesvirus 8 and oral health care: an update. Oral Surg Oral Med Oral Pathol Oral Radiol Endod 2000; 90: 694–704.

Lee DJ, Ahn HK, Koh ES, Rho YS, Chu HR. Necrotizing sialometaplasia accompanied by adenoid cystic carcinoma on the soft palate. Clin Exp Otorhinolaryngol 2009; 2: 48–51.

Markiewicz MR, Margarone 3rd JE, Aguirre A, Suresh L. Cavernous hemangioma of the palate. A review of etiology, pathogenesis and treatment options. N Y State Dent J 2006; 72: 40–2.

Marks R, Scarff CE, Yap LM, et al. Fungiform papillary glossitis: atopic disease in the mouth? Br J Dermatol 2005; 153: 740–5.

McKerrow WS. Inflammatory disorders of the tonsil. In: Gleeson M, et al., eds. Scott-Brown's Otorhinolaryngology: Head and Neck Surgery, 7th edn. London: Hodder Arnold, 2008.

Napier SS, Speight PM. Natural history of potentially malignant oral lesions and conditions: an overview of the literature. J Oral Pathol Med 2008; 37: 1–10.

Ojha J, Akers JL, Akers JO, et al. Intraoral cellular blue nevus: report of a unique histopathologic entity and review of the literature. Cutis 2007; 80: 189–92.

Osborne RF, Brown JJ. Carcinoma of the oral pharynx: an analysis of subsite treatment heterogeneity. Surg Oncol Clin N Am 2004; 13: 71–80.

Porter SR. Non-neoplastic salivary gland disease. In: Gleeson M, et al., eds. Scott-Brown's Otorhinolaryngology: Head & Neck Surgery, 7th edn. London: Hodder Arnold, 2008.

Poulopoulos A, Belazi M, Epivatianos A, Velegraki A, Antoniades D. The role of Candida in inflammatory papillary hyperplasia of the palate. J Oral Rehabil 2007; 34: 685–92.

Ravn T, Trolle W, Kiss K, Balle VH. Adenosquamous carcinoma of the larynx associated with necrotizing sialometaplasia—a diagnostic challenge. Auris Nasus Larynx 2009; 36: 721–4.

Reichart PA, Samaranayake LP, Philipsen HP. Pathology and clinical correlates in oral candidiasis and its variants: a review. Oral Dis 2000; 6: 85–91.

Rizkalla H, Toner M. Necrotizing sialometaplasia versus invasive carcinoma of the head and neck: the use of myoepithelial markers and keratin subtypes as an adjunct to diagnosis. Histopathology 2007; 51: 184–9.

Rohrmus B, Thoma-Greber EM, Bogner JR, Rocken M. Outlook in oral and cutaneous Kaposi's sarcoma. Lancet 2000; 356: 2160.

Rudnick EF, Sie KC. Velopharyngeal insufficiency: current concepts in diagnosis and management. Curr Opin Otolaryngol Head Neck Surg 2008; 16: 530–5.

Schwartz RH, Hayden GF, Rodriquez WJ, Shprintzen RJ, Cassidy JW. The bifid uvula: is it a marker for an otitis prone child? Laryngoscope 1985; 95(9 Pt 1): 1100–2.

Scully C, Eveson J. Sialosis and necrotising sialometaplasia in bulimia; a case report. Int J Oral Maxillofac Surg 2004; 33: 808–10.

Scully C, el-Kabir M, Samaranayake LP. Candida and oral candidosis: a review. Crit Rev Oral Biol Med 1994; 5: 125–57.

Scully C, Porter S. Orofacial disease: update for the dental clinical team: 4. Red, brown, black and bluish lesions. Dent Update 1999; 26: 169–73.

Scully C, Porter S. ABC of oral health. Swellings and red, white, and pigmented lesions. BMJ 2000; 321: 225–8.

Seah YH. Torus palatinus and torus mandibularis: a review of the literature. Aust Dent J 1995; 40: 318–21.

Shprintzen RJ, Marrinan E. Velopharyngeal insufficiency: diagnosis and management. Curr Opin Otolaryngol Head Neck Surg 2009; 17: 302–7.

Solomon LW, Merzianu M, Sullivan M, Rigual NR. Necrotizing sialometaplasia associated with bulimia: case report and literature review. Oral Surg Oral Med Oral Pathol Oral Radiol Endod 2007; 103: e39–42.

Stambuk HE, Karimi S, Lee N, Patel SG. Oral cavity and oropharynx tumors. Radiol Clin North Am 2007; 45: 1–20.

Stephenson P, Lamey PJ, Scully C, Prime SS. Angina bullosa haemorrhagica: clinical and laboratory features in 30 patients. Oral Surg Oral Med Oral Pathol 1987; 63: 560–5.

Suresh L, Aguirre A. Subacute necrotizing sialadenitis: a clinicopathological study. Oral Surg Oral Med Oral Pathol Oral Radiol Endod 2007; 104: 385–90.

Taybos G. Oral changes associated with tobacco use. Am J Med Sci 2003; 326: 179–82.

- aesthetic conditions
- bleeding
- blisters
- gingival attachment loss

- pigmented, red, purple or blue lesions
- soreness, ulceration and pain
- swellings and lumps
- white lesions

The gingivae in health are firm, pale pink, with a stippled surface, and have sharp gingival papillae reaching up between adjacent teeth to the tooth contact point. The gingivae consist of a free gingival margin overlapping the amelo-dentinal junction of the tooth and a strip of attached 'keratinized' gingiva bound down to the alveolar bone that supports the teeth. The attached gingiva (pale pink) is clearly demarcated from the non-keratinized vascular alveolar mucosa.

Bands of tissue which may contain muscle attachments (fraena) run from the labial mucosa centrally onto the alveolar mucosa and from the buccal mucosa in the premolar region onto the alveolar mucosa (Figs 2.5.1 and 2.5.2).

The dentogingival junction is a unique anatomical feature concerned with the attachment of the gingiva to the tooth. Non-keratinized gingival epithelium forms a cuff surrounding the tooth, and at its lowest point on the tooth is adherent to the enamel or cementum. This 'junctional' epithelium is unique in being bound both on its tooth and lamina propria aspects by basement membranes. Above this is a shallow sulcus or crevice (up to 2 mm deep), the gingival sulcus or crevice.

The tooth root is connected to the alveolar bone by fibres of the periodontal ligament, which run to the cementum.

Detailed description of periodontal examination techniques can be found in standard textbooks. Examine particularly for abnormalities such as gingival redness, swelling, ulceration or bleeding on gently probing the gingival margin, and for tooth mobility.

Most gingival and periodontal diseases are inflammatory and dental plaque-related, and others may be aggravated by the effects of plaque accumulation. Dental bacterial plaque is a complex biofilm containing various micro-organisms which forms rapidly on teeth, particularly between them, along the gingival margin and in fissures and pits. Plaque is not especially obvious clinically, although teeth covered with plaque lack the lustre of clear teeth. Various dyes (disclosing solutions) can be used to reveal the plaque.

Gingival and periodontal inflammatory disease is mainly evident on the gingival free margins. The attached gingivae may also show signs of other significant pathology [e.g. desquamative gingivitis (DG)] which may be overlooked or misinterpreted as inflammatory (plaque-related) periodontal disease.

A range of disorders can affect the gingivae; this chapter highlights only those that are seen particularly or exclusively in that location.

## AESTHETIC CONDITIONS
Acquired causes of gingival swellings include epulides and drug-induced swellings which can be unsightly. Swelling may also be congenital.

### Hereditary gingival fibromatosis
Hereditary gingival fibromatosis may cause considerable swelling with aesthetic consequences (Table 2.5.1; Fig. 2.5.3).

*Aetiology*
Hereditary gingival fibromatosis is an autosomal dominant condition due to chromosome 2 or 5 anomalies, resulting in transforming growth factor-alpha 1 autocrine stimulation of fibroblast proliferation with alteration in expression of matrix metalloproteinases (MMP)-1 and MMP-2.

*Clinical features*
The changes initially involve the gingival papillae and later the attached gingiva leading to generalized gingival enlargement, especially obvious over the anterior maxilla and during the transition from deciduous to permanent dentitions. The affected gingiva is usually of normal colour but firm in consistency, and the surface becomes coarsely stippled. If the enlargement becomes gross, it may move or cover the teeth and even protrude from the mouth.

Patients may also be hirsute (as may patients with drug-induced gingival hyperplasia). Although most patients otherwise have only gingival fibromatosis, there are also occasional associations with supernumerary teeth or with various syndromes (Table 2.5.1).

**Diagnosis**
Clinical.

*Management*
Gingival surgery is often indicated. Genetic counselling may be indicated.

## BLEEDING
### Chronic marginal gingivitis
*Aetiopathogenesis*
Most of the population has a degree of chronic gingivitis. Dental plaque accumulation and a change in the microflora may cause gingival inflammation (gingivitis). If plaque is not removed it calcifies to become calculus which aggravates the condition by facilitating plaque accumulation. If conditions are appropriate this may progress to damage the periodontal membrane (chronic periodontitis) and ultimately can lead to tooth loss.

*Clinical features*
Inflammation of the margins of the gingiva is painless and often the only features are gingival bleeding on eating or brushing, possibly some halitosis, erythema, swelling (Figs 2.5.4–2.5.6) and bleeding on probing.

*Diagnosis*
This is a clinical diagnosis.

*Management*
Plaque and calculus (tartar) must be removed by scaling and polishing. Root-planing and possible surgical removal of hyperplastic tissue and surgical recontouring of the gingivae may also be indicated.

Prevention of plaque-associated gingival and periodontal diseases is by:

- Oral hygiene, which can prevent periodontal disease and oral malodour (halitosis). The most important oral hygiene device is a toothbrush;

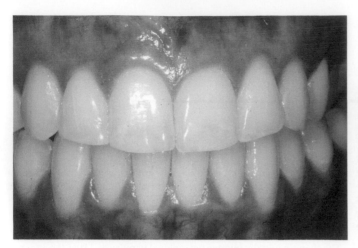

*Figure 2.5.1* Normal gingivae.

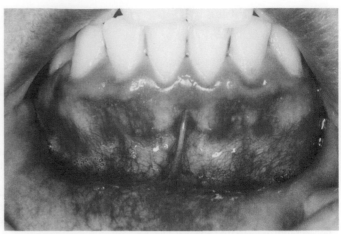

*Figure 2.5.2* Normal gingivae—showing racial pigmentation.

**Table 2.5.1** SYNDROMES ASSOCIATED WITH GINGIVAL FIBROMATOSIS

| Syndrome | Inheritance | Main features apart from gingival fibromatosis |
|---|---|---|
| Zimmermann–Laband | AD | Ears and nose thickened and enlarged<br>Nail dysplasia<br>Terminal phalanges hypoplastic<br>Joint hyper-extensibility<br>Hepatosplenomegaly |
| Murray–Puretic–Drescher | AR | Hyaline fibrous tumours over scalp, neck and limbs<br>Osteolysis of terminal phalanges<br>Recurrent infections |
| Rutherfurd | AD | Retarded tooth eruption<br>Corneal opacities |
| Cowden | AD | Giant fibroadenoma of breast<br>Hypertrichosis<br>Multiple hamartomas |
| Cross | AR | Hypopigmentation<br>Microphthalmia with cloudy corneas<br>Learning disability<br>Athetoid cerebral palsy |
| Gingival fibromatosis | AD | Hypertrichosis<br>Epilepsy<br>Learning disability |
| Gingival fibromatosis with progressive deafness | AD | Progressive sensorineural deafness |

*Abbreviations*: AD, autosomal dominant; AR, autosomal recessive.

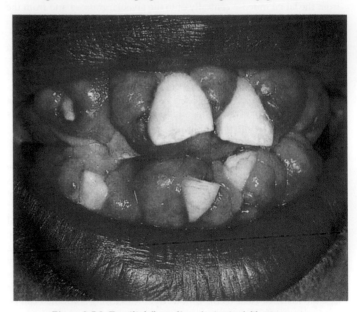

*Figure 2.5.3* Familial (hereditary) gingival fibromatosis.

many are available and most can be effective at removing plaque. Powered brushes may assist oral hygiene, especially in those with poor manual dexterity. Toothbrushing at least twice a day, only removes plaque from smooth dental surfaces and not from the depths of pits and fissures or interproximally; more effective interdental removal requires regular flossing (some flosses also contain fluoride).

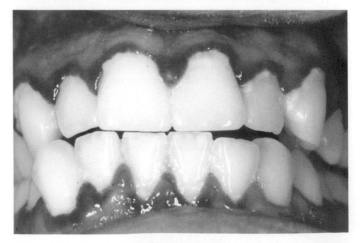

*Figure 2.5.4* Chronic gingivitis related to dental plaque accumulation.

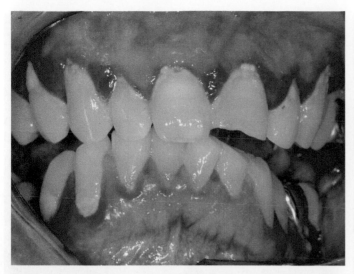

*Figure 2.5.5* Chronic gingivitis related to dental plaque accumulation.

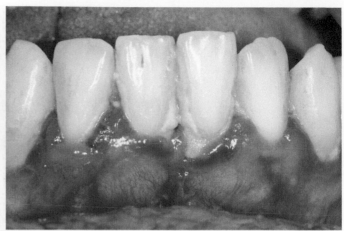

*Figure 2.5.6* Chronic periodontitis related to plaque.

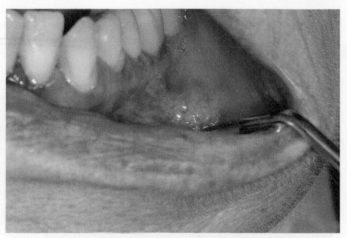

*Figure 2.5.7* Blister in mucous membrane pemphigoid.

- Antiseptics such as chlorhexidine and triclosan have anti-plaque activity. Dentifrices with calcium pyrophosphate have anti-calculus activity, inhibiting its accumulation.
- Mouthwashes are a more contentious issue; the most effective anti-plaque mouthwashes (e.g. chlorhexidine, triclosan) have prolonged retention on oral surfaces by adsorption, maintained activity once adsorbed, then slowly desorb, with continued activity. Chlorhexidine unfortunately binds tannins and thereby can cause dental staining if the patient drinks coffee, tea or red wine. This can be cleaned off by dental professionals.

Many other mouthwashes are subject to highly competitive advertising although legal constraints ensure that claims are never untrue, but the impression gained may be optimistic—many have only a transient antiseptic activity, some can be harmful by causing mucosal reactions, and there can be a danger to young children who might ingest the mouthwash.

### Leukaemia
Leukaemia (Chapter 1.4).

Gingival swelling is uncommon and most characteristic of acute myelomonocytic leukaemia, but has been reported in types of myelodysplasia and chronic lymphocytic leukaemia. Gingival involvement in leukaemia is most common in adults and is characterized by haemorrhage, swelling and ulceration. Petechiae, ecchymoses or haemorrhage is common.

## BLISTERS
Gingival blisters may be caused by burns or mucoceles, but bullous disorders should be excluded (Fig. 2.5.7).

## GINGIVAL ATTACHMENT LOSS
### Localized recession
Periodontitis and traumatic occlusion may cause recession (Figs 2.5.8–2.5.12). Self-induced ulcers of the gingival margin are not rare: the maxillary canine region seems a common site, and this may be a type of Munchausen syndrome (Chapter 1.9). Trauma can damage the periodontium, often through excessive occlusal stresses and sometimes through direct damage.

### Periodontitis
*Aetiopathogenesis*
*Chronic periodontitis* is common, related to plaque accumulation, and progresses from marginal gingivitis. Smoking, tobacco use and some other habits may contribute to periodontal disease, and immune defects may exacerbate the damage.

*Aggressive (accelerated) periodontitis* in pubertal and post-pubertal individuals (previously termed juvenile periodontitis or periodontosis) is seen especially in females, and in Afro-Asians and may be associated with minor defects of neutrophil function and micro-organisms such as *Aggregatobacter* (Actinobacillus) *actinomycetemcomitans* and capnocytophaga.

Aggressive periodontitis may also be related to a range of immune defects including HIV disease, diabetes mellitus and white cell dyscrasias including neutrophil defects and neutropenias. Similar periodontal

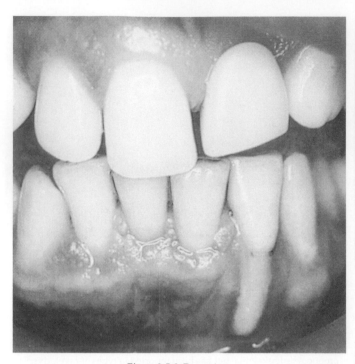

*Figure 2.5.8* Recession.

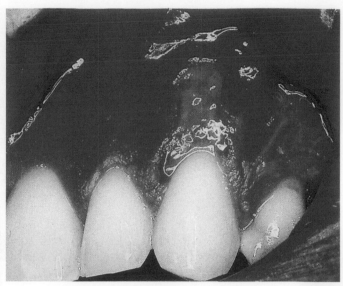

*Figure 2.5.9* Traumatic ulceration.

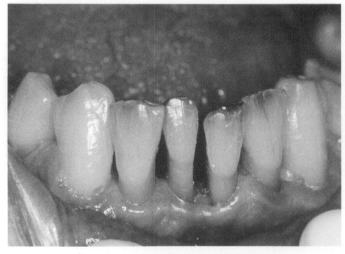

*Figure 2.5.10* Trauma—major gingival recession, lower anterior teeth.

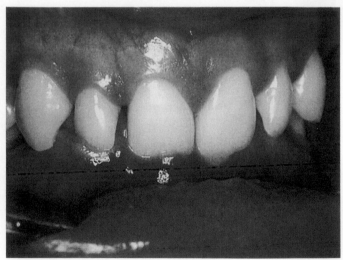

*Figure 2.5.11* Trauma—traumatic overbite in a class 2 division 2 occlusion.

destruction can be seen in Down syndrome, Ehlers–Danlos syndrome types III, VI and VIII, and hypophosphatasia.

### Clinical features
In chronic periodontitis, the gingiva detaches from the tooth neck, the periodontal membrane and alveolar bone are damaged, and an abnormal gap (pocket) develops between the tooth and gum. The tooth may slowly loosen and eventually be lost. The features are often those of marginal gingivitis but, with destruction of alveolar bone support, there is increasing tooth mobility, teeth may drift and there is deep pocket formation and attachment loss (Figs 2.5.13–2.5.16).

In aggressive (accelerated) periodontitis, despite good plaque control, patients develop periodontitis which varies from localized loss (such as around the incisors and first molars) to generalized involvement of most teeth.

### Diagnosis
Diagnosis is based on clinical features plus imaging. Periodontal breakdown in a person who is maintaining good oral hygiene almost invariably suggests aggressive periodontitis and an immune or other systemic defect.

### Management
Although chronic periodontitis has a bacterial component, systemic antibiotics have no place in routine treatment and management com-

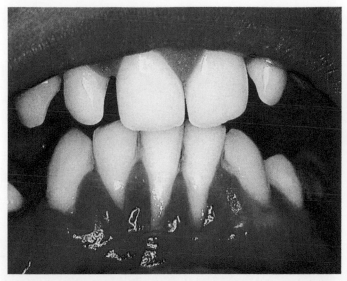

*Figure 2.5.12* Trauma—same patient as in Figure 2.5.11 showing periodontal damage.

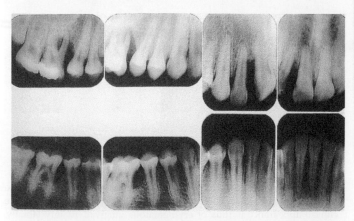

*Figure 2.5.14* Chronic periodontitis related to dental plaque accumulation.

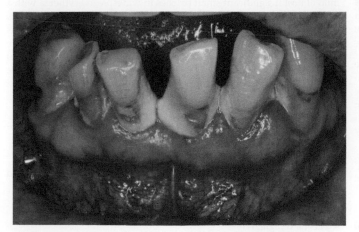

*Figure 2.5.16* Chronic periodontitis related to dental plaque accumulation and calculus.

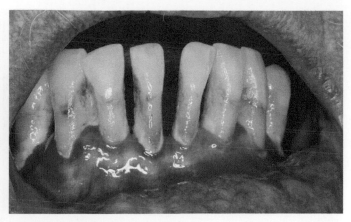

*Figure 2.5.13* Chronic periodontitis related to dental plaque accumulation.

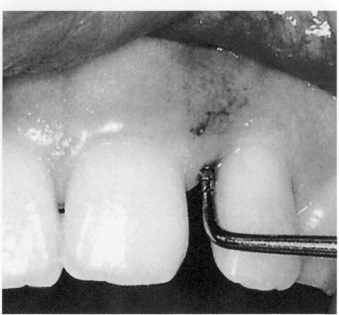

*Figure 2.5.15* Periodontitis.

prises improvement in oral hygiene, although in this case plaque accumulates below the gumline, within periodontal pockets. Toothbrushing and mouthwashes have little effect there, and are, therefore, ineffective alone in the treatment of periodontitis.

Surgical removal of the pocket wall and removal of diseased tissue may be needed to facilitate cleansing, and attempts to regenerate lost periodontal tissue (such as guided tissue regeneration) may be indicated. Periodontal specialist attention is, therefore, required.

## PIGMENTED, RED, PURPLE OR BLUE LESIONS
**Candidosis**
Candidosis (Chapter 1.8).

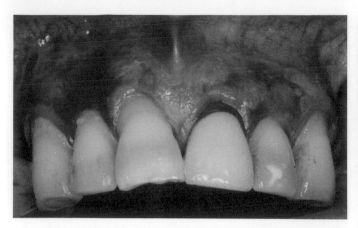

*Figure 2.5.17* Desquamative gingivitis due to lichen planus.

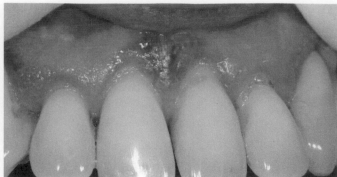

*Figure 2.5.18* Desquamative gingivitis due to lichen planus.

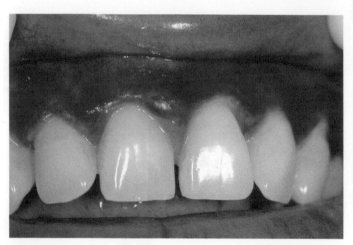

*Figure 2.5.19* Desquamative gingivitis due to pemphigoid.

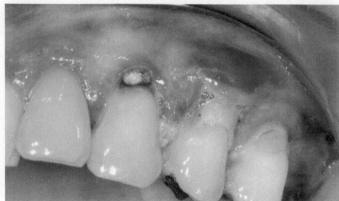

*Figure 2.5.20* Desquamative gingivitis due to pemphigoid.

## Desquamative gingivitis

### Aetiopathogenesis

Seen mainly in middle-aged women, desquamative gingivitis (DG) is caused by chronic desquamation which may be a manifestation of a variety of disorders ranging from vesiculobullous diseases to adverse reactions to chemicals or allergens. DG can be related to

* mucocutaneous disorders usually. Most gingival involvement in the vesiculobullous or skin diseases (dermatoses) is related to lichen planus or pemphigoid, but pemphigus, dermatitis herpetiformis: linear IgA disease, chronic ulcerative stomatitis, Kindler syndrome and other conditions may need to be excluded. Most of these conditions are acquired but a few are congenital with a strong hereditary predisposition, such as epidermolysis bullosa
* chemical damage
* allergic responses
* drug reactions.

### Clinical features

Some patients make no complaint, but the main complaint in others is of persistent soreness of the gingiva, worse when eating acidic foods such as tomatoes, citrus fruits and others.

DG differs from marginal gingivitis in that there is erythema involving the attached gingiva, and extending into the vestibule: indeed, the gingival margins themselves may be spared (Figs 2.5.17–2.5.24). The clinical appearance is thus of erythematous gingivae, mainly labially, the erythema and loss of stippling extending apically from the gingival margins to the alveolar mucosae. The desquamation may vary from mild almost insignificant small patches to widespread erythema with a glazed appearance. Erythema is most noticeable where oral hygiene is poor and there is superimposed plaque-related gingivitis. Most patients are seen only when with vesicles and bullae have broken down to leave desquamation, erosions or ulcers. Classically, the affected gingival epithelium is very fragile and the surface detaches easily in response to minor trauma, or this produces vesicles or bullae (Nikolsky sign).

### Diagnosis

Diagnosis is clinically supported by biopsy examination and appropriate histopathological and immunological investigations.

Conditions that should be excluded include:

* reactions to various mouthwashes, chewing gum, medications and dental materials
* candidosis
* lupus erythematosus
* plasma cell gingivitis
* Crohn disease, sarcoidosis and orofacial granulomatosis
* leukaemias

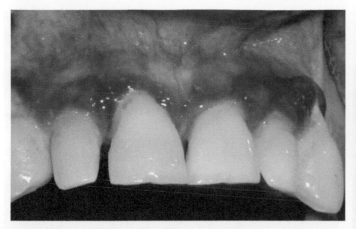

*Figure 2.5.21* Desquamative gingivitis due to pemphigoid.

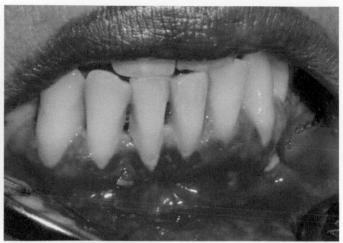

*Figure 2.5.22* Desquamative gingivitis due to pemphigus.

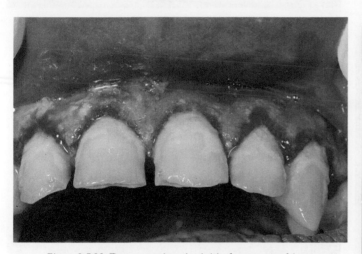

*Figure 2.5.23* Desquamative gingivitis due to pemphigus.

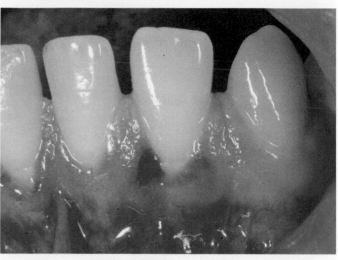

*Figure 2.5.24* Desquamative gingivitis due to pemphigus.

● factitial (self-induced) lesions.

*Management*
The treatment of DG consists of

● improving the oral hygiene
● minimizing irritation of the lesions
● specific therapies for the underlying disease where available
● often dapsone therapy or local or systemic immunosuppressive, notably corticosteroids. Topical corticosteroid creams are the mainstay of therapy and may be of particular benefit if applied during sleep in a polythene splint.

### Erythroplasia
Erythroplasia (Chapter 2.2).

### Haemangioma
Haemangioma (Fig. 2.5.25) (Chapter 2.1).

### Kaposi sarcoma
Kaposi sarcoma (Fig. 2.5.26) (Chapter 1.7).

### Macule
Macule (Figs 2.5.27 and 2.5.28) (Chapter 2.2).

### Naevus
Naevus (Fig. 2.5.29) (Chapter 2.2).

### Plasma cell gingivitis
Plasma cell gingivitis (allergic, atypical or plasma cell gingivostomatitis).

Diffusely red, swollen gingivae with or without oral ulceration may occasionally follow exposure to various allergens and other substances such as certain chewing gums, confectionery such as mints, and dentifrices and dental materials—particularly 'tartar control' dentifrices containing cinnamon or cinnamaldehyde (Fig. 2.5.30).

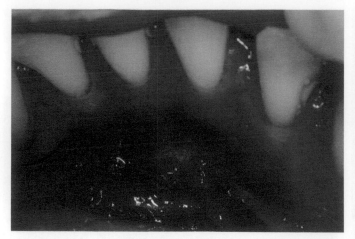

*Figure 2.5.25* Angioma.

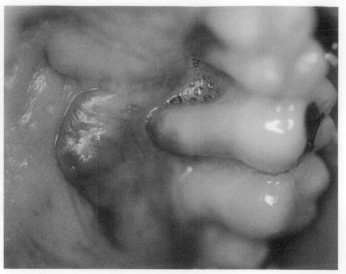

*Figure 2.5.26* Kaposi sarcoma.

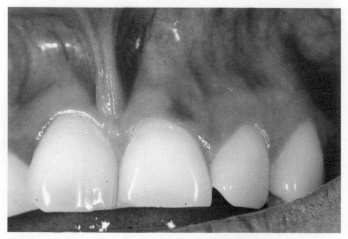

*Figure 2.5.27* Melanotic macule.

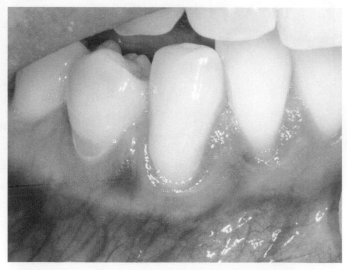

*Figure 2.5.28* Melanotic macule.

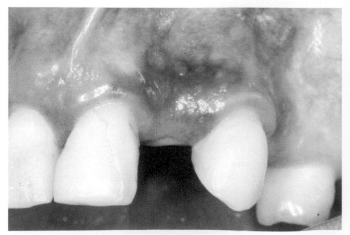

*Figure 2.5.29* Lentigo.

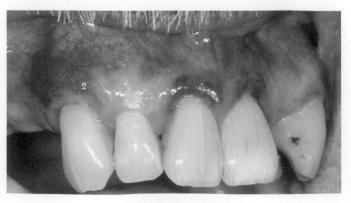

*Figure 2.5.30* Plasma cell gingivitis.

Plasma cell mucositis is a rare plasma cell proliferative disorder of the upper aerodigestive tract. Clinical features are an intensely erythematous mucosa with papillomatous, cobblestone, nodular or velvety surface changes. Symptoms include pain, dysphagia, hoarseness and pharyngitis. Most cases have a history of autoimmune or immunologically mediated disease. The histopathologic features of a dense, submucosal plasma cell infiltrate are not specific.

Patch testing is occasionally of value in diagnosis. It has been suggested that lesions resolve on withdrawal of any identifiable causal agent and reappear on rechallenge. However, often the causative agent is not identified; hence topical corticosteroids may be required. Biopsy is usually not indicated.

### Pregnancy gingivitis and epulis

Pregnancy gingivitis and epulis (Fig. 2.5.31) (Chapter 1.2).

### Racial

Racial (Figs 2.5.32–2.5.34).

Brown pigmentation is common, especially on the gingivae, in persons of Asian, African or Mediterranean origin. There is no direct correlation between skin colour and gingival or oral pigmentation.

### Tattoos

Tattoos (Figs 2.5.35–2.5.37) (Chapter 2.1).

### Telangiectasia

Telangiectasia (Fig. 2.5.38) (Chapter 1.1).

## SORENESS, ULCERATION AND PAIN
### Acute necrotizing ulcerative gingivitis

Acute necrotizing ulcerative gingivitis (ANUG) (acute ulcerative gingivitis, acute necrotizing gingivitis, ANUG, Vincent disease; trench mouth, ulceronecrotic gingivitis).

*Aetiopathogenesis*

ANUG is an uncommon, non-contagious anaerobic gingival infection associated with overwhelming proliferation of *Borrelia vincentii* and

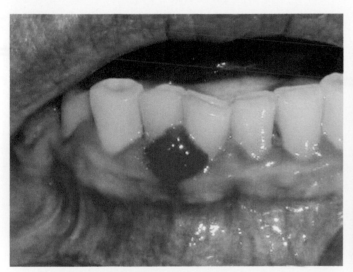

*Figure 2.5.31* Pregnancy epulis (pyogenic granuloma).

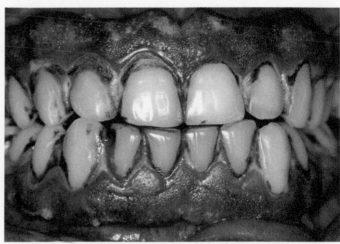

*Figure 2.5.32* Racial pigmentation.

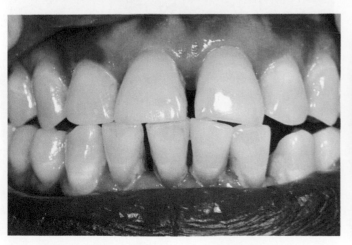

*Figure 2.5.33* Racial pigmentation.

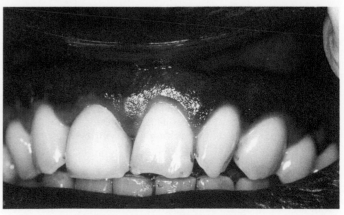

*Figure 2.5.34* Racial pigmentation.

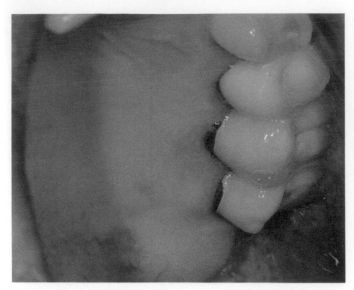

*Figure 2.5.35* Amalgam tattoo.

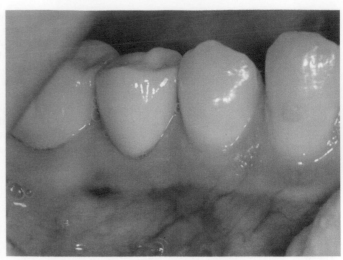

*Figure 2.5.36* Amalgam tattoo.

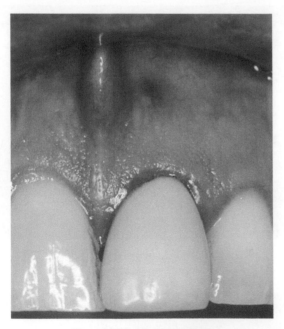

*Figure 2.5.37* Amalgam tattoo.

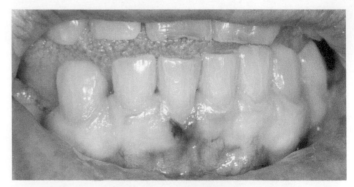

*Figure 2.5.38* Telangiectasis.

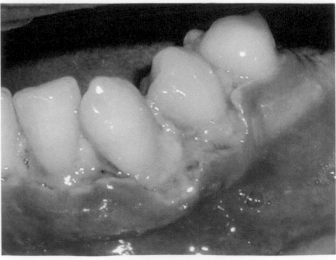

*Figure 2.5.39* Gingivitis—ulceronecrotic.

fusiform bacteria. Seen mainly in people of lower socio-economic status, this typically affects adolescents and young adults, especially in institutions, armed forces, etc. Predisposing factors include poor oral hygiene, smoking and immune defects such as may accompany viral respiratory or other infections and HIV/AIDS.

*Clinical features*
Characteristic features of ANUG include severe gingival soreness, profuse bleeding, halitosis and a bad taste. Interdental papillae are ulcerated with necrotic sloughs. Painful gingival ulceration occasionally spreads from the papillae to the gingival margins (Figs 2.5.39 and 2.5.40). Malaise,

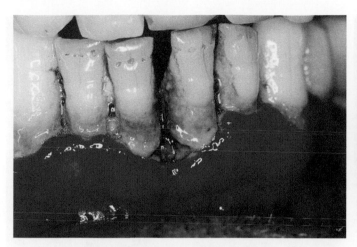

*Figure 2.5.40* Gingivitis—ulceronecrotic.

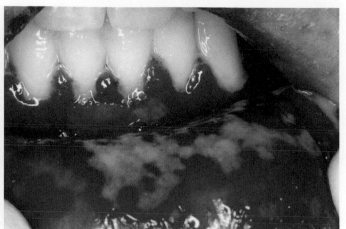

*Figure 2.5.41* Herpetic gingivitis.

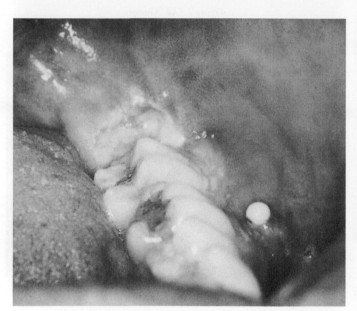

*Figure 2.5.42* Pericoronitis.

fever and/or cervical lymph node enlargement (unlike herpetic stomatitis) are rare. Necrotizing stomatitis and cancrum oris (noma) is a very rare complication, usually in debilitated children.

*Diagnosis*
Diagnosis of ANUG is usually clinical. Differentiation is from acute leukaemia or herpetic stomatitis and thus a smear for fusospirochaetal bacteria and a blood picture may be helpful.

*Management*
Management is by oral debridement, metronidazole (penicillin if pregnant) and improved oral hygiene.

**Desquamative gingivitis**
DG (Chapter 2.5).

**Herpetic stomatitis**
Herpetic stomatitis (Fig. 2.5.41) (Chapter 1.8).

**Pericoronitis**
*Aetiopathogenesis*
Acute pericoronitis is inflammation of the operculum over an erupting or impacted tooth, usually a partially erupted mandibular third molar. It appears in relation to the accumulation of plaque and trauma from the opposing tooth. A mixed flora is implicated and Fusobacterium and Bacteroides are recognized to be important. Immune defects may predispose.

*Clinical features*
Patients with acute pericoronitis complain of pain, trismus, swelling and halitosis. There may be fever and regional lymphadenitis, and the operculum is swollen, red and often ulcerated. Pus usually drains from beneath the operculum but may, in a migratory abscess of the buccal sulcus, track anteriorly (Fig. 2.5.42).

*Diagnosis*
Diagnosis is from clinical features. Radiology is usually indicated to confirm the position and root formation of the underlying partially erupted tooth.

*Management*
Initial management comprises local debridement and application of antiseptics such as chlorhexidine. Reduction of the occlusal surface of an opposing tooth may be helpful if there is local trauma; extraction of any opposing upper third molar may also be helpful, particularly if it is likely that the lower third molar will require extraction due to the degree of impaction. Rarely removal of the operculum (operculectomy) may be warranted if the impacted tooth is likely to erupt. Pyrexia, trismus or cervical lymphadenopathy may be indications for use of systemic antibiotics, typically metronidazole.

Long-term treatment may include extraction of the associated impacted tooth, particularly when this is a lower third molar.

## SWELLINGS AND LUMPS
**Abscesses**
*Aetiopathogenesis*
A gingival abscess may arise from gingival infection, or a foreign body.

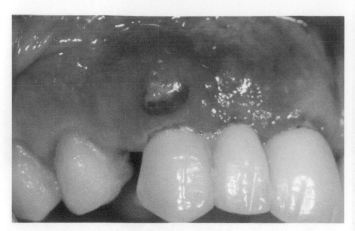

*Figure 2.5.43* Abscess.

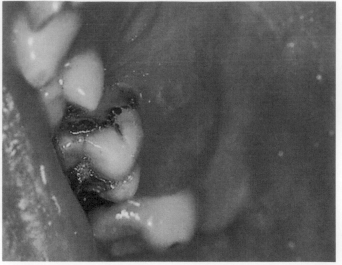

*Figure 2.5.44* Abscess.

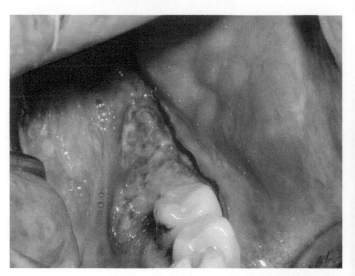

*Figure 2.5.45* Carcinoma.

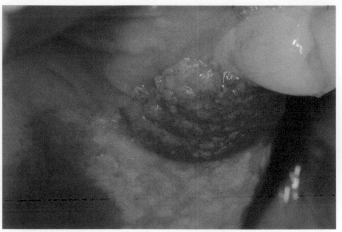

*Figure 2.5.46* Carcinoma.

A lateral periodontal abscess (parodontal abscess) is seen almost exclusively in patients with chronic periodontitis, but may follow impaction of a foreign body or, rarely, can be related to a lateral root canal on a non-vital tooth.

*Clinical features*
Erythema and swelling are the main features. Lateral periodontal abscesses may be painful, and eventually may discharge—either through the pocket or buccally, but more coronally than a periapical abscess (Figs 2.5.43 and 2.5.44).

*Diagnosis*
Clinical.

*Management*
Drainage, and sometimes antibiotics.

## Carcinoma
Carcinoma (Figs 2.5.45 and 2.5.46) (Chapter 2.3).

## Epulides
Epulides are localized gingival swellings but rarely true neoplasms.

*Aetiopathogenesis*
*Fibrous epulides* may result from local gingival irritation, leading to fibrous hyperplasia (Fig. 2.5.47).

*Pyogenic granulomas* are an exaggerated response to minor trauma, uncommon except in pregnancy or in some immunocompromised people (Figs 2.5.48–2.5.50).

*Giant cell epulides* may result from proliferation of giant cells persisting after resorption of deciduous teeth. It is most common in children (Fig. 2.5.51) after tooth extraction. The resorption of deciduous teeth and re-modelling of the alveolus at the mixed dentition stage indicate the osteoclastic potential of the area from which giant cell epulides arise. The swelling contains proliferating fibroblasts in a highly vascular stroma with many multinucleate giant cells.

*Neoplasms*—rarely, epulides prove to be neoplasms such as metastatic carcinomas.

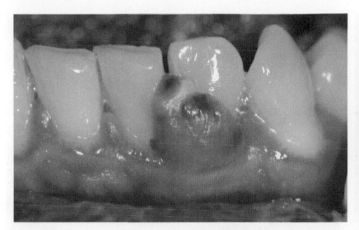

*Figure 2.5.47* Fibrous epulides.

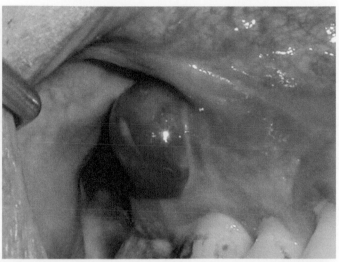

*Figure 2.5.48* Pyogenic granulomas.

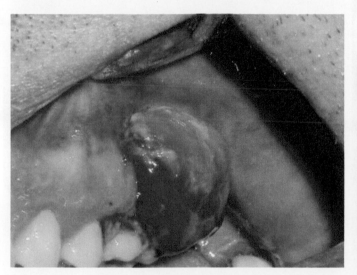

*Figure 2.5.49* Pyogenic granulomas.

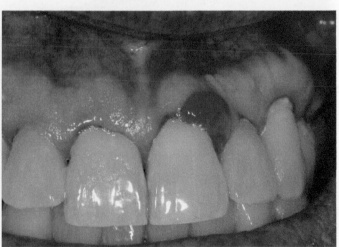

*Figure 2.5.50* Epulis.

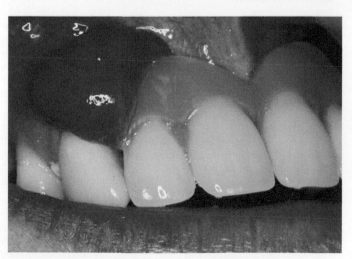

*Figure 2.5.51* Giant cell granuloma.

### Clinical features

Most epulides are seen in the anterior part of the mouth and most are fibrous epulides. *Fibrous epulides* typically form narrow, firm, pale swellings of an anterior interdental papilla and may ulcerate. *Pyogenic granulomas* are soft, fleshy, rough-surfaced vascular lesions that bleed readily, and are seen most commonly on the gingiva, often arising on the buccal aspect from the interdental papilla and especially where there is a slight malocclusion leading to plaque accumulation. Pregnancy predisposes to these, which are then termed 'pregnancy epulis'. Most pyogenic granulomas are seen in the maxilla, anteriorly. *Giant cell* epulides are uncommon, soft, deeper red or purple in colour. The giant cell epulis characteristically arises interdentally adjacent to permanent teeth which have had deciduous predecessors. Kaposi sarcoma and epithelioid angiomatosis may have a similar appearance.

### Diagnosis

Radiography is often indicated to supplement clinical observations. Giant cell granulomas are also a feature of hyperparathyroidism, and

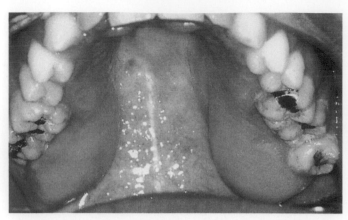

*Figure 2.5.52* Idiopathic gingival hyperplasia (fibromatosis).

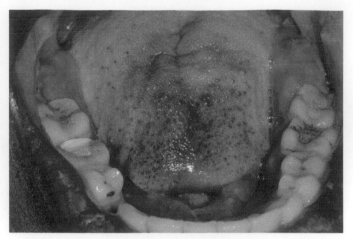

*Figure 2.5.53* Idiopathic gingival hyperplasia (fibromatosis).

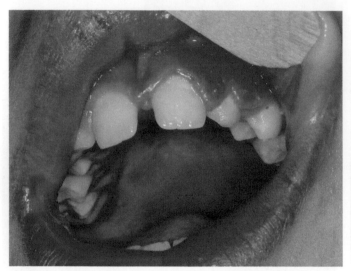

*Figure 2.5.54* Crohn disease—gingival lesions.

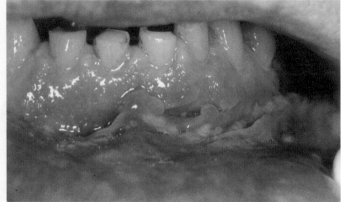

*Figure 2.5.55* Crohn disease—gingival lesions.

thus levels of plasma calcium, phosphate and alkaline phosphatase should be assayed and the area examined radiographically.

*Management*
Excision biopsy, and removal of local irritants (e.g. calculus).

### Gingival cysts in neonates
Small white nodules, sometimes termed Epstein pearls or Bohn nodules, are extremely common on the alveolar ridge and midline palate of the newborn. They usually disappear spontaneously by rupturing or involution within the first months of life.

### Gingival fibromatosis
Occasionally fibromatosis is found in the posterior maxillary or mandibular region (Figs 2.5.52 and 2.5.53).

### Granulomatous disorders
Granulomatous disorders (Crohn disease; orofacial granulomatosis; sarcoidosis) (Figs 2.5.54 and 2.5.55).

### Gingival hyperplasia
*Aetiopathogenesis*
Common in mouthbreathers (e.g. individuals with long-term nasal airway obstruction) and individuals who have persistent poor oral hygiene, gingival hyperplasia may also be congenital (Hereditary gingival fibromatosis; page 279) and is seen in those on some drugs. Histology shows marked thickening of epithelium with long overgrowths into the connective tissue. Fibroblasts show increased mitotic activity but are not increased in number, and the collagen fibre component is not increased.

*Clinical features*
*Drug-induced swelling (hyperplasia)* is usually aggravated by poor oral hygiene and starts interdentally, especially labially. Papillae are firm, pale and enlarge to form false vertical clefts (Figs 2.5.56 and 2.5.57; Chapter 1.6). This is associated with hypertrichosis. Causal drugs can include:

- *Phenytoin*, gingival enlargement characteristically affects the interdental tissues first but may later involve the marginal and even attached gingiva. The palatal and lingual gingiva are usually involved less than buccal and labial gingiva. The enlargement rarely affects edentulous sites.

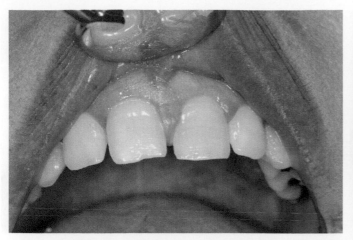

Figure 2.5.56 Drug-induced gingival swelling.

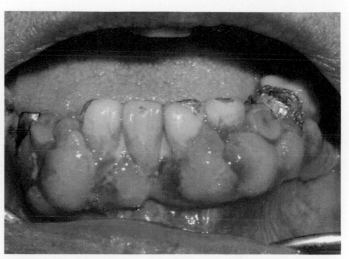

Figure 2.5.57 Drug-induced gingival swelling—from hydantoin (phenytoin).

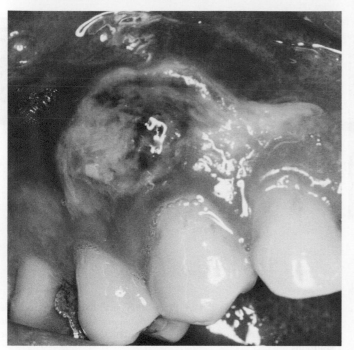

Figure 2.5.58 Lymphoma.

The enlargement in early lesions may be soft and red, sometimes giving the impression of 'bubbling up' behind the existing papillae but later characteristically becomes firm, pale and tough with coarse stippling. Older lesions may become red if inflamed. There is a positive correlation between the severity of gingival overgrowth and gingival inflammation, plaque score, calculus accumulation and pocket depths but there is no correlation with the dose of phenytoin, its serum level, or the age and sex of the patient.

- *Calcium-channel blockers* may induce gingival hyperplasia typically affecting the papillae which become red and puffy and tend to bleed. Increased numbers of fibroblasts containing strongly sulphated mucopolysaccharides may be demonstrated histochemically—their cytoplasm contains numerous secretory granules suggesting an increased production of acid mucopolysaccharides.

- *Ciclosporin* (cyclosporin) can cause gingival swelling initially affecting the gingival papillae. The occurrence may be influenced by the MRD1 gene. There have been small numbers of reports of Kaposi sarcoma or oral squamous cell carcinoma developing within ciclosporin-induced gingival enlargement.

*Diagnosis*
Diagnosis is clinical; biopsy is only occasionally needed.

*Management*
Treatment of drug-induced gingival hyperplasia is primarily that of chronic marginal gingivitis, although the management poses some problems. The physician may be willing to substitute another drug but, in any event, the patient's level of plaque control often needs considerable improvement and a chlorhexidine mouthwash may be helpful. Excision of enlarged tissue may be indicated but can be difficult if the tissue is very firm and fibrous. Healing may be slow, possibly hampered by infection of the large wound, and packs may require changing.

Unfortunately, the gingival enlargement readily recurs, although this is less likely with meticulous oral hygiene, particularly if the drug has been stopped.

**Lymphomas**
Lymphomas (Fig. 2.5.58) (Chapter 1.4).

**Papilloma**
Papilloma (Fig. 2.5.59) (Chapter 1.8).

**Torus mandibularis**
Torus mandibularis (Fig. 2.5.60) (Chapter 2.8).

# WHITE LESIONS
**Burns**
Burns (Chapter 2.1).

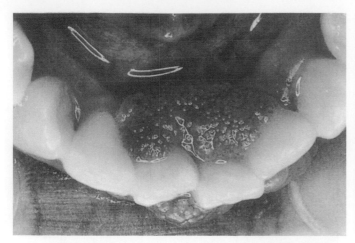

*Figure 2.5.59* Human papillomavirus.

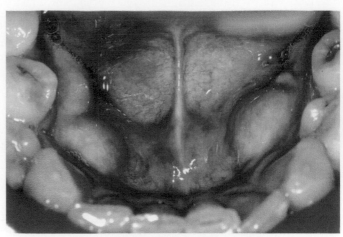

*Figure 2.5.60* Torus mandibularis.

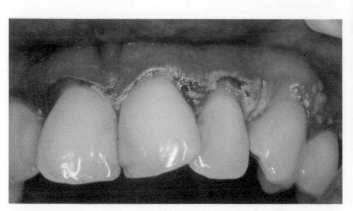

*Figure 2.5.61* Burn from use of chlorhexidine gel.

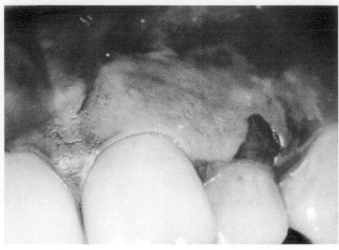

*Figure 2.5.62* Burn.

Burns to the gingivae can result from physical causes, or chemicals (Figs 2.5.61 and 2.5.62). Acidic dental material, for example, phosphoric acid may be implicated, as may the accidental ingestion of caustic solutions.

Cocaine is sometimes deliberately rubbed into the gingivae or vestibule. Gingival/ulceration and necrosis, accompanied by a brief 'high', can accompany local use of cocaine. The powerful vasoconstrictive effects of the cocaine are probably responsible for some of the local destruction. Tissue damage can develop within a few days of regular application of cocaine causing both soft- and hard-tissue destruction, although lesions usually heal when there is a cessation of the cocaine abuse. Crack cocaine (smoked) can cause ulceration of the palate and rarely oro-nasal fistulae. Oral neglect with caries and gingivitis are seen in juveniles who applied cocaine and amphetamine (mixed with sugar) to the maxillary gingiva, consequently with vestibular burns, and caries.

Natural products such as the houseplant Dieffenbachia, or the enzyme bromelin in pineapple may occasionally cause burns.

**Candidosis**

Candidosis (Chapter 1.8).

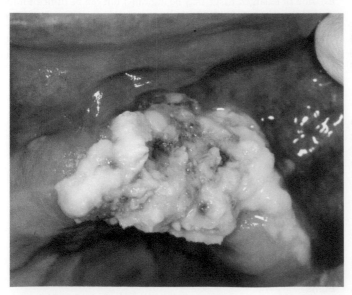

*Figure 2.5.63* Carcinoma.

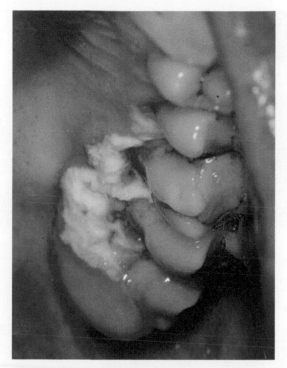

*Figure 2.5.64* Carcinoma.

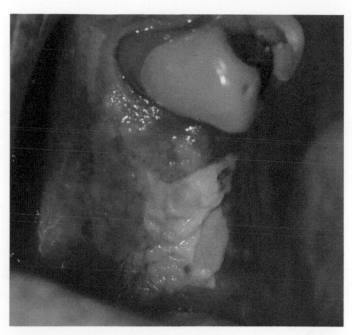

*Figure 2.5.65* Keratosis.

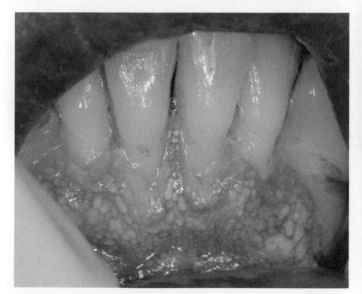

*Figure 2.5.66* Leukoplakia.

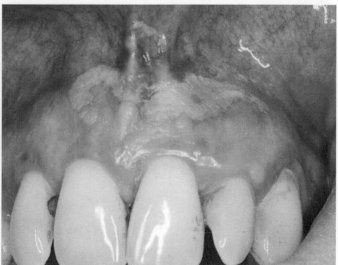

*Figure 2.5.67* Leukoplakia.

**Carcinoma**

Carcinoma (Figs 2.5.63 and 2.5.64) (Chapter 2.3).

**Keratoses**

Keratoses (Fig. 2.5.65) (Chapter 2.2).

**Leukoplakia**

Leukoplakia (Figs 2.5.66–2.5.70) (Chapter 2.2).

**Lichen planus**

Lichen planus (Figs 2.5.71–2.5.73) (Chapter 1.10).

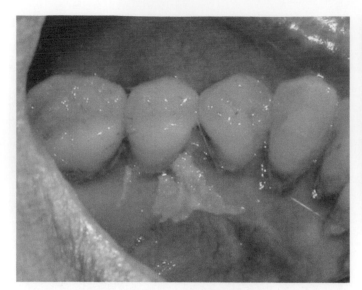

*Figure 2.5.68* Leukoplakia.

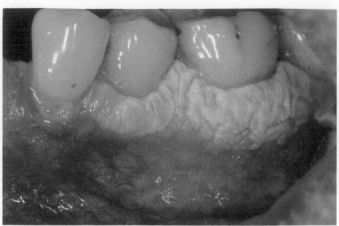

*Figure 2.5.69* Leukoplakia.

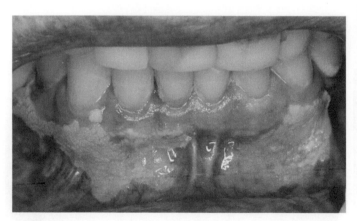

*Figure 2.5.70* Leukoplakia.

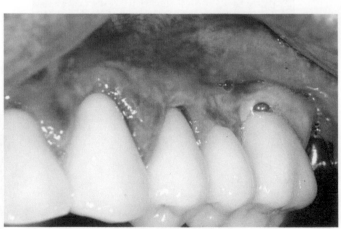

*Figure 2.5.71* Lichen planus.

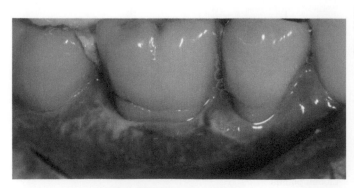

*Figure 2.5.72* Lichen planus.

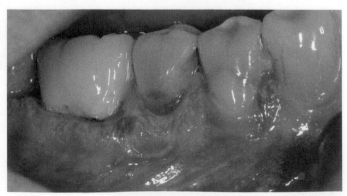

*Figure 2.5.73* Lichen planus.

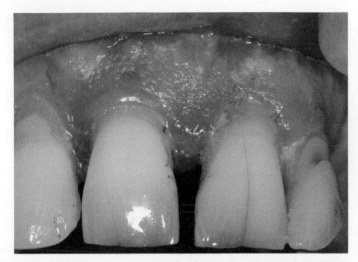

*Figure 2.5.74* Materia alba.

## Materia alba

Materia alba is the term given to the appearance of white debris on the gingivae resulting from lack of hygiene and the consequent accumulation of plaque and epithelial and other debris (Fig. 2.5.74).

## FURTHER READING

Al-Khateeb T, Ababneh K. Oral pyogenic granuloma in Jordanians: a retrospective analysis of 108 cases. J Oral Maxillofac Surg 2003; 61: 1285–8.

Anil S, Beena VT, Nair RG. Squamous cell carcinoma of the gingiva in an HIV-positive patient: a case report. Dent Update 1996; 23: 424–5.

Bagan JV, Jimenez Y, Sanchis JM, et al. Proliferative verrucous leukoplakia: high incidence of gingival squamous cell carcinoma. J Oral Pathol Med 2003; 32: 379–82.

Bakaeen G, Scully C. Hereditary gingival fibromatosis in a family with the Zimmermann-Laband syndrome. J Oral Pathol Med 1991; 20: 457–9.

Baptista IP. Hereditary gingival fibromatosis: a case report. J Clin Periodontol 2002; 29: 871–4.

Barrett AP. Leukemic cell infiltration of the gingivae. J Periodontol 1986; 57: 579–81.

Barros SP, Merzel J, de Araujo VC, de Almeida OP, Bozzo L. Ultrastructural aspects of connective tissue in hereditary gingival fibromatosis. Oral Surg Oral Med Oral Pathol Oral Radiol Endod 2001; 92: 78–82.

Bell RC, Chauvin PJ, Tyler MT. Gingival cyst of the adult: a review and a report of eight cases. J Can Dent Assoc 1997; 63: 533–5.

Bill TJ, Reddy VR, Ries KL, Gampper TJ, Hoard MA. Adolescent gingival squamous cell carcinoma: report of a case and review of the literature. Oral Surg Oral Med Oral Pathol Oral Radiol Endod 2001; 91: 682–5.

Binnie WH. Periodontal cysts and epulides. Periodontol 2000 1999; 21: 16–32.

Bittencourt LP, Campos V, Moliterno LF, Ribeiro DP, Sampaio RK. Hereditary gingival fibromatosis: review of the literature and a case report. Quintessence Int 2000; 31: 415–18.

Bouloux GF, Steed MB, Perciaccante VJ. Complications of third molar surgery. Oral Maxillofac Surg Clin North Am 2007; 19: 117–28.

Bozzo L, de Almedia OP, Scully C, Aldred MJ. Hereditary gingival fibromatosis. Report of an extensive four-generation pedigree. Oral Surg Oral Med Oral Pathol 1994; 78: 452–4.

Cairo F, Pagliaro U, Nieri M. Treatment of gingival recession with coronally advanced flap procedures: a systematic review. J Clin Periodontol 2008; 35(8 Suppl): 136–62.

Cairo F, Rotundo R, Ficarra G. A rare lesion of the periodontium: the gingival cyst of the adult—a report of three cases. Int J Periodontics Restorative Dent 2002; 22: 79–83.

Chimenos Kustner E, Finestres Zubeldia F, Huguet Redecilla P. Gingival squamous cell carcinoma: a clinical case and differential diagnosis. Med Oral 2001; 6: 335–41.

Clerehugh V, Tugnait A. Diagnosis and management of periodontal diseases in children and adolescents. Periodontol 2000 2001; 26: 146–68.

Craig RM Jr, Vickers VA, Correll RW. Erythroplastic lesion on the mandibular marginal gingiva. J Am Dent Assoc 1989; 119: 543–4.

Daley TD, Wysocki GP, Wysocki PD, Wysocki DM. The major epulides: clinicopathological correlations. J Can Dent Assoc 1990; 56: 627–30.

Dreizen S, McCredie KB, Keating MJ, Luna MA. Malignant gingival and skin "infiltrates" in adult leukemia. Oral Surg Oral Med Oral Pathol 1983; 55: 572–9.

Dummett CO. Normal and locally induced oral pigmentations. Int Dent J 1976; 26: 152–6.

Eisen D. The clinical manifestations and treatment of oral lichen planus. Dermatol Clin 2003; 21: 79–89.

Enwonwu CO, Falkler WA, Idigbe EO. Oro-facial gangrene (noma/cancrum oris): pathogenetic mechanisms. Crit Rev Oral Biol Med 2000; 11: 159–71.

da Fonseca MA, Feigal RJ, ten Bensel RW. Dental aspects of 1248 cases of child maltreatment on file at a major county hospital. Pediatr Dent 1992; 14: 152–7.

Genc A, Atalay T, Gedikoglu G, Zulfikar B, Kullu S. Leukemic children: clinical and histopathological gingival lesions. J Clin Pediatr Dent 1998; 22: 253–6.

Giunta JL. Gingival cysts in the adult. J Periodontol 2002; 73: 827–31.

Goette DK, Carpenter WM. Pyogenic granuloma of the oral cavity. South Med J 1977; 70: 1358–60.

Gomez D, Faucher A, Picot V, et al. Outcome of squamous cell carcinoma of the gingiva: a follow-up study of 83 cases. JJ Craniomaxillofac Surg 2000; 28: 331–5.

Graham RM. Pyogenic granuloma: an unusual presentation. Dent Update 1996; 23: 240–1.

Hart TC, Pallos D, Bozzo L, et al. Evidence of genetic heterogeneity for hereditary gingival fibromatosis. J Dent Res 2000; 79: 1758–64.

Jaber MA, Porter SR, Speight P, Eveson JW, Scully C. Oral epithelial dysplasia: clinical characteristics of western European residents. Oral Oncol 2003; 39: 589–96.

Jadwat Y, Meyerov R, Lemmer J, Raubenheimer EJ, Feller L. Plasma cell gingivitis: does it exist? Report of a case and review of the literature. SADJ 2008; 63: 394–5.

Jones AC, Gulley ML, Freedman PD. Necrotizing ulcerative stomatitis in human immunodeficiency virus-seropositive individuals: a review of the histopathologic, immunohistochemical, and virologic characteristics of 18 cases. Oral Surg Oral Med Oral Pathol Oral Radiol Endod 2000; 89: 323–32.

Kalpidis CD, Lysitsa SN, Lombardi T, et al. Gingival involvement in a case series of patients with acquired immunodeficiency syndrome-related Kaposi sarcoma. J Periodontol 2006; 77: 523–33.

Kamolmatyakul S, Kietthubthew S, Anusaksathien O. Long-term management of an idiopathic gingival fibromatosis patient with the primary dentition. Pediatr Dent 2001; 23: 508–13.

Kaugars GE, Burns JC, Gunsolley JC. Epithelial dysplasia of the oral cavity and lips. Cancer 1988; 62: 2166–70.

Kissel SO, Hanratty JJ. Periodontal treatment of an amalgam tattoo. Compend Contin Educ Dent 2002; 23: 930–2, 934, 936.

Lausten LL, Ferguson BL, Barker BF, Cobb CM. Oral Kaposi sarcoma associated with severe alveolar bone loss: case report and review of the literature. J Periodontol 2003; 74: 1668–75.

Leao JC, Ingafou M, Khan A, Scully C, Porter S. Desquamative gingivitis: retrospective analysis of disease associations of a large cohort. Oral Dis 2008; 14: 556–60.

Lee W, O'Donnell D. Severe gingival hyperplasia in a child with I-cell disease. Int J Paediatr Dent 2003; 13: 41–5.

Leston JM, Santos AA, Varela-Centelles PI, et al. Oral mucosa: variations from normalcy, part II. Cutis 2002; 69: 215–17.

Lodi G, Sardella A, Bez C, Demarosi F, Carrassi A. Interventions for treating oral leukoplakia. Cochrane Database Syst Rev 2001; (4): CD001829.

Lopez R, Fernandez O, Jara G, Baelum V. Epidemiology of necrotizing ulcerative gingival lesions in adolescents. J Periodontal Res 2002; 37: 439–44.

Makridis SD, Mellado JR, Freedman AL, et al. Squamous cell carcinoma of gingiva and edentulous alveolar ridge: a clinicopathologic study. Int J Periodontics Restorative Dent 1998; 18: 292–8.

Marciani RD. Third molar removal: an overview of indications, imaging, evaluation, and assessment of risk. Oral Maxillofac Surg Clin North Am 2007; 19: 1–13.

McGuff HS, Alderson GL, Jones AC. Oral and maxillofacial pathology case of the month. Gingival cyst of the adult. Tex Dent J 2003; 120: 108, 112.

Milano M, Flaitz CM, Bennett J. Pyogenic granuloma associated with aberrant tooth development. Tex Dent J 2001; 118: 166–72.

el-Mostehy MR, Stallard RE. The Sturge-Weber syndrome: its periodontal significance. J Periodontol 1969; 40: 243–6.

Murayama Y, Kurihara H, Nagai A, Dompkowski D, Van Dyke TE. Acute necrotizing ulcerative gingivitis: risk factors involving host defense mechanisms. Periodontol 2000 1994; 6: 116–24.

Naidoo S. A profile of the oro-facial injuries in child physical abuse at a children's hospital. Child Abuse Negl 2000; 24: 521–34.

Ogura I, Kurabayashi T, Amagasa T, Okada N, Sasaki T. Mandibular bone invasion by gingival carcinoma on dental CT images as an indicator of cervical lymph node metastasis. Dentomaxillofac Radiol 2002; 31: 339–43.

Otsubo H, Yokoe H, Miya T, et al. Gingival squamous cell carcinoma in a patient with chronic graft-versus-host disease. Oral Surg Oral Med Oral Pathol Oral Radiol Endod 1997; 84: 171–4.

Owens BM, Johnson WW, Schuman NJ. Oral amalgam pigmentations (tattoos): a retrospective study. Quintessence Int 1992; 23: 805–10.

Palmer RM. Acute lateral periodontal abscess. Br Dent J 1984; 157: 311–12.

Palmer RM, Eveson JW. Plasma-cell gingivitis. Oral Surg Oral Med Oral Pathol 1981; 51: 187–9.

Parry J, Porter S, Scully C, Flint S, Parry MG. Mucosal lesions due to oral cocaine use. Br Dent J 1996; 180: 462–4.

Perry HO. Idiopathic gingivostomatitis. Dermatol Clin 1987; 5: 719–22.

Petti S. Pooled estimate of world leukoplakia prevalence: a systematic review. Oral Oncol 2003; 39: 770–80.

Porter SR, Matthews RW, Scully C. Chronic lymphocytic leukaemia with gingival and palatal deposits. J Clin Periodontol 1994; 21: 559–61.

Ramon-Fluixa C, Bagan-Sebastian J, Milian-Masanet M, Scully C. Periodontal status in patients with oral lichen planus: a study of 90 cases. Oral Dis 1999; 5: 303–6.

Reibel J. Prognosis of oral pre-malignant lesions: significance of clinical, histopathological, and molecular biological characteristics. Crit Rev Oral Biol Med 2003; 14: 47–62.

Reichart PA. Oral manifestations in HIV infection: fungal and bacterial infections, Kaposi's sarcoma. Med Microbiol Immunol (Berl) 2003; 192: 165–9.

Reichart PA, Samaranayake LP, Philipsen HP. Pathology and clinical correlates in oral candidiasis and its variants: a review. Oral Dis 2000; 6: 85–91.

Robinson PG, Adegboye A, Rowland RW, Yeung S, Johnson NW. Periodontal diseases and HIV infection. Oral Dis 2002; 8(Suppl 2): 144–50.

Rosen PS, American Academy of Periodontology-Research, Science and Therapy Committee. Treatment of plaque-induced gingivitis, chronic periodontitis, and clinical conditions. Pediatr Dent 2008–2009; 30(7 Suppl): 253–62.

Rowland RW. Necrotizing ulcerative gingivitis. Ann Periodontol 1999; 4: 65–73.

Schreiber HR, Berla EA. Epithelial dysplasia of the gingiva. Report of a case. J Periodontol 1979; 50: 43–5.

Scully C, el-Kabir M, Samaranayake LP. Candida and oral candidosis: a review. Crit Rev Oral Biol Med 1994; 5: 125–57.

Scully C, Porter S. ABC of oral health. Swellings and red, white, and pigmented lesions. BMJ 2000; 321: 225–8.

Scully C, Porter S. Orofacial disease: update for the dental clinical team: 11. Cervical lymphadenopathy. Dent Update 2000; 27: 44–7.

Scully C, Porter S. Orofacial disease: update for the dental clinical team: 2. Ulcers, erosions and other causes of sore mouth. Part I. Dent Update 1998; 25: 478–84.

Scully C, Porter S. Orofacial disease: update for the dental clinical team: 3. White lesions. Dent Update 1999; 26: 123–9.

Scully C, Porter S. Orofacial disease: update for the dental clinical team: 4. Red, brown, black and bluish lesions. Dent Update 1999; 26: 169–73.

Scully C, Porter SR. The clinical spectrum of desquamative gingivitis. Semin Cutan Med Surg 1997; 16: 308–13.

Sela MN. Role of Treponema denticola in periodontal diseases. Crit Rev Oral Biol Med 2001; 12: 399–413.

Seward GR. Amalgam tattoo. Br Dent J 1998; 184: 470–1.

Shafer WG, Waldron CA. Erythroplakia of the oral cavity. Cancer 1975; 36: 1021–8.

Shashi V, Pallos D, Pettenati MJ, et al. Genetic heterogeneity of gingival fibromatosis on chromosome 2p. J Med Genet 1999; 36: 683–6.

Silverman S Jr, Lozada F. An epilogue to plasma-cell gingivostomatitis (allergic gingivostamtitis). Oral Surg Oral Med Oral Pathol 1977; 43: 211–17.

Slater LJ. Dentigerous cyst versus paradental cyst versus eruption pocket cyst. J Oral Maxillofac Surg 2003; 61: 149.

Smith RG, Davies RM. Acute lateral periodontal abscesses. Br Dent J 1986; 161: 176–8.

Solomon LW, Wein RO, Rosenwald I, Laver N. Plasma cell mucositis of the oral cavity: report of a case and review of the literature. Oral Surg Oral Med Oral Pathol Oral Radiol Endod 2008; 106: 853–60.

Stansbury DM, Peterson DE, Suzuki JB. Rapidly progressive acute periodontal infection in a patient with acute leukemia. J Periodontol 1988; 59: 544–7.

Stefanova M, Atanassov D, Krastev T, Fuchs S, Kutsche K. Zimmermann-Laband syndrome associated with a balanced reciprocal translocation t(3;8)(p21.2;q24.3) in mother and daughter: molecular cytogenetic characterization of the breakpoint regions. Am J Med Genet 2003; 117A: 289–94.

Telang GH, Ditre CM. Blue gingiva, an unusual oral pigmentation resulting from gingival tattoo. J Am Acad Dermatol 1994; 30: 125–6.

Terezhalmy GT, Riley CK, Moore WS. Pyogenic granuloma (pregnancy tumor). Quintessence Int 2000; 31: 440–1.

Timms MS, Sloan P. Association of supraglottic and gingival idiopathic plasmacytosis. Oral Surg Oral Med Oral Pathol 1991; 71: 451–3.

Vélez I, Mintz SM. Soft tissue plasmacytosis. A case report. N Y State Dent J 2005; 71: 48–50.

van der Waal I. The diagnosis and treatment of precancerous lesions. FDI World 1995; 4: 6–9.

Zain RB, Fei YJ. Fibrous lesions of the gingiva: a histopathologic analysis of 204 cases. Oral Surg Oral Med Oral Pathol 1990; 70: 466–70.

# 2.6 NECK

- skin and fascia
- lymph nodes

- lymph node swelling
- other lesions in the neck

Lesions in the neck may arise mainly from skin, subcutaneous tissues, the cervical lymph nodes, thyroid gland, salivary glands and heterotopic salivary tissue, muscle, nerve or other tissues.

Lesions arising from the skin can usually be moved with the skin and are generally readily recognizable.

## SKIN AND FASCIA
### Cervicofacial actinomycosis
Actinomycosis is a chronic infection caused by bacteria of the genus Actinomyces from the normal oropharyngeal flora.

Most cervicofacial actinomycosis follows tooth extractions, other oral surgical procedures, or trauma to the jaws/face. The most common pathogen is *Actinomyces israelii*, but other actinomycetes have been implicated and Actinobacillus spp., Prevotella spp. and Fusobacterium spp. may be found in the lesions.

*Clinical features*
Lesions present as a small, flat hard swelling in the mouth or on the neck or jaw (subperiosteal) (Figs 2.6.1–2.6.4) which enlarges to produce a purplish swelling with abscess formation and sinuses that discharge sulphur-like granules containing the micro-organisms. Rare complications include involvement of nearby soft tissues and bones and cerebral, pulmonary and abdominal infections.

*Diagnosis*
Diagnosis is confirmed by examination of pus or biopsy specimens for the presence of sulphur granules (pathognomonic) and Gram-positive filaments.

*Management*
Adequate surgical debridement and early treatment with antibiotics produces the best results, but response is slow and treatment must be prolonged—even as long as for up to 1 year. Actinomycetes are usually susceptible to penicillins, doxycycline and other tetracyclines, erythromycin, clindamycin and ciprofloxacin.

### Dermoid cysts
A dermoid cyst is a cystic teratoma, usually present from birth, and typically containing developmentally mature skin complete with hair follicles and sweat glands (Figs 2.6.5 and 2.6.6). Dermoid cysts grow slowly and are not tender unless ruptured. They usually occur on the face, inside the skull, on the lower back and in the ovaries. Superficial dermoid cysts on the face or neck usually can be removed surgically without complications.

### Fascial space infections
Fascial spaces are potential spaces lined/covered/defined by sheets of connective tissue. Infections may occasionally enter and spread in the fascial spaces of the neck. Odontogenic infections, periodontal infections or infections from penetrating wounds may cause fascial space infections.

Fascial space infections have the potential to obstruct the airway, or spread intracranially or to the mediastinum and are, therefore, potentially lethal serious infections. Thus infections complicated with signs of neck swelling, especially bilaterally or close to the airway (Figs 2.6.7–2.6.9) or systemic involvement such as pyrexia, tachypnoea, tachycardia, sweating or dehydration must be taken very seriously. Complications may include:

- Ludwig angina
- Cavernous sinus thrombosis
- Periorbital oedema
- Airway embarrassment
- Toxaemia and septicaemia
- Erosion into vital structures
- Mediastinitis
- Subperiosteal abscess
- Dysphagia.

*Diagnosis*
Diagnosis is confirmed by specimens for Gram stains and culture/sensitivity tests.

*Management*
Management is by removal of cause, drainage and high-dose antimicrobials.

## LYMPH NODES
Palpate for the lymph nodes in a systematic fashion, starting from the head and working down the neck. Most areas are examined easier if the examiner stands behind the patient and ask them to relax their head, letting it drop slightly forward. The posterior groups can then be palpated from the front. It is helpful to use all the fingers (except the thumb), moving them in a circular pattern and trying to press any nodes against hard surfaces like the lower border of the mandible.

The cervical lymph nodes are mostly deep and small, and should not be readily palpable. Any lymph nodes felt are usually abnormal and should be described carefully.

Lymphatic regions of the neck:

- Waldeyer ring
  - Pharyngeal tonsil (adenoids)
  - Palatine tonsils
  - Lingual tonsil.
- Transitional lymph nodes (between the head and the neck)
  - Sublingual
  - Submental
  - Submandibular
  - Buccal
  - Preauricular (parotid)
  - Retroauricular
  - Suboccipital
  - Retropharyngeal.
- Cervical lymph nodes
  - Lateral
    - Superficial (along the external jugular vein)
    - Deep (1. along the internal jugular vein including the jugulo-digastric and the jugulo-omohyoid; 2. along the accessory nerve; and 3. supraclavicular chain)

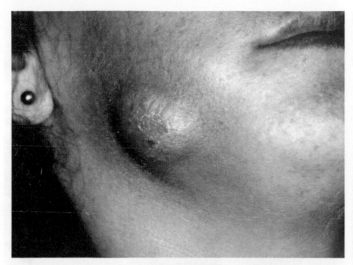

*Figure 2.6.1* Actinomycosis—cervico-facial.

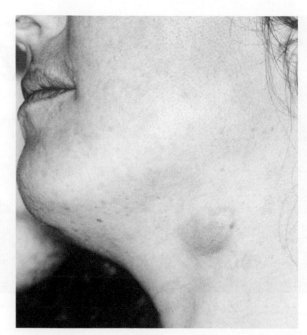

*Figure 2.6.2* Actinomycosis—cervico-facial.

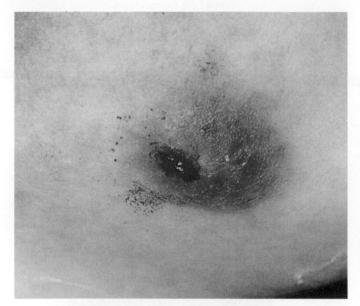

*Figure 2.6.3* Actinomycosis—cervico-facial showing the dusky purplish colour of the swelling.

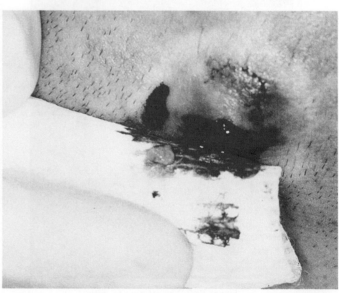

*Figure 2.6.4* Actinomycosis—cervico-facial pus showing sulphur granules.

o Anterior
o Superficial (along anterior jugular vein)
o Deep (prelaryngeal, prethyroidal, pretracheal and paratracheal)
o Posterior (in the posterior triangle).

Enlargement of certain lymph nodes can be characteristic for the area drained. For example, the jugulo-digastric nodes seem to react mainly to pathology in the palatine tonsils, while enlarged supraclavicular nodes may be due to lung or upper digestive tract neoplasms (Virchow node).

Lymphadenitis is common, presents with swelling and tenderness and usually is related to infection in the drainage area. Infective lymph nodes are more common in children and young people; they usually follow dental, nasal, tonsillar or ear infections. Systemic infective causes include glandular fever [infectious mononucleosis caused by the Epstein–Barr virus (EBV); or by cytomegalovirus], HIV infection, toxoplasmosis and many other infections.

Enlarged lymph nodes may arise from metastatic malignant disease or malignancies of the lymphatic system and may present in the neck nodes.

Painless cervical lymphadenopathy may also be a feature of connective tissue, granulations or other disease.

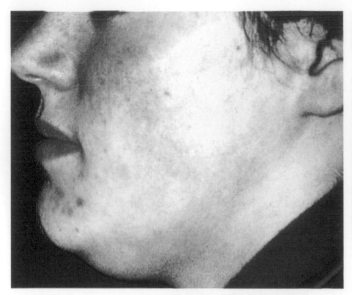

*Figure 2.6.5* Dermoid cyst.

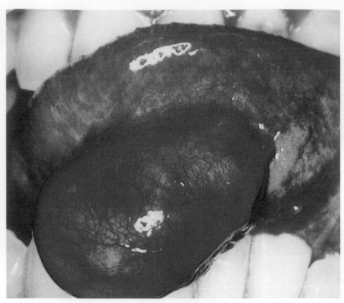

*Figure 2.6.6* Dermoid cyst.

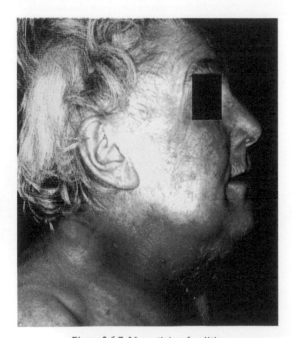

*Figure 2.6.7* Necrotizing fasciitis.

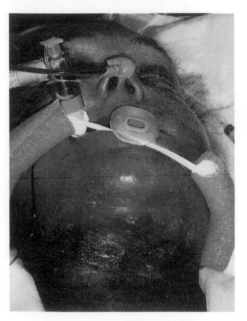

*Figure 2.6.8* Necrotizing fasciitis.

# LYMPH NODE SWELLING

## Lymphadenitis

*Aetiopathogenesis and clinical features*

Lymphadenitis is an infection in a lymph node, usually a consequence of spread of infection from a focus in the drainage area. Nodes tend to be swollen, tender or painful.

Parotid, or facial lymph nodes may occasionally become infected—typically from a cutaneous lesion which may be hidden in the scalp or ear.

Cervical lymphadenitis is common in persons with

- bacterial infections
  - o dental abscess
  - o pericoronitis
  - o mycobacterioses (tuberculosis and non-tuberculous mycobacteria)
  - o syphilis
  - o others (staphylococci, brucellosis, cat scratch disease, rickettsioses, tularaemia).

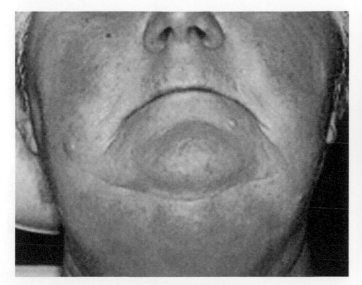

Figure 2.6.9  Fascial space infection—Ludwig angina.

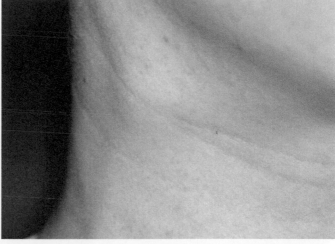

Figure 2.6.10  Lymphadenitis—from viral respiratory infection.

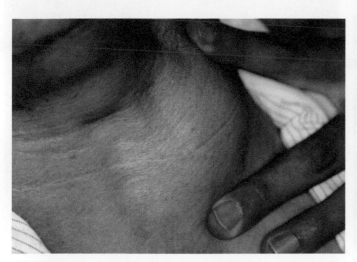

Figure 2.6.11  Lymphadenopathy.

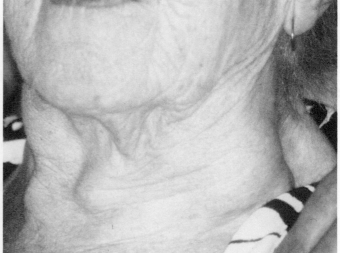

Figure 2.6.12  Lymph node enlargement.

- viral stomatitides, and many systemic viral infections such as
  o primary herpetic gingivostomatitis
  o HIV infection
  o EBV infection [infectious mononucleosis, etc. (Chapter 1.8)]
  o cytomegalovirus infection
  o mucocutaneous lymph node syndrome.
- parasitic infections, for example, toxoplasmosis, leishmaniasis, trypanosomiasis.

Occasionally the source of an infected facial, submandibular or other lymph node remains unidentified. Such *idiopathic* abscesses are usually seen in pre-school children who are apparently healthy but *Staphylococcus aureus* is usually implicated and it is presumed that a small lesion in the nose, mouth or scalp is the focus. Lymph nodes may also be infected and enlarged in this way in the non-tuberculous (atypical) mycobacterioses.

Cervical lymph nodes may also be enlarged in the absence of an obvious identifiable local infective lesion in connective tissue diseases, in sarcoidosis, in human herpesvirus-6 infection and for other uncommon reasons (Figs 2.6.10–2.6.19).

*Diagnosis*
Diagnosis is clinical, sometimes supplemented with serology, culture, imaging and biopsy. It is important to search the drainage area carefully for an infective focus.

*Management*
Management depends on the aetiology.

**Metastatic neoplasms**
*Aetiopathogenesis*
Metastatic lymphatic spread is a particular feature of carcinomas of the oral and perioral regions, and is a poor prognostic finding. Metastatic

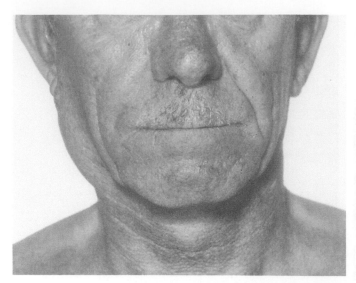

Figure 2.6.13 Lymph node—metastatic carcinoma.

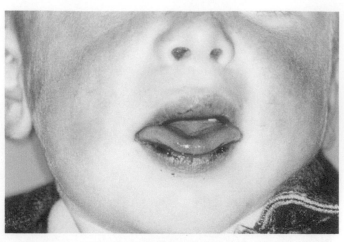

Figure 2.6.14 Lymphadenitis—cat scratch disease.

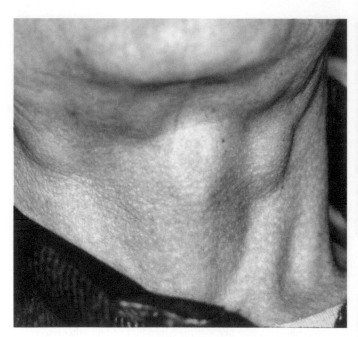

Figure 2.6.15 Lymphadenopathy—chronic lymphatic leukaemia.

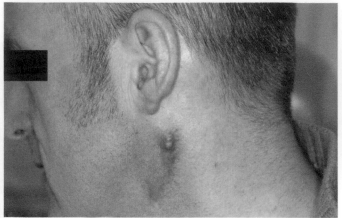

Figure 2.6.16 Lymphadenitis—tuberculous (scrofula).

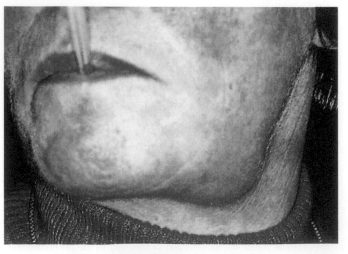

Figure 2.6.17 Lymphadenitis—facial node.

spread to the cervical region can arise particularly from salivary, oesophageal, thyroid, gastric, pancreatic, breast and pulmonary malignancies.

*Clinical features*

Enlarged lymph nodes from metastatic malignant disease are hard, fixed, and may or may not be tender and are seen mainly in older people.

*Diagnosis*

Diagnosis is clinical, sometimes supplemented with serology, culture, imaging and biopsy. It is imperative to search carefully for the site of primary malignancy; the usual culprits are the lateral border of the

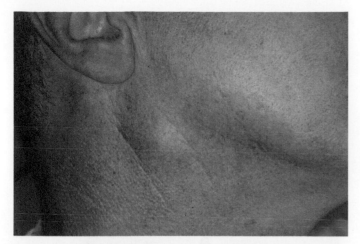

*Figure 2.6.18* Lymphadenitis—cervical node.

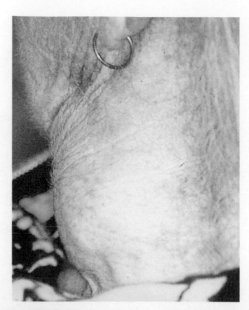

*Figure 2.6.19* Lymph node—metastatic carcinoma.

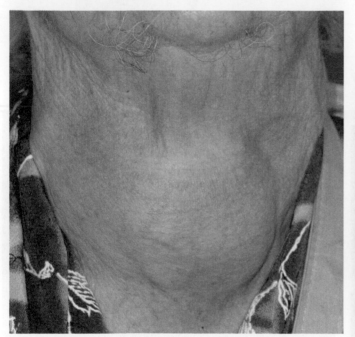

*Figure 2.6.20* Thyroid gland enlargement.

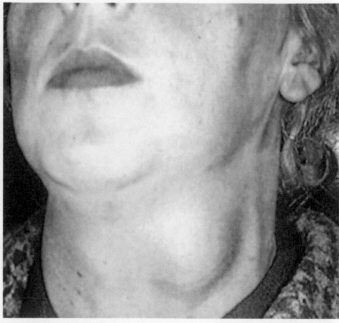

*Figure 2.6.21* Branchial cyst.

tongue, the floor of mouth, the retromolar region, the palatine tonsils, the pharynx, the larynx and the skin of the head.

*Management*
Management depends on the aetiology.

### Lymphoproliferative disease
Lymph node swelling is common in leukaemias, lymphomas, multiple myeloma and post-transplant lymphoproliferative disorder. Cervical lymphadenopathy may also be seen as part of a number of conditions that may be mistaken for a malignant process such as lymphoma, including

- *Castleman disease*—a benign condition curable with complete surgical resection.

- *Kikuchi–Fujimoto disease* (cervical subacute necrotizing lymphadenitis)—another important benign disease characterized by fever, neutropenia and cervical lymphadenopathy, seen mainly in young women of Asian descent.
- *Reactive haemophagocytic lymphohistiocytosis*—a severe hyperinflammatory condition with prolonged fever, cytopenias, hepatosplenomegaly and haemophagocytosis by activated, morphologically benign macrophages.
- *Lymphomatoid granulomatosis*—an EBV-associated and chemotherapy-resistant disorder, with polymorphic lymphoid infiltrates involving lung, skin and central nervous system.

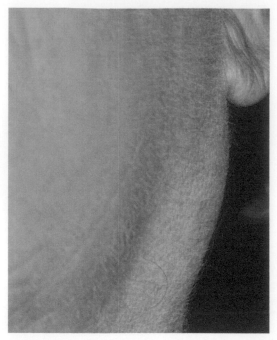

*Figure 2.6.22* Salivary gland swelling—neoplasm (pleomorphic salivary adenoma).

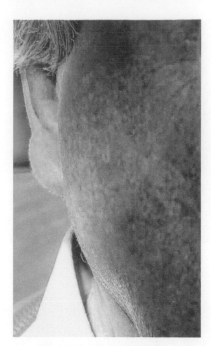

*Figure 2.6.23* Sialadenitis.

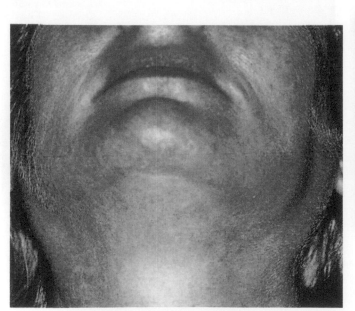

*Figure 2.6.24* Sjögren syndrome.

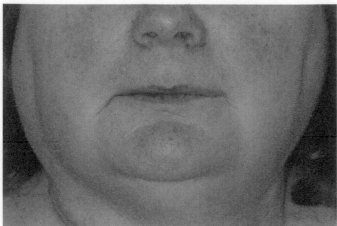

*Figure 2.6.25* Sialosis.

- *Langerhans cell histiocytosis* (Chapter 1.4).
- *Rosai–Dorfman disease*—a rare, non-neoplastic histiocytosis characterized by painless, massive cervical lymphadenopathy.

**Other causes**

Cervical lymphadenopathy may also be a feature of connective tissue or granulomatous disease (e.g. Crohn disease or orofacial granulomatosis), thyroiditis or drug therapy (drug-induced hypersensitivity syndrome, caused, e.g. by phenytoin).

## OTHER LESIONS IN THE NECK

*Thyroid gland swellings* are attached to the anterior aspect of the upper trachea and move characteristically with it during swallowing. This should be observed from the front and palpated from behind the patient (Fig. 2.6.20).

*Branchial (cervical lymphoepithelial) cyst* (Fig. 2.6.21) usually presents as a unilateral, soft-tissue fluctuant swelling—typically in the lateral aspect of the neck, anterior to the sternocleidomastoid muscle. It becomes clinically evident late in childhood or in early adulthood. Imaging is indicated to assess the extent of the lesion before definitive surgical treatment. Alternatively, therapy is with Picibanil—a lyophilized preparation of a low-virulence strain of *Streptococcus pyogenes* inactivated by heating with benzylpenicillin.

Salivary swellings (Figs 2.6.22–2.6.25) are discussed in Chapter 2.7. Heterotopic salivary tissue in peri-parotid and upper cervical lymph nodes is more common than traditionally recognized and occasionally undergoes neoplastic change.

## FURTHER READING

Brady-West DC, Buchner-Daley LM, McGrowder DA, Taylor-Houston J, West KA. Multiple myeloma presenting as cervical lymphadenopathy in a 16-year-old boy. J Natl Med Assoc 2009; 101: 810–12.

Bruce IA, Roper AJ, Gayed SL, Dabrowski M, Morar P. Syphilitic cervical lymphadenopathy: return of an old foe. Am J Otolaryngol 2009; 30: 347–9.

Chitadze N, Kuchuloria T, Clark DV, et al. Water-borne outbreak of oropharyngeal and glandular tularemia in Georgia: investigation and follow-up. Infection 2009; Oct 13. [Epub ahead of print].

Daniel E, McGuirt Sr WF. Neck masses secondary to heterotopic salivary gland tissue: a 25-year experience. Am J Otolaryngol 2005; 26: 96–100.

Díaz Manzano JA, Cegarra Navarro MF, Medina Banegas A, López Meseguer E. Diagnostic and treatment of necrotizing cervical fascitis. Clinical course after a Ludwig angina. An Otorrinolaringol Ibero Am 2006; 33: 317–22.

Glosser JW, Pires CA, Feinberg SE. Branchial cleft or cervical lymphoepithelial cysts: etiology and management. J Am Dent Assoc 2003; 134: 81–6.

Kim MG, Lee NH, Ban JH, et al. Sclerotherapy of branchial cleft cysts using OK-432. Otolaryngol Head Neck Surg 2009; 141: 329–34.

Kremer MJ, Blair T. Ludwig angina: forewarned is forearmed. AANA J 2006; 74: 445–51.

Lee DH, Lee JH, Shim EJ, et al. Disseminated Kikuchi–Fujimoto disease mimicking malignant lymphoma on positron emission tomography in a child. J Pediatr Hematol Oncol 2009; 31: 687–9.

Leung AK, Davies HD. Cervical lymphadenitis: etiology, diagnosis, and management. Curr Infect Dis Rep 2009; 11: 183–9.

Liang J, Newman JG, Frank DM, Chalian AA. Cervical unicentric Castleman disease presenting as a neck mass: case report and review of the literature. Ear Nose Throat J 2009; 88: E8.

Nakamura I, Imamura A, Yanagisawa N, Suganuma A, Ajisawa A. Medical study of 69 cases diagnosed as Kikuchi's disease. Kansenshogaku Zasshi 2009; 83: 363–8.

Paksoy N, Yazal K. Cervical lymphadenopathy associated with Hashimoto's thyroiditis: an analysis of 22 cases by fine needle aspiration cytology. Acta Cytol 2009; 53: 491–6.

Papadopouli E, Michailidi E, Papadopoulou E, et al. Cervical lymphadenopathy in childhood epidemiology and management. Pediatr Hematol Oncol 2009; 26: 454–60.

Pramanik S, Pal P, Das PK, et al. Reactive haemophagocytic lymphohistiocytosis. Indian J Pediatr 2009; 76: 643–5.

Primrose WJ, Napier SS, Primrose AJ. Kikuchi-Fugimoto disease (cervical subacute necrotising lymphadenitis): an important benign disease often masquerading as lymphoma. Ulster Med J 2009; 78: 134–6.

Scully C, Porter S. Orofacial disease: update for the dental clinical team: 11. Cervical lymphadenopathy. Dent Update 2000; 27: 44–7.

Vassilakopoulos TP, Pangalis GA, Siakantaris MP, et al. Kikuchi's lymphadenopathy: a relatively rare but important cause of lymphadenopathy in Greece, potentially associated with the antiphospholipid syndrome. Rheumatol Int 2009; Aug 20.

# 2.7 SALIVARY GLANDS

- history related to salivary problems
- diagnosis
- investigations
- drooling
- dry mouth

- swellings and lumps
- sarcoidosis
- sialosis (sialadenosis)
- Sjögren syndrome

The major salivary glands are the parotids, submandibular and sublingual glands. Minor salivary glands are found elsewhere in the mouth—especially in the lips, ventrum of tongue and soft palate. The major salivary glands should be inspected and palpated noting any swelling or tenderness, and the character and volume of saliva exuding from the salivary ducts.

Early enlargement of the parotid gland is characterized by outward deflection of the lower part of the ear lobe, which is best observed by inspecting the patient from behind. This simple sign may allow distinction of parotid enlargement from simple obesity. Swelling of the parotid sometimes causes trismus. The parotid duct (Stensen duct) is most readily palpated with the jaws clenched firmly since it runs horizontally across the upper masseter where it can be gently rolled. The duct opens at a papilla on the buccal mucosa opposite the upper molars. The submandibular gland is best palpated bimanually with a finger of one hand in the floor of the mouth lingual to the lower molar teeth, and a finger of the other hand placed over the submandibular triangle. The submandibular duct (Wharton duct) runs anteromedially across the floor of the mouth to open at the side of the lingual fraenum.

Examine intraorally for normal salivation from Stensen duct (Fig. 2.7.1) and Wharton duct, and pooling of saliva in the floor of the mouth. Any exudate obtained by milking the ducts should be noted.

Examine for signs of xerostomia (a mirror placed in contact with the buccal mucosa draws a string of thick saliva, or sticks, as it is slowly moved away).

Disorders which affect the salivary glands may appear to be unilateral, but the other glands should always be examined, and it is important to consider the possibility of related systemic disorders especially sarcoidosis, and those affecting

- joints or the skeleton/connective tissue, such as rheumatoid arthritis
- endocrine glands (diabetes)
- the liver (alcoholic cirrhosis)
- nutrition (eating disorders such as bulimia).

## HISTORY RELATED TO SALIVARY PROBLEMS
The history related to salivary problems should include:

- date of onset of symptoms
- swelling details such as duration and character
- xerostomia details
- pain details such as duration, daily timing, character, radiation, aggravating and relieving factors, relationship to meals and associated phenomena
- mouth opening restriction
- fever
- history of dry eyes or dryness of other mucosae
- personal or family history of arthritis

- occupation such as glass blowing or trumpet playing, which might introduce air into the gland (pneumoparotid).

## DIAGNOSIS
Salivary disorders are diagnosed mainly from history and examination findings. The salivary glands should be examined by

- inspecting
  - facial symmetry
  - for evidence of enlarged glands
  - salivary ducts for evidence of salivary flow
  - saliva
- palpating the glands
  - parotids
    - using fingers placed over the glands in front of the ears, to detect pain, or swelling
  - submandibulars
    - by bimanual palpation between fingers inside the mouth and extraorally
- examining the eyes
- examining the mucosa; note particularly angular cheilitis, dryness and lingual depapillation or erythema.

## INVESTIGATIONS
Investigations required may include

- Plasma viscosity or erythrocyte sedimentation rate (ESR).
- Antibodies
  - antinuclear antibodies for lupus or rheumatoid arthritis
  - rheumatoid factor for rheumatoid arthritis
  - Sjögren syndrome (SS)-A (Ro) and SS-B (La) antibodies for SS (and allied autoantibodies, e.g. anti-mitochondrial antibodies for primary biliary cirrhosis)
  - mumps, HIV or other viral antibodies.
- Radiology of the salivary glands may be achieved using
  - orthopantomogram and reverse orthopantomogram
  - oblique lateral views
  - lateral skull views
  - occlusal views
  - three-dimensional information may be gained from:
    - tomography in both the coronal and sagittal planes
    - CT scan.
- Other investigations can include the following:
  - Ultrasound.
  - Sialography. The ductal tree can be revealed by injecting radio–opaque dye into the duct.
  - Scintiscanning; using technetium pertechnetate can visualize all the glands.

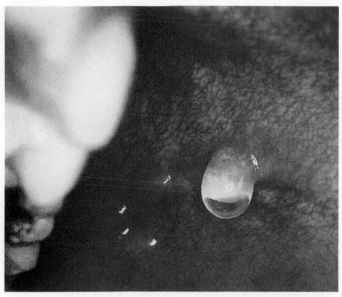

*Figure 2.7.1* Normal saliva visible secreting from Stensen (parotid) duct.

○ MRI, which avoids irradiating the patient and can be helpful. Diffusion-weighted imaging allows the apparent diffusion coefficient (ADC) to be calculated, determined which can help in staging and detection of small nodal metastasis. The ADC value also discriminates carcinomas from lymphomas, benign lesions from malignant tumours and tumour necrosis from abscesses. Low pretreatment ADC values typically predict a favourable response to chemoradiation therapy.
○ Biopsy.

## DROOLING

### Aetiopathogenesis

Drooling is caused either by increased saliva flow (sialorrhoea; ptyalism) that cannot be compensated for by swallowing, by poor oral and facial muscle control in patients with swallowing dysfunction (secondary sialorrhoea), or by anatomic or neuromuscular anomalies. Drooling is a particular problem for many children with cerebral palsy, intellectual disability, and other neurological conditions, and in adults with these conditions or who have Parkinson disease, stroke, pseudobulbar palsy or bulbar palsy.

### Clinical features

Saliva soils the clothing of the patient, peers, siblings, parents, and care-givers, and furniture, carpets, teaching materials, communicative devices and toys. Affected persons are at increased risk of skin maceration with repeated perioral skin breakdown and infections, and aspiration -related respiratory and pulmonary complications.

### Diagnosis

Quantitative measurements can be helpful for guiding management decisions. Apart from examination of tongue size and control, tonsil and adenoid size, gag reflex and intraoral tactile sensitivity, it is helpful to assess:

- nasal passage upon anterior rhinoscopy
- swallowing efficiency
- neurologic examination.

### Management

- Medical therapy:
  ○ oral motor training exercises
  ○ behaviour therapy
  – pharmacotherapeutics, either systemically (e.g. atropine-related oral anticholinergics) or more locally (e.g. sublingual ipratropium spray; clonidine patch or botulinum toxin type A injected into the salivary glands).
- Radiotherapy: but this has the potential risk of late malignancy.
- Surgery
  ○ gland excision
  ○ duct re-routing
  ○ duct ligation
  ○ nerve sectioning or
  ○ combinations of the above.

## DRY MOUTH

Dry mouth (xerostomia).

### Aetiopathogenesis

The main causes of dry mouth are drugs (those with anticholinergic or sympathomimetic activity), irradiation of the salivary glands, SS (see page 178), HIV disease, sarcoidosis and dehydration. Many patients complain of a dry mouth and yet lack objective evidence of xerostomia.

### Clinical features

Oral complaints (often the presenting feature) can include:

- Xerostomia: often the most frequent and obvious clinical component, although not all patients complain of dry mouth (Figs 2.7.2 and 2.7.3).
- Soreness or burning sensation.
- Difficulty eating dry foods, such as biscuits (the cracker sign).
- Difficulties in controlling dentures.
- Difficulties in speech: there may be a clicking quality of the speech as the tongue tends to stick to the palate.
- Difficulties in swallowing.
- Complications such as unpleasant taste or loss of sense of taste, oral malodour, caries, candidosis and sialadenitis.

In xerostomia there is reduced salivation (hyposalivation), and the dry mucosa may become tacky and the lips can adhere one to another. An examining dental mirror may often stick to the mucosa. There may be lack of salivary pooling in the floor of the mouth: any saliva present tends to be viscous and appear frothy and saliva flows poorly, if at all, from the ducts of the major glands on stimulation or palpation.
There may be:

- tendency of the mucosa to stick to a dental mirror
- food residues
- lack of salivary pooling

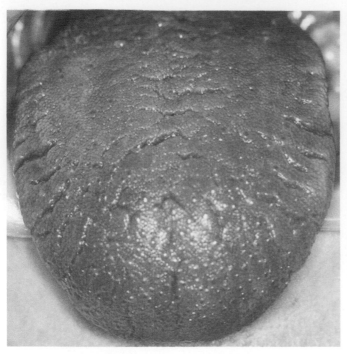

*Figure 2.7.2* Dry mouth showing lobulated dry tongue.

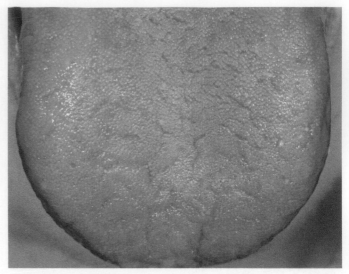

*Figure 2.7.3* Dry mouth—there are food residues on the dry tongue.

- frothiness of saliva, particularly in the lower sulcar reflection, and absence of frank salivation from major gland duct orifices
- a characteristic tongue appearance; lobulated, usually red, surface with partial or complete depapillation
- in advanced cases—obviously dry and glazed oral mucosae.

### Complications

- Unpleasant taste (dysgeusia), or loss of sense of taste.
- Malodour is common.
- Candidosis is common and may cause soreness with or without redness of the oral mucosa and/or angular cheilitis.
- Dental caries tends to be severe, affect smooth surfaces and is difficult to control (Figs 1.15.61 and 1.15.62).
- Ascending (suppurative) sialadenitis, particularly of the parotid glands (Fig. 2.7.4) is a hazard.

### Diagnosis

A subjective feeling of dry mouth (xerostomia) is common, although reduced salivary flow (hyposalivation) is not always confirmed by objective studies. Indeed, in the older age groups, 16–25% complain of xerostomia—usually caused by drugs.

Autoantibody assays can be extremely helpful in diagnosis, and are readily available, inexpensive and fairly non-invasive. SS-A (Ro) and SS-B (La) antibodies are found especially in primary SS, may have diagnostic value in patients with unexplained parotid swelling and may antedate clinical evidence of SS by months or years.

Blood tests may be indicated to

- examine for SS-A and SS-B and autoantibodies seen in other connective tissue diseases
- assess ESR, C reactive protein or plasma viscosity
- exclude anaemia
- examine IgA immune complexes
- exclude similar syndromes seen in infection with hepatitis C virus, Epstein–Barr virus (EBV), human T-lymphotropic virus-1 or HIV
- exclude diabetes and hypercalcaemia.

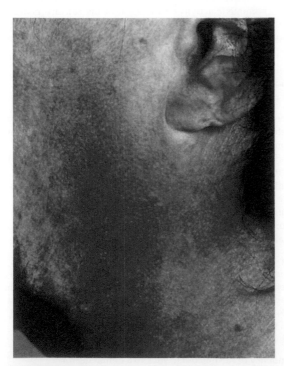

*Figure 2.7.4* Sialadenitis—acute bacterial sialadenitis showing swelling and erythema.

## Salivary gland examination
Salivary gland functional studies, imaging and biopsy which may be indicated include:

- Salivary flow measurements (sialometry)
- Salivary gland biopsy
- Sialograph and CT scan
- Salivary scintiscanning
- Ultrasonography
- Magnetic resonance imaging.

If SS is suspected, specialist referral is warranted since investigations may be needed, and the differential diagnosis may include:

- Viral infections:
  ○ hepatitis C virus
  ○ HIV
  ○ HTLV-1
  ○ EBV.
- Sarcoidosis and Heerfordt syndrome.
- Glandular deposits in:
  ○ haemochromatosis
  ○ lipoproteinaemias
  ○ amyloidosis.
- Lymphomas.

## Management
The management of xerostomia due to salivary gland dysfunction remains unsatisfactory. Simple measures such as the patient sipping water or other fluids throughout the day, protecting the lips with lip salve, and modifying their eating behaviour (e.g. small bites of food; eaten slowly) and diet [creamy foods (casseroles, soups) or cool foods with a high liquid content (melon, ice cream)] are advantageous as well as moistening foods with water, gravies, sauces, extra oil, dressings, sour cream, mayonnaise or yoghurt.

It is wise for the patient to avoid: mouth-breathing; any drugs that may produce xerostomia (e.g. tricyclic antidepressants), alcohol (including in mouthwashes), smoking, caffeine (coffee, some soft drinks), dry foods such as biscuits (or moisten in liquid first), spicy foods and oral healthcare products containing sodium lauryl sulphate, which may irritate the mucosa.

Salivation may be stimulated by using: chewing gums (containing xylitol or sorbitol, not sucrose), diabetic sweets, cholinergic drugs such as pilocarpine or cevimeline that stimulate salivation (sialogogues) and transglossal electrical stimulation.

Mouth wetting agents (salivary substitutes) may help symptomatically. Various apart from water are available, including: methylcellulose, Saliva Orthana and Oralbalance are particularly useful since they contain fluoride and mucin. However, there may be religious or cultural objections to use of mucin by some Muslims, Hindus, Jews and Rastafarians: products containing carboxymethylcellulose (e.g. Glandosane or Luborant) may, therefore, be preferred by some individuals.

Complications should be avoided or managed by:

- avoiding sugary foods
- keeping the mouth clean
- using fluorides
- using mouthwashes of chlorhexidine.

Dental caries is best controlled by dietary control of sucrose intake, and the daily use of fluorides as toothpastes, mouthwashes and gels (1% sodium fluoride gels or 0.4% stannous fluoride gels).

Candidosis may cause soreness or burning and thus should be treated with antifungals until there is neither erythema nor symptoms. Topical antifungals in liquid form such as nystatin or amphotericin suspension are effective and acceptable since the mouth is dry. Other preparations such as miconazole or fluconazole are also effective. Dentures should be left out of the mouth at night and stored in sodium hypochlorite solution, chlorhexidine or benzalkonium chloride to disinfect. An antifungal such as miconazole gel or amphotericin or nystatin ointment should be spread on the denture before reinsertion.

Bacterial sialadenitis may be best treated with a penicillinase-resistant antibiotic such as flucloxacillin.

# SJÖGREN SYNDROME
SS (Chapter 1.15).

# SWELLINGS AND LUMPS
## Mikulicz disease
Mikulicz disease (MD)—once thought to be SS-1 (Chapter 1.15), it is now recognized to be a unique condition with persistent lacrimal and salivary gland enlargement associated with prominent infiltration of IgG4-expressing plasmacytes, raised serum immunoglobulin G4 (IgG4), few autoimmune reactions and good responsiveness to glucocorticoids. MD is, therefore, now termed systemic IgG4-related plasmacytic disease. Diagnostic features include:

- Symmetrical and persistent swelling in more than two lacrimal and major salivary glands.
- Prominent mononuclear cell infiltration of lacrimal and salivary glands. IgG4-related sclerosing sialadenitis involving the submandibular glands may be seen.
- Exclusion of SS, sarcoidosis and lymphoproliferative disease.

Complications of MD include autoimmune pancreatitis, retroperitoneal fibrosis, tubulo-interstitial nephritis, autoimmune hypophysitis and Riedel thyroiditis, in all of which IgG4 is involved.

## Mikulicz syndrome
Leukaemic infiltration of the parotids and lacrimal glands is sometimes termed Mikulicz syndrome (Chapter 1.15).

## Mucocele
Mucocele (Chapter 2.1).

*Aetiopathogenesis*
Extravasation mucoceles are the most common type and are usually seen in the lower labial mucosa or ventral lingual mucosa, usually resulting from the escape of mucus into the lamina propria from a damaged minor salivary gland duct. These are not lined by epithelium, and, therefore, not true cysts.

Occasional deep mucoceles are retention cysts, seen particularly in the sublingual gland (see below). Cysts may rarely develop within salivary neoplasms.

*Clinical features*
Mucoceles are common. Most are dome-shaped, fluctuant, bluish, non-tender, submucosal swellings with a normal over lying mucosa (Figs 2.7.5–2.7.9). Extravasation mucoceles arising from the sublingual gland are termed ranulas because of their resemblance to a frog's belly (Figs 2.7.10 and 2.7.11). Rarely, such a ranula extends through the

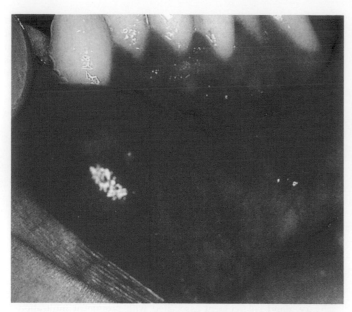

Figure 2.7.5 Mucocele.

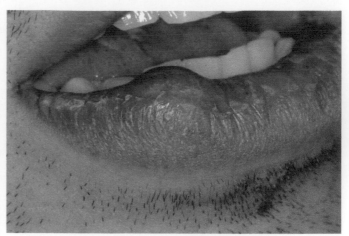

Figure 2.7.6 Mucocele.

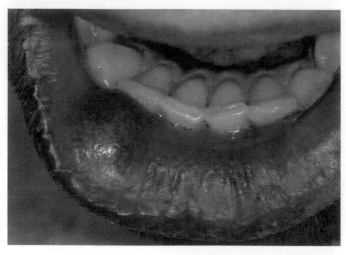

Figure 2.7.7 Mucocele.

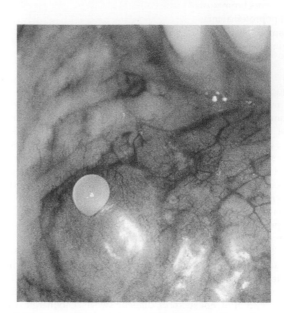

Figure 2.7.8 Mucocele—mucopus leaking from perforated mucocele.

mylohyoid muscle—a plunging ranula. Superficial mucoceles are caused by small extravasations intraepithelially or occasionally sub-epithelially and seen mainly in lichen planus; palatal lesions are most commonly seen (Fig. 2.7.12).

*Diagnosis*

Clinical mainly but histology is helpful; mucoceles are strongly periodic acid Schiff positive and diastase resistant. Care should be taken to ensure that the lesion is not a salivary gland tumour with cystic change, especially when dealing with an apparent mucous cyst in the upper lip.

*Management*

Mucoceles can be excised but they also respond well to cryosurgery, using a single freeze–thaw cycle.

Superficial mucoceles can be left alone.

## Neoplasms

Salivary gland neoplasms are uncommon and most are benign and affect the parotid—presenting as a unilateral swelling. The 'rule of nines' is an approximation that states that 9 out of 10 salivary gland neoplasms

- affect the parotid;
- are benign;
- are pleomorphic salivary adenomas (PSAs).

Neoplasms

- of major salivary glands are usually PSAs but sometimes monomorphic adenomas [such as adenolymphomas (Warthin tumour)], mucoepidermoid tumours or acinic cell tumours.
- in the parotid glands are usually PSAs but the next most common neoplasm is carcinoma.

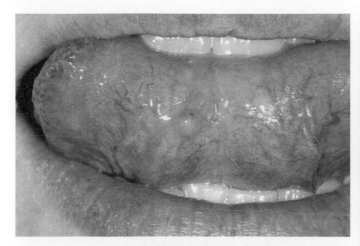

*Figure 2.7.9* Mucocele.

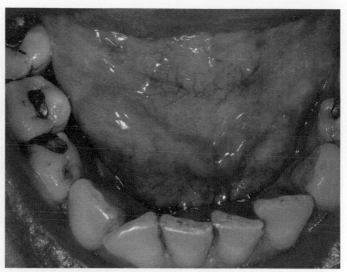

*Figure 2.7.10* Mucocele (ranula).

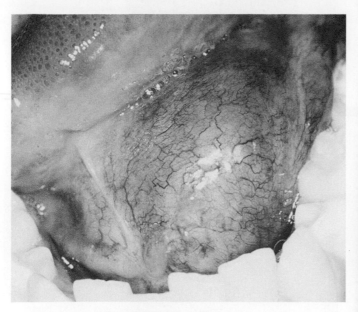

*Figure 2.7.11* Mucocele (ranula).

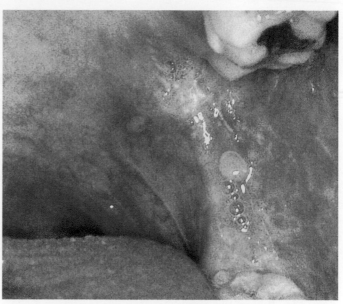

*Figure 2.7.12* Mucocele—superficial mucocele.

- in the submandibular glands are usually PSAs but malignant neoplasms contribute up to one-third.
- in the sublingual gland are exceedingly rare but virtually all are malignant.
- in the minor salivary glands most commonly are pleomorphic adenomas but carcinomas and adenoid cystic carcinomas account for about 50% of all neoplasms.

Apart from the above epithelial neoplasms, the next most common neoplasms found in salivary glands are lymphomas. SS is recognized as predisposing to lymphomas which have arisen in up to 6% of patients over 10 years in some studies.

### Aetiopathogenesis
Salivary gland neoplasms have an increased incidence in:

- survivors of the atomic explosions in Japan
- the use of 131-iodine in the treatment of thyroid cancer
- patients following radiotherapy to the head and neck
- patients with HIV/AIDS.

Salivary gland neoplasms are also more common in certain geographical locations: inuits (Eskimos), for example, have an increased prevalence and this has been suggested to be related to EBV infection. There is a correlation between salivary gland and breast cancer. Warthin tumour has a relationship with smoking.

### Clinical features
A long history of gradual gland enlargement suggests a benign process while pain or facial nerve palsy is ominous and suggests carcinoma (see above). Warthin tumours account for 70% of all bilateral salivary gland neoplasms; they are bilateral in 10–15%.

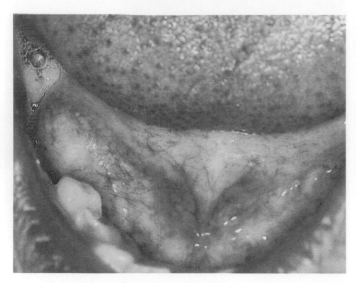

*Figure 2.7.13* Neoplasm.

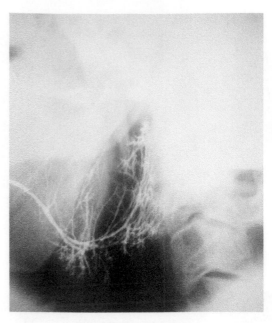

*Figure 2.7.14* Neoplasm.

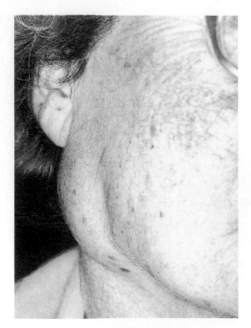

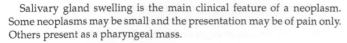

*Figure 2.7.15* Neoplasm—parotid pleomorphic salivary adenoma.

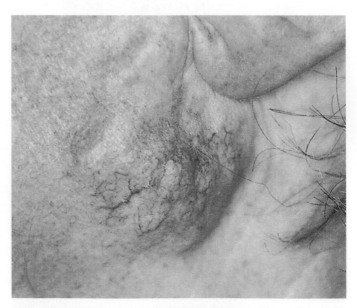

*Figure 2.7.16* Neoplasm—parotid malignant pleomorphic salivary adenoma showing swelling and abnormal vasculature.

Salivary gland swelling is the main clinical feature of a neoplasm. Some neoplasms may be small and the presentation may be of pain only. Others present as a pharyngeal mass.

*Diagnosis*
Clinical examination may reveal an obvious swelling in the case of the parotid outlining the gland anteriorly to the ear, and causing eversion of the ear lobe (Figs 2.7.13–2.7.30). Diagnosis is from clinical features supported by imaging and histology.

MRI scans are particularly helpful. Sialography may reveal an obvious filling defect or displacement of the gland but is a relatively imprecise means of neoplasm detection. CT alone, or in conjunction with sialography, is a more sensitive means of neoplasm detection.

Radionuclides such as technetium, selenomethionine or gallium have been reported to be selectively taken up by some or excluded by other neoplasms but in fact both false positive and negative results make the current techniques unsatisfactory. Ultrasonography may have a limited application.

The diagnosis can only be firmly established by fine needle, core or open biopsy.

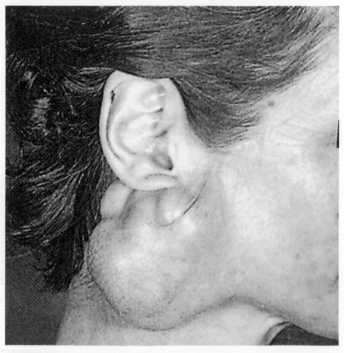

Figure 2.7.17 Neoplasm—parotid pleomorphic salivary adenoma.

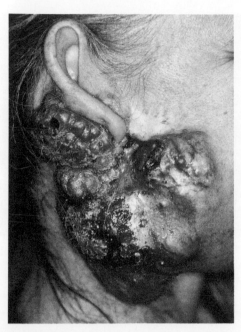

Figure 2.7.18 Neoplasm—parotid pleomorphic salivary adenoma showing ulcerating mass.

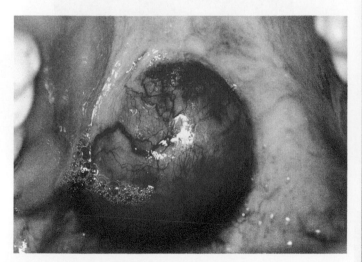

Figure 2.7.19 Neoplasm—minor salivary gland.

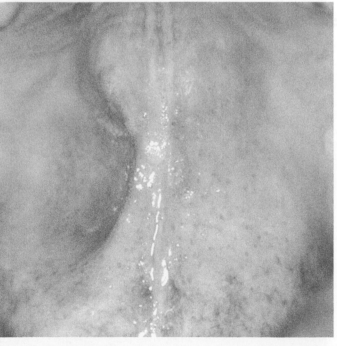

Figure 2.7.20 Neoplasm—minor salivary gland.

*Management*
The treatment of choice for salivary gland neoplasms of either major or minor gland origin is surgical excision. Most are relatively radioresistant but radiotherapy is sometimes used as an adjunct. Chemotherapy is used only on a very limited basis and for some malignant salivary gland neoplasms such as adenocarcinoma or adenoid cystic carcinoma and is usually used along with surgery and/or radiotherapy.

Parotidectomy complications may include facial palsy, wound dehiscence or necrosis, post-operative bleeding, fever or wound infection, sialoceles and Frey syndrome.

## SARCOIDOSIS
Sarcoidosis (Chapter 1.14).

**Sialadenitis**
Bacterial ascending sialadenitis (acute suppurative sialadenitis).

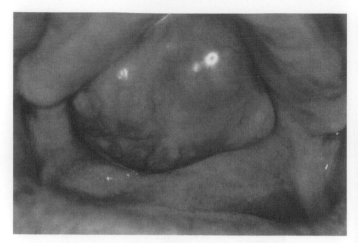

*Figure 2.7.21* Neoplasm—minor salivary gland pleomorphic salivary adenoma.

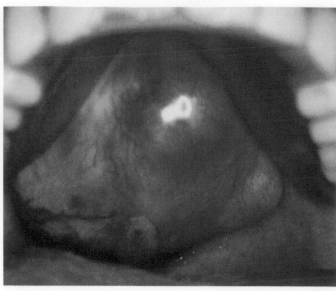

*Figure 2.7.22* Neoplasm—minor salivary gland pleomorphic salivary adenoma as in Figure 2.7.21.

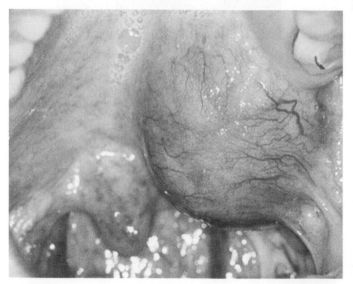

*Figure 2.7.23* Neoplasm—minor salivary gland mucoepidermoid tumour.

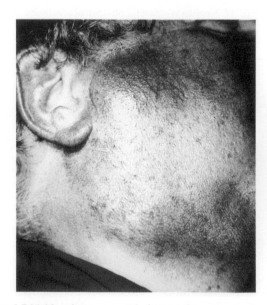

*Figure 2.7.24* Neoplasm—parotid pleomorphic salivary adenoma.

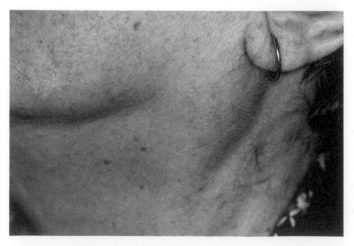

*Figure 2.7.25* Neoplasm—parotid neoplasm.

*Aetiopathogenesis*

The parotid salivary glands are more commonly affected by ascending sialadenitis than are the submandibulars.

The underlying causes include:

- Xerostomia—for example in SS and radiotherapy
- Prematurity and orogastric feeding in newborns
- HIV disease and other immunodeficiencies (selective IgA deficiency may predispose to recurrent parotitis of childhood)
- Dehydration—a post-surgical complication, uncommon nowadays
- Ductal abnormalities—such as calculi, mucus plugs and strictures.

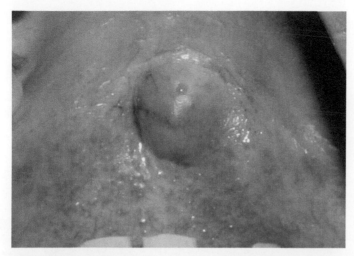

*Figure 2.7.26* Neoplasm—minor salivary gland pleomorphic adenoma.

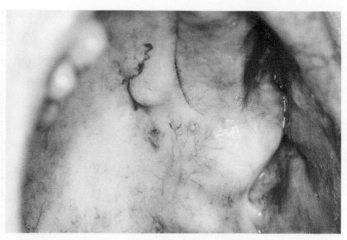

*Figure 2.7.27* Neoplasm—minor salivary gland adenoid cystic carcinoma.

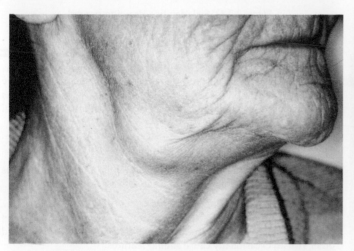

*Figure 2.7.28* Neoplasm—submandibular adenoid cystic carcinoma.

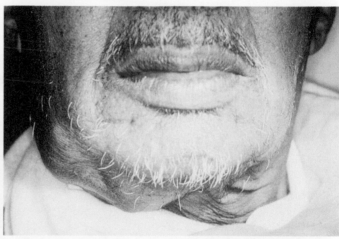

*Figure 2.7.29* Neoplasm—submandibular adenoid cystic carcinoma.

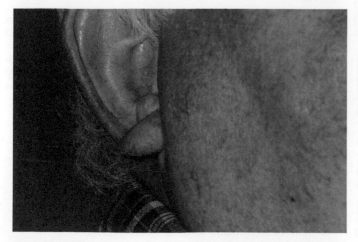

*Figure 2.7.30* Neoplasm—parotid showing ear lobe eversion and parotid swelling.

Acute bacterial sialadenitis is usually a mixed infection, involving *Streptococcus viridans* and penicillin-resistant *Staphylococcus aureus* that ascend the duct from the mouth because of such an underlying problem. Enteric Gram-negative rods have a high oropharyngeal colonization in hospitalized persons and have been implicated in a few cases.

*Clinical features*
Acute suppurative sialadenitis of the parotid gland presents as

- a painful parotid enlargement (Figs 2.7.31–2.7.33), tender to palpation. A single parotid gland is usually involved and the overlying skin may be reddened. Intraorally, pus may be seen exuding from the parotid duct orifice, thus giving rise to dysgeusia and oral malodour. If the infection localizes as a parotid abscess it may point externally through the overlying skin or, rarely, into the external acoustic meatus.
- trismus
- pyrexia
- cervical lymphadenopathy.

Chronic bacterial sialadenitis may develop after acute sialadenitis particularly if inappropriate antibiotics are used or predisposing factors

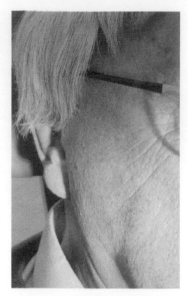

*Figure 2.7.31* Sialadenitis.

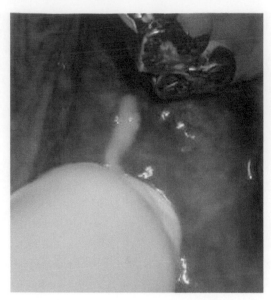

*Figure 2.7.32* Sialadenitis—draining parotid.

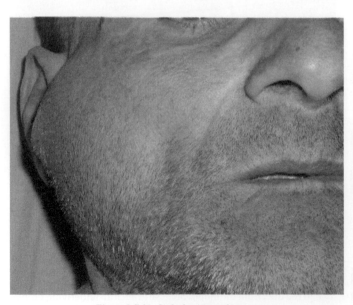

*Figure 2.7.33* Sialadenitis—abscess.

are not eliminated. Unfortunately, serous acini may atrophy when salivary outflow is chronically obstructed and this further reduces salivary function.

*Diagnosis*

Diagnosis is on clinical grounds but, after resolution of the infection, investigations may be needed to exclude an underlying cause. Ultrasonography can be useful, particularly if abscess formation is likely, as can magnetic resonance imaging.

*Management*

Pus should be sent for culture and sensitivity. Prompt antimicrobial therapy and surgical drainage are required where there is fluctuation.

The antibiotic of choice is flucloxacillin, with erythromycin as an alternative if the patient is penicillin–allergic. The antibiotic prescribed may be guided by the results of sensitivity tests. Supportive therapy, such as ensuring an adequate fluid intake, analgesics and attention to good oral hygiene are important.

## Mumps

Mumps (acute viral sialadenitis: epidemic parotitis) is an acute infectious disease which affects principally the major salivary salivary glands.

*Aetiopathogenesis*

Mumps is caused by an RNA paramyxovirus transmitted by direct contact or by droplet spread from saliva but some Coxsackie, ECHO- and other viruses occasionally cause similar features.

*Clinical features*

A longish incubation period of 2–3 weeks is followed by an acute onset of

- painful salivary swelling (parotitis) usually bilaterally, although in the early stages only one parotid gland may appear to be involved (Fig. 2.7.34). In approximately 10% of cases the submandibular glands are also affected and rarely these may be the only glands involved. The salivary swelling persists for about 7 days and then gradually subsides. The most obvious intraoral feature is swelling and redness at the duct orifice of the affected gland (papillitis)
- trismus
- fever
- malaise.

Mumps less commonly and mainly in adults has extrasalivary manifestations which can include:

- orchitis (ensuing infertility is rare)
- pancreatitis
- meningoencephalitis
- oophoritis and thyroiditis (ensuing infertility is rare)
- glomerulonephritis—especially in immunocompromised persons.

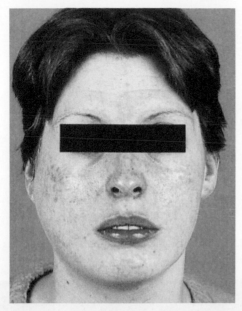

Figure 2.7.34 Mumps.

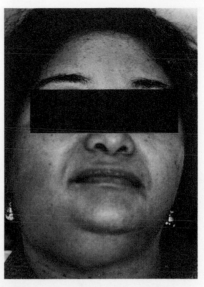

Figure 2.7.35 Sialolithiasis—submandibular swelling.

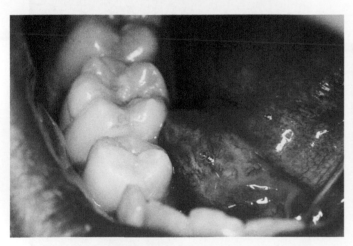

Figure 2.7.36 Sialolithiasis.

*Diagnosis*

The diagnosis is on clinical grounds but confirmation, if needed, is by demonstrating a four–fold rise in serum antibody titres to mumps S and V antigens between acute serum and convalescent serum taken 3 weeks later.

A similar clinical picture can arise with radioactive iodine therapy ('iodine mumps'), as salivary gland swelling and possible xerostomia that lasts for about 7 days. Rarely these features persist and cause permanent loss of function of one or more gland.

*Management*

No specific antiviral agents are available. Treatment is, therefore, symptomatic involving

- analgesics
- adequate hydration
- reducing the fever.

## Obstructive sialadenitis

*Aetiopathogenesis*

Major salivary ducts may be obstructed intraductally (within the lumen), such as by a calculus (sialolithiasis) or mucus plug; ductally (stenosis of the duct wall) or extraductally (pressure from outwith) such as by a neoplasm.

The most common cause is a sialolith. Over 80% of sialoliths arise in the submandibular glands. The precise cause of these calculi is not known, although associations with diabetes mellitus, hypertension and/or chronic liver disease, and possibly nephrolithiasis (but not to water hardness) have been suggested. Chronic sialadenitis may develop if a salivary obstruction is not removed. Rarely, 'physiological' duct obstruction either due to duct spasm or oedema from trauma, or an abnormal passage of the parotid duct through the buccinator (buccinator window anomaly) or in relation to the masseter muscles can be responsible.

Prolonged duct obstruction can produce gland atrophy particularly of serous acini.

*Clinical features*

Sometimes asymptomatic, the typical presentation is a history of painful salivary gland swelling just before, or at, mealtimes but, in older patients, this history is not always obtained. There may be dull pain over the affected gland, or referred elsewhere (Figs 2.7.35–2.7.48).

Quite large calculi can form, and calculi may be multiple.

*Diagnosis*

Calculi can sometimes be seen in the duct and are usually yellow or white, or may be palpable. Otherwise, it is rarely possible clinically to determine the cause of major duct obstruction. Plain radiographs may reveal a calculus if it is radio-opaque but not all are radio-opaque and hence ultrasonography may be helpful.

Sialography or sialoendoscopy may help differentiate the various causes of major duct obstruction: intraductal or ductal causes are usually readily seen, but 'physiological' obstructions, such as the buccinator window anomaly, require pressure-monitored sialographic techniques

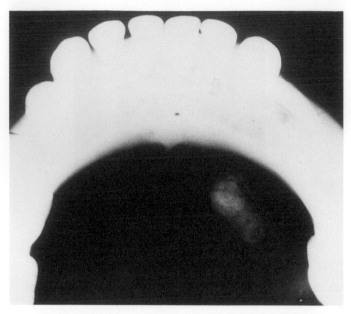

*Figure 2.7.37* Sialolithiasis—occlusal radiograph showing a radiopaque mass.

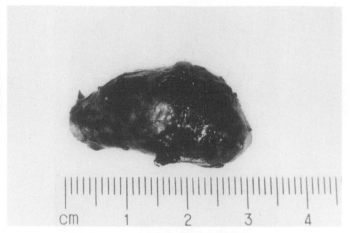

*Figure 2.7.38* Sialolithiasis—excised calculus (same patient as Fig. 2.7.37).

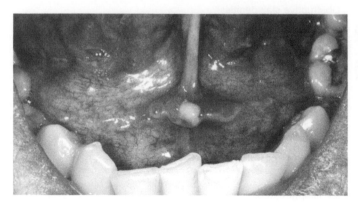

*Figure 2.7.39* Sialolithiasis.

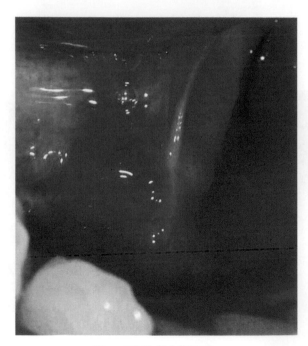

*Figure 2.7.40* Sialolithiasis.

for detection. Extraductal causes of obstruction may be clinically obvious or apparent only on sialography or combined CT sialography, ultrasound or MRI.

*Management*
Intraductal and ductal causes of duct obstruction are usually correctable by the removal of the cause (e.g. mucus plug or calculi) or in a benign stricture by repeated duct dilatation. Lithotripsy, aided by fluoroscopically guided basket retrieval of fragments, is effective for calculi less than 7 mm in diameter.

### Recurrent parotitis of childhood (juvenile recurrent parotitis)
*Aetiopathogenesis*
In children, an uncommon form of recurrent parotitis that is of uncertain aetiology, possibly viral, may be seen—mainly seen in boys. Peak

incidence is between ages 5 and 7 years. The condition may be due to EBV infection, selective IgA deficiency or IgG subclass deficiency.

*Clinical features*
Recurrent parotitis is characterized by recurrent painful parotid swelling, usually unilaterally. The number of attacks vary from 1 to 5 per year, although some individuals may have up to 20 episodes per annum.

*Diagnosis*
The diagnostic procedures indicated are similar to those for acute suppurative sialadenitis. Sialectasis is seen on sialography.

*Management*
Antimicrobials may be given but are not always helpful; analgesics, however, may reduce painful symptoms and any associated pyrexia.

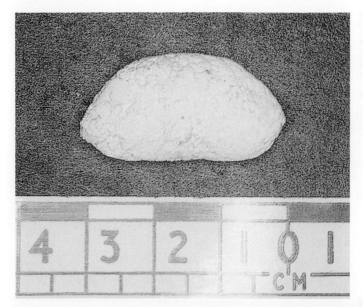

*Figure 2.7.41* Sialolithiasis.

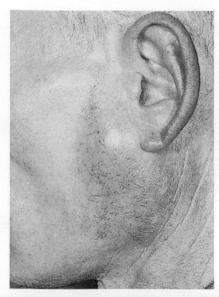

*Figure 2.7.42* Sialolithiasis—rare in parotid.

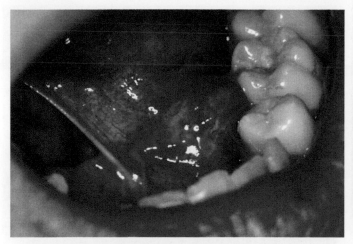

*Figure 2.7.43* Sialolithiasis.

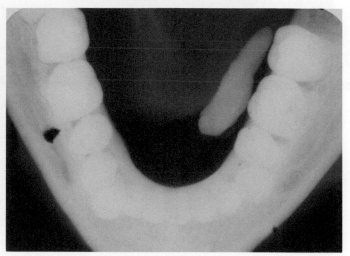

*Figure 2.7.44* Sialolithiasis.

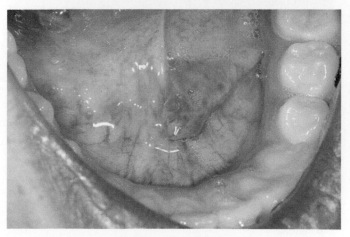

*Figure 2.7.45* Sialolithiasis.

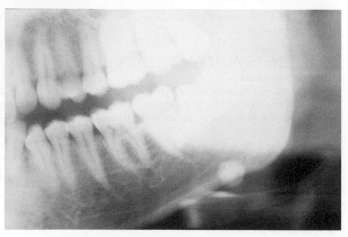

*Figure 2.7.46* Sialolithiasis.

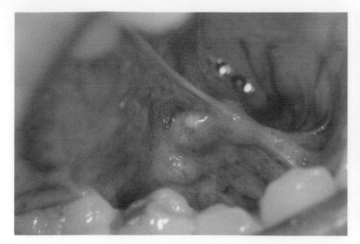

*Figure 2.7.47* Sialolithiasis.

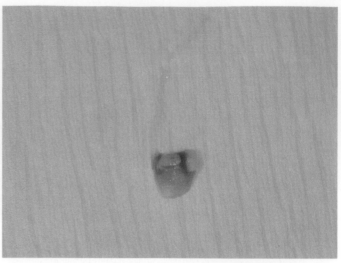

*Figure 2.7.48* Sialolithiasis—calculus from Figure 2.7.47.

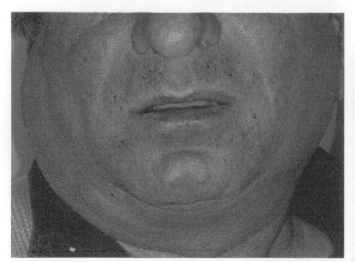

*Figure 2.7.49* Sialosis.

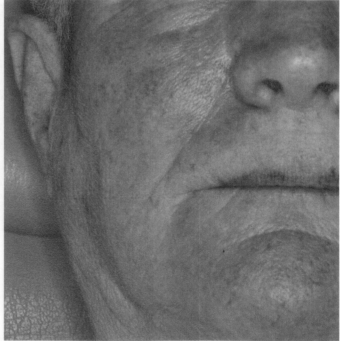

*Figure 2.7.50* Sialosis.

Most instances of recurrent parotitis of childhood resolve spontaneously by about puberty.

## SIALOSIS (SIALADENOSIS)
### Aetiopathogenesis
The affected glands show acinar hypertrophy which appears related to an autonomic neuropathy with serous cell hypertrophy and striated duct atrophy. A variety of causes recognized include:

- Drugs
  - alcohol abuse with or without accompanying liver cirrhosis
  - sympathomimetic agents such as isoprenaline
  - phenylbutazone, isoprenaline, anti–thyroid drugs and phenothiazines
  - methyl dopa
  - valproic acid.
- Liver cirrhosis (alcoholic or non-alcoholic).
- Endocrine conditions
  - diabetes mellitus
  - pregnancy
  - acromegaly
  - following oophorectomy.
- Nutritional disorders
  - malnutrition
  - anorexia nervosa
  - bulimia
  - cystic fibrosis and pancreatitis.

### Clinical features

Sialosis is painless bilaterally symmetrical chronic swelling of the salivary glands, typically the parotids (Figs 2.7.49 and 2.7.50) without xerostomia. There is soft painless general enlargement of the involved glands. A useful guide to whether the patient is simply obese or has parotid enlargement is to observe the outward deflection of the ear lobe which is seen in true parotid swelling.

### Diagnosis

The diagnosis of sialosis is one of exclusion, based mainly on history and clinical examination. Although sialosis is benign and usually idiopathic, it is important to exclude underlying causes and therefore investigations indicated may include:

- Serology; for raised glucose levels (possibly also glucose tolerance testing) or abnormal liver function.
- Sialography; salivary secretion is not impaired and sialographic examination reveals enlarged but otherwise normal glands. Rarely, a bilateral space-occupying lesion such as a salivary neoplasm, cyst or lymphoid neoplasm may present difficulties in differentiation from sialosis, and then sialography may help.
- Ultrasonography; rarely, a bilateral space-occupying lesion such as a salivary neoplasm, cyst or lymphoid neoplasm may present difficulties in differentiation from sialosis, and then ultrasound may help.
- Biopsy; rarely needed.
- Sialochemistry; raised potassium and calcium levels which are not found in other causes of parotid enlargement (although sialochemistry is rarely available in most centres).

### Management

No treatment is available. In alcoholism or diabetes, sialosis may resolve when alcohol intake is reduced or glucose control is instituted.

## SJÖGREN SYNDROME

SS (Chapter 1.15).

## FURTHER READING

Abe T, Sato T, Tomaru Y, et al. Immunoglobulin G4-related sclerosing sialadenitis: report of two cases and review of the literature. Oral Surg Oral Med Oral Pathol Oral Radiol Endod 2009; 108: 544–50.

Arduino PG, Carrozzo M, Pentenero M, Bertolusso G, Gandolfo S. Non-neoplastic salivary gland diseases. Minerva Stomatol 2006; 55: 249–70.

Baas MC, van Donselaar KA, Florquin S, et al. Mumps: not an innocent bystander in solid organ transplantation. Am J Transplant 2009; 9: 2186–9.

Capodiferro S, Scully C, Lacaita MG, et al. Bilateral intraosseous adenoid cystic carcinoma of the mandible. Report of a case with lung metastases at first clinical presentation. Oral Dis 2005; 11: 1–4.

Cascarini L, McGurk M. Epidemiology of salivary gland infections. Oral Maxillofac Surg Clin North Am 2009; 21: 353–7.

Chawla S, Kim S, Wang S, Poptani H. Diffusion-weighted imaging in head and neck cancers. Future Oncol 2009; 5: 959–75.

Dougherty NJ. A review of cerebral palsy for the oral health professional. Dent Clin North Am 2009; 53: 329–38, x.

Fox PC. Autoimmune diseases and Sjogren's syndrome: an autoimmune exocrinopathy. Ann N Y Acad Sci 2007; 1098: 15–21.

Fox RI. Sjögren's syndrome. Lancet 2005; 366: 321–31.

Guggenheimer J, Close JM, Eghtesad B. Sialadenosis in patients with advanced liver disease. Head Neck Pathol 2009; 3: 100–5.

Guggenheimer J, Moore PA. Xerostomia: etiology, recognition and treatment. J Am Dent Assoc 2003; 134: 61–9.

Hegde AM, Pani SC. Drooling of saliva in children with cerebral palsy-etiology, prevalence, and relationship to salivary flow rate in an Indian population. Spec Care Dentist 2009; 29: 163–8.

Lee YY, Wong KT, King AD, Ahuja AT. Imaging of salivary gland tumours. Eur J Radiol 2008; 66: 419–36.

Little SA, Kubba H, Hussain SS. An evidence-based approach to the child who drools saliva. Clin Otolaryngol 2009; 34: 236–9.

Mathews SA, Kurien BT, Scofield RH. Oral manifestations of Sjögren's syndrome. J Dent Res 2008; 87: 308–18.

Oulis P, Masdrakis VG, Karakatsanis NA, Kouzoupis AV, Papadimitriou GN. Quetiapine-induced dose-dependent hypersalivation in mania. Clin Neuropharmacol 2009; 32: 56–7.

Porter SR. Non-neoplastic salivary gland disease. In: Gleeson M, et al., eds. Scott-Brown's Otorhinolaryngology: Head & Neck Surgery, 7th edn. London: Hodder Arnold, 2008.

Porter SR, Scully C, Hegarty AM. An update of the etiology and management of xerostomia. Oral Surg Oral Med Oral Pathol Oral Radiol Endod 2004; 97: 28–46.

Praharaj SK, Jana AK, Sinha VK. Aripiprazole-induced sialorrhea. Prog Neuropsychopharmacol Biol Psychiatry 2009; 33: 384–5.

Schreiber A, Hershman G. Non-HIV viral infections of the salivary glands. Oral Maxillofac Surg Clin North Am 2009; 21: 331–8.

Scully C. The role of saliva in oral health problems. Practitioner 2001; 245: 841–56.

Scully C. Drug effects on salivary glands; dry mouth. Oral Dis 2003; 9: 165–76.

Scully C, Bagan J, Turner F, Barnard N, Eveson JW. Sialosis: 35 cases of persistent parotid swelling from two countries. Br J Oral Maxillofac Surg 2008; 46: 468–72; Mar 14. [Epub ahead of print].

Scully C, Limeres J, Gleeson M, Tomás I, Diz P. Drooling. J Oral Pathol Med 2009; 38: 321–7.

Shebl FM, Bhatia K, Engels EA. Salivary gland and nasopharyngeal cancers in individuals with acquired immunodeficiency syndrome in United States. Int J Cancer 2009; Oct 6. [Epub ahead of print].

Yamamoto M, Takahashi H, Ohara M, et al. A new conceptualization for Mikulicz's disease as an IgG4-related plasmacytic disease. Mod Rheumatol 2006; 16: 335–40. [Epub 2006 Dec 20].

# 2.8 JAWS

- history related to jaw problems
- diagnosis
- jaw anatomical and morphological defects and non-odontogenic cystic lesions
- jaw pain
- jaw swellings

## HISTORY RELATED TO JAW PROBLEMS

The history should include:

- date of onset of symptoms
- precipitating factors (e.g. trauma)
- swelling details, such as duration and character
- pain details, such as site of maximum intensity, onset, duration, severity, daily timing, character, radiation, aggravating and relieving factors, relationship to meals and associated phenomena
- mouth-opening restriction
- history of dry eyes or dryness of other mucosae
- personal or family history of arthritis
- occupation.

**Examination** in patients with suspected disorders of the jaws or temporomandibular joints should include the following.

### Face

Morphology: some genetic conditions (Down syndrome), endocrine and other conditions (e.g. 'moon face' in corticosteroid therapy or Cushings syndrome) have characteristic facies. There is wide normal individual variation in face morphology but usually of a minor degree that cannot be regarded as abnormal.

Symmetry: as possible variations are limitless, comparing with the opposite side should make it easier to recognize localized abnormalities. Most individuals have some facial asymmetry but usually of a minor degree that cannot be regarded as abnormal.

### Cranial vault

The cranial size and shape may indicate a genetic abnormality (e.g. microcephaly, hydrocephalus, Down syndrome, Crouzon syndrome, Apert syndrome, Treacher–Collins syndrome or cleidocranial dysplasia).

### Nose and sinuses

The nose and to some extent the frontal sinuses show wide variation between individuals, and between ethnic groups. The nose is not infrequently deformed from injury (or surgical trauma). The nose and the frontal sinuses may be enlarged and prominent in acromegaly, or saddle-shaped due to a septal defect (congenital syphilis, cocaine-sniffing or post-traumatic).

Nasal inspection through a speculum or nasendoscope can assess the presence of pathology such as polyps, discharge from the maxillary sinus or obstruction of its opening.

Maxillary or frontal sinus inflammation may be confirmed by palpating for tenderness over these structures. Transillumination or endoscopy can be helpful.

### Jaws

The jaws should be palpated to detect swelling or tenderness. Maxillary, mandibular or zygomatic deformities, fractures or lumps may be more reliably confirmed by inspection from above (maxillae/zygomas) or behind (mandible).

Following trauma, all borders and sutures should be palpated for tenderness or a step deformity (at the infraorbital rim, the lateral orbital rim, the zygomatic arch and the zygomatic buttress intraorally).

Disorders which affect the jaws may appear to be unilateral, but the other jaw should always be examined, and it is important to consider the possibility of related systemic disorders especially those affecting:

- the skeleton/connective tissue—such as rheumatoid arthritis
- endocrine glands (e.g. hyperparathyroidism).

The jaws should be examined then by

- inspecting
  - facial symmetry
  - jaw margins
  - jaw opening and movements (Fig. 2.8.1)
- palpating the bones and joints
  - temporomandibular joint
    - using fingers placed over the joints in front of the ears, to detect pain, or swelling
  - mandible and maxilla
- examining the teeth and occlusion
- examining the mucosa.

## DIAGNOSIS

Jaw disorders are diagnosed mainly from history and examination findings.

Investigations required may include:

- full blood picture
- plasma viscosity or erythrocyte sedimentation rate or C reactive protein
- blood biochemistry
  - calcium
  - phosphate
  - alkaline phosphatase
  - parathyroid hormone levels
- antibodies
  - antinuclear antibodies—for lupus or rheumatoid arthritis
  - rheumatoid factor—for rheumatoid arthritis
  - extractable nuclear antibodies including SS-A and SS-B antibodies—for Sjogren syndrome
- plain radiography of the jaws may be achieved largely using extraoral films, for example,
  - orthopantomogram
  - oblique lateral views
  - three-dimensional information may be gained from:
    - tomography in both the coronal and sagittal planes
    - CT scan with cone beam and T1 and T2 weighting

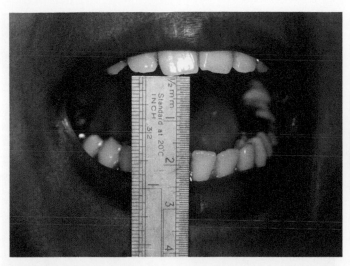

Figure 2.8.1 Oral submucous fibrosis—showing restricted oral opening.

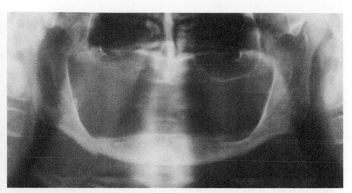

Figure 2.8.2 Radiograph showing alveolar atrophy and fractured mandible.

- other investigations can include
  - MRI—which avoids irradiating the patient
  - biopsy
  - radionuclide scanning.

## JAW ANATOMICAL AND MORPHOLOGICAL DEFECTS AND NON-ODONTOGENIC CYSTIC LESIONS

### Alveolar atrophy

The alveolar bone of the jaw normally bears the teeth but, when these are removed, or exfoliate, it atrophies and can eventually become so thin so that denture retention is impaired and, in extreme cases, the mandible can fracture under relatively little stress (Fig. 2.8.2).

Osteoporosis may affect the jaws as other bones and is seen particularly in post-menopausal women and patients taking systemic corticosteroids. It is also seen in the short-bowel syndrome.

### Aneurysmal bone cyst

Aneurysmal bone cysts are seen mainly in the mandible, mostly in younger and female patients. Often, but not always, these lesions appear in association with other bone lesions, such as unicameral (traumatic bone) cyst, dentigerous cyst, osteoclastoma, central giant cell tumour, fibrous dysplasia or osteosarcoma.

#### Clinical features

Aneurysmal bone cysts may displace but rarely resorb teeth, and sensory disturbances are rare.

#### Diagnosis

Aneurysmal bone cysts appear as cystic, honeycomb or soap bubble radiolucencies with excentric expansion. Cortical bone may be thinned or destroyed, and a periosteal reaction may be present.

Histologically, there are many cavernous or sinusoidal blood-filled spaces in a lesion that is otherwise almost identical to the central giant cell granuloma.

#### Management

Complete removal of the lesion with aggressive curettage.

### Focal osteoporotic bone marrow defect

Bone marrow stimulated in response to unusual demands for increased blood cell production, may present as focal jaw radiolucencies. Around 85% of jaw lesions are found in the mandible, and 75% are seen in female patients.

#### Aetiopathogenesis

These lesions present as ill-defined radiolucencies most commonly in edentulous areas, suggesting that some represent failure of normal bone regeneration post-extraction.

#### Clinical features

The lesions are almost always asymptomatic and discovered as incidental findings on radiographs taken for other reasons.

#### Diagnosis

The radiographic appearance is not pathognomonic so biopsy is indicated. Histologically, the tissue in these areas is composed primarily of red marrow, yellow marrow, or a combination of both with long thin irregular trabeculae that are missing the osteoblastic layer.

#### Management

No specific treatment is required.

### Stafne bone cavity

Stafne bone cavity (latent bone cyst: Stafne 'cyst').

#### Aetiopathogenesis

Heterotopic salivary gland tissue can develop in non-salivary locations, and a Stafne bone cavity is a common example of this; there is salivary tissue usually within the medial aspect of the lower border of the posterior mandible. Although the Stafne bone cavity is classically seen in the posterior mandible, a rare anterior variant presents as a round or ovoid radiolucency between the central incisors and first premolars.

#### Clinical features

Stafne bone cavity is a radiological finding only.

#### Diagnosis

A well-demarcated radiolucency is seen at the lower border of the mandible, always inferior to the inferior alveolar canal (Fig. 2.8.3).

#### Management

Malignant transformation of heterotopic salivary gland tissue is possible, but exceedingly rare. Therefore, reassurance and periodic radiographic observation seem prudent.

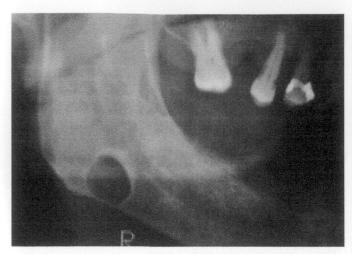

*Figure 2.8.3* Stafne bone cavity—typically lies inferior to the inferior alveolar canal.

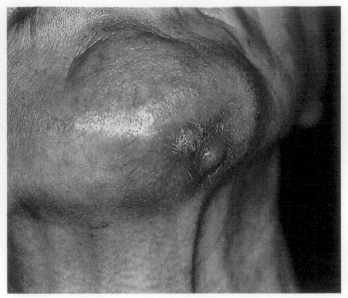

*Figure 2.8.4* Osteomyelitis of the mandible, discharging on to chin.

### Traumatic bone cyst

Traumatic bone cyst (solitary bone cyst, haemorrhagic cyst, extravasation cyst, unicameral bone cyst, simple bone cyst, idiopathic bone cavity).

*Aetiopathogenesis*

The traumatic bone cyst is a relatively frequent lesion and, despite its name, is of unproven aetiopathogenesis. The most widely accepted hypothesis, however, is that the lesion originates from intramedullary haemorrhage caused by trauma, the clot eventually degenerating, leaving an empty bone cavity.

*Clinical features*

The traumatic bone cyst is far more commonly seen in the mandible than maxilla. It is most commonly found in young persons (median age, 18 years); the male-to-female incidence ratio is 3:2. The lesions are usually symptomless incidental findings on radiographs.

*Diagnosis*

The traumatic bone cyst appears as a smoothly outlined radiolucency that scallops around the roots of the teeth and lies above the inferior alveolar canal. The lesions do not expand the cortex, displace teeth or resorb roots, and the lamina dura is left intact. They may range from very small (<1 cm) to very large (involving most of the mandible).

The lesions are usually surgically explored to establish a diagnosis, which is made upon finding a cavity which is either empty or filled with a small amount of straw-coloured fluid. Histologically, these cysts may have a thin connective tissue membrane lining or no lining at all.

*Management*

No further treatment is generally necessary because surgical manipulation causes the cavity to fill with blood, and the lesion resolves.

## JAW PAIN

Inflammation, fracture and tumour are the main causes of jaw pain but pain may also occasionally arise in, for example, angina, infarction in sickle cell diseases or from the effects of some drugs (e.g. vinca alkaloids).

### Dry socket

Dry socket (Chapter 2.8).

### Odontogenic infections

Odontogenic infections (see periapical abscess; fascial space infections).

### Osteomyelitis

*Aetiopathogenesis*

Most odontogenic infections are localized by the host immune defences but, if sufficiently virulent, micro-organisms may defeat defences to produce osteomyelitis.

### Acute osteomyelitis

In most cases, acute osteomyelitis arises where the bone vascularity has been compromised (as after radiation, bisphosphonates, osteopetrosis, Paget disease of bone and malignancy), or where the patient is immuno-compromised. The mandible receives its major blood supply from the inferior alveolar artery. A secondary source is the periosteal supply giving off nutrient vessels that penetrate the cortical bone and anastomose with branches of the inferior alveolar artery. Osteomyelitis of the mandible is more frequent than that of the maxilla, presumably because the maxillary blood supply is far more extensive.

*Clinical features*

Osteomyelitis starts commonly as a bacterial infection and inflammation of the jaw bone medulla, with eventually, pus formation in the medullary cavity or beneath the periosteum the pressure of which obstructs the blood supply, causing necrosis (Figs 2.8.4–2.8.11). Early acute osteomyelitis is usually characterized by intense pain, high intermittent fever, hypoaesthesia or paraesthesia of the mental nerve and a clearly identifiable cause.

In the absence of effective treatment, teeth in the area involved become sensitive to percussion and begin to loosen and pus may exude from the gingival sulcus or through fistulae. In osteomyelitis, periosteal new bone apposition causes cortical thickening and mandibular enlargement, most common on the buccal plate of the mandibular angle or body, especially in young people.

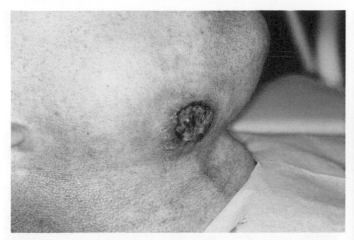

Figure 2.8.5 Osteomyelitis—skin swelling, erythema and sinus.

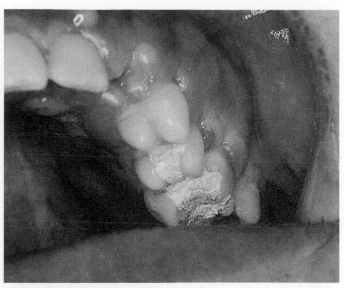

Figure 2.8.6 Osteomyelitis 1 early stages showing swelling. The premolars and molar were then extracted.

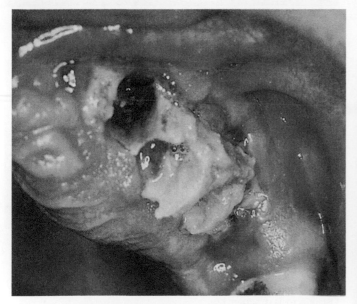

Figure 2.8.7 Osteomyelitis—showing sequestration 2 months later.

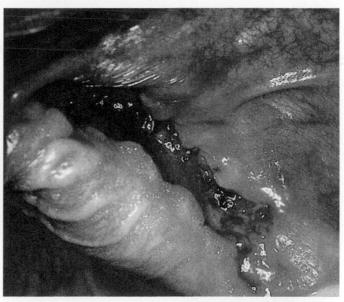

Figure 2.8.8 Osteomyelitis—after sequestrotomy 2 weeks later.

## Diagnosis and management

Imaging shows no findings until the acute inflammatory reaction leads to significant osteolysis. Bone density has to fall by 30–50% to show on plain radiography—and this usually takes 2–3 weeks. Plain radiographs, and more accurately CT [either multidetector CT (MDCT) or Cone Beam (CBCT)] can then demonstrate the osteopaenia and cortical lysis (including the inferior alveolar canal and mental foramen), sequestra and periosteal new bone formation. MRI has high sensitivity in detecting cancellous marrow abnormalities. Swelling of masseter and medial pterygoid muscles is common and both CT and MRI show the soft-tissue inflammation especially in the masticatory and submandibular spaces.

Bone scintigraphy (bone scan) is highly sensitive in detecting acute osteomyelitis but requires anatomical correlation. Technetium-labelled compounds depict bone turnover and radiolabelled leukocyte scans can confirm that this represents infection.

## Management

Osteomyelitis usually requires both medical and surgical treatment but in the early stages, immediate antibiotic therapy may prevent progression to involvement of the periosteum. Intravenous or parenteral antibiotics and supportive measures are indicated. Expeditious drainage of pus from the bone is required to prevent spread of infection and the formation of sequestra. Extremely loose teeth and sequestra should be removed (sequestrectomy), with debridement, decortication, resection of infected bone, and immediate or late bone graft reconstruction. It may also be necessary to maintain the integrity of the mandible using pin fixation into the normal bone adjacent to the osteomyelitic areas.

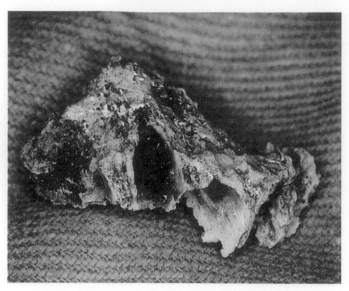

*Figure 2.8.9* Osteomyelitis sequestrum—necrotic bone.

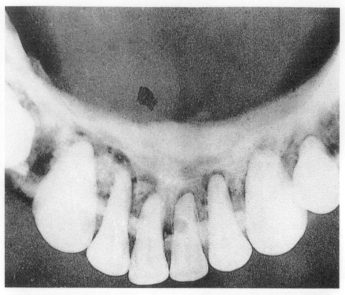

*Figure 2.8.10* Osteomyelitis—moth-eaten radiographical appearance.

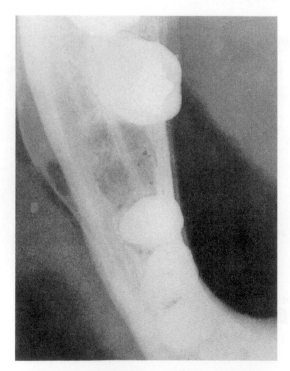

*Figure 2.8.11* Osteomyelitis—proliferative periostitis.

Chronic osteomyelitis includes:

- Primary chronic osteomyelitis—shows extensive and diffuse sclerosis sometimes with secondary chronic osteomyelitis—shows a mixed radiolucent and radiopaque appearance
- Focal sclerosing osteomyelitis (condensing osteitis)
- Chronic diffuse sclerosing osteomyelitis
- Specific osteomyelitis—tuberculosis, syphilis, actinomycosis
- Garré osteomyelitis (children).

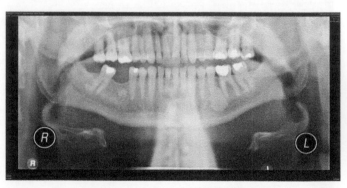

*Figure 2.8.12* Idiopathic osteosclerosis.

### Osteonecrosis
Osteonecrosis (Chapter 1.6).

### Osteoradionecrosis
Osteoradionecrosis (Chapter 1.6).

### Osteosclerosis
Idiopathic osteosclerosis (dense bone island) is an area of dense bone in the jaw without apparent cause, signs or symptoms, typically seen in the mandibular premolar/molar area, which may be associated with root resorption and occasionally Gardner syndrome (Fig. 2.8.12).

### Periapical abscess
Periapical abscess (dental abscess, odontogenic abscess).

*Aetiopathogenesis*
A periapical abscess is often a sequel to pulpitis caused by dental caries, but may arise in relation to any non-vital tooth. A mixed bacterial flora is implicated, especially anaerobes such as Fusobacterium and Bacteroides (Porphyromonas) species.

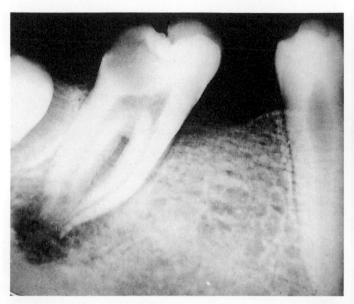

Figure 2.8.13 Abscess—periapical abscess related to carious mandibular molar.

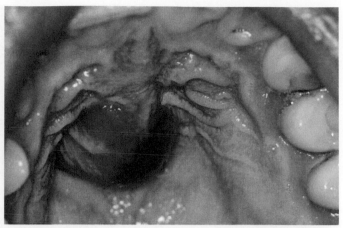

Figure 2.8.14 Periapical dental abscess from a lateral incisor.

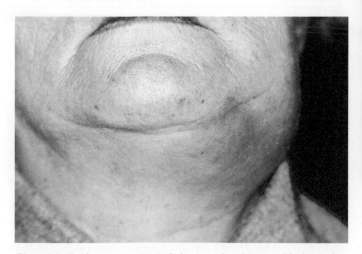

Figure 2.8.15 Abscess—periapical abscess related to mandibular molar.

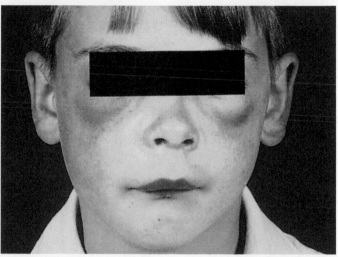

Figure 2.8.16 Abscess—periapical abscess related to maxillary canine.

*Clinical features*
Pain and facial swelling are characteristic (Figs 2.8.13–2.8.19). Most dental abscesses also produce an intraoral swelling, typically on the labial or buccal gingiva. Abscesses arising from maxillary lateral incisors and those from the palatal roots of the first molar tend to present palatally. The causal tooth is non-vital but tender to palpation. Once the abscess discharges, the acute inflammation, pain and swelling resolve and a chronic abscess develops discharging from a sinus—usually buccally. Occasionally, abscesses—especially those of lower incisors or molars—discharge extraorally.

*Diagnosis*
Clinical plus imaging.

*Management*
Extraction or endodontic therapy of a tooth affected with a periapical abscess with or without apicectomy removes the source of infection; this is essential to prevent recurrence. Antimicrobials may also be required.

## JAW SWELLINGS
Jaw swellings may be due to infections, cysts and tumours of odontogenic origin; or to bone disorders; fibro-osseous lesions and maxillary sinus conditions.

### Cysts and tumours of odontogenic origin
Odontogenic cysts and tumours:

- arise from tissue with the potential for differentiation into tooth or periodontal ligament structures [odontogenic ectoderm, mesenchyme

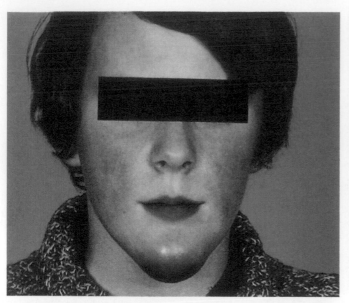

*Figure 2.8.17* Abscess—periapical abscess related to mandibular incisor.

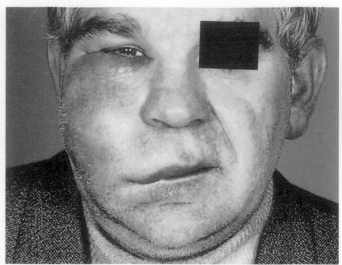

*Figure 2.8.18* Abscess—periapical abscess related to maxillary premolar tooth.

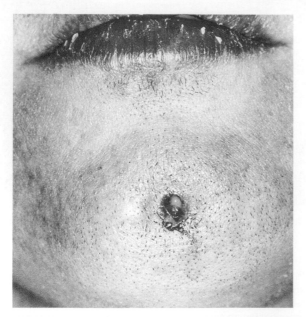

*Figure 2.8.19* Abscess—periapical abscess related to mandibular incisor, discharging on to skin.

### Table 2.8.1 ODONTOGENIC CYSTS

| Inflammatory | Developmental |
|---|---|
| Buccal bifurcation cyst | Calcifying odontogenic cyst |
| Periapical granuloma and cyst | Dentigerous cyst |
| Residual cyst | Eruption cyst |
| | Glandular odontogenic cyst |
| | Lateral periodontal cyst |

or a combination (ectomesenchyme)]. They may thus replace a tooth germ, or be associated with a tooth
- are, therefore, found predominantly in tooth-bearing sites
- vary widely in their degree of differentiation. There is a rough correlation between the degree of differentiation and the biologic behaviour: in general, the less-differentiated lesions (the immature ones) are more likely to have indistinct radiographic borders, invasive growth patterns and aggressive clinical behaviour, while mature or well-differentiated lesions are more likely to be well circumscribed, and self-limiting

- rarely undergo true malignant transformation or develop malignancy de novo.

Odontogenic cysts are quite common—most are inflammatory (55% of all) or dentigerous (related to a tooth—22%). Most odontogenic cysts are defined more by their location than by histological characteristics. The mandible is affected three times as common as the maxilla.

Cysts are generally benign, slow-growing and may reach large sizes before they give rise to symptoms such as swelling, pain or discharge and most are found as an incidental finding on imaging. There is initially a smooth bony hard lump with normal mucosa but, as bone thins, it may crackle on palpation like an egg shell. The cyst may resorb bone to show as a bluish fluctuant swelling.

MDCT, CBCT or MRI can help distinguish solid and cystic lesions. Other investigations may include pulp vitality testing, aspiration and analysis of cyst fluids, and histopathology. Before the biopsy of any such lesions, the area should be aspirated to exclude a vascular lesion.

Cysts are generally best managed by enucleation (complete removal of the cyst) as all tissue is then available for histological examination, and the cavity usually heals uneventfully with minimal aftercare but, unfortunately, enucleation may render adjacent teeth non-vital. Marsupialization (partial removal of the cyst lining and decompression of the cyst contents)—which is the alternative treatment—requires considerable aftercare and patient cooperation in maintaining the cavity, healing may take months and not all lining is available for histopathology (Table 2.8.1).

A few odontogenic cysts can be problematic because of a tendency to recurrence and/or aggressive growth—this includes especially the calcifying odontogenic, and glandular odontogenic cysts (GOCs).

## Table 2.8.2 MAIN ODONTOGENIC CYSTS

| Type | Decade at presentation | Commonest location | Usual management |
|---|---|---|---|
| Dentigerous | 3rd and 4th | Lower third molars, maxillary canines | Enucleation or marsupialization |
| Eruption | 1st | Anterior to permanent molars | Nil unless impeding eruption |
| Radicular | 3rd and 4th | Anterior maxilla | Enucleation |
| Residual | 4th and 5th | Anterior maxilla | Enucleation or marsupialization |

Odontogenic tumours are rare lesions derived from primordial tooth-forming tissues and can present in many histologic patterns (Table 2.8.2). They include a wide range of lesions but:

- Most are benign though they may infiltrate bone, presenting a problem in that they can recur after surgical removal.
- Some, such as ameloblastoma, are true neoplasms which should be diagnosed and treated as such.
- Some other, particularly odontomas, are developmental malformations (hamartomatous lesions)—rather than true neoplasms.

Most odontogenic tumours (>50%) are odontomas, or ameloblastomas (around 10%). Benign odontogenic tumours are 100 times more common than malignant ones.

Odontogenic tumours are generally slow-growing and may reach a large size before becoming symptomatic and, as with cysts, are often discovered incidentally on imaging. Swelling, may be because the tumour expands and/or destroys bone. Pain though not a feature of benign odontogenic tumours is common in malignant tumours. Before the biopsy of any such lesions, the area should be aspirated to exclude a vascular lesion.

Management can be enucleation, dentoalveolar segmental resection with lower border of mandible preservation, segmental resection or composite resection (Table 2.8.3).

### Adenomatoid odontogenic tumour

Adenomatoid odontogenic tumour (AOT: adeno-ameloblastoma).

*Aetiopathogenesis*
AOT is an uncommon and benign lesion, more a hamartoma than a neoplasm.

*Clinical features*
Clinically, the AOT presents as a gradually increasing intrabony swelling which is occasionally painful. The AOT may be remembered as the 'two-thirds tumour' since:

- it most commonly occurs in the second and third decades of life
- two-thirds of cases are seen in females
- two-thirds of cases occur in the anterior maxilla
- two-thirds of cases are associated with an impacted tooth (usually the maxillary canine) and generally attached to the tooth further apical on the root than is a dentigerous cyst.

*Diagnosis*
AOT can usually be readily identified from its clinical and radiographic appearance. There is typically a unilocular radiolucency and in some lesions there are radiopaque foci. AOT should always be considered in

## Table 2.8.3 MAIN ODONTOGENIC TUMOURS

| Benign | Malignant |
|---|---|
| *Odontogenic epithelium with mature, fibrous stroma without odontogenic ectomesenchyme* | *Odontogenic carcinomas* |
| Ameloblastoma | Metastasizing (malignant) ameloblastoma |
| Squamous odontogenic tumour | Ameloblastic carcinoma |
| Calcifying epithelial odontogenic tumour | Primary intraosseous squamous cell carcinoma |
| Adenomatoid odontogenic tumour | Clear cell odontogenic carcinoma |
| Keratocystic odontogenic tumour | Ghost cell odontogenic carcinoma |
| *Odontogenic epithelium with odontogenic ectomesenchyme, with or without hard tissue formation* | *Odontogenic sarcomas* |
| Ameloblastic fibroma | Ameloblastoma fibrosarcoma |
| Ameloblastic fibrodentinoma | Ameloblastic fibrodentino- and fibro- odontosarcoma |
| Ameloblastic fibro-odontoma | |
| Odontoma (odontome) | |
| Odontoameloblastoma | |
| Calcifying cystic odontogenic tumour | |
| Dentinogenic ghost cell tumour | |
| *Mesenchyme and/or odontogenic ectomesenchyme with or without odontogenic epithelium* | |
| Odontogenic fibroma | |
| Odontogenic myxoma/myxofibroma | |
| Cementoblastoma | |

*Source*: Adapted from WHO classification of odontogenic tumours 2005.

the differential diagnosis of a radiolucent lesion around the crown of an impacted maxillary canine.

*Management*
The treatment of choice is enucleation and curettage, after which AOT rarely if ever recurs.

### Ameloblastic fibroma

Ameloblastic fibroma is usually well-defined, pericoronal multiloculated radiolucent and associated with an impacted tooth, often in the posterior mandible.

### Ameloblastoma

Ameloblastoma (adamantinoma).

*Aetiopathogenesis*
The ameloblastoma is the most common odontogenic neoplasm, and is an entirely epithelial tumour arising from the dental lamina, Hertwig sheath, the enamel organ or the lining of dental follicles/dentigerous cysts. The Fos and TNFRSF genes are overexpressed.

The tumour is not uncommon in people of African heritage compared to a lower incidence in white people.

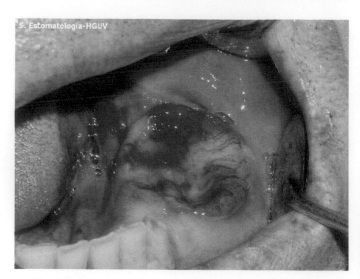

*Figure 2.8.20* Ameloblastoma presenting with intraoral swelling.

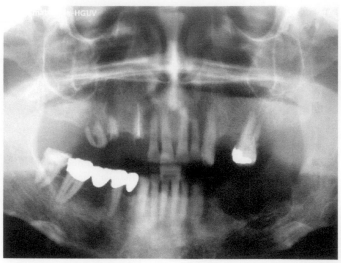

*Figure 2.8.21* Ameloblastoma—radiography from patient in Figure 2.8.20.

*Clinical features*

Ameloblastomas usually appear between ages 20 and 40 years, affect the mandible four times more frequently than the maxilla, and 75% are seen at the mandibular angle. A unicystic variant most often occurs in adolescents (early lesions usually appear unilocular while established ones have generally become multi-locular).

The initial detection of an ameloblastoma is likely to be a 'chance finding' but, when the tumour is evident clinically, there is a slow-growing, painless, expansile swelling of bone. The lesion expands and invades to produce progressive facial swelling and intraorally there may be evidence of malocclusion and mobile teeth. Bony expansion may be seen, especially lingually. Eventually the bone is perforated and soft tissues involved. The ameloblastoma grows insidiously, however, rarely causing neuropathy or mucosal breakdown. Swelling and ulceration (Figs 2.8.20 and 2.8.21) may, however, be caused by trauma from a denture.

*Diagnosis*

The plain radiographic appearance of ameloblastoma is generally of a cystic expansile radiolucency usually in the area of the lower third molar. Approximately 20% of ameloblastomas appear in a dentigerous relationship to unerupted teeth. Ameloblastomas are never radiopaque. The lesions may be unilocular when small, later multi-locular, and they often resorb the teeth and/or roots they contact.

Diagnosis is confirmed by histological examination of a biopsy specimen.

*Management*

Ameloblastoma, though it is regarded as generally benign, may recur or, very rarely, metastasize. Metastatic dissemination is rare and usually occurs by aspiration to the lungs following longstanding local disease or previous surgical intervention. The treatment of choice, therefore, is surgical excision of the tumour together with removal of a margin of normal bone and retention of the lower border of the mandible. All patients with ameloblastoma, regardless of surgical treatment method or histologic type, must be monitored radiographically for life.

**Buccal bifurcation cyst**

Buccal bifurcation cyst is centred on the first or second mandibular molar, often presenting with delayed tooth eruption.

**Calcifying epithelial odontogenic tumour**

Calcifying epithelial odontogenic tumour (CEOT: Pindborg tumour) is a rare, benign but aggressive tumour (though less so than the ameloblastoma), usually seen in the mandibular premolar or molar regions associated with the crown of an impacted tooth, CEOT is radiolucent with scattered calcified components. Conservative resection is the treatment of choice.

**Calcifying odontogenic cyst**

Calcifying odontogenic cyst (Gorlin cyst) is most common in the anterior jaw, as a unilocular radiolucency. In one-third of cases, an impacted tooth is involved. It may occasionally be aggressive/recurrent.

**Cementoblastoma**

Cementoblastoma is a neoplasm of cementum typically seen in patients under 25 years. Usually fused to a root (typically mandibular premolar or first molar), it is a well-defined radiopacity with a radiolucent margin. It may cause pain which responds to nonsteroidal anti-inflammatory drugs.

Hypercementosis in contrast, is smoother, less nodular, and has a thin radiolucent margin continuous with the periodontal ligament space.

**Cemento-osseous dysplasia**

Cemento-osseous dysplasia (COD) [periapical cemental or cemento-osseous dysplasia (PCD); cementoma is an older term].

COD is a fibro-osseous lesion now often termed osseous dysplasia. Particularly common in black females during the fourth and fifth decades, it presents as radiolucent and radiopaque lesions often at the apices of vital teeth (periapical type), which may be isolated (focal) or multi-quadrant (florid). Lesions usually involve the mandibular anterior teeth and start as well-circumscribed radiolucent lesions which progressively become radiopaque centrally, although a thin radiolucent margin is usually visible [helpful in distinguishing from enostosis (idiopathic osteosclerosis)]. The lesions are asymptomatic, usually incidental radiographic findings, and crucially, the related teeth are vital (Fig. 2.8.22).

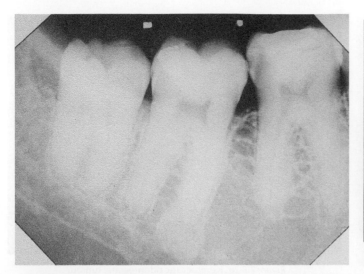

*Figure 2.8.22* Cementoma.

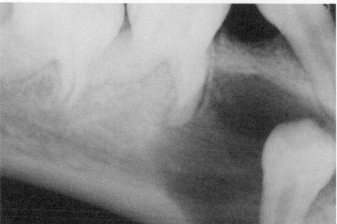

*Figure 2.8.23* Dentigerous cyst.

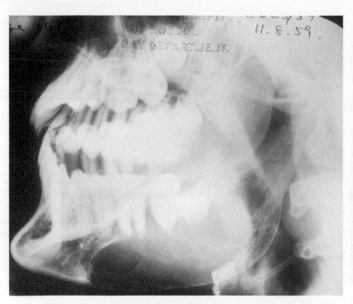

*Figure 2.8.24* Dentigerous cyst.

Florid COD is probably a widespread form, also occurring mainly in black females but usually affecting three or more quadrants. Bone expansion may occur, and the lesions may present with pain. Bone cysts may develop, and there is a liability to osteomyelitis.

Sometimes COD occurs as isolated lesions unassociated with teeth (focal COD).

COD is self-limiting, so treatment is best limited to symptomatic relief of active infection and localized sequestration. In cases of florid COD, surgical removal may be required.

## Dentigerous cyst
Dentigerous cyst (follicular cyst).

### Aetiopathogenesis
Dentigerous cyst—the second most common odontogenic cyst after dental cyst—develops within the normal dental follicle that surrounds an unerupted tooth, or from degeneration of the stellate reticulum, or an accumulation of fluid between the layers of the reduced enamel epithelium. A dentigerous cyst thus envelops the crown of an unerupted tooth and is attached to its neck. The dentigerous cyst is most frequently found in areas where unerupted teeth are most commonly found—mandibular third molars, maxillary canines and maxillary third molars, in decreasing order of frequency (Figs 2.8.23 and 2.8.24).

Multiple dentigerous cysts can be a feature of cleidocranial dysplasia (see page 169).

### Clinical features
These cysts are usually asymptomatic but may grow to a large size and may produce an intraoral swelling and occasionally an extraoral swelling, or may displace the tooth with which they are associated, or rarely cause resorption of adjacent tooth roots.

### Diagnosis
Diagnosis is usually made by clinical and radiographic assessment. Follicular cysts are unilocular, radiolucent, and may become extremely large (more so than the radicular cyst) but, in contrast to a malignant lesion, cortical bone is usually preserved.

The typical radiographic appearance is a well-demarcated radiolucent lesion attached at an acute angle to the cervical area of an unerupted tooth. The border of the lesion may be radiopaque. The radiographic differentiation between a dentigerous cyst and a normal dental follicle is based mainly on size; a hyperplastic follicle is <5 mm, but it also neither displaces the tooth nor causes cortical expansion. A 2–3 mm follicle can be considered normal, whilst the hyperplastic variant is a little larger.

The dental follicle is normally lined by reduced enamel epithelium while the dentigerous cyst lining is stratified squamous non-keratinizing epithelium sometimes with dystrophic calcification and clusters of mucous cells. Dentigerous cysts may be mimicked radiologically by the keratocystic odontogenic tumour (KCOT, odontogenic keratocyst) and ameloblastoma. Aspiration may be helpful in differentiating these lesions but biopsy is required: occasionally, more ominous lesions including mucoepidermoid carcinoma arising from mucous cells, ameloblastoma (17% of ameloblastomas arise within a dentigerous cyst), or squamous cell carcinoma may arise from a dentigerous cyst.

### Management
Treatment may be either marsupialization, allowing the tooth to erupt, or enucleation, often with removal of the associated tooth.

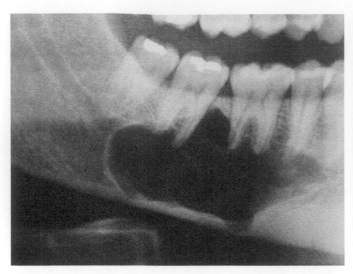

*Figure 2.8.25* Keratocystic odontogenic tumour.

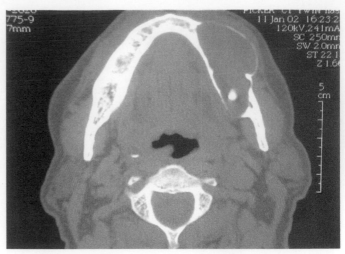

*Figure 2.8.26* Keratocystic odontogenic tumour.

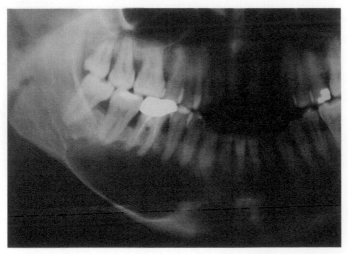

*Figure 2.8.27* Keratocystic odontogenic tumour.

### Eruption cyst

*Aetiopathogenesis*

The eruption cyst is a type of dentigerous cyst.

*Clinical features*

The eruption cyst often presents clinically as a smooth, rounded swelling with a bluish appearance if there is no overlying bone.

*Diagnosis*

Clinical. Radiographs will demonstrate the location of the erupting tooth.

*Management*

The eruption cyst usually bursts spontaneously before eruption of the associated tooth, and only requires excision if it impedes normal eruption. If thought necessary, a narrow window can be excised over the erupting tooth.

### Glandular odontogenic cyst

GOC (sialo-odontogenic cyst) is rare but may superficially mimic a central mucoepidermoid carcinoma. GOC tend to be aggressive and may recur following curettage.

### Keratocystic odontogenic tumour

KCOT: odontogenic keratocyst.

*Aetiopathogenesis*

The KCOT is one of the least common but most dangerous odontogenic lesions, being aggressive and difficult to remove. By definition, KCOTs develop instead of a tooth, arising from the dental lamina or remnants which may harbour patch PTCH1 mutations on chromosome 9, leading to constitutive activity of the embryonic Hedgehog signalling pathway, while some KCOTs, particularly in the posterior mandible, may develop from basal cell off-shoots or hamartomas from the overlying gingival epithelium.

KCOTs can be associated with the naevoid basal cell carcinoma syndrome (Gorlin syndrome) (Chapter 1.10).

*Clinical features*

KCOT are typically seen in young persons, especially in the mandibular molar region, and they can expand rapidly to occupy most of the ramus and may resorb the cortical plates, expand into the soft tissues and may produce an intraoral swelling and occasionally an extraoral swelling (Figs 2.8.25–2.8.27). KCOTs are generally painless, and often grow to a large size before giving rise to symptoms, unless they become secondarily infected. They may envelop unerupted teeth giving a dentigerous appearance, or they may displace teeth but do not resorb teeth.

*Diagnosis*

Clinical plus imaging. KCOT is a radiolucent lesion, sometimes multilocular. However, the KCOT is a great mimic; it may have any appearance, and may be seen over a wide age range. About 40% of KCOTs appear in a dentigerous relationship, and about 9% of what appear to be dentigerous cysts on radiography prove to be KCOTs. Sometimes aspiration of cyst fluid for analysis is helpful: a protein level of <4 g/100 ml suggests KCOT, whereas a value >5 g/100 ml suggests a radicular or dentigerous cyst, or rarely a cystic ameloblastoma. The demonstration of keratin squames in an aspirate is virtually diagnostic but the diagnosis of KCOT is essentially confirmed on histological grounds.

KCOTs in young patients or if bilateral should suggest the basal cell naevus (Gorlin–Goltz) syndrome.

A variant of KCOT that contains only orthokeratin is almost always are found in a dentigerous association, usually located the mandibular third molar, and is much less aggressive and not associated with basal cell nevus syndrome.

### Management
The KCOT cyst lining should be meticulously removed. Small unilocular lesions should be thoroughly enucleated. Large or multiloculated cysts should be excised with a margin of surrounding bone. However, KCOTs rates of recurrence (or perhaps new disease) following removal can be as high as 60%, so that adjuvant therapy with cryotherapy or Carnoy solution (ethanol/chloroform/acetic acid) is often considered advisable. Long-term clinical and radiographic follow-up is mandatory as recurrences may occur many years after initial treatment.

### Lateral periodontal cyst
Lateral periodontal cyst is a small cyst which develops from the post-functional dental lamina lateral to the root of a vital tooth, often a mandibular canine or premolar (botryoid odontogenic cyst is similar except that it is polycystic).

The lateral periodontal cyst is not inflammatory and is rarely clinically evident, rather being detected through radiographic examination.

### Gingival cysts
Gingival cysts of newborns originate from dental lamina remnants and are typically multiple and found on the alveolar ridges of newborns or young infants, occasionally, large enough to be noticeable as discrete white swellings. They are asymptomatic and do not require treatment.

Bohn nodules—keratin-filled cysts scattered over the palate, most obvious at the junction of the hard and soft palate, and Epstein pearls—cystic keratin-filled nodules along the midpalatine raphe—are also symptomless and need no treatment.

Gingival cysts of adults are found only in the lower premolar areas as tense, fluctuant, vesicular, or bullous lesions, histologically resembling lateral periodontal cysts.

### Odontomes
Odontomas (odontomes)—are 'hamartomas' consisting of dentine and enamel, which can appear in the tooth bearing area either in the maxilla or mandible. Typically, they can behave like teeth: they can grow and tend to erupt, or may displace adjacent teeth or impede their eruption, thus are usually discovered during adolescence. Odontomes are more common in females than males.

Odontomes are classified as the:

- Compound type (compound composite odontome)—which consists of multiple small simple denticles embedded in fibrous connective tissue within a capsule (Fig. 2.8.28) is most commonly found in the maxillary anterior alveolus. Multiple odontomes may be seen in Gardner syndrome (Chapter 1.3).
- Complex type (complex composite odontome)—which consists of disorganized irregular masses of all dental tissues (Fig. 2.8.29) are common lesions with a predilection for the mandibular molar regions.

Odontomes are treated by local excision and do not recur. Orthodontic therapy may be needed for any associated malocclusion.

### Periapical cyst
Periapical cysts (radicular or dental cysts) are the most common odontogenic cysts.

### Aetiopathogenesis
A radicular granuloma may arise at the apex of a non-vital tooth and may occasionally develop into an inflammatory cyst from proliferation of epithelial cell rests of Malassez in the area. The capsule of collagenous fibrous connective tissue causes bone resorption from activity of NFkappaB ligand and osteoprotegerin. The Runx2 [core-binding protein (cbfa)1/polyoma enhancer-binding protein (pebp)2alphaA] a DNA-binding transcriptional

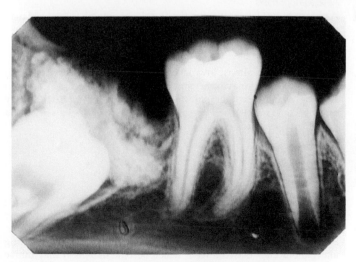

*Figure 2.8.28* Odontome.

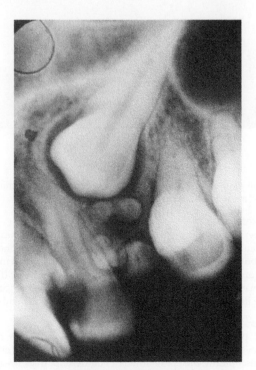

*Figure 2.8.29* Odontome.

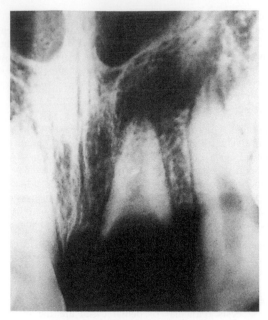

*Figure 2.8.30* Periapical dental cyst.

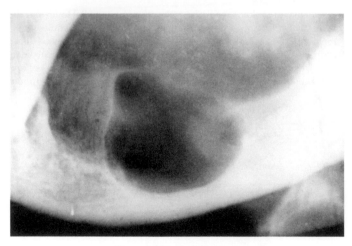

*Figure 2.8.32* Residual cyst.

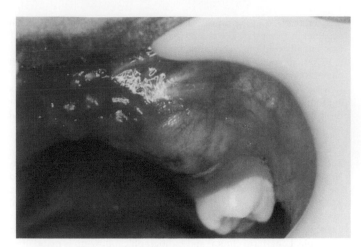

*Figure 2.8.31* Cyst showing a blue-tinged swelling in the jaw.

changes may be observed in the cyst wall, and these changes, in turn, may lead to epithelial changes (e.g. ulceration, atrophy, hyperplasia). There may be areas of chronic inflammation, or acute inflammation with abscess formation. Cholesterol crystal clefts are often present and mucous cells and/or foamy macrophages may be found. The cyst fluid is usually watery but may be thick and viscid with cholesterol crystals giving a shimmering appearance.

*Management*
A small periapical cyst may resolve with endodontic therapy, or remain attached to, and be extracted with, the causal root or tooth. Any cyst that remains after surgery is termed a residual cyst—most arise from periapical cysts.

Lesions that fail to resolve with such therapy should be surgically removed and histopathologically examined; enucleation is the standard therapy.

Although periapical cysts are typically benign, carcinoma occasionally may arise de novo, and thus all tissues removed should be histopathologicaly examined.

**Residual cyst**
*Aetiopathogenesis*
A periapical cyst left in situ after the causal root or tooth is removed may continue to expand and is then termed a residual cyst.

*Clinical features*
A residual cyst is almost invariably unilocular but may expand to an appreciable size. It may be asymptomatic, may be detected as a bluish swelling, a chance radiographic finding (Figs 2.8.31 and 2.8.32), or may rarely become infected and present as an abscess, or may give rise to a pathological fracture.

*Diagnosis*
Clinical plus imaging.

*Management*
Enucleation or, if large, marsupialization.

**Squamous odontogenic tumour**
Squamous odontogenic tumour usually presents as a painless swelling and radiolucency between teeth which become mobile. It may mimic periodontal disease. Conservative excision is the treatment of choice.

molecule expressed in osteoprogenitor cells, and transforming growth factor-β2 are involved in reactive new bone formation.

*Clinical features*
Many periapical cysts involve upper lateral incisors since these teeth not infrequently become carious or traumatized or have invaginated odontomes, but they can be found on any tooth. A periapical cyst may well be asymptomatic and often is a chance radiographic finding (Fig. 2.8.30) but it may present as a swelling (usually in the labial sulcus) or may become infected and present as an abscess with swelling and pain.

*Diagnosis*
Clinical plus imaging. Radiography, cannot distinguisha granuloma from a cyst, but if the lesion is large it is more likely to be a cyst.

Microscopically, the epithelium is a non-descript thick irregular stratified squamous epithelium without keratin formation. Inflammatory

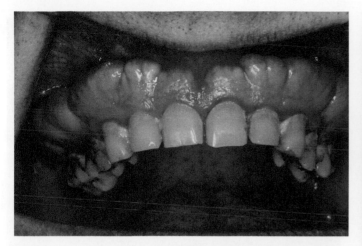

Figure 2.8.33 Exostoses.

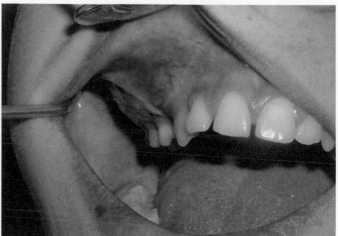

Figure 2.8.34 Fibrous dysplasia.

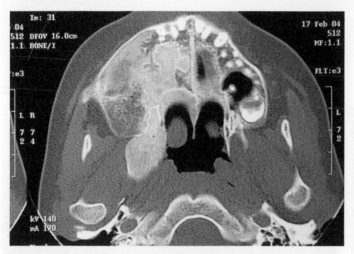

Figure 2.8.35 Fibrous dysplasia.

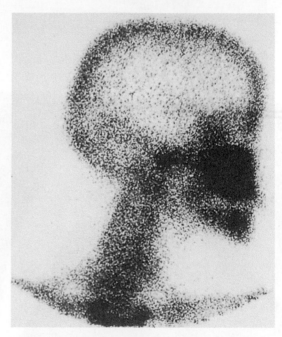

Figure 2.8.36 Fibrous dysplasia.

## Exostoses

Exostoses buccal to the maxillary posterior teeth are fairly common (Fig. 2.8.33) but the possibility of osteomas and Gardner syndrome should be considered (Chapter 1.3).

## Fibrous dysplasia

### Aetiopathogenesis

Fibrous dysplasia is a fibro-osseous lesion caused by mutation in the gene encoding G protein (GNAS1).

### Clinical features

Fibrous dysplasia usually affects only one bone (monostotic: about 70%) but occasionally several (polyostotic) (Figs 2.8.34–2.8.37). Bone enlarges but the morphology is preserved, distinguishing it from a neoplasm.

### Diagnosis

Fibrous dysplasia lesions vary from radiolucent to radiopaque (often a 'ground-glass appearance') with ill-defined margins—a feature helpful to distinguish it radiologically from other lesions. CT can best assess the extent in the facial skeleton. Biopsy may be indicated.

### Management

Growth of lesions in the jaws tends to be self limiting at the end of the growth period. Typically therefore, no treatment is needed as fibrous dysplasia is self-limiting. Bisphosphonates can help and surgery may be indicated if there is major deformity or pressure on nerves, or for example, if the frontal bone starts to grow after puberty and cause eye displacement.

Mazabraud's syndrome is fibrous dysplasia with intramuscular myxoma.

McCune–Albright's syndrome is fibrous dysplasia with skin hyper-pigmentation and endocrinopathy (precocious puberty in females and hyperthyroidism in males).

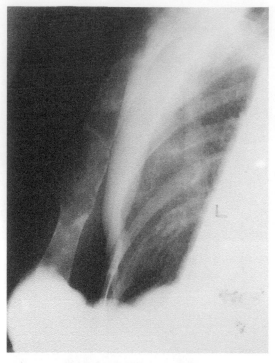

*Figure 2.8.37* Fibrous dysplasia.

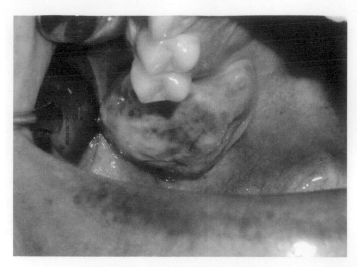

*Figure 2.8.38* Central giant cell granuloma.

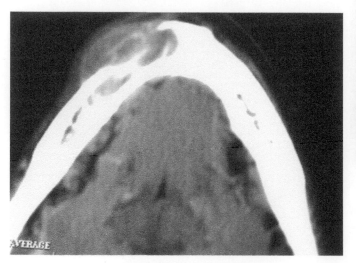

*Figure 2.8.39* Central giant cell granuloma.

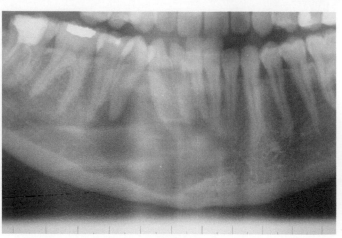

*Figure 2.8.40* Central giant cell granuloma.

## Giant cell granuloma

Giant cell granuloma (central giant cell granuloma or giant cell reparative granuloma).

### Aetiopathogenesis

Central giant cell granulomas often contain abundant giant cells in a vascular matrix but not granulomas and, despite having histopathological features identical to those of the bony lesions of hyperparathyroidism, the affected patients do not have hyperparathyroidism.

### Clinical features

Central giant cell granuloma is an uncommon lesion that tends to arise in the anterior mandible as a painless swelling (Figs 2.8.38–2.8.43).

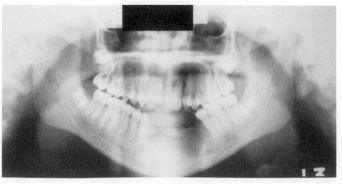

*Figure 2.8.41* Giant cell granuloma.

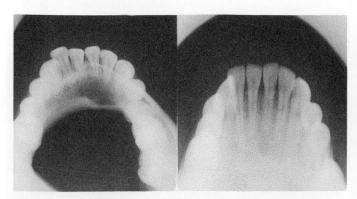

*Figure 2.8.42* Giant cell granuloma.

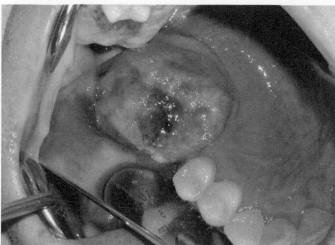

*Figure 2.8.43* Giant cell granuloma.

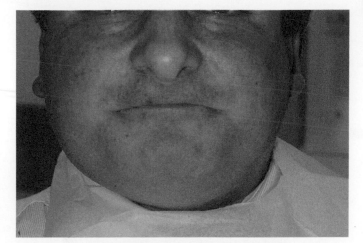

*Figure 2.8.44* Masseteric hypertrophy.

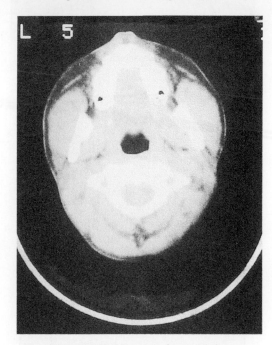

*Figure 2.8.45* Masseteric hypertrophy.

*Diagnosis*
Radiologically there is a well-defined unilocular or multilocular radiolucency.

*Management*
Curettage is the typical treatment but calcitonin and intralesional steroids may help.

### Masseteric hypertrophy
*Aetiopathogenesis*
Masseteric hypertrophy may be associated with an increase in the number of muscle fibres as well as their size. It is usually consequent on a clenching or bruxing habit such as may especially be seen in patients with a learning impairment, Rett syndrome, or amphetamine or ecstacy abuse—when dental attrition and temporomandibular joint pain dysfunction syndrome may also be present.

*Clinical features*
Masseteric hypertrophy manifests as painless enlargement of one or both masseter muscles. When bilateral, the face can take on a rather square appearance. There may also be some enlargement of the inferior and posterior borders of the mandible (enlarged mandibular angle) on  the affected sides (Figs 2.8.44–2.8.46).

*Diagnosis*
This is a clinical diagnosis. An orthopantomogram often shows accentuation of the antegonial notch of the mandible. Computed tomography, magnetic resonance imaging or ultrasonography can delineate the extent of the muscle enlargement.

*Management*
There is often no requirement for treatment but if it is really unaesthetic, it may be treated by surgery or botulinum toxoid injections, along with attention to the underlying cause.

### Metastases
Metastases (Chapter 1.11).

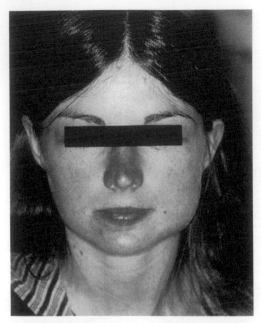

*Figure 2.8.46* Masseteric hypertrophy.

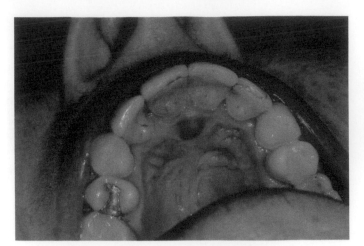

*Figure 2.8.47* Nasopalatine cyst.

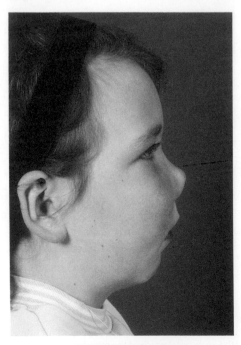

*Figure 2.8.48* Ossifying fibroma.

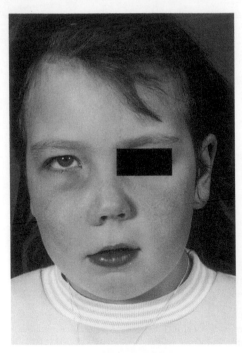

*Figure 2.8.49* Ossifying fibroma.

### Myeloma

Myeloma (Chapter 1.4).

### Nasopalatine cyst

The nasopalatine duct cyst (NPDC) is the most common non-odontogenic cyst. NPDC is a developmental cyst, unique in that it is found only in the midline anterior maxilla (Fig. 2.8.47).

### Ossifying fibroma (cemento-ossifying fibroma)

Ossifying fibroma is a benign, slow-growing, painless bone neoplasm, typically monostotic and seen in the third and fourth decades in the posterior mandible as a radiolucent, radiopaque, or mixed opacity (Figs 2.8.48–2.8.51). Ossifying fibroma has a fibro-osseous microscopic appearance not easily differentiated histopathologically from focal COD.

Juvenile ossifying fibroma is an aggressive variant with a rapid growth pattern seen mainly in boys aged under 15 years.

Traditionally, the initial treatment for ossifying fibroma has been simple curettage. More definitive resection has been reserved for recurrent disease.

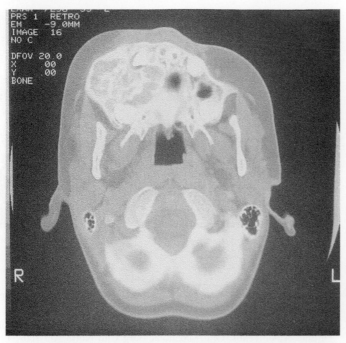

Figure 2.8.50 Ossifying fibroma.

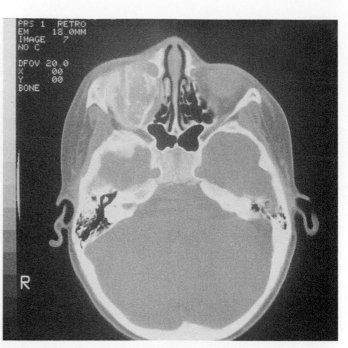

Figure 2.8.51 Ossifying fibroma.

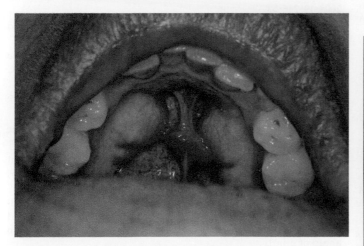

Figure 2.8.52 Torus mandibularis.

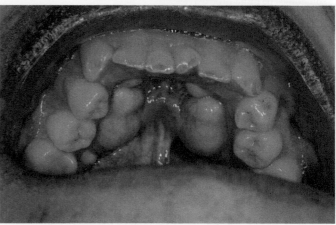

Figure 2.8.53 Torus mandibularis.

### Osteoma
Osteoma (Chapter 1.11).

### Paget disease of bone
Paget disease of bone (Chapter 1.15).

### Torus mandibularis
*Aetiopathogenesis*
Tori are bony exostoses of developmental origin which are fairly common (about 60% of the population) but especially seen in Mongoloid races. They are also said to be more common in parafunctional states.

*Clinical features*
Mandibular tori are uni- or bilateral, single or multiple bony lumps lingual to the lower premolars (Figs 2.8.52 and 2.8.53).

*Diagnosis*
Clinical.

*Management*
Tori are benign. Reassurance only is necessary unless surgery is indicated because the tori interfere with a prosthesis.

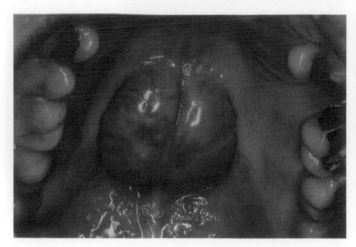

*Figure 2.8.54* Torus palatinus.

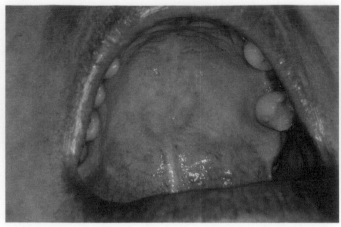

*Figure 2.8.55* Torus palatinus.

## Torus palatinus

*Aetiopathogenesis*

Palatal tori are congenital exostoses, seen in up to 20% of the population, most common in Mongoloid races.

*Clinical features*

Palatal tori are bony lumps typically seen in the midline vault of palate (Figs 2.8.54 and 2.8.55). They vary in size and morphology but can sometimes be quite protrusive.

*Diagnosis*

Clinical.

*Management*

Tori are benign and usually require no treatment unless interfering with the construction of an appliance.

## FURTHER READING

Al-Muharraqi MA, Fedorowicz Z, Al Bareeq J, Al Bareeq R, Nasser M. Botulinum toxin for masseter hypertrophy. Cochrane Database Syst Rev 2009; CD007510.

Arias-Irimia O, Barona Dorado C, Santos Marino JA, Martínez-Rodriguez N, Martínez-González JM. Meta-analysis of the etiology of odontogenic maxillary sinusitis. Med Oral Patol Oral Cir Bucal 2009; 15: 70–3.

Baqain ZH, Newman L, Hyde N. How serious are oral infections? J Laryngol Otol 2004; 118: 561–5.

Bevin CR, Inwards CY, Keller EE. Surgical management of primary chronic osteomyelitis: a long-term retrospective analysis. J Oral Maxillofac Surg 2008; 66: 2073–85.

Bouloux GF, Steed MB, Perciaccante VJ. Complications of third molar surgery. Oral Maxillofac Surg Clin North Am 2007; 19: 117–28.

Bronner MP. Gastrointestinal polyposis syndromes. Am J Med Genet 2003; 122A: 335–41.

Bruce I, Ndanu TA, Addo ME. Epidemiological aspects of oral tori in a Ghanaian community. Int Dent J 2004; 54: 78–82.

Chen Y, Wang JM, Li TJ. Ameloblastic fibroma: a review of published studies with special reference to its nature and biological behavior. Oral Oncol 2007; 43: 960–9.

Costello BJ, Betts NJ, Barber HD, Fonseca RJ. Preprosthetic surgery for the edentulous patients. Dent Clin North Am 1996; 40: 19–38.

Coviello V, Stevens MR. Contemporary concepts in the treatment of chronic osteomyelitis. Oral Maxillofac Surg Clin North Am 2007; 19: 523–34.

Cundy T, Bolland M. Paget disease of bone. Trends Endocrinol Metab 2008; 19: 246–53.

Dahlén G. Microbiology and treatment of dental abscesses and periodontal-endodontic lesions. Periodontol 2000 2002; 28: 206–39.

Davies DR, Armstrong JG, Thakker N, et al. Severe Gardner syndrome in families with mutations restricted to a specific region of the APC gene. Am J Hum Genet 1995; 57: 1151–8.

DelBalso AM. Lesions of the jaws. Semin Ultrasound CT MR 1995; 16: 487–512.

Favia GF, Di Alberti L, Scarano A, Piattelli A. Squamous odontogenic tumour: report of two cases. Oral Oncol 1997; 33: 451–3.

Fedele S, Kumar N, Davies R, et al. Dental management of patients at risk of osteochemonecrosis of the jaws: a critical review. Oral Dis 2009; Jul 13. [Epub ahead of print].

García-García AS, Martínez-González JM, Gómez-Font R, Soto-Rivadeneira A, Oviedo-Roldán L. Current status of the torus palatinus and torus mandibularis. Med Oral Patol Oral Cir Bucal 2009; Sep 21. [Epub ahead of print].

Garner JM, Wein RO. Use of the palatal flap for closure of an oronasal fistula. Am J Otolaryngol 2006; 27: 268–70.

Hyun HK, Hong SD, Kim JW. Recurrent keratocystic odontogenic tumor in the mandible: a case report and literature review. Oral Surg Oral Med Oral Pathol Oral Radiol Endod 2009; 108: e7–10.

Jainkittivong A, Langlais RP. Buccal and palatal exostoses: prevalence and concurrence with tori. Oral Surg Oral Med Oral Pathol Oral Radiol Endod 2000; 90: 48–53.

Jones K, Korzcak P. The diagnostic significance and management of Gardner's syndrome. Br J Oral Maxillofac Surg 1990; 28: 80–4.

Koga DH, Salvajoli JV, Alves FA. Dental extractions and radiotherapy in head and neck oncology: review of the literature. Oral Dis 2008; 14: 40–4.

Ladeinde AL, Ajayi OF, Ogunlewe MO, et al. Odontogenic tumors: a review of 319 cases in a Nigerian teaching hospital. Oral Surg Oral Med Oral Pathol Oral Radiol Endod 2005; 99: 191–5.

de Lange J, van den Akker HP, van den Berg H. Central giant cell granuloma of the jaw: a review of the literature with emphasis on therapy option. Oral Surg Oral Med Oral Pathol Oral Radiol Endod 2007; 104: 603–15.

Lietman SA, Schwindinger WF, Levine MA. Genetic and molecular aspects of McCune-Albright syndrome. Pediatr Endocrinol Rev 2007; 4(Suppl 4): 380–5.

MacDonald-Jankowski DS. Fibro-osseous lesions of the face and jaws. Clin Radiol 2004; 59: 11–25.

Mandel L, Kaynar A. Masseteric hypertrophy. N Y State Dent J 1994; 60: 44–7.

Manfredi M, Vescovi P, Bonanini M, Porter S. Nevoid basal cell carcinoma syndrome: a review of the literature. Int J Oral Maxillofac Surg 2004; 33: 117–24.

Mehra P, Murad H. Maxillary sinus disease of odontogenic origin. Otolaryngol Clin North Am 2004; 37: 347–64.

Mendenhall WM, Werning JW, Fernandes R, Malyapa RS, Mendenhall NP. Ameloblastoma. Am J Clin Oncol 2007; 30: 645–8.

Michal M, Boudova L, Mukensnabl P. Gardner's syndrome associated fibromas. Pathol Int 2004; 54: 523–6.

Parks ET, Caldemeyer KS, Mirowski GW. Gardner syndrome. J Am Acad Dermatol 2001; 45: 940–2.

Payne M, Anderson JA, Cook J. Gardner's syndrome–a case report. Br Dent J 2002; 193: 383–4.

Philipsen HP, Reichart PA. Adenomatoid odontogenic tumour: facts and figures. Oral Oncol 1999; 35: 125–31.

Philipsen HP, Reichart PA. Calcifying epithelial odontogenic tumour: biological profile based on 181 cases from the literature. Oral Oncol 2000; 36: 17–26.

Pitak-Arnnop P, Sader R, Dhanuthai K, et al. Management of osteoradionecrosis of the jaws: an analysis of evidence. Eur J Surg Oncol 2008; 34: 1123–34.

Poeschl PW, Baumann A, Russmueller G, et al. Closure of oroantral communications with Bichat's buccal fat pad. J Oral Maxillofac Surg 2009; 67: 1460–6.

Pogrel MA. The use of liquid nitrogen cryotherapy in the management of locally aggressive bone lesions. J Oral Maxillofac Surg 1993; 51: 269–73.

Regezi JA. Odontogenic cysts, odontogenic tumors, fibroosseous, and giant cell lesions of the jaws. Mod Pathol 2002; 15: 331–41.

Reichart PA, Philipsen HP, Sonner S. Ameloblastoma: biological profile of 3677 cases. Eur J Cancer B Oral Oncol 1995; 31B: 86–99.

Riminucci M, Robey PG, Bianco P. The pathology of fibrous dysplasia and the McCune-Albright syndrome. Pediatr Endocrinol Rev 2007; 4(Suppl 4): 401–11.

Sadeghi EM, Sewall SR, Dohse A, et al. Odontogenic tumours that mimic a dentigerous cyst. Compend Contin Educ Dent 1995; 16: 500, 502, 504 passim.

Sampson DE, Pogrel MA. Management of mandibular ameloblastoma: the clinical basis for a treatment algorithm. J Oral Maxillofac Surg 1999; 57: 1074–9.

Sayan NB, Ucok C, Karasu HA, Gunhan O. Peripheral osteoma of the oral and maxillofacial region: a study of 35 new cases. J Oral Maxillofac Surg 2002; 60: 1299–301.

Seoane J, Aguirre-Urizar JM, Esparza-Gómez G, et al. The spectrum of plasma cell neoplasia in oral pathology. Med Oral 2003; 8: 269–80.

Shibata Y, Asaumi J, Yanagi Y, et al. Radiographic examination of dentigerous cysts in the transitional dentition. Dentomaxillofac Radiol 2004; 33: 17–20.

Shimizu M, Osa N, Okamura K, Yoshiura K. CT analysis of the Stafne's bone defects of the mandible. Dentomaxillofac Radiol 2006; 35: 95–102.

Silverman SL. Paget disease of bone: therapeutic options. J Clin Rheumatol 2008; 14: 299–305.

Thakker N, Davies R, Horner K, et al. The dental phenotype in familial adenomatous polyposis: diagnostic application of a weighted scoring system for changes on dental panoramic radiographs. J Med Genet 1995; 32: 458–64.

Worthington P, Rubenstein JE. Problems associated with the atrophic mandible. Dent Clin North Am 1998; 42: 129–60.

# 2.9 TEMPOROMANDIBULAR JOINT DISORDERS

- mandibular pain-dysfunction syndrome [temporomandibular joint (TMJ) dysfunction syndrome]
- temporomandibular ankylosis
- temporomandibular joint subluxation

## MANDIBULAR PAIN-DYSFUNCTION SYNDROME [TEMPOROMANDIBULAR JOINT (TMJ) DYSFUNCTION SYNDROME]

### Aetiopathogenesis

Seen predominantly in young adult females, the aetiology is unclear but hypotheses are many, and facts are few. Trauma and stress appear to predispose as may psychogenic and/or occlusal factors. There is no neurophysiological evidence to support a primary aetiological role for the occlusion: many people with gross malocclusions have no TMJ dysfunction; there is neither significant difference in the incidence of occlusal abnormalities between patients and controls subjects, nor any evidence for a relationship between orthodontic treatment (or the wearing of orthodontic headgear) and TMJ dysfunction.

TMJ dysfunction is a symptom complex of multifactorial aetiology which may sometimes have a traumatic element but almost certainly usually represents a psychological response to stress that becomes chronic through increasing activity of the muscles of mastication (temporalis, masseter and pterygoid muscles).

#### Trauma

- Trauma including from road accidents, sports injuries, fights and dental extractions can be followed very rarely by TMJ dysfunction.
- TMJ dysfunction can be secondary to microtrauma and subsequent muscle hyperactivity, which can result from prolonged mouth opening, as in dental treatment sessions. Other causes of prolonged and/or excessive mandibular opening: for example, general anaesthesia, choir singing or wind instrument playing, or parafunctions such as day-time jaw clenching or night-time tooth grinding (bruxism), and habits such as chewing a pen, can also lead to TMJ dysfunction.

#### Stress and muscle hyperactivity

- Approximately 50–70% of patients (twice as common as controls) have experienced stressful life events in the 6 months before onset (e.g. problems concerning work, money, health, loss and interpersonal relationships).
- Psychological stress can cause muscle hyperactivity. Depression and shortage of sleep are considered important risk indicators.
- Muscle hyperactivity has been demonstrated in TMJ patients during activities such as school examinations and watching horror films.
- In TMJ dysfunction patients, the lower head of the lateral pterygoid muscle contracts during the closing phase (when it should be relaxed) and it has been suggested that anterior displacement of the TMJ meniscus, perhaps from a tear of the posterior capsule, prevents the superior head from acting effectively. The lower head perhaps attempts to help stabilize the meniscus. This might explain why this muscle is tender on palpation in TMJ dysfunction patients. Anterior meniscus displacement has been demonstrated by radiology and found at operation in some patients.

### Clinical features

Symptoms are highly variable, but dysfunction is characterized by:

- Recurrent clicking in the TMJ: either on attempted opening or closing. Clicks are not diagnostic, however, since they are common in normal TMJs.
- Limitation of jaw movement: may affect opening, with jaw 'locking'. The jaw may deviate to the affected side on attempted opening. Limitation may be more obvious on waking, especially after nocturnal grinding. In some others, the limitation increases throughout the day.
- Pain in the joint and surrounding muscles and elsewhere: usually preauricularly, but discomfort can radiate to the mouth, neck or temple. Pain may range from a vague dull ache to an acute pain. Patients with a night-time clenching or grinding habit (bruxism) may awake with joint pain which abates during the day. The symptoms of individuals who clench or grind during working hours tend to worsen towards evening, and sometimes have a psychogenic basis. There is often diffuse tenderness over masseters and temporalis muscles which may be tender to palpation. Some patients may also complain of headaches, neck aches and lower back pain. Female patients have significantly fewer children and are more likely to have never been pregnant, possibly due to fibromyalgia.

### Diagnosis

Diagnosis is mainly on clinical grounds. Self-ratings for psychological factors are helpful and the occlusion and any dental appliances should also be assessed.

#### Imaging

Radiographic changes are uncommon in TMJ dysfunction, and the condylar position as seen on plain or tomographic radiographic views is unreliable for diagnosis (and does not indicate meniscus displacement). CT or MRI is rarely indicated. Imaging is recommended for diagnosis, only if there is:

- a trauma history
- significant movement limitation
- sensory or motor alteration
- a likelihood of organic joint or other disease.

CT is then most useful.

### Management

TMJ dysfunction rarely leads to any long-term joint damage, and most patients spontaneously remit. There is no indication for attempting treatment for symptomless TMJ clicks; however, for persons in pain, treatment may be worthwhile. The level of placebo response and the response from reassurance is impressive and conservative measures are at least partially successful in up to 90%, usually within 6 months. Of the other 10%, half may be functional and respond to psychotropic medication—and the rest are chronic pain sufferers.

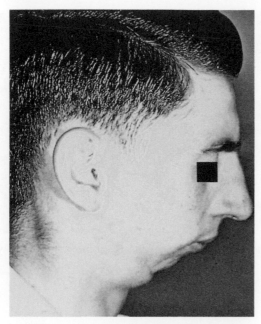

*Figure 2.9.1* Temporomandibular joint arthritis.

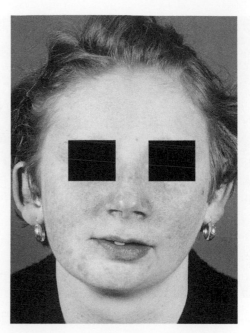

*Figure 2.9.2* Condylar ankylosis.

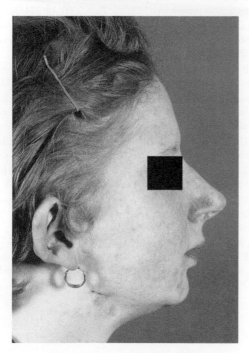

*Figure 2.9.3* Condylar ankylosis.

The aims of treatment, therefore, are to:

- control immediate pain
- lower psychological stress (reassure)
- eliminate TMJ damage.

TMJ dysfunction patients mostly respond to simple measures such as:

- Avoidance of trauma, clenching, excessively chewy foods such as nuts or steak, and wide opening (e.g. to bite an apple) and abnormal habits (e.g. pencil-chewing).
- Warmth, massage and remedial jaw exercises; analgesics; non-steroidal anti-inflammatory agents such as aspirin can be helpful. Injection of local analgesics into painful sites, or the spraying of coolants such as trichloro-fluoromethane onto the areas, can ease pain and break the cycle. Muscle relaxants such as clonazepam or baclofen daily can help provide relief.
- Hard plastic splints or vinyl splints on the occlusal surfaces (occlusal splints) can benefit at least 40% symptomatically.

## TEMPOROMANDIBULAR ANKYLOSIS

TMJ intra-articular (true) ankylosis mostly follows trauma or infection, including middle ear infection, but it can be congenital or result from rheumatoid arthritis.

When ankylosis impairs condylar growth, facial asymmetry is common (Figs 2.9.1–2.9.3). Chronic, painless limitation of movement is seen.

Extra-articular (false) ankylosis can be caused by a depressed zygomatic fracture, coronoid hypertrophy or tumour, or scarring from surgery, irradiation or infection.

Diagnosis is assisted by TMJ radiography. In most cases of true ankylosis, joint radiography shows loss of normal bony architecture.

Management may include condylectomy if the ankylosis is intra-articular or a ramus ostectomy if the coronoid process and zygomatic arch are also affected.

## TEMPOROMANDIBULAR JOINT SUBLUXATION
### Aetiopathogenesis

Subluxation can follow severe trauma but is especially liable to occur in hypermobility syndromes, such as Ehlers–Danlos syndrome (Figs 2.9.4 and 2.9.5; see page 160).

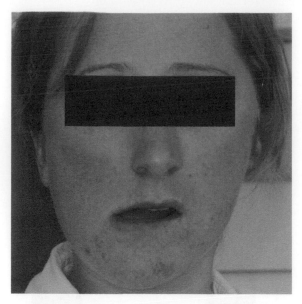

*Figure 2.9.4* Temporomandibular joint dislocation.

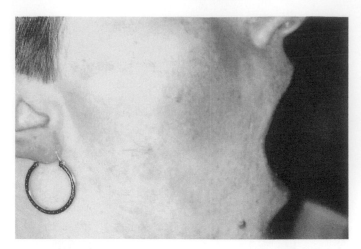

*Figure 2.9.5* Temporomandibular joint pain–release of ankylosis.

### Clinical features

There may be a history of repeated subluxation or dislocation of the mandible. It may also be possible to easily induce subluxation. Patients often report that they are able to manipulate the mandible back to its correct position.

### Diagnosis

Patients may have other features of hypermobility syndromes (e.g. 'double jointed', easy bruising, cardiac valvular defects, as well as aggressive periodontitis and absence of labial fraenae) and possible pain over one or both temporomandibular joints.

### Management

Surgery may be warranted.

## FURTHER READING

Israel HA, Diamond B, Saed-Nejad F, et al. The relationship between parafunctional masticatory activity and arthroscopically diagnosed temporomandibular joint pathology. J Oral Maxillofac Surg 1999; 57: 1034–9.

Kamisaka M, Yatani H, Kuboki T, et al. Four-year longitudinal course of TMD symptoms in an adult population and the estimation of risk factors in relation to symptoms. J Orofac Pain 2000; 14: 224–32.

MacFarlane TV, Blinkhorn AS, Davies RM, et al. Association between female hormonal factors and oro-facial pain: study in the community. Pain 2002; 97: 5–10.

Madland G, Feinmann C, Newman S. Factors associated with anxiety and depression in facial arthromyalgia. Pain 2000; 84: 225–32.

Meldolesi G, Picardi A, Accivile E, et al. Personality and psychopathology in patients with temporomandibular joint pain-dysfunction syndrome: a controlled investigation. Psychother Psychosom 2000; 69: 322–8.

Nassif NJ, Talic YF. Classic symptoms in temporomandibular disorder patients: a comparative study. Cranio 2001; 19: 33–41.

Reston JT, Turkelson CM. Meta-analysis of surgical treatments for temporomandibular articular disorders. J Oral Maxillofac Surg 2003; 61: 3–10.

Truelove EL, Sommers EE, LeResche L, et al. Clinical diagnostic criteria for TMD: new classification permits multiple diagnoses. J Am Dent Assoc 1992; 123: 47–54.

Yamada K, Hanada K, Fukui T, et al. Condylar bony change and self-reported parafunctional habits in prospective orthognathic surgery patients with temporomandibular disorders. Oral Surg Oral Med Oral Pathol Oral Radiol Endod 2001; 92: 265–71.

# 2.10 TEETH

- history related to dental problems
- dental examination
- diagnosis
- aesthetics
- early tooth loss

- eruption disorders
- tooth number variations
- tooth size, shape and structural anomalies
- tooth surface loss

The teeth develop from neuroectoderm, and development (odontogenesis) begins at about 28 days *in utero*, with proliferation of areas of oral ectoderm to form the dental lamina. At each of the locations where a tooth will be formed, a downgrowth from the dental lamina forms the early enamel organ. Together, the enamel organ, dental papilla and dental sac are the formative structures for the entire tooth and supporting structures.

All the deciduous and some of the permanent dentition commence development in the foetus. Each enamel organ eventually produces tooth enamel, and the mesenchyme, which condenses beneath the enamel organ, forms a dental papilla that produces the dentine and pulp of the tooth.

Odontogenesis proceeds through a series of stages:

Bud stage—initiation and formation of the enamel organs.

Cap stage—the cuboidal peripheral cells are termed the outer enamel epithelium, and the tall columnar cells in the concavity are termed the inner enamel epithelium (IEE). The polygonal cells between outer and inner enamel epithelia form the delicate cellular network known as the stellate reticulum, the spaces of which are filled with a mucoid fluid. The cells of the dental papilla eventually form tooth pulp and dentine. The cells of the dental sac eventually form cementum and the periodontal ligament.

Bell stage—the IEE induces the adjacent cells of the dental papilla to differentiate into odontoblasts, which form dentine which, in turn, induces the IEE to differentiate into ameloblasts, which produce enamel matrix.

The enamel organ also forms Hertwig epithelial root sheath, which determines the root shape and initiates root dentine formation and apposition–deposition of the enamel and dentine matrices. These structures then calcify.

Mineralization of the primary dentition commences at about 14 weeks *in utero* and all primary teeth are mineralizing by birth. Permanent incisor and first molar teeth begin to mineralize at, or close to, the time of birth; mineralization of other permanent teeth starting later. Tooth eruption occurs after crown formation when mineralization is largely complete but before the roots are fully formed.

The fully developed tooth comprises a crown of insensitive enamel, surrounding sensitive dentine, and a dentine root which has a cementum rather than enamel covering. Teeth contain a vital pulp (nerve). The fibres of the periodontal ligament run from the alveolus to attach through cementum to the dentine surface and thus attach the tooth to the jaw.

The first or primary (deciduous or milk) dentition comprises two incisors, a canine and two molars in each of the four mouth quadrants. There are 10 deciduous (primary or milk) teeth in each jaw: all are fully erupted by the age of about 3 years.

The secondary or permanent teeth begin to erupt at about the age of 6–7 years and the deciduous teeth are slowly lost by normal root resorption. The full permanent (adult) dentition consists of 16 teeth in each jaw: two incisors, a canine, two premolars and three molars in each quadrant

(Table 2.10.1). Normally most teeth have erupted by about 12–14 years of age. However, some milk teeth may still be present at the age of 12–13 years. The last molars (third molars or wisdom teeth), if present, often erupt later or may impact and never appear in the mouth.

## HISTORY RELATED TO DENTAL PROBLEMS

The history related to dental problems should include:

- date of onset of symptoms
- swelling details such as duration and character
- xerostomia details
- pain details such as duration, site of maximum intensity, severity, onset, daily timing, character, radiation, aggravating and relieving factors, relationship to meals and associated phenomena
- mouth opening restriction
- changes in the occlusion of the teeth
- dietary history
- occupation.

## DENTAL EXAMINATION

Detailed description of dental examination techniques can be found in standard textbooks. All findings should be charted using one of various systems of tooth notations. The system most widely used worldwide is the Federation Dentaire Internationale system.

Inspection: the dentition should be checked to make sure that the expected complement of teeth is present for the patient's age (Figs 2.10.1 and 2.10.2). Deficiency of teeth (oligodontia, hypodontia or anodontia) as well as abnormalities of size, shape, colour or structure may be features of many syndromes, but teeth are far more frequently missing because they are unerupted, or lost as a result of caries or periodontal disease. Extra teeth (hyperdontia) are supplemental if part of the normal series or supernumerary if abnormal morphology.

Look for carious, mobile, heavily or poorly restored teeth, retained roots or other signs that could explain extensive local (e.g., facial abscess) or systemic (e.g. infective endocarditis) pathology.

Palpation: feel for tenderness or swelling of the alveolar process adjacent to apical areas of suspicious teeth (feel the buccal/labial and lingual/palatal sides of the alveolus).

Percussion: use a long metal instrument (like the handle of a dental mirror) to tap on suspicious teeth (warn the patient and start gently, or rapport may be lost in a second!). Any tenderness elicited may signify pulpal or periodontal/periapical inflammation. Finally, the occlusion of the teeth should be checked.

Vitality testing: non-vital teeth are primary suspects of local pain and infections, occasionally even when they are root-treated. In such cases, the patient should report no sensation of hot (melting gutta percha), cold (ethyl chloride on a cotton bud) or electric (special apparatus; pulp vitality tester) stimuli.

**Table 2.10.1** NORMAL TOOTH ERUPTION TIMES

|  | Upper | Lower |
|---|---|---|
| *Deciduous (primary) teeth* | *Months* | *Months* |
| Central incisors | 8–13 | 6–10 |
| Lateral incisors | 8–13 | 10–16 |
| Canines (cuspids) | 16–23 | 16–23 |
| First molars | 13–19 | 13–19 |
| Second molars | 25–33 | 23–31 |
| *Permanent teeth* | *Years* | *Years* |
| Central incisors | 7–8 | 6–7 |
| Lateral incisors | 8–9 | 7–8 |
| Canines (cuspids) | 11–12 | 9–10 |
| First premolars (bicuspids) | 10–11 | 10–12 |
| Second premolars (bicuspids) | 10–12 | 11–12 |
| First molars | 6–7 | 6–7 |
| Second molars | 12–13 | 11–13 |
| Third molars | 17–21 | 17–21 |

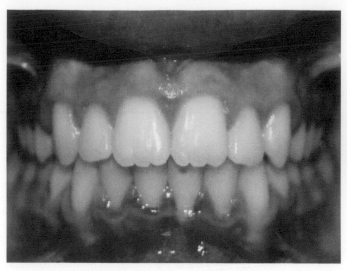

*Figure 2.10.1* Normal young adult dentition.

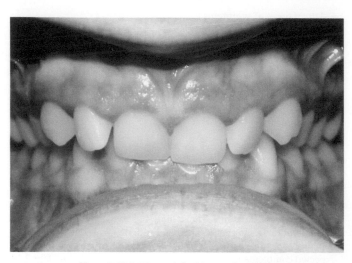

*Figure 2.10.2* Normal deciduous dentition.

Disorders which affect the teeth may appear to be unilateral, but the other teeth should always be examined, and it is important to consider the possibility of related systemic disorders especially those affecting

- the skeleton/connective tissue
- neurological system (e.g., epilepsy)
- nutrition (eating disorders such as bulimia).

## DIAGNOSIS

Disorders affecting teeth are diagnosed mainly from history and examination findings.

Investigations required may include:

- Plain radiography of the teeth may be achieved using
  - ○ periapical radiographs
  - ○ bitewings
  - ○ oblique lateral views.
- Tomographic views
  - ○ dental pan-oral tomographic views
  - ○ other tomographic views.

- Three-dimensional information may be gained from:
  - ○ tomography in both the coronal and sagittal planes
  - ○ CT scan.
- Other investigations can include:
  - ○ vitality testing
  - ○ electronic caries detectors.

Disorders affecting teeth, except caries and trauma, are not common. Most disorders are present with pain.

## AESTHETICS

Aesthetics can be compromised by genetic or acquired abnormalities of tooth crown size, shape, colour or position or missing teeth.

### Body art

The grinding of teeth to a different shape, the placement of anterior gold or other crowns or inserts in intact teeth or the wearing of dental grills (grillz of the hip-hop culture) on teeth are fashions regarded by some as body art (see Fig 2.10.100).

### Discolouration

Teeth may be discoloured most commonly from superficial (extrinsic) staining or internally from caries, trauma or tooth restorations. In these latter instances, the discolouration usually affects one or a few teeth or only parts of the teeth.

### Extrinsic tooth discolouration

*Aetiopathogenesis*

Extrinsic staining usually affects several if not all, teeth, is seen mainly where oral hygiene is lacking and at interproximal areas and the cervical areas and can be of various colours (Figs 2.10.3–2.10.8).

Brown stain is most common and usually caused by poor oral hygiene and habits such as beverages (e.g. tea, coffee and wine), smoking tobacco

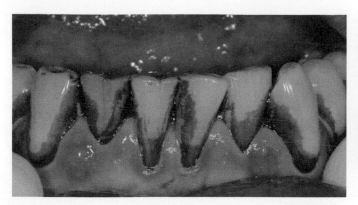

*Figure 2.10.3* Stain.

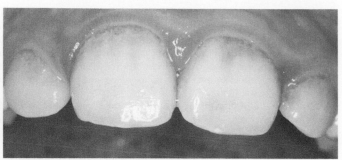

*Figure 2.10.4* Stain.

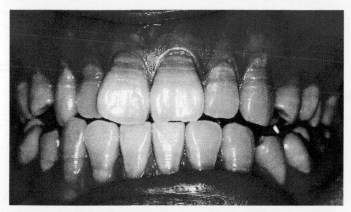

*Figure 2.10.5* Stain—tetracycline induced.

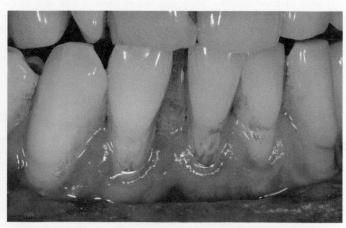

*Figure 2.10.6* Stain from inability to cleanse the instanding incisor.

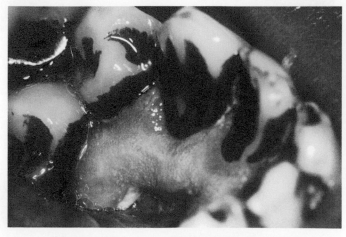

*Figure 2.10.7* Stain from very heavy tobacco smoking.

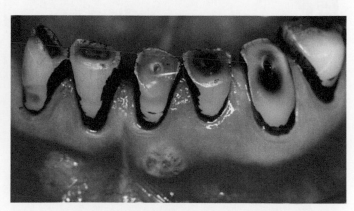

*Figure 2.10.8* Stain from paan (betel) use. There is also a sinus related to a dental abscess on the lower incisor (non-vital because of the severe attrition).

or cannabis, chewing tobacco, betel or khat. Foods, and drugs such as iron, chlorhexidine or long-term oral antimicrobials or stannous fluoride, can cause similar staining. Chlorhexidine binds to dental pellicle where it can produce discolouration, especially from tannins found in tea or coffee or red wine. Cetylpyridinium may have a similar effect. Some systemic medications (e.g. minocycline and doxycycline) can cause extrinsic staining.

Orange stain is believed to be caused by chromogenic bacteria such as *Serratia marcescens* and *Flavobacterium lutescens*. Similar effects can result from prolonged antimicrobial exposure or from chromic acid fumes.

Green stain is most common in children with poor oral hygiene, and may result from breakdown of blood pigment after gingival haemorrhage, or from chromogenic micro-organisms such as Penicillium and Aspergillus species. Mercury and lead dust can cause a blue-green stain; copper and nickel, green to blue-green stain. Copper-containing mouthwashes may have similar effect.

Black stain is of unknown aetiology and is unusual in that it seems to be associated, by an unknown mechanism, with caries-resistance. It is seen in clean mouths. Black-staining of teeth is also carried out deliberately for cosmetic reasons in some communities. The Si La ethnic peoples from Laos and Vietnam paint their teeth; women paint their teeth black and the men paint their teeth red. Silver nitrate can stain black. Potassium permanganate mouthwash can produce a violet-black stain.

In contrast, many people in the West strive for white teeth, and bleach them to try to achieve this.

### Clinical features

Superficial tooth discolouration is typically seen where plaque accumulates—mainly on the interproximal and cervical surfaces, and in pits and fissures—and is more likely to appear where oral hygiene is poor or where coloured foods/drinks are taken.

### Diagnosis

Clinical. The Nathoo classification system describes three types of extrinsic dental stain as follows:

- N1: coloured material (chromogen) binds to tooth surfaces. The chromogen colour is similar to that of stains caused by tea, coffee, wine, chromogenic bacteria and metals.
- N2: coloured material changes colour after binding to the tooth. The stains are N1-type food stains that darken with time.
- N3: colourless material or prechromogen binds to the tooth and undergoes a chemical reaction to cause a stain. These include carbohydrate-rich foods (e.g. apples and potatoes), stannous fluoride and chlorhexidine.

### Management

Tooth cleansing; extrinsic staining can be cleaned away by dental staff.

### Intrinsic tooth discolouration

The primary dentition is generally whiter than the permanent dentition. Younger people characteristically have lighter teeth, but teeth tend to darken with age partly because of the laying down of secondary dentine, and gradual enamel loss. Teeth are typically composed of a number of colours and there is in an individual tooth a gradation of colour from the gingival margin, which often has a darker appearance because of the close approximation of the dentine below the enamel, to the incisal edge. Canine teeth are generally darker than incisors. Intrinsic tooth staining is uncommon (Figs 2.10.9–2.10.32). Pink, brown or black discolouration of a single tooth is most common and usually arises because the tooth is non-vital, heavily filled or carious. The brown colour of caries is possibly due to the formation of Maillard pigments (reaction between proteins and small aldehydes from cariogenic bacteria), melanins, lipofuscins and uptake of various food colours and bacterial pigments. Dental materials that can cause intrinsic discolouration include eugenol, formocresol, root canal sealers and polyantimicrobial pastes. Enamel erosion can lead to a yellow tooth discolouration. In patients with anorexia or bulimia, a yellow discolouration often appears on lingual tooth surfaces where the acid reflux material makes contact with the teeth. The discolouration of teeth following severe trauma is due to the accumulation of haemoglobin or other haematin molecules

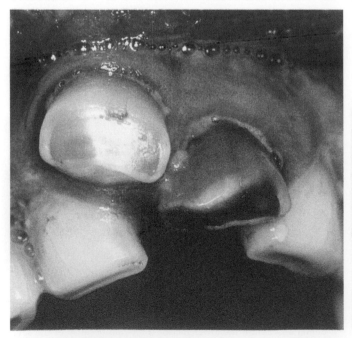

*Figure 2.10.9* Trauma causing the incisor to lose vitality and darken.

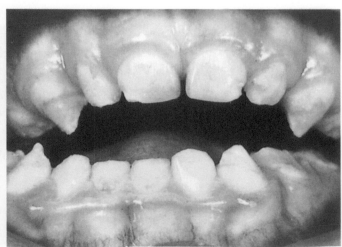

*Figure 2.10.10* Amelogenesis imperfecta in the primary dentition.

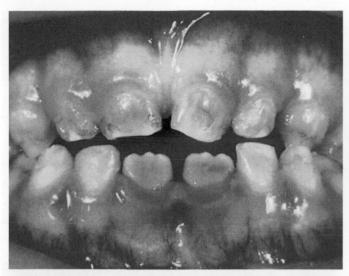

Figure 2.10.11 Amelogenesis imperfecta in the primary dentition of a sibling on patient in Figure 2.10.10.

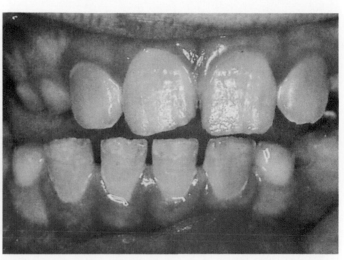

Figure 2.10.12 Amelogenesis imperfecta of the hereditary enamel hypoplasia type.

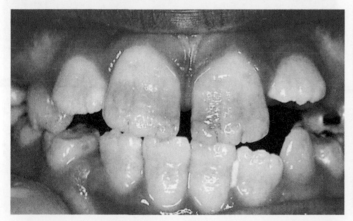

Figure 2.10.13 Amelogenesis imperfecta of the hereditary enamel hypoplasia type.

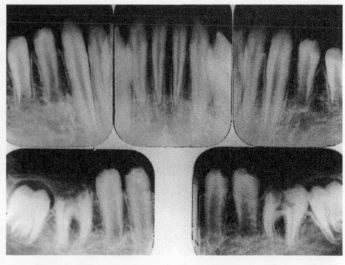

Figure 2.10.14 Amelogenesis imperfecta of the hereditary enamel hypoplasia type.

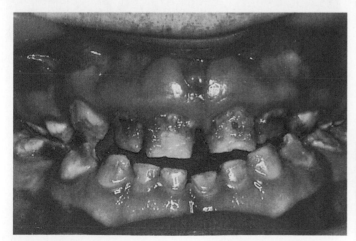

Figure 2.10.15 Amelogenesis imperfecta of the hereditary enamel hypocalcification type.

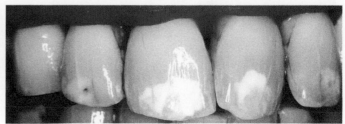

Figure 2.10.16 Amelogenesis imperfecta—snow-capped incisors.

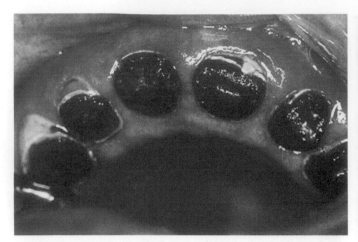

*Figure 2.10.17* Caries.

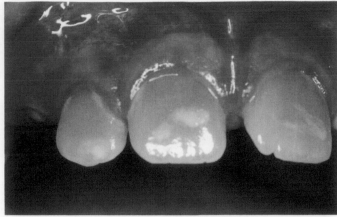

*Figure 2.10.18* Dentinogenesis imperfecta.

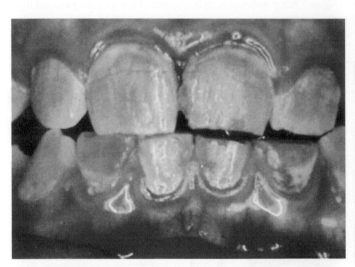

*Figure 2.10.19* Dentinogenesis imperfecta type 1.

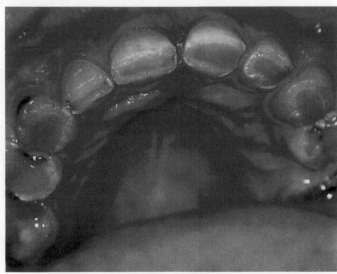

*Figure 2.10.20* Dentinogenesis imperfecta.

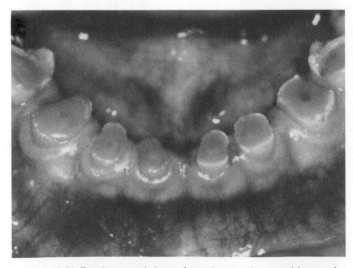

*Figure 2.10.21* Dentinogenesis imperfecta showing how attrition can be severe.

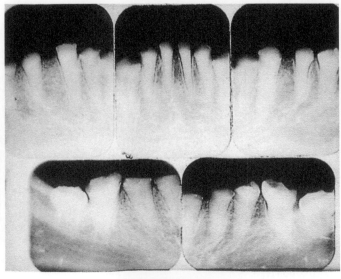

*Figure 2.10.22* Dentinogenesis imperfecta showing pulpal obliteration.

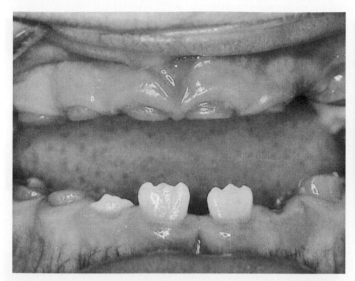

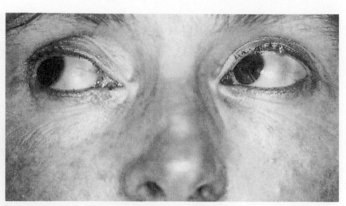

*Figure 2.10.24* Dentinogenesis imperfecta may be associated with osteogenesis imperfecta—showing here as blue sclerae.

*Figure 2.10.23* Dentinogenesis imperfecta type II showing the more profound abnormality in the deciduous dentition.

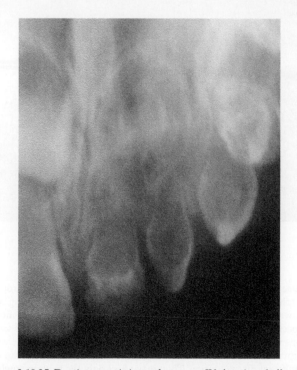

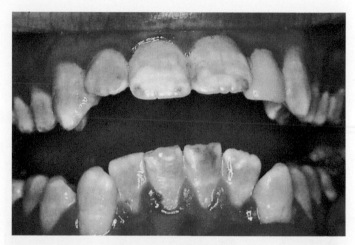

*Figure 2.10.26* Fluorosis.

*Figure 2.10.25* Dentinogenesis imperfecta type IV showing shell teeth.

and may disappear in 2–3 months if the tooth becomes revascularized. The discolouration related to dental amalgam restorations appears due to the contained tin leaching into the dentine. Occasionally tooth resorption may produce pink discolouration.

Generalized intrinsic tooth staining can arise mainly where there is a congenital or systemic cause operative during odontogenesis. Brown discolouration can be caused by tetracyclines (Chapter 1.6). Blue or brown discolouration may occur with alkaptonuria due to the build up of homogentisic acid. Erythroblastosis fetalis and biliary atresia may

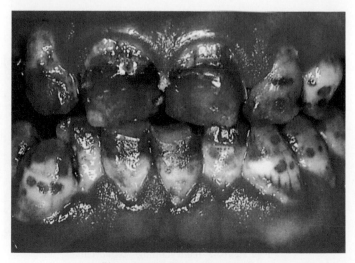

*Figure 2.10.27* Fluorosis (severe).

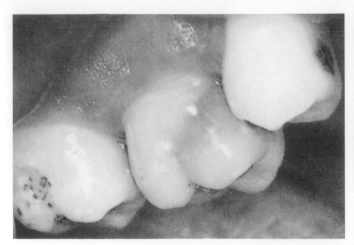

Figure 2.10.28 Internal resorption—pink spot.

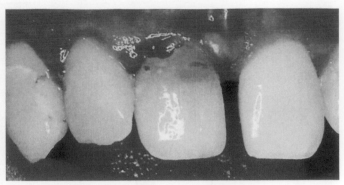

Figure 2.10.29 External resorption.

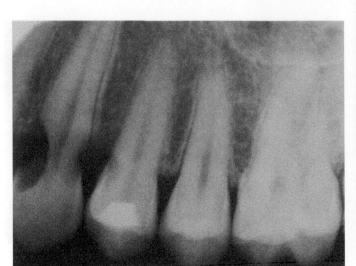

Figure 2.10.30 External resorption.

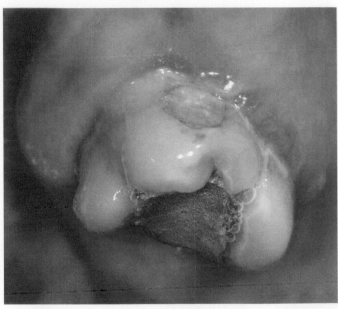

Figure 2.10.31 Trauma—cracked tooth.

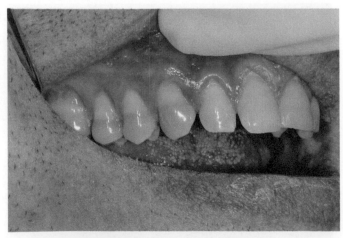

Figure 2.10.32 Teeth staining—tetracycline.

cause green teeth from biliverdin deposition. Congenital erythropoietic porphyria causes porphyrins to be deposited in teeth, causing a red-brown colouration. Generalized pink staining can arise post-mortem, especially after carbon monoxide poisoning. Pink and red discolourations may also be seen in patients with lepromatous leprosy.

Enamel and dentine defects of genetic origin are rare but can cause significant discolouration. They may affect only the teeth in amelogenesis imperfecta (enamel defective) or dentinogenesis imperfecta (dentine defective), but the latter may also be associated with osteogenesis imperfecta. In dentinogenesis imperfecta, newly erupted teeth may appear brownish and translucent—an appearance also seen in some patients with osteogenesis imperfecta.

Tooth hypoplasia and discolouration is only part of the disorder in rare conditions such as epidermolysis bullosa dystrophica and Ehlers–Danlos syndrome.

Generalized intrinsic tooth staining can arise from excessive fluoride ingestion during early life (fluorosis)—with white enamel opacities and sometimes yellow or brown discolouration. With the exception of those

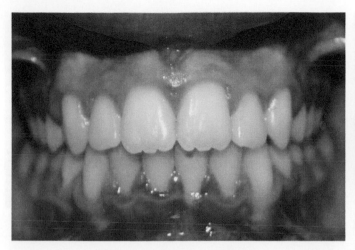

*Figure 2.10.33*  Class 1 occlusion.

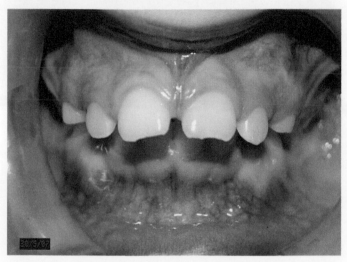

*Figure 2.10.35*  Class 2 division 1 malocclusion.

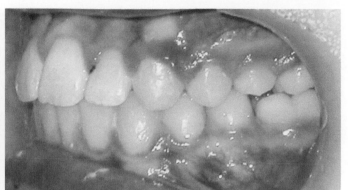

*Figure 2.10.34*  Class 1 occlusion.

parts of the world where water supplies contain very high levels of fluoride (e.g. parts of the Middle East, India and Africa), this is most often extremely mild. Fluorosis varies in severity:

- Mildest form: white flecks or spotting or diffuse cloudiness in the mildest form may not produce a cosmetic defect.
- More severe form: yellow-brown or darker patches. Mottling of the enamel may be seen where the fluoride in drinking water exceeds about 2 ppm or excess fluoride is taken via other sources.
- Most severe form: opacity and yellow-brown or darker brown patches, and white staining and pitting of the entire enamel.

### Internal resorption

In internal resorption (pink spot) dentine is spontaneously resorbed from within and the pulp granulation tissue shows through the enamel and is eventually exposed.

### External resorption

Resorption may progress from the external surface, eventually to involve the pulp. Possible causes include unerupted teeth, cysts and tumours.

*Clinical features*

Intrinsic tooth discolouration, unless caused by caries (or a restoration) or trauma, often affects all surfaces of many or all of the teeth, or occurs in bands.

*Diagnosis*

Clinical; intrinsic staining does not reduce with professional cleaning.

*Management*

Intrinsic staining may be ameliorated by tooth bleaching or other cosmetic dental procedures, or restorative procedures such as veneers or crowns.

### Malocclusion

*Aetiopathogenesis*

A wide spectrum of disorders can give rise to malocclusion. These range from congenital disease such as cleft palate and associated disorders, to genetically mediated abnormal skeletal growth ('the long face', 'the short face') and local disorders such as the presence of odontomes and habits such as thumb sucking.

*Clinical features*

These are highly variable and reflect the underlying cause (Figs 2.10.33–2.10.45). Mandibular retrusion produces a typical bird face. Mandibular protrusion (class III malocclusion) shows the Hapsburg chin, the teeth often show reverse overjet with the upper incisors occluding lingual to the lowers. Another form of malocclusion is open bite—the posterior teeth are in occlusion but the incisors fail to meet. Anterior open bites may be caused by increased height of the lower face, tongue posture, dentoalveolar factors, trauma or thumb sucking. The upper lateral incisors are also congenitally absent in this patient. Finally, the permanent canine normally erupts slightly later than the premolar and lateral incisor and, if there is lack of space in the dental arch (dentoalveolar disproportion), it is crowded out. Second premolars and third molars are the other teeth that may suffer this fate. Any of these teeth, especially lower third molars, may then impact.

*Diagnosis*

The diagnosis is usually based upon the clinical and radiological features. There may also be a need for clinical genetic and surgical expertise.

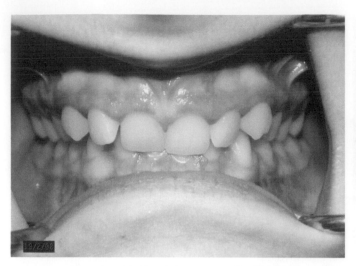

*Figure 2.10.36* Class 2 division 2 malocclusion.

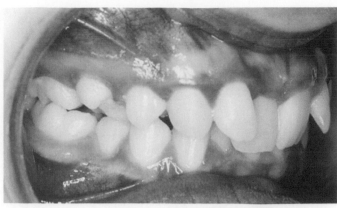

*Figure 2.10.37* Class 2 molars.

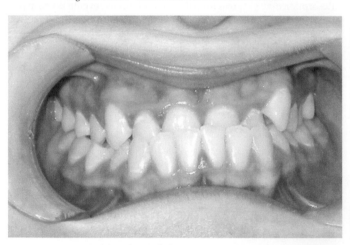

*Figure 2.10.38* Class 3.

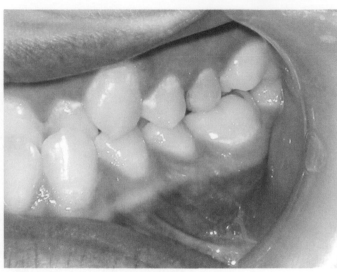

*Figure 2.10.39* Class 3 molars.

*Management*

Treatment of malocclusion usually requires referral to specialists in orthodontics, and sometimes also maxillofacial surgical teams.

# EARLY TOOTH LOSS

Early tooth loss usually has an obvious cause such as trauma (in sports, assaults or other injuries, extraction as a result of dental caries) or for orthodontic reasons or, in adults, periodontal disease.

Unexplained early tooth loss in children or adults may be a feature in non-accidental injury or immune defects (e.g. Down syndrome, diabetes mellitus and HIV/AIDS), or rare conditions such as eosinophilic granuloma, hypophosphatasia or cathepsin C deficiency (this includes Papillon–Lefevre syndrome, palmo-plantar hyperkeratosis or leukocyte adhesion defects).

# ERUPTION DISORDERS

## Ankylosis

*Aetiopathogenesis*

Deciduous molars may be retained in infraocclusion and ankylosed ('submerged') because the permanent successor is absent. Teeth that are

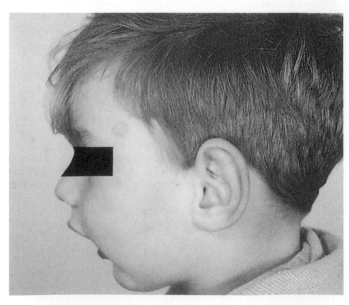

*Figure 2.10.40* Malocclusion—bird face of mandibular retrusion.

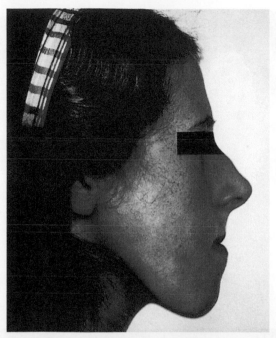

*Figure 2.10.41* Malocclusion—Hapsburg chin of mandibular prognathism.

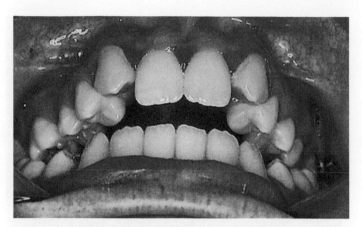

*Figure 2.10.42* Malocclusion—open bite.

### Diagnosis
Clinical features plus radiological investigation. The latter will demonstrate whether there a permanent successor is absent.

### Management
The affected tooth is usually extracted, and there may be a need for orthodontic and restorative treatment.

### Early tooth eruption
Teeth, mainly in the mandibular central incisor region, may erupt prematurely and be present at birth (natal teeth) or appear within the first few days or weeks of life (neonatal teeth). This rare event is usually of unknown cause. Occasionally there is a familial or obvious genetic basis: the Tlinget Indians in Alaska show a high prevalence.

There are correlations between natal teeth and various syndromes (e.g. Jadassohn–Lewandowsky–syndrome, Ellis–van Creveld syndrome, Hallermann–Streiff syndrome). Environmental factors, especially polychlorinated biphenyls (PCB) appear to increase the incidence of natal teeth.

Such teeth occasionally cause ulceration of the infant's tongue or mother's nipple but usually they can best be safely left *in situ* since they are part of the normal series and are not additional teeth.

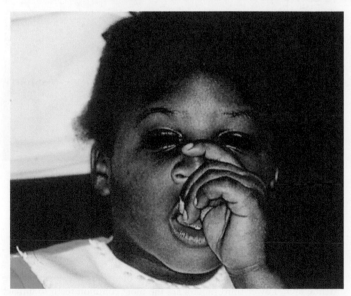

*Figure 2.10.43* Malocclusion—the thumb habit.

single-standing molars are often ankylosed as are those that are hypercementosed (Fig. 2.10.46).

### Clinical features
Ankylosis often affects second primary molars. The tooth becomes gradually infraoccluded, and occasionally can become covered by gingival tissue. The adjacent permanent teeth may tip into the resultant space.

### Failed or late tooth eruption
Teeth missing from the normal series may have failed to erupt usually because of tooth impaction, or they may have failed to develop (hypodontia), or rarely because of systemic disease. A delay in tooth eruption of up to 12 months may be of little or no significance in an otherwise healthy child.

Localized delayed eruption often arises from impaction due to local factors such as obstruction from a tooth in the path of eruption or insufficient space in the dental arch, or dental infection. Ectopic positioning and impaction most often affect the third molar, second premolar and canines, perhaps because these are the last teeth normally to erupt.

More generalized delay in eruption is rare but can be associated with a variety of systemic causes, such as Down syndrome, or cleidocranial dysplasia, or may be due to damage from irradiation or chemotherapy.

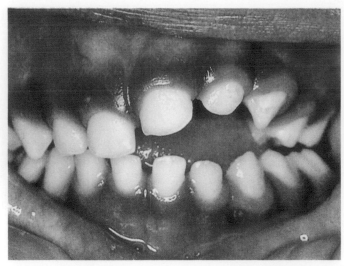

*Figure 2.10.44* Malocclusion—open bite from thumb habit as in Figure 2.10.43.

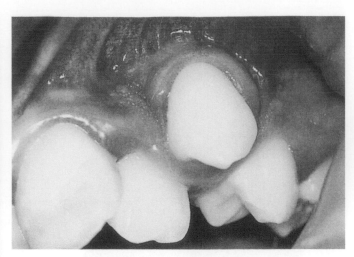

*Figure 2.10.45* Malocclusion—tooth crowding.

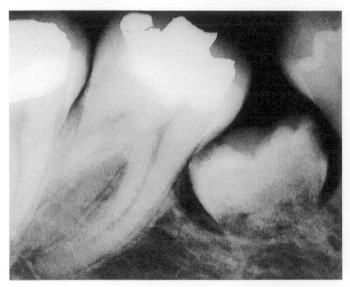

*Figure 2.10.46* Ankylosis (infraocclusion or submergence).

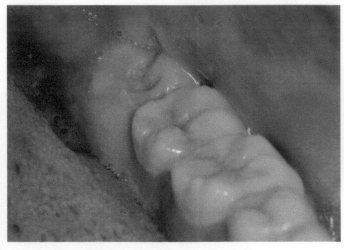

*Figure 2.10.47* Impacted partially erupted third molar.

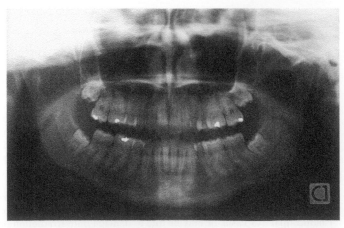

*Figure 2.10.48* Unerupted third molars.

## Impaction

### Aetiopathogenesis

Teeth impact (fail to erupt fully) because of insufficient space in the dental arch. Lower third molars are the most common teeth to impact (Figs 2.10.47 and 2.10.48). Canines, second premolars and second molars, as well as other teeth may also impact.

### Clinical features

Impacted teeth are often asymptomatic. There is no evidence they contribute to malocclusion but occasionally they may cause pain (from caries or pericoronitis), or are the site of dentigerous cyst formation.

### Diagnosis

Clinical and imaging.

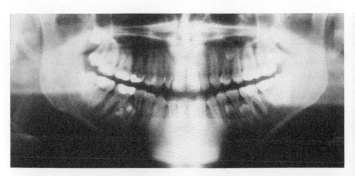

*Figure 2.10.49* Hyperdontia—several supernumerary teeth.

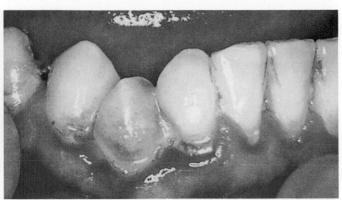

*Figure 2.10.50* Hyperdontia.

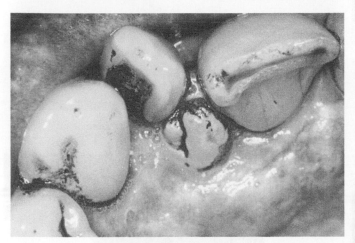

*Figure 2.10.51* Hyperdontia.

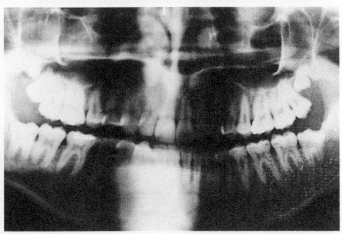

*Figure 2.10.52* Hyperdontia (supplemental molars).

*Management*
Orthodontics and sometimes surgery.

### Pericoronitis
Pericoronitis (Chapter 2.5).

### Teething
Tooth eruption may be associated with irritability, disturbed sleep, cheek flushing, drooling, sometimes a small rise in temperature and/or a circumoral rash but does not cause diarrhoea, or bronchitis (these may occur coincidentally).

## TOOTH NUMBER VARIATIONS
### Hyperdontia
Hyperdontia (additional teeth).

When normal permanent teeth erupt before the deciduous incisors have exfoliated (i.e. the mixed dentition), it is not uncommon to see what appear to be two rows of teeth in the lower incisor region, particularly when there is inadequate space to accommodate the larger permanent teeth. The situation usually resolves as primary incisors are lost and the mandible grows.

Additional teeth are uncommon (in 0.8% of primary dentitions and in 2.1% of permanent dentitions) but often occur alone in otherwise healthy individuals. They are more common in the relatives of affected people than in the general population.

Multiple additional teeth are typically seen in association with cleft lip/palate, cleidocranial dysplasia or rare syndromes such as Apert, Crouzon, Ehlers–Danlos, Gardner and Sturge–Weber syndromes.

Additional teeth may be of normal morphology (supplemental) but are more often small and/or conical, or tuberculate (Figs 2.10.49–2.10.53).

Additional teeth of normal form (supplemental teeth) are uncommon. Of unknown cause, they are most frequently seen in the maxillary lateral incisor region, sometimes in the premolar and third molar regions. Extra maxillary molars are sometimes termed distodens.

Most other additional teeth are conical and seen in the maxillary midline where they may remain unerupted and may cause a permanent incisor to impact (mesiodens). Although a mesiodens may erupt, sometimes it is inverted.

Tuberculate supernumeraries are uncommon, often paired, usually located palatal to the central incisors and they rarely erupt and so are frequently associated with delayed eruption of the incisors.

Additional teeth often erupt in an abnormal position and may cause malocclusion, occasionally impede tooth eruption, or, rarely, are the site of dentigerous cyst formation. Removal of the supernumerary tooth is usually recommended where:

- a central incisor has been displaced, or eruption delayed or inhibited;
- there is associated pathology;

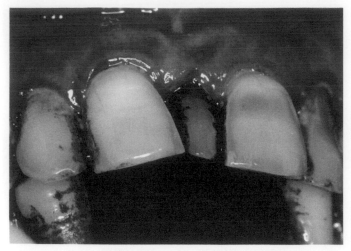

*Figure 2.10.53* Hyperdontia—mesiodens which is non-vital and discoloured, and all teeth are stained by betel use. Lower incisors have been lost because of periodontitis.

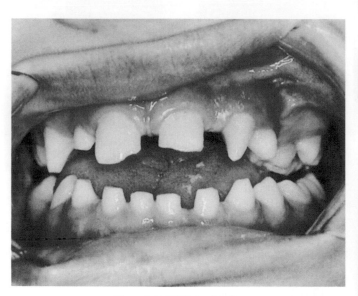

*Figure 2.10.54* Hypodontia.

• active treatment envisaged includes orthodontic alignment of an incisor in close proximity to the supernumerary; secondary alveolar bone grafting is needed in cleft lip and palate patients; the supernumerary is present in bone designated for implant placement.

## Hypodontia

Teeth missing from the normal series may have failed to erupt, may have been lost prematurely or may have failed to develop—hypodontia.

Hypodontia is the term used when some teeth have failed to develop and the germ is not present on radiography (used more specifically when less than six teeth apart from third molars are missing).

Oligodontia is the term also used when some teeth have failed to develop but is usually used when there are more extreme numbers absent (more than six teeth).

### Table 2.10.2 DENTAL RADIOGRAPHIC FINDINGS AT VARIOUS AGES

| Age (years) | Should be visible on radiography |
| --- | --- |
| Birth | All primary teeth |
| | Crypts of first molars |
| 2 | Crowns of premolars and second molars |
| 6 | Crowns of all permanent teeth except third molars |
| 18 | All permanent teeth |

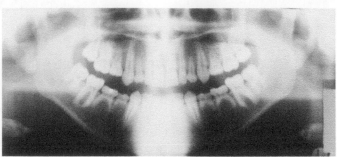

*Figure 2.10.55* Hypodontia—missing premolars.

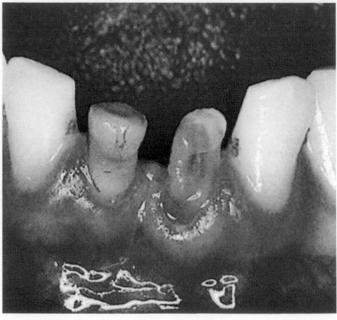

*Figure 2.10.56* Hypodontia—the retained deciduous incisors have been worn down and become non-vital.

Anodontia is the term used when all teeth have failed to develop. Anodontia is rare, and typically seen in ectodermal dysplasia.

Table 2.10.2 shows approximate ages at which tooth elements are visible on radiographs.

Hypodontia is not uncommon: non-syndromic hypodontia affects the permanent dentition in 2–8% of the population, while non-syndromic oligodontia affects about 0.1%. Hypodontia is more common in the second dentition but, where it affects the primary dentition, the permanent dentition is usually also affected (Figs 2.10.54–2.10.60).

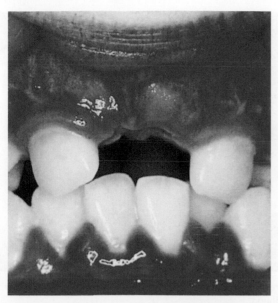

*Figure 2.10.57* Hypodontia.

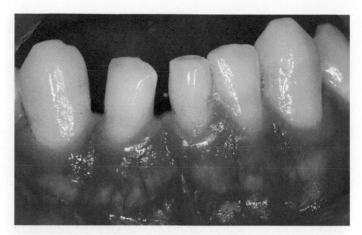

*Figure 2.10.58* Hypodontia.

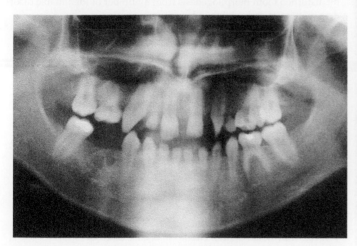

*Figure 2.10.59* Hypodontia.

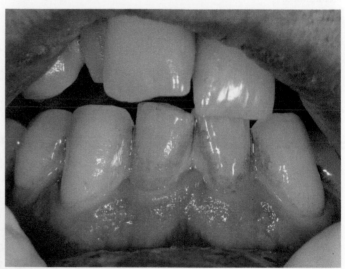

*Figure 2.10.60* Hypodontia.

Hypodontia most often affects permanent third molars; up to 10–30% of the population may miss these teeth. After that, incisor–premolar hypodontia is most common, affecting mainly, mandibular second premolars and then maxillary lateral incisors. Maxillary second premolars and maxillary and mandibular first molars and canines are then affected.

Hypodontia is usually seen in otherwise apparently healthy people. However, it can also be a feature of local growth disorders such as after radiotherapy to the area, chemotherapy or thalidomide exposure, in cleft palate or in several systemic disorders (e.g. ectodermal dysplasia, incontinentia pigmenti and syndromes such as Crouzon, Down, Ehlers–Danlos and Gorlin). Genes MSX1 and PAX9 are associated with some familial cases. Hypodontia in other families has been associated with epithelial ovarian cancer and those with gene *AXIN2* mutations with colorectal cancer.

Hypodontia is often associated with retention of the deciduous predecessor, and may be associated with delayed eruption, reduction in size of teeth, ectopic teeth, short roots, taurodontism, tooth rotation or hypocalcification.

# TOOTH SIZE, SHAPE AND STRUCTURAL ANOMALIES

A variety of local and generalized factors may act during the period of tooth formation and/or mineralization. Although tooth development in utero is generally well protected, it may be affected by maternal disease and intrauterine infection, and by systemic disturbance during early life.

### Enamel hypoplasia

Tooth abnormalities caused during tooth development have long-lasting effects with inadequate enamel formation causing hypoplasia, with pits or fissures in the teeth. Enamel and dentine do not regenerate after they mineralize initially, so the defects are permanent.

Enamel hypoplasia affecting multiple deciduous teeth is rare but may be seen as genetic disorders (amelogenesis imperfecta; dentinogenesis

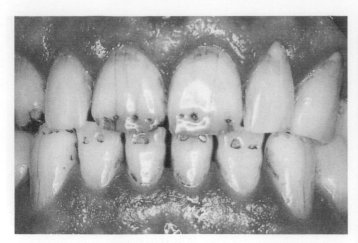

*Figure 2.10.61* Enamel hypoplasia due to developmental disturbance in childhood.

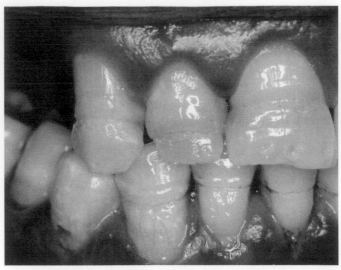

*Figure 2.10.62* Enamel hypoplasia due to developmental disturbance in childhood.

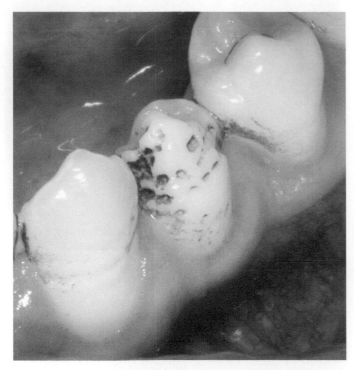

*Figure 2.10.63* Turner tooth in chronic granulomatous disease.

imperfecta), in intrauterine infections such as rubella, or in metabolic disturbances such as jaundice, producing a linear pattern of defects corresponding to the site of amelogenesis at the time ('chronological' hypoplasia).

Enamel hypoplasia affecting multiple permanent teeth is more common since systemic disturbances are especially common during the first year of life, and defects then usually affect the tips of permanent incisors and canines. It arises from influences affecting the developing dentition and often also causes tooth discolouration (Figs 2.10.61–2.10.63). Between birth and six years of age, the permanent teeth, particularly those of cosmetic importance, may be damaged. Enamel hypoplasia may appear in the absence of any identifiable cause but may be caused

by disturbed tooth morphogenesis from a number of identifiable disorders in utero or early childhood, such as:

- amelogenesis imperfecta
- chemotherapy involving developing dentition
- cleidocranial dysplasia
- congenital hypoparathyroidism
- Down and other syndromes
- endocrinopathies (especially hypoparathyroidism)
- epidermolysis bullosa
- intrauterine infections (e.g. syphilis)
- jaundice (kernicterus-neonatal hyperbilirubinaemia; or biliary atresia)
- neonatal hypoxia or hypocalcaemia
- nephrotic syndrome
- prematurity
- radiotherapy involving developing dentition
- severe fluorosis
- severe infections
- severe nutritional deficiencies (as in coeliac disease)
- trauma or infection of developing teeth
- vitamin D resistant rickets (hypophosphataemia).

Molar–incisor hypoplasia may result from PCB/dioxin exposure; there is weak evidence for the role of nutrition, birth and neonatal factors, and acute or chronic childhood illness/treatment; and very weak evidence to implicate fluoride or breastfeeding. Enamel hypoplasia of single permanent teeth (Turner tooth) is uncommon and typically caused usually by disturbed odontogenesis from periapical infection of a deciduous predecessor. Malformed lower premolars secondary to periapical infection of their deciduous predecessors are not uncommon, especially mandibular (Fig 2.10.63). Upper permanent incisors may show defects as a consequence of trauma to the primary predecessor. The crown is opaque, yellow-brown and hypoplastic.

### Cusps or tubercules

Cusp of Carabelli is an anatomical variant—a palatal cusp on the upper first molar (Fig. 2.10.64). Teeth are occasionally malformed with a large palatal cusp, to the extent that they have a talon cusp configuration (Fig. 2.10.65).

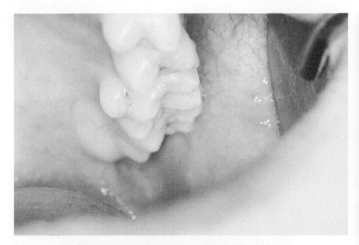

*Figure 2.10.64* Carabelli cusp.

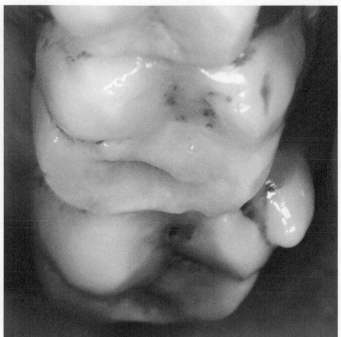

*Figure 2.10.65* Paramolar.

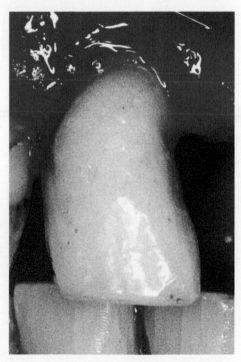

*Figure 2.10.66* Dilacerations.

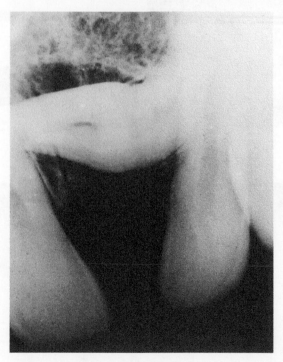

*Figure 2.10.67* Dilaceration.

## Dilaceration

Trauma to a developing tooth may produce distortion and dilaceration—a bend (Figs 2.10.66 and 2.10.67).

## Microdontia

Microdontia (small teeth) is largely genetic and is common in patients with hypodontia, and in Down syndrome. Microdontia most often affects lateral incisors which also are conical or peg-shaped (Figs 2.10.68 and 2.10.69). All teeth, however, especially third molars, may genetically vary in size, form and structure.

## Macrodontia

Macrodontia (large teeth).

Teeth larger than normal (megadont) are uncommon (Figs 2.10.70–2.10.72). They may be seen in hemifacial hyperplasia.

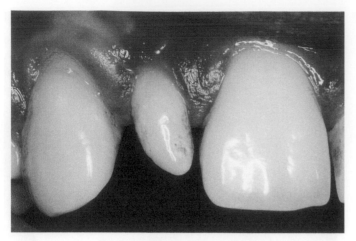

*Figure 2.10.68* Peg-shaped tooth.

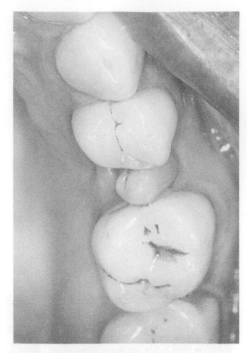

*Figure 2.10.69* Peg-shaped tooth.

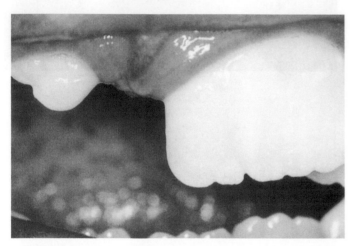

*Figure 2.10.70* Fusion.

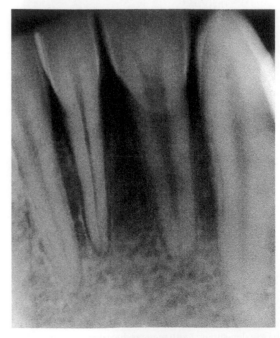

*Figure 2.10.71* Fusion.

Double teeth may result from the fusion of two teeth and occur most often in the primary dentition, when they are likely to be followed by extra tooth elements in the succeeding permanent dentition.

**Odontomes**

Odontomes (this chapter).

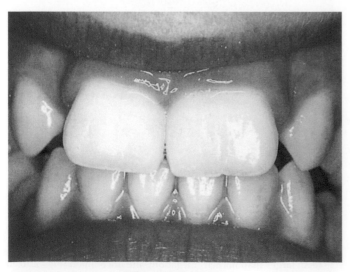

*Figure 2.10.72* Fusion.

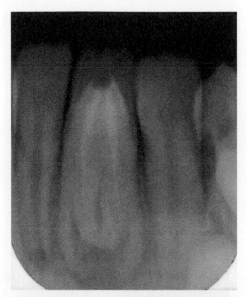

*Figure 2.10.73* Odontome—dilated invaginated.

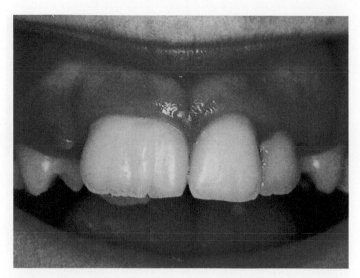

*Figure 2.10.74* Odontome—geminated.

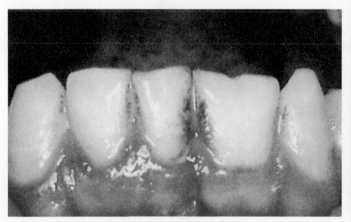

*Figure 2.10.75* Odontome.

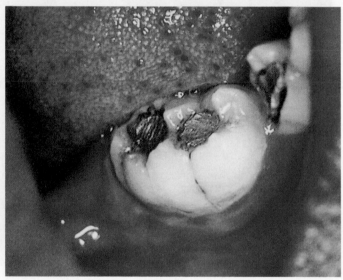

*Figure 2.10.76* Odontome—double tooth.

## Hypercementosis and cementoma

Cementum is normally deposited on tooth roots throughout life to compensate for occlusal wear. An excess of such physiological deposition is termed 'hypercementosis', commonly caused by chronic periapical infection, a functionless tooth, a reaction to increased stress on the tooth or Paget disease. Hypercementosis is often symptomless and cause complications only during exodontia. It should be differentiated from cementoblastoma.

A cementoma is when cementum is deposited neoplastically, lesions including:

- benign cementoblastoma
- gigantiform cementoma
- periapical cemental dysplasia
- cementifying fibroma.

## Dens invaginatus

Dens invaginatus arises because, during odontogenesis, a portion of the enamel organ protrudes, or invaginates, into the dental papilla. The resultant affected and distorted tooth (dilated odontome) contains a cavity that is completely or partially lined by enamel, radiographically resembling a tooth within a tooth (dens in dente) (Figs 2.10.73–2.10.80). The degree of invagination may be mild to severe, presents as a small pit on the palatal surface of the affected tooth, and the defect collects plaque and food debris, as a result of which there is often caries and consequently pulpitis and periapical infection.

Dens invaginatus occurs in children and adolescents, shows no gender predilection, commonly affects teeth of the permanent dentition (usually the upper lateral incisor or an upper anterior tooth) and is not infrequently bilateral.

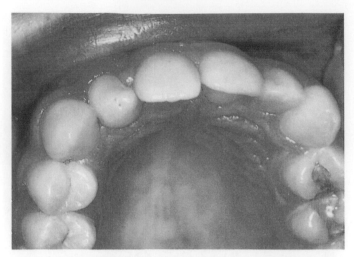

*Figure 2.10.77* Odontome—dilated invaginated.

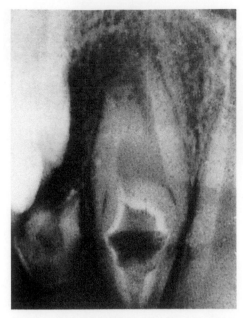

*Figure 2.10.78* Odontome—dilated invaginated.

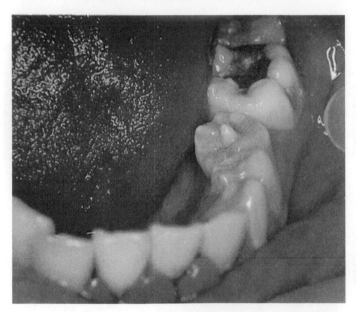

*Figure 2.10.79* Odontome—evaginated.

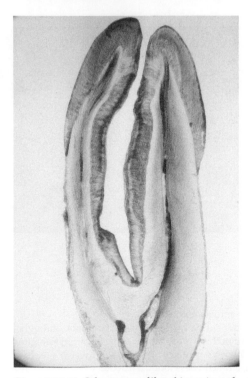

*Figure 2.10.80* Odontome—dilated invaginated.

Routine conservation is adequate for mild defects but, in more severe cases, particularly where there is pulpitis or periapical infection, extraction is needed.

### Dens evaginatus
Dens evaginatus causes a nodule on the occlusal surface. It is most common in Mongoloid races.

### Dentinoma
Dentinoma is a focal deposit of dentine or osteodentine overlying the crown of unerupted mandibular molar teeth in young adults. The lesions are usually asymptomatic and appear as chance findings, as opacities on radiographic examination.

### Enamel clefts
Enamel cleft is a small cleft at the tooth cervical margin (Fig. 2.10.81).

### Enamel pearls
Enamel pearls (enamelomas) are small enamel deposits between the roots of the first permanent molars (Fig. 2.10.82).

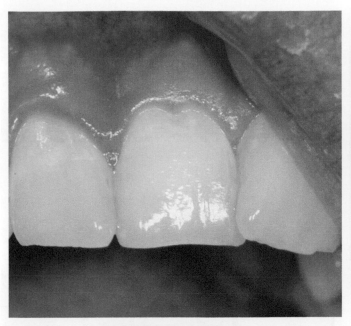

*Figure 2.10.81* Enamel cleft.

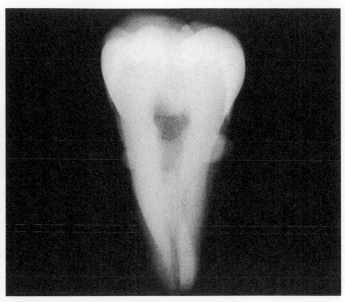

*Figure 2.10.82* Enamel pearl.

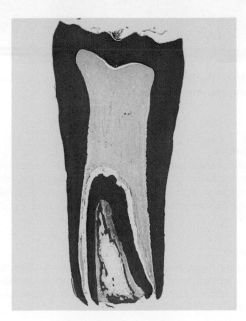

*Figure 2.10.83* Taurodont.

Taurodont teeth are genetically determined with an enlarged pulp chamber and a more inferiorly placed root furcation in posterior teeth, resulting in a long crown and short roots. Taurodontism is generally most obvious in molars and premolars of both deciduous and permanent dentitions, and may be found in single or several teeth. Lack of constriction of the tooth at the neck may be suggestive of taurodontism but they are most easily diagnosed on radiographs (Fig. 2.10.83).

Taurodontism is genetically determined. Most studies have shown an overall prevalence of the order of 2% with no sex predilection, but oriental people and some other racial groups are especially affected. Taurodontism occurs in syndromes, particularly in those having an ectodermal defect. Taurodontism may be associated with hypodontia, the tricho-dento-osseous syndrome and syndromes with additional X chromosomes such as Klinefelter (XXY) and XXX, as well as some other chromosomal anomalies.

## TOOTH SURFACE LOSS

Teeth may be damaged mainly by dental caries or trauma, but abfraction, abrasion, attrition and erosion may also cause tooth surface loss. Any of the dental tissues can be affected and often, more than one of these causes is at play.

### Abfraction

Abfraction may be the loss of tooth structure from flexural forces which separate enamel rods especially at the amelocemental junction and lead to tooth hypersensitivity.

### Abrasion

*Aetiopathogenesis*

Abrasion is tooth surface loss caused by mechanical forces from a foreign element, such as from a habit such as toothbrushing with a hard brush and coarse dentifrice, which may abrade the neck of the tooth.

### Geminated odontome

Geminated odontome is a large abnormal tooth seen mainly anteriorly that is composed of two joined teeth, resulting either from partial division of a tooth germ, or from the fusion of adjacent tooth germs. The crowns may be separate or divided by a groove; the roots may be fused or separate.

### Taurodontism

Taurodontism ('bull like' teeth).

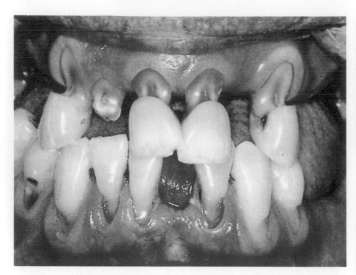

*Figure 2.10.84* Tooth surface loss—abrasion.

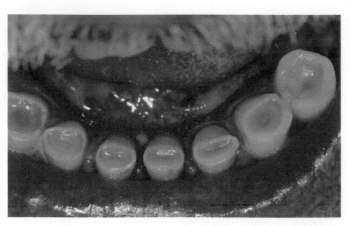

*Figure 2.10.86* Tooth surface loss—severe attrition.

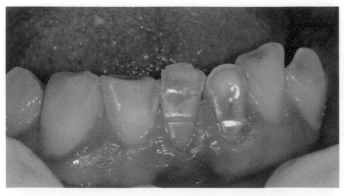

*Figure 2.10.88* Tooth surface loss—attrition.

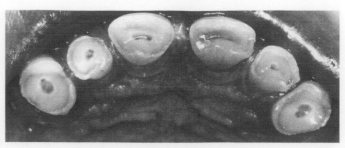

*Figure 2.10.85* Tooth surface loss—attrition.

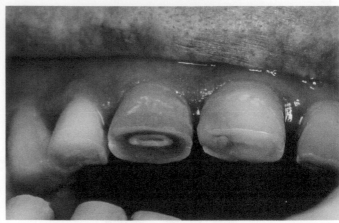

*Figure 2.10.87* Tooth surface loss—attrition with pulp exposure causing the incisor to become non-vital.

*Clinical features*
The gingiva recedes but is otherwise healthy. The cementum and dentine wear but the harder enamel survives, resulting in a notch, and it can lead to exposure of dentine, and, therefore, sensitivity to hot and cold. There may in extreme cases be eventual tooth fracture (Fig. 2.10.84).
*Diagnosis*
Clinical.

*Management*
Desensitizing toothpastes are available but dental attention may be needed. Soft brushes and silica-based toothpastes are less abrasive than those with calcium carbonate or aluminium trihydrate bases. Restorative dentistry may be required.

**Attrition**
*Aetiopathogenesis*
Attrition is the mechanical wearing down of tooth surfaces by tooth–tooth contact. The wearing away of tooth biting (occlusal) surfaces by mastication is most obvious where there is excessive occlusal forces/movements such as in a parafunctional habit such as bruxism (seen especially in profound vegetative states, Rett syndrome or Fragile X syndrome), where the diet is particularly coarse as in some unrefined diets, or where the teeth are of less strong composition such as amelogenesis imperfecta or dentinogenesis imperfecta. Interproximal attrition is less common.

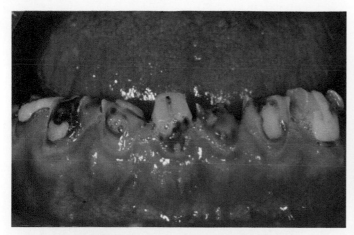

Figure 2.10.89 Tooth surface loss—attrition.

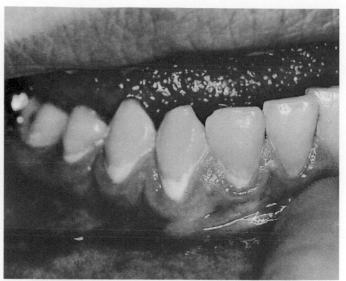

Figure 2.10.90 Caries—decalcification white lesions.

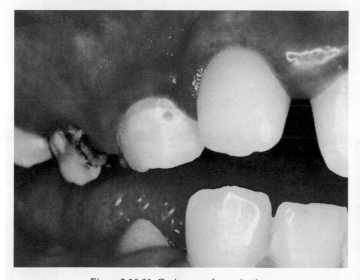

Figure 2.10.91 Caries—early cavitation.

## Clinical features

The incisal edges, cusps and occlusal surfaces wear and there is more loss of dentine than enamel, leading to a flat or hollowed surface—a facet (Figs 2.10.85–2.10.89). Characteristically, opposing tooth facets will match perfectly in occlusion.

Unless attrition is rapid, the pulp is generally protected by obliteration with secondary dentine formation.

## Diagnosis
Clinical.

## Management
Restorative dentistry.

## Caries

### Aetiopathogenesis
Caries is one of the most prevalent oral diseases, a result of the activity of dental bacterial plaque. Fermentation of sucrose and other non-milk extrinsic sugars by plaque bacteria to lactic and other acids causes tooth decalcification and with proteolysis results in caries (decay). The main causal organisms are *Streptococcus mutans*.

### Clinical features
Decalcification beneath the bacterial plaque that accumulates in stagnation areas, such as within fissures of the occlusal surface or sites close to the gingival margin, produces an opaque whitish band (Figs 2.10.90–2.10.97). At this early stage, where there is no cavitation, the lesion is reversible if diet is changed and fermentable carbohydrates reduced or excluded. Fluoride aids remineralization. The carious enamel eventually breaks down to form a cavity, the enamel becomes undermined and caries progresses in dentine. Change in dietary habits (particularly a reduction in frequency of fermentable carbohydrate intake), fluoride treatment and improved oral hygiene can arrest the progress of caries.

Once caries reaches the dentine, pain may result on stimulation thermally or with sweet/sour. Pain may also occur when dentine is exposed by trauma, erosion or abrasion; this subsides within seconds of removing the stimulus, and may be poorly localized often only to an approximate area within 2–3 teeth adjacent to the affected tooth. The tooth should be restored, as untreated, caries can progress through dentine to the pulp which becomes inflamed (pulpitis). Within the rigid confines of the pulp chamber this produces severe persistent pain (toothache) and the pulp eventually undergoes necrosis when inflammation can spread around the tooth apex (apical periodontitis), eventually forming an abscess, granuloma or cyst (Chapter 2.8).

Only when the coronal pulp is widely exposed and there is a very good blood supply does the pulp survive trauma or infection, a situation that can occur in young persons, when the pulp becomes hyperplastic and epithelialized (hyperplastic pulpitis; pulp polyp).

Caries has been declining for some years, mainly because of the protective effect of fluoride but caries is now more prevalent in the disadvantaged and deprived, especially in pre-school children. Rampant caries, affecting mainly the upper incisors is typically seen in children using a sugar/fruit juice mix in a bottle to aid sleep at night. Xerostomia for any reason significantly predisposes to caries.

Caries protection is increased by improved oral hygiene but mainly by diet, fluorides and fissure sealants.

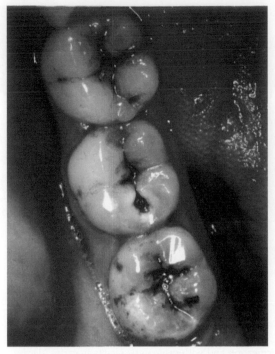

*Figure 2.10.92* Caries.

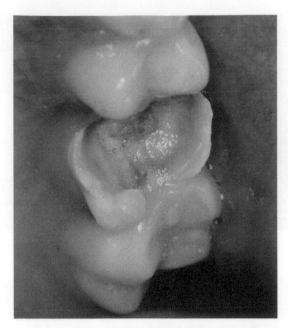

*Figure 2.10.93* Caries—with pulpal involvement.

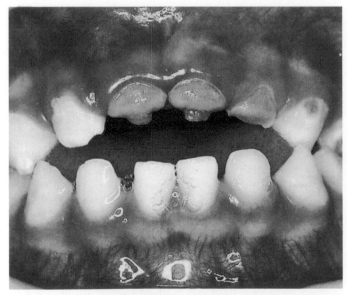

*Figure 2.10.94* Caries—rampant from using a sweetened bottle feeder.

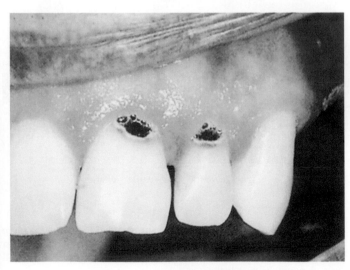

*Figure 2.10.95* Caries—arrested caries after diet change.

### Diet

Sugars, particularly non-milk sugars in items other than fresh fruits and vegetables, are the major dietary factors in caries aetiology. The frequency of intake is more important than the amount. Similarly the more sticky the sugary agent is, the greater the risk of caries.

Dietary advice should begin with emphasis on appropriate infant feeding and weaning practice. Drinks other than milk and water should not be given in feeding bottles and should be confined to main meals.

Children should be introduced to a cup at about 6 months and should have ceased using bottles by 1 year. Weaning foods should be free of or very low in sugars other than those present in fresh milk, raw fruits or vegetables. For older children and adults snack foods and drinks especially should be free of sugars. Because of the risk of erosion as well as of caries, frequent consumption of carbonated and cola type drinks should be discouraged. Grapefruit, apple, orange and other fruit juices can also cause tooth erosion. For children tap water and milk are preferred options.

Saliva buffers may counter plaque acids and thus chewing sugar-free gum or cheese after meals may be of value.

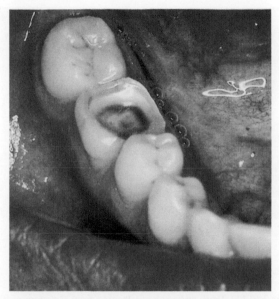

Figure 2.10.96 Caries—arrested caries after cusp has fractured.

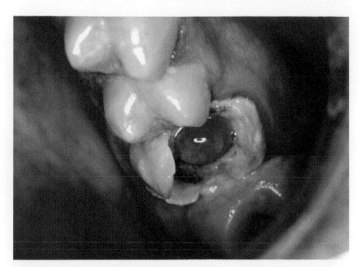

Figure 2.10.97 Pulp polyp.

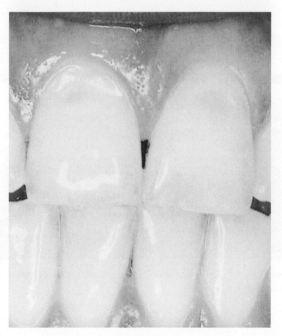

Figure 2.10.98 Tooth surface loss—erosion.

## Fluorides

Fluorides are protective against caries by reducing formation of plaque acids, inhibiting mineral loss, and promoting remineralization of decalcified tooth substance. In practical terms, water fluoridation has consistently has been shown to be the most effective, safe and equitable means of preventing caries, resulting in a decrease of approximately 50%.

Where the water supply contains fluoride less than 700 µg/l (0.7 ppm) fluoride, infants and children over the age of 6 months who are at high risk may be given daily fluoride drops or tablets, as fluoride supplements to reduce caries. However, many toothpastes contain added fluoride, which is probably largely responsible for the decline in caries in many countries. Children under about 6 years of age may ingest toothpaste, so only a pea-sized amount of a paste with less than 1000 ppm of fluoride should be used and in supervised brushing, or there is a possibility of producing fluorosis.

High fluoride content toothpastes, fluoride rinses and gels are useful mainly for patients with special needs or those at high risk of caries such as people with dry mouths.

### Fissure sealants

Plastic coatings placed by the dental professional in the pits and fissures of the permanent teeth can also help reduce caries.

## Erosion

### Aetiopathogenesis

Erosion is tooth surface loss of substance caused by acids other than those produced in the carious process. Most erosion has an extrinsic cause. Citrus fruits or drinks, carbonated beverages, wines, ciders and alco-pops are mostly responsible. Even flavoured waters can be as erosive as some fruit juices. Some medications such as vitamin C, aspirin and some iron preparations are acidic and may contribute towards tooth erosion.

Rarely, occupational exposure to acids may produce erosion, and even the low pH of indoor swimming pools may be a cause.

Erosion may also be due to intrinsic causes (perimolysis) and is seen where there is gastric regurgitation such as in gastro-oesophageal reflux disease, in alcoholism or anorexia nervosa/bulimia.

### Clinical features

In most cases there is little more than a loss of normal enamel contour but, in more severe cases, dentine or pulp may become involved (Figs 2.10.98 and 2.10.99). Early on the incisal edges become transparent. Then the teeth develop a yellowish tint and a change in shape with a broad rounded concavity, and the gaps between teeth enlarge. There can be evidence of wear on surfaces of teeth not expected to be in contact with one another. Amalgam restorations in the mouth may be clean and non-tarnished and may also appear to be rising out of the tooth. The most severe signs are cracking, and pain when eating hot, cold or sweet foods or drinks.

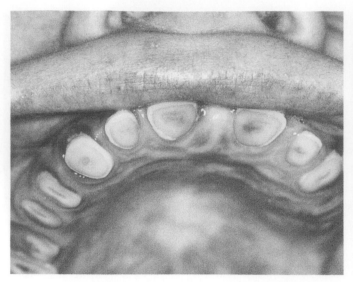

*Figure 2.10.99* Tooth surface loss—erosion.

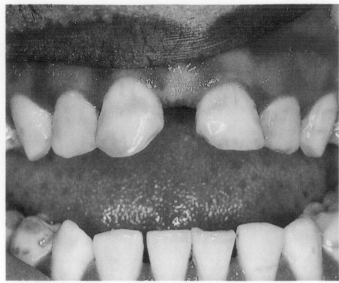

*Figure 2.10.100* Tooth surface loss—trauma from a custom of filing the incisors.

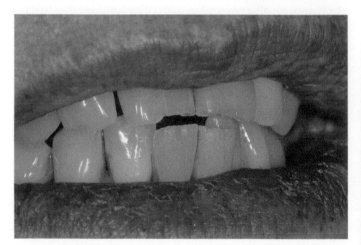

*Figure 2.10.101* Tooth surface loss—trauma from holding objects between the teeth.

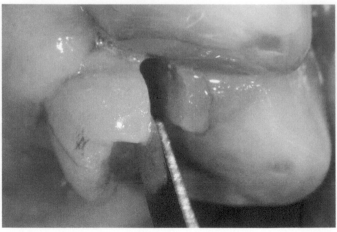

*Figure 2.10.102* Tooth surface loss—trauma from occlusion causing fracture.

*Diagnosis*
Clinical.

*Management*
Restorative dentistry.

**Trauma**

Trauma is common in sport, road accidents, violence and epilepsy and is seen mainly in males, affecting the maxillary incisors. Teeth can be cracked, fractured, devitalized, subluxated or lost. Cracked teeth are more common than often believed, can result from extreme occlusal stresses in clenching and may cause severe pain (Figs 2.10.100–2.10.102).

Localized tooth damage can occur from habits or occupation, for example, the known rare 'seamstress' notch: holding pins, nails, etc.

between the teeth can produce a variety of lesions. Localized damage may be produced for aesthetic reasons, according to custom.

## FURTHER READING

Daniel E, McCurdy EA, Shashi V, McGuirt Jr WF. Ectodermal dysplasia: otolaryngologic manifestations and management. Laryngoscope 2002; 112: 962–7.

De Coster PJ, Marks LA, Martens LC, Huysseune A. Dental agenesis: genetic and clinical perspectives. J Oral Pathol 2009; 38: 1–17.

Donahue JP, Shea CJ. Hidrotic ectodermal dysplasia with corneal involvement. J Am Assoc Pediatr Ophthalm Strabis 1999; 3: 372–5.

Ettinger RL. Epidemiology of dental caries. A broad review. Dent Clin North Am 1999; 43: 679–94.

Fejerskov O, Kidd E, eds. Dental Caries. The Disease and Its Clinical Management, 1st edn. Oxford: Blackwell Munksgaard, 2003.

Garvey MT, Barry HJ, Blake M. Supernumerary teeth—an overview of classification, diagnosis and management. J Can Dent Assoc 1999; 65: 612–16.

Haskova JE, Gill DS, Figueiredo JA, Tredwin CJ, Naini FB. Taurodontism—a review. Dent Update 2009; 36: 235–6, 239–40, 243.

Hemmings K, Griffiths B, Hobkirk J, Scully C. ABC of oral health 8. Improving occlusion and orofacial aesthetics; tooth repair and replacement. Br Med J 2000; 321: 438–41.

Holt R, Roberts G, Scully C. ABC of oral health 1. Oral health and disease. Br Med J 2000; 320: 1652–5.

Holt R, Roberts G, Scully C. ABC of oral health 2. Dental disease prevention and sequelae. Br Med J 2000; 320: 1717–19.

Kerr AR. Tooth discoloration. Available from: [http://emedicine.medscape.com/article/1076389-overview].

Koch G, Kreiborg S. Eruption and shedding of teeth. In: Koch G, Poulsen S, eds. Pediatric Dentistry. A Clinical Approach, 1st edn. Oxford: Blackwell Munksgaard, 2003: 301–19.

Noffke CE, Chabikuli NJ, Nzima N. Impaired tooth eruption: a review. SADJ 2005; 60: 422, 424–5.

Peres KG, Armenio MF, Peres MA, Traebert J, De Lacerda JT. Dental erosion in 12-year-old schoolchildren: a cross-sectional study in Southern Brazil. Int J Paediatr Dent 2005; 15: 249–55.

Pinheiro M, Freire-Maia N. Ectodermal dysplasias: a clinical classification and a causal review. Am J Med Genet 1994; 53: 153–62.

Priolo M, Silengo M, Lerone M, Ravazzolo R. Ectodermal dysplasias: not only "skin" deep. Clin Genet 2000; 58: 415–30.

Rajab LD, Hamdan MAM. Supernumerary teeth: review of the literature and a survey of 152 cases. Int J Paediatr Dent 2002; 12: 244–54.

Rees J, Loyn T, Hunter L, Sadaghiani L, Gilmour A. The erosive potential of some flavoured waters. Eur J Dent 2007; 1: 5–9.

Robinson S, Connell J, Kirkham SJ, et al. The effect of fluoride on the developing tooth. Caries Res 2004; 38: 268–76.

Seow WK. Biological mechanisms of early childhood caries. Commun Dent Oral Epidemiol 1998; 26 (Suppl 1): 8–27.

Winter GB. Anomalies of tooth formation and eruption. In: Welbury RR, ed. Paediatric Dentistry. Oxford: Oxford University Press, 1997: 199–220.

# 2.11 MAXILLOFACIAL NEUROLOGICAL DISORDERS AND PAIN

- history related to pain and neurological problems
- general features
- sensory system
- motor system
- cranial nerve examination
- diagnosis

- investigations
- involuntary movements
- pain
- paralysis in the maxillofacial region
- sensory loss in the maxillofacial region

---

Facial pain or maxillofacial pain is a common complaint; most is of local (odontogenic) cause. Neurological and vascular disorders also often present with pain, and pain may have a psychogenic basis or may be referred from elsewhere.

Medical advice may well be indicated and specialist advice should always be sought if a neurological lesion is at all possible. Medical advice should urgently be sought if pain is:

- accompanied by pain elsewhere (chest, shoulder, neck or arm—may be angina)
- accompanied by other unexplained symptoms or signs (numbness, weakness, headaches, neck stiffness, nausea or vomiting—may be intracerebral disease)
- focused in the temple on one side (may be giant cell arteritis).

Examination findings and imaging using radiography, CT, MRI or ultrasonography are important not to miss detecting organic disease and thus mislabelling the patient as having psychogenic pain. Even patients with psychogenic disorders can suffer organic pain: 'hypochondriacs can be ill'! MRI of the entire trigeminal nerve gives better resolution of brain stem and cranial nerves than CT and is recommended for all patients, and is certainly mandatory if atypical features, sensory or motor disturbances are present.

Neurological disorders may present with sensory or motor disturbances or pain and most are important but, except trigeminal neuralgia, facial palsy and dyskinesias, they are not common.

## HISTORY RELATED TO PAIN AND NEUROLOGICAL PROBLEMS

The history should include at least:

- date of onset of symptoms
- symptom details such as duration and character
- pain details such as duration, daily timing, character, radiation, aggravating and relieving factors, relationship to meals and associated phenomena
- movement disorders
- sensory loss, including visual changes
- medical history, including drug use
- family history
- occupation.

## GENERAL FEATURES

- Check the vital signs.

- Look for abnormal posture or gait (broad based in cerebellar deficit, shuffling in parkinsonism, high stepping in peripheral leg neuropathy, swinging leg in hemiparesis, etc.).
- Assess the mental state and level of consciousness (Glasgow Coma Scale) and, if necessary.
- Assess speech:
  o dysarthria (oropharyngeal, neurological or muscular pathology),
  o dysphonia (respiratory pathology) or
  o dysphasia (abnormal speech content due to damage in the brain language areas).
- Check for neck stiffness (meningeal inflammation).

## SENSORY SYSTEM

There are several different sensory modalities, conducted by axons following different pathways in the posterior (dorsal) and lateral spinal cord (spinothalamic):

- Dorsal columns: consist of large fast-conducting axons that have not yet decussated and serve the following sensory modalities:
  o touch (tested with cotton wool)
  o vibration (tested with a tuning fork)
  o proprioception (move a joint slightly with the patient's eyes closed and ask them to recognize the direction of the movement).
- Spinothalamic tracts are in the lateral spinal cord, consist of small slow-conducting axons that have decussated at their entry into the cord and serve:
  o pain (pin-prick testing)
  o temperature (test with a warm object).

### Sensory defects

- Higher lesions can cause an endless variety of sensory deficits.
- Lesions of the posterior spinal cord cause ipsilateral loss of touch, vibration and proprioception sense beyond the level of the lesion.
- Lesions of the lateral spinal cord cause a contralateral loss of pain and temperature sensation.
- Lesions of the nerve root cause dermatomal pain or hypoaesthesia.
- Lesions of peripheral nerves (peripheral neuropathies, e.g. diabetes) cause a characteristic 'glove or stocking' pattern of sensory loss (all modalities affected).

## MOTOR SYSTEM

Look for muscle:

- tremor [anxiety, drugs, coffee, alcohol or drug withdrawal, cerebro-vascular accident (CVA), hyperthyroidism, parkinsonism]

- tics (partially controlled repetitive movements), maxillofacial dyskinesias (involuntary tic-like movements involving the lips and the tongue—a long term side-effect of antipsychotics), etc.
- fasciculations (involuntary twitches of groups of muscle fibres, e.g. in motor neurone disease)
- dystonia (e.g. torticollis), myoclonus (sudden jerky muscle movements)
- wasting (motor neurone disease or myopathy).

## Test tone, power, coordination and reflexes

Move the patient's limbs at various joints and in various random directions, noting tone and any abnormal resistance.

- Reduced tone can be a sign of a lower motor neurone (LMN) lesion or a recent upper motor neurone (UMN) lesion (CVA).
- Increased tone is seen in an established UMN lesion or Parkinson disease.

*Test muscle power*

Test movement; coordination is usually lost due to cerebellar dysfunction (e.g. alcohol intoxication), and can be revealed by examining:

- eye movements (nystagmus)
- speech (dysarthria)
- finger–nose test (look for intention tremor and past pointing)
- posture (difficulty in standing may also be due to visual, vestibular or proprioceptive defects)
- gait (ataxic)
- heel–toe walk
- heel–shin test.

Testing the spinal reflexes (biceps, triceps, supinator, knee and ankle jerks) tests the LMN integrity, the cerebellum and the UMN (reflexes reduced initially, but increased later). Hyper-reflexia follows the pattern of hypertonia in UMN disease. Another important reflex is the plantar reflex, where by scratching the lateral aspect of the sole induces flexion and adduction of the toes in the normal subject: if the toes extend and abduct (Babinski response), a UMN lesion is present.

## CRANIAL NERVE EXAMINATION

Specific neurological disease may be encountered, and the dental surgeon should be adept in examining the cranial nerves, as outlined:

### Olfactory (cranial nerve number I)

- Function: smell.
- Examination: odiferous substances are passed before each nostril in turn.
- Lesions: upper respiratory infections; nasal obstruction; tumours; fracture of cribriform plate (head injury).
- Abnormal finding: anosmia.

### Optic (II)

- Function: vision.
- Examination: visual acuity; pupillary reflexes; visual fields; fundoscopy.
- Lesions: trauma to the orbit; brain tumours; CVAs.

- Abnormal findings: impaired visual acuity; loss of direct and consensual pupillary responses (when shining a light at the affected eye, neither eye will react); visual field defects; abnormalities on fundoscopy.

### Oculomotor (III)

- Function: motor for most extraocular muscles (medial, superior and inferior recti, inferior oblique, and levator palpebrae superioris); visceral motor (parasympathetic fibres) for pupillary sphincter and ciliary muscle (lens accommodation).
- Examination: test eye movements and focusing of lens.
- Lesions: neuropathy (orbital trauma or disease is usually the cause of abnormal eye movements).
- Abnormal findings: eye points downwards and outwards (because of retained IV and VI nerve action); diplopia; movements impaired; ptosis (of upper eyelid); dilated pupils; loss of direct pupillary response (but consensual response preserved, i.e. the opposite eye will react while shining light at the affected).

### Trochlear (IV)

- Function: motor for superior oblique muscle.
- Examination: check inferolateral eye movement.
- Lesions: as for III.
- Abnormal findings: difficulty looking downwards (particularly from the adducted position); strabismus; diplopia.

### Trigeminal (V)

- Function: sensation from head and face and mouth; motor (muscles of mastication, mylohyoid, anterior belly of digastric, tensor veli palatini and tensor tympani).
- Examination: test light touch (with cotton wool); pain (with pin prick); corneal reflex (touch the cornea with a wisp of cotton wool); open and close jaw against resistance; jaw jerk.
- Lesions: brain lesions; facial bone fractures (orbital floor, mandible, etc.); surgical trauma, connective tissue disease, others.
- Abnormal findings: facial hypoaesthesia or paraesthesia; abnormal reflexes; weakness and wasting of masticatory muscles.

### Abducens (VI)

- Function: motor for lateral rectus muscle.
- Examination: check eye movement to the affected side.
- Lesions: as for III.
- Abnormal findings: impaired eye movement to affected side; diplopia.

### Facial (VII)

- Function: motor (muscles of facial expression, stylohyoid, posterior belly of digastric, and stapedius); secretomotor (parasympathetic fibres to lacrimal, submandibular and sublingual salivary, nasal and

palatine glands); taste (from anterior two-thirds of tongue via the chorda tympani).
- Examination: test facial movements (eye shutting, smiling, etc.); Schirmer test (lacrimation); check for xerostomia; test taste sensation (apply salty, sweet, sour and bitter substances to the tongue) and hearing for hyperacusis. The nerve can be tested by asking the patient to close their eyes and lips tightly—the strength of closure can be felt by manually trying to open them; asking the patient to show their teeth; asking the patient to look upwards, elevating the eyebrows and creasing the forehead; and also asking the patient to whistle or fill their cheeks with air with their lips tightly pursed—if the face is weak, the patient will find it difficult to hold in the air. Tapping each inflated cheek reveals the weakness.
- Lesions: UMN lesions (brain lesions);LMN lesions (e.g. Bell palsy, parotid surgery, etc.).
- Abnormal findings: contralateral facial weakness with partial sparing of the upper face (bilateral innervation) in UMN lesions; ipsilateral facial weakness, impaired lacrimation, salivation and taste in LMN lesions.

### Vestibulo-cochlear (VIII)

- Function: balance and hearing.
- Examination: nystagmus tests; Rinne and Webber tests.
- Lesions: acoustic neuroma (vestibular schwannoma), local malignancy or destruction (e.g. cholesteatoma).
- Abnormal findings: impaired balance; nystagmus; impaired hearing (tests will differentiate from conduction deficit).

### Glossopharyngeal (IX) and vagus (X)

- Function:
  o IX serves motor (stylopharyngeus); secretomotor (parasympathetic fibres to parotid gland); sensory (pharynx); and taste (posterior third of tongue).
  o X serves motor (pharynx, palate and larynx); taste (palate and epiglottis) and autonomic innervation of heart, lungs and intestines.
- Examination: examine the soft palate while the patient says 'aah'; test gag reflex.
- Lesions: brainstem lesions or injury.
- Abnormal findings: deviation of uvula to unaffected side; impaired gag reflex, taste, speech and cough.

### Accessory (XI)

- Function: motor (sternocleidomastoid and trapezius).
- Examination: test head flexion/rotation and shoulder elevation.
- Lesions: neck lacerations; radical neck dissection.
- Abnormal findings: weakness and wasting of muscles; shoulder drop.

### Hypoglossal (XII)

- Function: motor (intrinsic and extrinsic muscles of tongue).
- Examination: test tongue protrusion.
- Lesions: neck lacerations; other neurological disorders.
- Abnormal findings: with LMN—wasting; dysarthria; deviation of protruded tongue towards affected side; UMN may give rise to fasciculation without wasting.

## DIAGNOSIS

The cranial nerves should be examined as above and by:

- inspecting
  o facial symmetry and movement
  o ocular movements
- sensory testing with cotton wool and pin-prick
- hearing
- examining the eyes
- testing taste sensation. Gustometry uses stimuli on a cotton bud, including: citric acid or hydrochloric acid (sour taste), caffeine or quinine hydrochloride (bitter), sodium chloride (salty), saccharose (sweet), monosodium glutamate (umami taste). Electrogustometry examines taste sensitivity by means of electric excitability thresholds determined through the response to the irritation of taste buds area with electrical current of different intensity.

Trigeminal functions that should be tested include:

- Corneal reflex (this tests V and VII cranial nerves); touching the cornea gently with sterile cotton wool should produce a blink.
- Skin sensation, by using:
  o light touch (cotton wool)
  o pin point (sterile needle)
  o temperature
  o vibration
  o two-point discrimination.
- Motor function by jaw jerk, and palpating:
  o muscles of mastication during function
  o masseters during clenching
  o temporalis during clenching
  o pterygoids during jaw protrusion.

Neurological disorders may appear to be unilateral, but the other cranial nerves should always be examined, as should there be a general neurological examination. It is important to consider drug use and the possibility of related systemic disorders especially:

- cardiovascular system
- respiratory system (sarcoidosis)
- connective tissues, such as rheumatoid arthritis
- endocrine glands (diabetes)
- mental health
- nutrition (eating disorders such as bulimia).

## INVESTIGATIONS

Investigations required may include:

- Plasma viscosity or erythrocyte sedimentation rate (ESR) or C-reactive protein (CRP).
- Full blood count, serum angiotensin converting enzyme and random glucose.
- Antibodies
  o antinuclear antibodies for lupus or rheumatoid arthritis
  o rheumatoid factor for rheumatoid arthritis
  o Sjögren syndrome (SS)-A (Ro) and SS-B (La) antibodies for SS
  o ribonucleoprotein (RNP) antibodies for mixed connective tissue disease (MCTD)
  o viral antibodies.

- Other investigations can include:
  - imaging
    - radiography
    - CT
    - MRI, which avoids irradiating the patient, has almost completely replaced CT as the modality of choice for investigating trigeminal neuropathy, though CT still plays a role in the assessment of skull base foramina and facial skeleton
    - ultrasound
  - biopsy
  - urinalysis.

# INVOLUNTARY MOVEMENTS

One of the most common involuntary movements is a tremor but there are many other types and a range of causes (Table 2.11.1).

Facial muscles are subject to the same movement disorders as muscles of the trunk or limbs. Craniofacial tremor may be seen in association with essential tremor, parkinsonism, hyperthyroidism or electrolyte disturbances. Conditions such as cerebral palsy, epilepsy are also characterized by abnormal involuntary movements that can involve the

## Table 2.11.1 MOTOR ABNORMALITIES: TERMS, FEATURES AND MAIN CAUSES

| Disorder | Features | Main causes |
|---|---|---|
| Akathisia | Restlessness | Neuroleptic drugs |
| Akinesia | Lack of movement | Parkinsonism |
| Athetosis | Dystonia of limbs | Athetoid cerebral palsy |
| Chorea | Continual flow of jerky movements | Huntington chorea Sydenham chorea (rheumatic fever) |
| Clonus | Rhythmic contractions | Upper motor neurone lesions |
| Dyskinesia | Involuntary chewing or grinding | L-dopa, phenothiazines and other neuroleptic drugs |
| Dystonia | Sustained spasms causing abnormal posture | Phenothiazines and other neuroleptic drugs |
| Fasciculation | Spontaneous contractions of muscle fibres | Lower motor neurone lesions |
| Hemiballismus | Chorea affecting half the body | Subthalamic lesions |
| Nystagmus | Repeated eye movements | Cerebellar disease |
| Rigidity | Limbs resist passive movement | Parkinsonism |
| Spasticity | Excess tone in arm flexors, leg extensors | Cerebral palsy; upper motor neurone lesion |
| Tonus | Excess muscle tone | Epilepsy |
| Tremor | Rhythmic movements of a part; at rest | Parkinsonism, anxiety, alcohol, drugs, liver disease, thyrotoxicosis, benign or brain lesion |
| | Rhythmic movements of a part; on intention to move | Essential tremor, cerebellar disease |

maxillofacial region. Facial chorea may occur in systemic chorea (e.g. Huntington disease and Sydenham chorea).

## Dystonias

Dystonias are uncommon conditions characterized by abnormal movements and muscle spasm, probably emanating from a lesion in the basal ganglia. They can be focal or generalized, and primary (a neurological disorder cannot be identified) or secondary to a defined organic brain disease.

Oromandibular dystonia refers to recurrent spasmodic episodes of lower facial muscles—causing lip movements, tongue protrusion and retraction, and jaw clenching or opening. It may be associated with blepharospasm (then called Meige syndrome), the respiratory muscles and speech may be impaired and over one-third of patients may suffer from depression. Benzodiazepines, or antimuscarinics such as benztropine or levodopa may be helpful.

Acute oromandibular dystonia (drug-induced parkinsonism) can appear within hours or days of starting treatment with neuroleptics such as phenothiazines and butyrophenones. It may resolve after withdrawal of the drug or be improved with antimuscarinics. However, it is made worse by levodopa, which in large dose can itself also cause involuntary spasmodic movements.

Torticollis (Latin torti—twisted and collis—neck) refers to the neck being held in a twisted or bent position. Idiopathic spasmodic torticollis (acute wryneck) or acquired torticollis, is the more common type, and is an example of focal dystonia. It develops overnight in young and middle-aged adults who present with painful neck spasms. Symptoms usually resolve within weeks with use of heat, massage, cervical collar, muscle relaxants and analgesics.

Congenital torticollis due to birth trauma or intrauterine malpositioning and an injured sternocleidomastoid, presents after birth over days to weeks, with a soft-tissue swelling over the muscle, which may be confused with a branchial cyst, regresses and leaves a fibrous band in place of the muscle, causing neck contracture.

## Dyskinesias

Dyskinesia is a difficulty or distortion in performing voluntary movements (Greek: dys-, trouble and kinesis, movement), as in tic, chorea, spasm or myoclonus.

Orofacial dyskinesias are abnormal movements of tongue or facial muscles, sometimes with abnormal jaw movements, bruxism or dysphagia. Common dyskinesias are involuntary tongue protrusion and retraction, and facial grimacing (Figs 2.11.1–2.11.3). Orofacial dyskinesias are seen in older edentulous patients and may be a consequence of ill-fitting dental prostheses.

Tardive dyskinesia is usually a late complication of long-term neuroleptic treatment similar to oromandibular dystonia but it rarely responds to withdrawal of the offending drug, is usually made worse by giving antimuscarinics and may be resistant to any treatment.

## Myoclonus

Myoclonus refers to a quick, abnormal, involuntary muscle jerk, caused by sudden muscle contractions. In severe cases, myoclonus can distort movement and limit the abilities to walk, talk and eat. Myoclonus can be normal [e.g. a hiccup or if it only affects persons as they fall asleep (hypnic jerks)] but otherwise it can be a sign of:

- Drug adverse effects (e.g. amitryptiline)
- Central nervous system (CNS) disorders

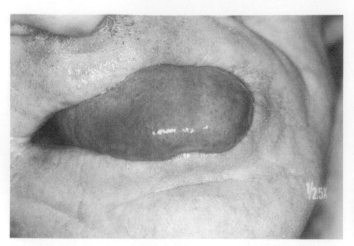

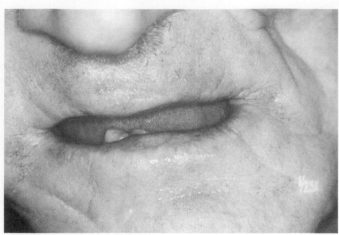

*Figure 2.11.1* Dyskinesia—Figures 2.11.1–2.11.3 show involuntary tongue, jaw and lip movements in the same patient.

*Figure 2.11.2* Dyskinesia.

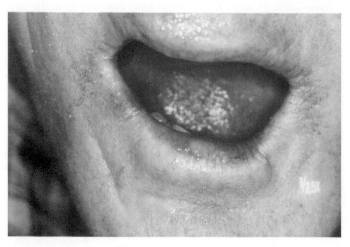

*Figure 2.11.3* Dyskinesia.

o Infection, e.g. encephalitis or Creutzfeldt–Jakob disease
o Damage (trauma or stroke)
o Multiple sclerosis
o Epilepsy
o Parkinsonism
o Alzheimer disease
• Metabolic disorders, such as hepatic or renal failure or hyponatraemia.

Treatment is usually with anticonvulsants.

Jerking leg movements while the person is at rest, used to be called myoclonus, but is now referred to as periodic leg movements (restless legs syndrome).

Types of myoclonus include: *Hemifacial spasm* (clonic facial spasm)—a type of myoclonus that mainly affects older people, presenting with unilateral facial spasm that affects especially the angle of the mouth or the eyelid and worsens towards the evening. Many cases are idiopathic but some herald a cerebellopontine angle other lesion irritating the facial nerve (e.g. tumour, arteriovenous malformation and Paget disease of bone) and other lesions (e.g. stroke, multiple sclerosis and basilar meningitis), and some follow facial palsy. Occasionally facial paralysis or

trigeminal neuralgia ensue. Hemifacial spasm may respond for up to 3 months to local injections of botulinum toxin into affected muscles.

*Hemimasticatory spasm*—analogous to hemifacial spasm, but occurs with irritation to the motor trigeminal nerve.

*Palatal myoclonus* (palatal tremor)—a rapid rhythmic contraction of the soft palate, which may persist during sleep and may be accompanied by myoclonus in other muscles (e.g. face, tongue, throat and diaphragm). The cause may be unidentified (primary or essential myoclonus) but even then it may be secondary to latent CNS lesions such as cerebrovascular disease, multiple sclerosis, tumours, trauma, infection, Behçet disease and vertebral artery aneurysm. A neurological opinion is mandatory.

### Tics

Tics are brief, *repetitive*, coordinated, semi-purposeful movements.

Facial tics include blinking, grimacing, shaking the head, clearing the throat, coughing or shrugging. Most are benign habit spasms usually seen in children. Some drugs appear to produce tics (e.g. anticonvulsants, caffeine, methylphenidate and anti-parkinsonian drugs), but emotion or fatigue intensify tics.

The natural history is of spontaneous remission but, if persistent, the dopamine receptor blocker haloperidol may be helpful.

*Blepharospasm* is a spasm of both eyelids that may be seen in older people, in isolation or along with hemifacial spasm. Blepharospasm is usually benign (benign essential blepharospasm) and often aggravated or precipitated by anxiety, stress or fatigue. Blepharospasm can also be caused by hormone replacement therapy, and anti-parkinsonian agents, or by benzodiazepines or their withdrawal . More seriously, blepharospasm can occasionally arise from basal ganglia lesions (when a neurological opinion is essential).

Injections of botulinum toxin into affected muscles in benign essential blepharospasm may give relief for up to 3 months.

*Facial myokymia* is a rare but serious condition, in which there are continuous fine, worm-like contractions of one or more of the facial muscles, especially the perioral or periorbital muscles. Facial myokymia starts suddenly, lasts for variable periods and is unaffected by voluntary movements. It is associated with any brainstem lesion, frequently multiple sclerosis, or neoplasm, or posterior cranial fossa tumours or other neurological disorders.

Facial myokymia must be distinguished from benign fasciculation and myokymia of the lower eyelid, and from facial hemispasm, facial tics or blepharospasm (which involves several muscles synchronously)—all of which are quite innocuous. Neurological assessment is mandatory.

*Gilles de la Tourette syndrome* is a familial early onset syndrome, seen mainly in males, in which chronic motor tics involve the head and neck and are associated with compulsive vocal tics and sometimes swearing (coprolalia). Tongue thrusting and lip smacking are common and sometimes regarded as lewd (copropraxia). Intelligence is usually normal but many of those affected have obsessive–compulsive tendencies or attention-deficit hyperactivity.

Temporomandibular or other oral pain may result and self-mutilation such as tongue and lip biting may be associated.

Haloperidol is usually effective, suggesting that there is basal ganglia overactivity. Pimozide and/or clonidine may also be used.

# PAIN

Maxillofacial pain most often has a local cause—usually odontogenic. Pain can also be caused by neurological disorders, vascular disease or can be referred. This section discusses maxillofacial pain rather than headache, causes of which are noted in Table 2.11.2.

Psychogenic causes may underlie various clinical facial pain presentations but can only be suggested once all possibility of organic disease has been excluded. Persistent pain, in the absence of identifiable organic disease, is seen in some psychiatric disorders, such as depression and, in others may be a monosymptomatic hypochondriasis. Many patients affected with this type of facial pain are females of middle age or older. A feature sometimes seen in examination of tense or anxious patients is a remarkable degree of tongue protrusion to the extent that the epiglottis can be seen. Others have pronounced occlusal lines, and/or crenation of the lateral border of the tongue.

Patients with psychogenically related maxillofacial symptoms not infrequently bring in diaries, graphs or notes outlining their complaints, which are often of pain, bad taste in the mouth, non-existent slime, lumps, dry or wet mouth, and are often multiple. A 'syndrome of oral complaints' has even been described.

## Burning mouth syndrome

Burning mouth syndrome (oral dysaesthesia, glossopyrosis, glossodynia, stomatodynia) (Chapter 2.3).

## Persistent idiopathic facial pain (PIFP)

PIFP (atypical facial pain).

### Aetiopathogenesis

PIFP, formerly termed atypical facial pain, is a medically unexplained symptom but, since positron emission tomography shows enhanced cerebral activity, an enhanced alerting mechanism in response to peripheral stimuli may be the underlying cause leading to neuropeptide and free radical release causing cell damage, and release of pain-inducing eicosanoids (e.g. prostaglandins).

Most sufferers are otherwise normal individuals who are stressed or have been under extreme stress, such as bereavement or concern about cancer. However, some have personality traits such as hypochondriasis or neuroses (usually depression), and a few are psychotic.

### Clinical features

Pain persists for much or all of the day, but does not waken the patient from sleep. It is often poorly localized, deep, dull boring or burning and chronic, often in the upper jaw but unrelated to the anatomical distribution of trigeminal nerve innervation, sometimes crossing the midline, or moving elsewhere.

Pain is frequently longstanding and unchanging often associated with multiple oral and/or other psychogenic related complaints, such as:

- dry mouth
- bad taste
- chronic back pain
- headaches
- irritable bowel syndrome
- dysmenorrhoea.

PIFP affects both genders approximately equally, but more women than men seek care. Patients only uncommonly use analgesics to try and control the pain but may consult many health care professionals.

### Diagnosis

PFIP is a diagnosis by exclusion. The clinical history is often highly suggestive, but very careful dental, oral, otolaryngological and neurological examination, and imaging (tooth/jaw/sinus/skull radiography and MRI/CT scan with particular attention to the skull base) are mandatory in order to exclude organic disease such as space-occupying or demyelinating diseases. Chronic daily headache syndromes, including hemicrania continua, temporomandibular joint (TMJ) syndrome, migraine, migrainous neuralgia, short-lasting, unilateral, neuralgiform headache attacks with conjunctival injection and tearing, trigeminal neuralgia and other conditions also need excluding.

Examination and investigation findings exclude:

- erythema, tenderness or swelling in the painful area
- obvious odontogenic or other local cause for the pain
- objective physical (including neurological) signs
- abnormal imaging results
- abnormal blood test results.

### Management

Few patients have spontaneous remission and thus treatment is indicated.

Cognitive behavioural therapy or a specialist referral may be indicated as antidepressants (e.g. amitriptyline, doxepin, dosulepin, fluoxetine, moclobemide or nortriptyline), anxiolytics (e.g. clonazepam) or analgesics, for example, gabapentin may be indicated.

## Post-herpetic neuralgia (PHN)

PHN is more likely to develop, and more likely to be severe, in people aged over 60, when about 25% develop neuralgia lasting over 30 days (Fig. 2.11.4) (Chapter 1.8).

## Trigeminal neuralgia

Trigeminal neuralgia [paroxysmal trigeminal neuralgia (PTN)].

### Aetiopathogenesis

PTN cause is unclear, but one hypothesis is that there is compression around the trigeminal root entry into the pons with demyelination, due to an atherosclerotic posterior superior cerebellar artery.

### Clinical features

Paroxysmal attacks of facial pain which last a few seconds to less than 2 minutes; occurring especially in the morning, rarely during sleep. Most patients are entirely asymptomatic between paroxysms. Patients

**Table 2.11.2** CAUSES OF HEADACHE AND MAXILLOFACIAL PAIN

| Condition | Pain character | Pain location | Other features | Management |
|---|---|---|---|---|
| Sluder, or cluster headache (migrainous neuralgia) | Severe, boring and burning | Often retro-orbital | May be precipitated by alcohol. Episodes last 30–180 minutes awaken the patient from sleep and do not improve with rest. Ipsilateral conjunctival injection, tearing and nasal congestion | Preventative treatment includes verapamil, lithium, divalproex sodium and topiramate Abortive treatment includes oxygen, sumatriptan and/or dihydroergotamine |
| Cluster-tic syndrome | Mimics cluster headache or trigeminal neuralgia | | | AEDs, TCAs and SSRIs/NeRIs |
| Giant cell arteritis (Horton disease, granulomatous, cranial or temporal arteritis) | Burning pain | Usually over the temple | Sometimes associated with polymyalgia rheumatica. Rarely, tongue or lip pain or 'jaw claudication', or ischaemic necrosis. ESR and interleukin-6 raised Artery biopsy Ultrasound MRI | May cause retinal artery spasm and blindness, or stroke, so corticosteroids as an emergency treatment |
| Hemicrania continua | Daily head aches | Unilateral headache and facial pain | Continuous (24 hour/day, 7 day/week), with pain exacerbation periods that occur with varying frequency from multiple times per week to every third month or less | Responds to indomethacin, which aids in diagnosis |
| Migraine | Throbbing quality and feels as if associated with a pulse | Headache unilateral but can be bilateral | Patient may or may not experience aura. Photophobia, phonophobia, osmophobia and nausea. Pain worsens with exertion and improves with sleep | Preventative agents include AEDs, beta-blockers, calcium channel blockers, TCAs, SSRIs/NeRIs and angiotensin receptor blocking agents Abortive agents include serotonin agonists, ergotamine, isometheptene and anti-inflammatories |
| Post-herpetic neuralgia (pain persists for 1–6 months after acute herpes zoster infection) | Variable | Trigeminal nerve branches most commonly V1 | Associated with allodynia and hyperalgesia | AEDs, TCAs and SSRIs |
| Raeder syndrome | Unilateral burning | V1 distribution | Associated with hyperaesthesia, ptosis and miosis | May be caused by sinusitis, trauma, middle cranial fossa mass lesion or syphilis but in absence of underlying conditions, pain is self-limited |
| SUNCT syndrome | Unilateral burning, stabbing or electric | Eyes, temple or face | Brief (15–120 seconds) and frequent in a 24-hour period (>100 episodes). Neck movements can trigger pain. Ipsilateral conjunctival injection and lacrimation | Lamotrigine has recently been reported as an effective first line therapy. Otherwise, refractory to drugs |
| TMJ pain-dysfunction syndrome | Dull, usually aggravated by chewing, talking and jaw movement | Side of face | Focal tenderness to one or both TMJs and masticatory muscles | Directed at relaxing masseters and temporalis muscles |
| Thalamic pain syndrome | Burning dysaesthesias | Unilateral facial | Attributed to a lesion of the *ventral-medial thalamic nuclei*. Severe burning, or aching pain to the contralateral side of the face | AEDs, TCAs, SSRIs, NeRIs |
| Trigeminal neuralgia | Lancinating pain | Trigeminal nerve branches | Severe bursts of pain, seconds in duration, often with a trigger | Carbamazepine, other AEDs, nerve blocks and/or surgical |

*Abbreviations*: AEDs, antiepileptic drugs; TCAs, tricyclics antidepressants; SSRIs, selective serotonin reuptake inhibitors; NeRIs, norepinephrine reuptake inhibitors; ESR, erythrocyte sedimentation rate; SUNCT, short-lasting, unilateral, neuralgiform headache attacks with conjunctival injection and tearing; TMJ, temporomandibular joint.

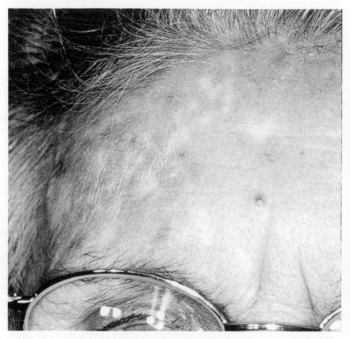

*Figure 2.11.4* Herpes zoster causes pain and may leave post-herpetic neuralgia and scarring.

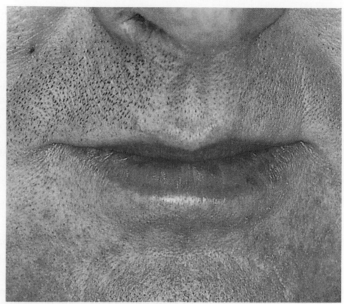

*Figure 2.11.5* Trigeminal neuralgia may lead to avoidance of washing or shaving in a trigger zone.

can localize precisely the pain as unilateral and can identify with the following main characteristics:

- distribution along one or more divisions of the trigeminal nerve
- a sudden intense, sharp superficial, stabbing, lancinating or burning quality
- intense severity: during attacks, patients may grimace—hence the term 'tic douloureux'
- precipitation from trigger areas, such as in eating, talking, washing the face (Fig. 2.11.5), shaving or cleaning the teeth.

'Atypical trigeminal neuralgia', which causes less intense, constant, dull burning or aching pain, sometimes with occasional electric-shock-like stabs, usually unilaterally, may be an early feature of MCTD. Trigeminal neuralgia may also be caused by space-occupying lesions such as neoplasms or aneurysms, vascular anomalies, cerebrovascular disease, demyelination (e.g. multiple sclerosis) and inflammatory infiltrates about the trigeminal central areas or Gasserian ganglion, or lesions irritating the trigeminal nerve roots along the pons or at the cerebellar pontine angle such as acoustic neuromas (vestibular schwannomas), trigeminal neuromas, cerebral aneurysms and meningiomas, Thus it is essential to exclude organic lesions (secondary trigeminal neuralgia).

*Diagnosis*
History, physical examination and special investigations are needed to exclude secondary trigeminal neuralgia, which is much more likely when pain:

- is associated with trigeminal nerve hyperaesthesia or hypoaesthesia
- is observed with other cranial neuropathies
- occurs in patients with onset when younger than 40 years
- is predominantly forehead and/or orbit pain (i.e. first division of the trigeminal nerve)

- is bilateral, or
- where there is bilateral sensory loss or weakness of the facial muscles or jaw.

Other less common syndromes with paroxysmal lancinating head pain to be ruled out include migraine, migrainous neuralgia, giant cell arteritis, glossopharyngeal neuralgia, occipital neuralgia and paroxysmal hemicrania.

Magnetic resonance imaging is essential in many if not all instances, as well as blood tests including:

- ESR—to exclude vasculitides such as giant cell arteritis
- anti-RNP antibodies—to exclude MCTD
- serology—to exclude Lyme disease or, rarely, HIV/AIDS.

*Management*
Trigeminal neuralgia is managed with anticonvulsants, especially carbamazepine. Some use a trial of baclofen since it has fewer adverse effects; the synergistic combination of carbamazepine and baclofen may also provide relief. Carbamazepine is contraindicated in people of Chinese or Thai origin who are HLA-B1502 positive—as they may develop Stevens–Johnson syndrome. In others carbamazepine must be given continuously prophylactically for long periods and under strict medical surveillance—a baseline test and then monthly tests of blood levels of carbamazepine and:

- balance (disturbed—ataxia)
- blood pressure (may increase)
- blood urea and electrolytes; liver function; bone marrow function (full blood cell count).

Other potential therapies include baclofen, clonazepam, gabapentin, lamotrigine, oxcarbazepine, phenytoin, pregabalin, sumatriptan, topiramate and valproate.

Should medications be ineffective, or give rise to excessive undesirable adverse effects, surgical options available include:

- Peripheral procedures (e.g. nerve blocks using glycerol, 10% phenol in glycerol, 10% lidocaine, tetracaine–glycerin or tetracaine in bupivacaine; cryotherapy or surgery).
- Open surgical posterior cranial fossa procedures such as microvascular decompression (MVD) of the trigeminal root and retrogasserian rhizotomy.
- Percutaneous approaches to trigeminal gangliolysis by inserting a needle into the skull through the face. Radiofrequency lesioning (RFL: percutaneous radiofrequency trigeminal gangliolysis) is the most commonly performed of these. Percutaneous Fogarty balloon microcompression, and percutaneous retrogasserian glycerol rhizotomy are also used.
- Stereotactic gamma knife radiosurgery is the least invasive and with the fewest adverse effects.

In younger patients, the other first choice treatment is MVD. For older patients, RFL is recommended.

# PARALYSIS IN THE MAXILLOFACIAL REGION

Paralysis is especially noticeable when it affects the facial nerve. Paralysis of the eyelid (ptosis) may also be evident in some conditions, usually caused by either a weakness of the levator palpebrae superioris (muscle that raises the eyelid), or a problem with the nerve supply from the oculomotor or sympathetic nerves. Hypoglossal nerve palsy is often obvious because of the consequent dysarthria.

### Facial palsy

Facial palsy can result from a lesion affecting any part of the facial nerve. UMN lesions are usually a consequence of a CVA (stroke). The facial nerve LMN begins at the facial motor nucleus in the pons. Damage to this nucleus is not common but because of the proximity of other sensory and motor pathways in the brain stem, there are then almost always other signs of neurological damage (hemiplegia, hemihypoaesthesia, gaze palsy, etc.). LMN lesions are only rarely congenital (Moebius syndrome); most are acquired through damage to the facial nerve in the pons, internal auditory of facial canal (e.g. infection, tumour, cholesteatoma or trauma) or extracranially (e.g. trauma). Bell palsy is one cause of LMN facial palsy.

Thus the causes of facial palsy can range from

- Stroke
- Tumours affecting the facial nerve in the pons (e.g. metastasis) or peripherally (e.g. acoustic neuroma, vestibular schwannoma or cholesteatoma). The classic presentation of an acoustic neuroma in the internal auditory canal, is unilateral progressive hearing loss, vestibular dysfunction and tinnitus but, as the tumour enlarges, hearing loss and disequilibrium increase and compression of other structures may lead to facial pain or to hypoaesthesia due to trigeminal involvement. However, despite the tumour pressing on the facial nerve, facial weakness is uncommon.
- Trauma, including surgery (e.g. parotidectomy; cochlear implant surgery, mastoid surgery) and lacerations affecting the facial nerve (e.g. in the parotid region or to the base of the skull), or by underwater diving (barotrauma).
- Diabetes
- Lymphoma

- Inflammatory disorders affecting the facial nerve:
  o Bell palsy
  o multiple sclerosis
  o middle ear infections
  o connective tissue diseases
  o granulomatous diseases (sarcoidosis, Melkersson–Rosenthal syndrome/orofacial granulomatosis/Crohn disease, Wegener granulomatosis).

### Bell palsy
*Aetiopathogenesis*
Bell palsy is a primary facial nerve palsy (FNP)—an acute LMN paralysis of the face, which represents about 75% of all non-traumatic facial palsies. Usually seen in the young adult, there is an equal male to female ratio and a greater incidence in pregnant females. The cause is unknown but it is presumed to involve oedema affecting the facial nerve within its bony canal—usually in the stylomastoid canal—probably due to a virally mediated neuritis. Herpes simplex virus (HSV) has been demonstrated by serologic, animal and human studies. Rarely, facial palsy is associated with another infection, such as other herpesviruses (varicella-zoster virus; Epstein–Barr virus; cytomegalovirus; human herpesviruses 6); a retrovirus (HIV; human T-cell lymphotropic virus-1); other viruses (Coxsackie, influenza); or bacteria [otitis media; *Borrelia burgdorferii* infection (Lyme disease); Listeriosis; *Mycoplasma pneumoniae*]. Kawasaki disease (mucocutaneous lymph node syndrome) is an occasional cause.

Up to 10% of patients have a positive family history and up to 10% suffer recurrent episodes.

Inferior dental (alveolar) regional nerve local analgesic injections, if misplaced, may track through the parotid gland to reach the facial nerve and cause transient facial palsy.

*Clinical features*
Bell palsy affects young or middle-aged patients mainly and is acute and unilateral, often preceded by mild pain around the ear region and sometimes a degree of hypoaesthesia. Although usually a mononeuropathy, Bell palsy may occasionally be part of a more widespread cranial or even peripheral polyneuropathy.

There is:

- Acute onset of paralysis over a few hours, maximal within 48 hours.
- Usually only unilateral facial paralysis affecting both upper and lower face (Figs 2.11.6–2.11.9).
- Diminished blinking and absence of tearing.

Occasionally:

- Pain in the ear or jaw preceding the palsy by a day or two; almost 50% of patients experience post-auricular pain in the mastoid region.
- Complaints of facial numbness, but sensation is intact on testing.
- Hyperacusis (reduced damping activity of the stapedius because of loss of function of the nerve to the stapedius) or loss of taste (loss of function of the chorda tympani), or loss of lacrimation if the lesion is located proximal to the stylomastoid canal. One-third of patients complain about taste disorders, and 80% show a reduced sense of taste. Two-thirds of patients complain about epiphora due to the reduced function of the orbicularis oculi in transporting the tears.

*Diagnosis*
The minimum diagnostic criteria for facial palsy include paralysis or paresis of all muscle groups on one side of the face, sudden onset and absence of CNS disease. Bell palsy is not synonymous with lower FNP,

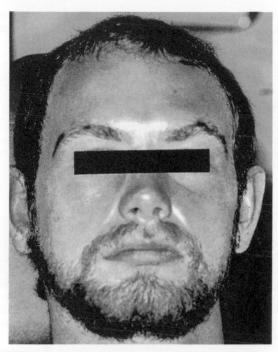

*Figure 2.11.6* Bell palsy—patient at rest showing right-sided palsy.

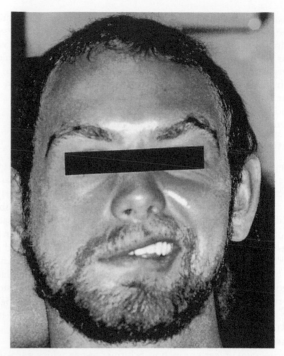

*Figure 2.11.7* Bell palsy—patient attempting a smile—more obviously showing the right sided palsy.

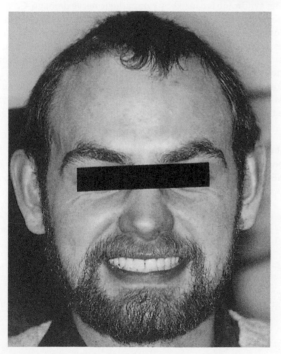

*Figure 2.11.8* Bell palsy—patient smiling after recovery.

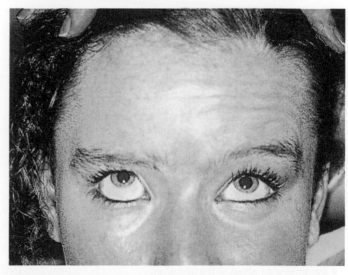

*Figure 2.11.9* Bell sign—eyes roll upwards as patient attempts to close eyelids.

- there are features consistent with multiple sclerosis
- there are signs of neoplasia
- viral vesicles are present in the palate or ear
- the paralysis is slowly progressive or chronic.

The examination should include:

- A full neurological examination, especially to exclude a stroke, and to exclude organic lesions involving the facial and related cranial nerves (especially abducens and vestibulocochlear).

and this should be diagnosed only when other causes (e.g. infection, tumour, cholesteatoma or trauma) have been excluded. Idiopathic Bell palsy is less likely to be the diagnosis if:

- trauma has occurred
- multiple cranial nerves are involved

- Facial nerve examination; weakness is demonstrated by testing the corneal reflex and asking the patient to close the eyes against resistance, raise the eyebrows, raise the lips to show the teeth and try to whistle.
- Ear and mouth examination to exclude Ramsay–Hunt syndrome; herpes zoster of the facial nerve ganglion (geniculate ganglion), which causes lesions in the palate and ipsilateral ear, and facial palsy.
- Ear and peri-aural examination, for discharge and other signs of middle ear disease, or mastoid or parotid disease/surgery.
- General and neurological examination.

Investigations which may be indicated include:

- Magnetic resonance imaging or computed tomography imaging of the internal auditory meatus, cerebellopontine angle and mastoid to exclude organic lesions—particularly in progressive facial palsy. Bone changes are best shown by CT, soft tissue best by MRI. The ability to scan direct coronal and sagittal planes makes MRI more versatile. CT is often the study of first choice because it is less dependent on patient co-operation. If questions are raised by CT, then MRI should also be performed. Chest radiography may be prudent in older patients.
- A test for the degree of nerve damage; facial nerve stimulation or needle electromyography may be useful, as may electrogustometry, nerve excitability tests, electromyography and electroneuronography.
- Assessment of hearing loss—pure tone audiometry is often—used.
- Assessment of taste loss.
- Assessment of balance.
- Assessment of tear production. Schirmer test, in which a strip of filter paper is placed in the lower conjunctival fornix, is usually used.
- Blood pressure measurement to exclude hypertension.
- Haematology/serology may include:
  o fasting blood sugar levels (to exclude diabetes mellitus, this may also warrant glucose tolerance test)
  o tests for HSV or other virus infections such as HIV may need to be considered
  o serum angiotensin converting enzyme levels to exclude sarcoidosis (although not a very sensitive investigation)
  o antinuclear antibodies (and others) to exclude connective tissue disease
  o in some areas, Lyme disease (tick-borne infection with *Borrelia burgdorferi*) should be assessed by determining presence of specific antibodies.

Occasionally, a lumbar puncture is required.

*Management*

Most patients with Bell palsy (up to 85%) improve spontaneously within a few weeks. However, the after-effects in the others can be so severe and distressing, that active treatment is warranted. The prognosis can be assessed on several factors:

Favourable prognostic signs include:

- incomplete paralysis in the first week
- persistence of the stapedial reflex, measured by electroneurography.
- Bad prognostic signs include:
  o an initially complete paralysis (then only 50% recover completely within a week, and few who have not recovered by 2 weeks will do so)
  o hyperacusis
  o severe taste impairment
  o diminished lacrimation or salivation, especially if in older, diabetic or hypertensive patients.

During the acute phase, the cornea should be protected with an eye pad.

There is a lack of large, randomized, controlled, prospective treatment studies but there are indications that corticosteroids or antiviral agents are beneficial though there are also some studies which show no benefit. Systematic reviews support the efficacy of corticosteroids but not antivirals. Treatment may, therefore, include:

- Anti-inflammatory medication. A short course of prednisolone.
- Antiviral medication (controversial). Aciclovir or valaciclovir or famciclovir.
- Massage. Facial massage may help prevent permanent contractures.

In chronic cases surgical decompression of the nerve in the stylomastoid canal may be attempted or fascial suspensory slings inserted.

Botulinum toxin injection may restore some facial contour (but not function) in instances of longstanding, irreversible facial muscle weakness.

### Cerebrovascular accident (stroke)

CVA (stroke) (Chapter 1.13).

Pure motor strokes cause partial or complete weakness in the face, arm and leg on one side of the body and, by definition, there is no loss of sensation, visual or speech symptoms. The weakness can be in any of these parts alone, or in combination with either of the other two. Most commonly, there is either a combination of arm and leg weakness, sparing the face, or a combination of arm, leg and face weakness. However, paralysis can also be seen in only one of these parts. Sensory strokes are also recognized (see below).

### Horner syndrome

Horner syndrome is caused by sympathetic nerve damage. Compression of the sympathetic chain by a lung tumour (e.g. Pancoast tumour—at the lung apex) is the most common cause. Damage to the post-ganglionic fibres, for example, a cavernous sinus tumour, may also be seen. Central lesions that damage the spinothalamic pathway (e.g. transection of the cervical spinal cord) are a rare cause.

Horner syndrome manifests with ipsilateral ptosis, enophthalmos, anhydrosis and facial flushing (Fig. 2.11.10). In children, Horner syndrome sometimes leads to a difference in eye colour between the two eyes.

### Hypcoglossal nerve palsy

Hypoglossal nerve (cranial nerve XII) palsy is uncommon, damage usually producing unilateral atrophy of the tongue muscles (Fig. 2.11.11).

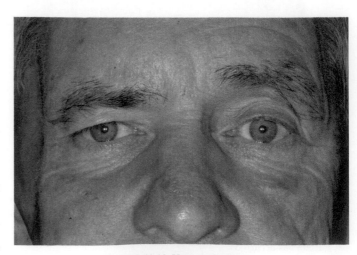

*Figure 2.11.10* Horner syndrome.

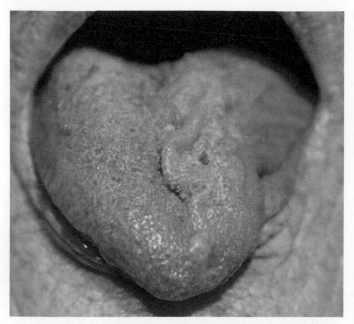

*Figure 2.11.11* Hypoglossal (XII) nerve palsy on the left side.

The hypoglossal nerve is liable to damage from lesions at the medullary, cisternal, skull base, nasopharyngeal space, parapharyngeal space, carotid space and lingual levels. Hypoglossal nerve palsy may be accompanied by other cranial nerve palsies (typically IX, X and XI) and by long tract signs, when malignant neoplasms are the most common cause. Other causes may include trauma, infarctions, multiple sclerosis, Guillain–Barré syndrome and infections.

Isolated hypoglossal nerve palsy is rare but may be caused by tumours at the skull base (nasopharyngeal and metastatic carcinomas—mostly from breast, kidney and prostate), Chiari malformation and dural arteriovenous fistulae. Direct compression of the hypoglossal nerve in the parapharyngeal space by a pseudoaneurysm or compression of small nutrient vessels can occasionally lead to palsy. Isolated hypoglossal nerve palsy is also rarely caused by internal carotid artery dissection (ICAD) and is then accompanied by pain in the head, neck or face ipsilateral to the dissected artery, and a partial Horner syndrome, followed hours or days later by cerebral or retinal ischaemia.

## SENSORY LOSS IN THE MAXILLOFACIAL REGION

The trigeminal nerve supplies sensation to most of the maxillofacial region, and the most common causes of sensory losses in the region are acquired—especially trauma to a division or branch of the nerve.

Trigeminal pathology may cause ipsilateral sensory loss as well as pain, in the trigeminal trophic syndrome (TTS) caused mainly by trigeminal neuralgia surgery, lateral medullary infarction (Wallenberg syndrome) or zoster.

Numb chin syndrome is unilateral chin numbness which may be caused by inferior alveolar nerve malignant infiltration; compression by jaw metastases (mainly lymphomas or breast cancer); osteomyelitis; metastatic or other deposit at the base of skull involving the mandibular division; metastasis to the meninges or as part of a paraneoplastic syndrome.

Bilateral chin numbness, or circumoral numbness may be caused by hyperventilation, hypocalcaemia or syringobulbia, vitamin B deficiency, ciguatera poisoning or drugs such as protease inhibitors or acetazolamide.

### Diagnosis

Blood tests may be needed to exclude connective tissue. Imaging is invariably indicated; dental panoramic tomogram (DPT) and CT or MRI of brain and skull base and mandibular division may be appropriate. Lumbar puncture may be necessary to exclude carcinomatous meningitis or leptomeningeal metastases.

### Extracranial causes of facial sensory loss

Extracranial causes of facial sensory loss are more common than intracranial, and include damage to the trigeminal nerve from the following causes.

Trauma—the usual cause—seen especially after orthognathic or cancer surgery. For example, after orthognathic sagittal split osteotomy, sensory loss affects 60–85% and, by 1 year follow-up is still seen in 12–18%. If the nerves are stretched or compressed (neuropraxia), there is often only hypoaesthesia, and recovery of sensation is speedy, typically within days. However, if the nerves are severed (neurotmesis), anaesthesia is profound and recovery is delayed for months and accompanied by paraesthesia or hyperaesthesia. Recovery is sometimes not complete.

Other causes of trauma to the mandibular division include:

- inferior alveolar local analgesic injections
- fractures of the mandibular body or angle
- surgery (particularly surgical extraction of lower third molars) or even endodontics or implants. Injuries to trigeminal nerves during endosseous implant placement in the posterior mandible may affect up to 5–15 of cases.

Other causes of damage to the mental nerve include:

- surgery in the region
- trauma from a denture—the mental foramen is close beneath a lower denture and there is ipsilateral anaesthesia of the lower lip.

Other causes of damage to the lingual nerve include lower third molar removal, particularly when the lingual split technique is used. Ipsilateral lingual hypoaesthesia or anaesthesia usually result.

Other causes of damage to branches of the maxillary division of the trigeminal nerve include trauma (usually Le Fort II or III middle-third facial fractures).

*Bone disease*

- Osteomyelitis (and now increasingly bisphosphonate-related osteonecrosis) in the mandible may affect the inferior alveolar nerve to cause ipsilateral labial anaesthesia.
- Paget disease.
- Osteopetrosis.

Diabetes may produce a neuropathy.

*Neoplastic disease*

- Trigeminal neuromas are the second most common form of schwannomas.
- Leukaemia, myeloma or metastases (usually from breast, lung, stomach or colon cancer) may cause deposits in the mandible and labial hypoaesthesia. Bone malignancies such as osteosarcoma may produce a similar pattern.
- Nasopharyngeal carcinomas may invade the pharyngeal wall to infiltrate the mandibular division of the trigeminal nerve, causing

pain and sensory loss in the region of the inferior alveolar, lingual and auriculotemporal nerve distributions; the levator palati to cause soft palate immobility; occlude the Eustachian tube, to cause deafness (Trotter syndrome).
- Oral carcinomas may invade the jaws to cause anaesthesia.
- Carcinoma of the maxillary antrum may produce ipsilateral upper labial hypoaesthesia or anaesthesia.

### Intracranial causes of facial sensory loss

Intracranial causes of facial sensory loss are uncommon but serious and may include:

*Sensory strokes*

Lacunar strokes (Chapter 1.13) affecting the thalamus may result in pure sensory changes (e.g. anaesthesia, hypoaesthesia, unusual perception of pain, temperature or pressure or changes in vision, hearing and taste). Most sensory lacunar strokes result in loss or abnormal sensation on one side of the body—affecting the face, arm, leg, thorax, genitals and anus. In some cases, these different body parts are affected in isolation. Thalamic syndrome (Dejerine–Roussy) is a rare disorder in which the body becomes hypersensitive to pain as a result of damage to the thalamus by pure sensory lacunar stroke.

Lower brainstem strokes such as lateral medullary infarcts may lead to facial sensory abnormalities as part of hemisensory loss of the spinothalamic type limited to the whole hemibody.

Ventroposteromedial nucleus stroke can lead to isolated facial sensory loss.

Sensorimotor lacunar stroke results from a lesion in the thalamus and also the adjacent posterior internal capsule and results in both sensory loss (thalamic damage) and motor loss—ipsilateral hemiplegia (internal capsule damage).

Stroke secondary to ICAD is seen usually under 40 years of age, in Marfan syndrome, after trauma to the neck, after certain medical procedures involving the carotid artery (e.g. arteriogram) and sometimes spontaneously. Ipsilateral headache, Horner syndrome and lower cranial neuropathies (especially XII but also sometimes the glossopharyngeal, vagal and the accessory nerves) may suggest carotid dissection. The wide range of features may include:

- Neck pain which may radiate to the eye
- Horner syndrome
- Pulsatile tinnitus
- Paresis
- Sensory changes
- Visual defects
- Vertigo
- Problems talking or understanding speech
- Inability in recognizing or identifying sensory stimuli (agnosia)
- Loss of memory and coordination
- Dysphagia
- Reduced taste sensation
- Personality, mood and emotion changes
- Changes in consciousness.

Cheiro-oral syndrome is a usually unilateral sensory disturbance at the commissure of the mouth and the ipsilateral palm of hand, due usually to a frontal, thalamic, midbrain or pontine (when there is often a cheiro-oral-pedal syndrome) lesion.

Complete hemisensory syndrome may be due to a sensory stroke where there is a thalamic lacunar infarction.

Trauma including surgical treatment of trigeminal neuralgia.

Drugs occasionally produce hypoaesthesia.

Multiple sclerosis may cause sensory loss.

Inflammatory disorders:

- sarcoidosis
- infections (e.g. HIV, syphilis)
- connective tissue disorders.

Neoplasms, such as brain tumours [often a metastasis or acoustic neuroma (vestibular schwannoma)].

- Since other cranial nerves are anatomically close, there may be associated neurological deficits in intracranial causes of facial sensory loss.
- In posterior cranial fossa lesions, for example, there may be cerebellar features such as ataxia.
- In middle cranial fossa lesions there may be associated neurological deficits affecting cranial nerve VI and thus mediolateral eye movements.
- Syringobulbia:

This may result from congenital abnormality, trauma or neoplasm, and is characterized by fluid- filled cavities (syrinxes), in the brainstem which can affect cranial nerves, resulting in facial palsies or sensory or motor nerve defects. It may lead to sensory loss spreading from the periphery of the face inwards towards the nose, plus a lower motor nerve lesion of the vagus, hypoglossal and accessory nerves, leading to disturbances of speech and swallowing, and bilateral UMN lesions affecting all limbs. A 'syringomyelia-like' syndrome has been infrequently reported in neurological disorders such as Tangiers disease, lepromatous leprosy and a novel syndrome termed facial onset sensory and motor neuronopathy, or FOSMN syndrome.

*Benign trigeminal neuropathy*

This is a longstanding sensory loss in one or more divisions of the trigeminal nerve of unknown cause. It seldom occurs until the second decade or affects the corneal reflex. The aetiology is unknown although it is important to exclude intracranial and extracranial causes before considering this to be the final diagnosis.

*Diabetes mellitus*

Diabetes mellitus (as part of a peripheral neuropathy).

*Psychogenic causes*

Hysteria, and particularly hyperventilation syndrome, may underlie some causes of facial anaesthesia/hypoaesthesia. Typically then, the 'anaesthesia' is bilateral and associated with bizarre neurological complaints.

*Congenital causes*

Rare cases of facial sensory loss are congenital, and may be associated with anhidrosis [congenital insensitivity to pain with anhidrosis (hereditary sensory and autonomic neuropathy type IV)], or with autonomic neuropathy [hereditary sensory and autonomic neuropathy (Riley–Day syndrome)].

*Clinical features*

Clinical tests for trigeminal nerve function include applying gentle touch, pinpricks or warm or cold objects to areas supplied by the nerve—these are reduced in trigeminal sensory loss. The jaw jerk and eye and corneal reflexes should also be examined. The patient's ability to chew and work against resistance tests motor function (Figs 2.11.12–2.11.15).

*Diagnosis*

In view of the potential seriousness of facial sensory loss, a full neurological assessment must be undertaken, unless the loss is unequivocally related to local trauma.

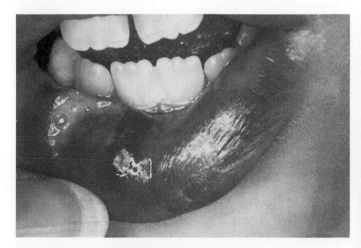

*Figure 2.11.12* Traumatic ulcer.

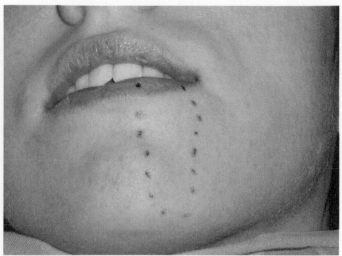

*Figure 2.11.13* Outline of area of mental nerve paraesthesia/hypoaesthesia in numb chin syndrome.

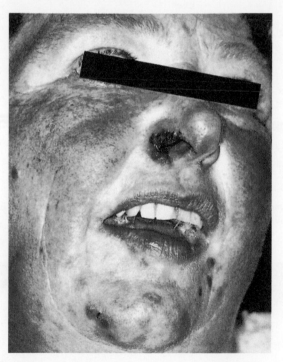

*Figure 2.11.14* Traumatic ulcer in cerebral neoplasm.

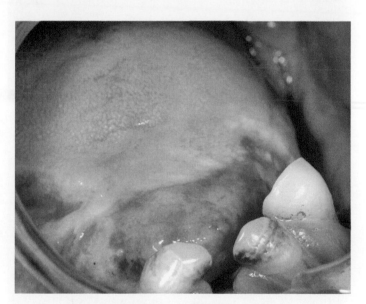

*Figure 2.11.15* Trauma in Riley–Day syndrome.

Possible investigations include:

- imaging (panoral, occipitomental, lateral and postero-anterior skull, and MRI/CT)
- a full blood count, ESR or CRP, random sugar, syphilis and HIV serology, autoantibody screen, electrophoresis, plasma calcium, phosphate and alkaline phosphatase
- lumbar puncture may be required if multiple sclerosis is suspected.

*Management*

If there has been neurotmesis, surgical correction can achieve good results. In benign, reversible causes, the underlying cause should be corrected, and the patient reassured that there should be some if not full return of sensation over the subsequent 18 months. Facial hypoaesthesia results in the loss of protective reflexes and a TTS with facial ulceration can follow. If the cornea is anaesthetic or hypoaesthetic, an eye pad should be worn over the closed eyelids, since the protective corneal reflex is lost and the cornea may be damaged.

### Frey syndrome

Frey syndrome (gustatory sweating).

*Aetiopathogenesis*

Gustatory sweating and flushing is a rare clinical problem that may occur after trauma to skin overlying a salivary gland. The syndrome follows between 6% and 60% of parotidectomies but it may follow damage in the parotid region by trauma, mumps, infection orthognathic or TMJ surgery and has also been recorded after submandibular gland surgery, thoracic sympathectomy (for hyperhidrosis), thyroidectomy, neck dissection and carotid endarterectomy. Less commonly, gustatory sweating follows facial injury or infection. Diabetes mellitus is a rare cause.

During nerve regeneration after the damage, parasympathetic fibres are misdirected down previously sympathetic pathways such that normal parasympathetic stimulation results in a sympathetic-driven vasomotor effect of sweating and flushing of the skin. The disorder usu-

ally involves the area of skin innervated by the auriculotemporal nerve and is often termed the auriculotemporal syndrome (Frey syndrome) but it may involve the lesser occipital nerve, the long buccal nerve, or any cutaneous branch of the cervical plexus. Onset is usually 12–18 months following the trauma but may be delayed for several years. Some cases are congenital and probably due to birth trauma. The term 'auriculotemporal syndrome' is misleading, as the skin innervated by the greater auricular nerve, may be involved.

### Clinical features

Gustatory sweating is characterized by sweating, flushing, a sense of warmth and occasional mild pain over an area of skin of the face while eating foods that produce a strong salivary stimulus. Sweating of the skin over the area of innervation can easily be induced by the patient sucking on a piece of orange.

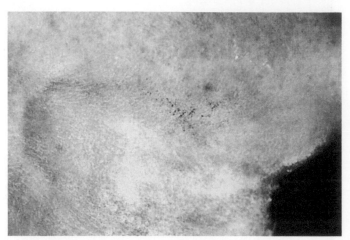

*Figure 2.11.16* Frey syndrome—after painting with starch iodine.

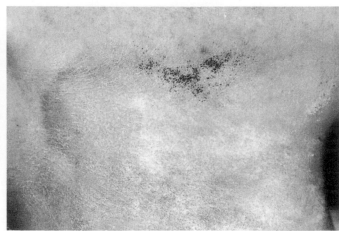

*Figure 2.11.17* Frey syndrome—after painting with starch iodine—colour change.

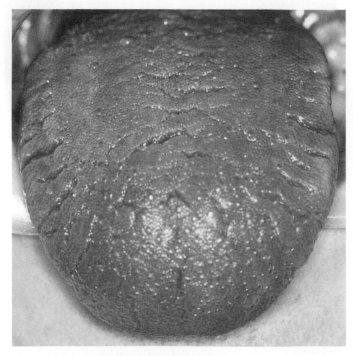

*Figure 2.11.18* Autonomic nerve dysfunction causing xerostomia in a patient with cholinergic dysautonomia.

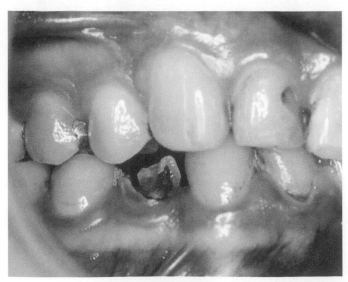

*Figure 2.11.19* Autonomic nerve dysfunction causing xerostomia in a patient with cholinergic dysautonomia.

*Diagnosis*

Frey syndrome is characterized by warmth and sweating of the face in the territory of the facial nerve initiated by any gustatory stimulus such as thinking or talking about food, or by eating foods that produce a strong salivary stimulus. Flushing is more prevalent in females, sweating in males. The diagnosis is confirmed either by applying an oral stimulus such as lemon or a positive starch–iodine test (Figs 2.11.16 and 2.11.17).

*Management*

Topical antiperspirants (e.g. alcoholic solution of aluminium hydroxide), anticholinergics (topical hyoscine as ointment or patch, topical glycopyrrolate or systemic clonidine, oxybutynin chloride, or propantheline bromide) or botulinum toxin injections are the most useful agents for the treatment of gustatory sweating.

### Autonomic neuropathy

Autonomic neuropathy (Figs 2.11.18 and 2.11.19) may be idiopathic or autoimmune (AAN; autoimmune autonomic neuropathy) when it is typically associated with autoantibodies against ganglionic acetylcholine receptors. Most patients have sicca complex (dry eyes and dry mouth), abnormal pupillary light response, orthostatic hypotension, upper gastrointestinal symptoms and neurogenic bladder.

# FURTHER READING

Adhikary SD, Korula PJ. The role of monitoring the depth of anesthesia in a case of hereditary sensory and autonomic neuropathy (Riley Day syndrome). Paediatr Anaesth 2007; 17: 402–3.

Ahn JY, Kwon SO, Shin MS, Joo JY, Kim TS. Chronic granulomatous neuritis in idiopathic trigeminal sensory neuropathy. Report of two cases. J Neurosurg 2002; 96: 585–8.

Alore PL, Jay WM, Macken MP. SUNCT syndrome: short-lasting unilateral neuralgiform headache with conjunctival injection and tearing. Semin Ophthalmol 2006; 21: 9–13.

Becker M, Kohler R, Vargas MI, Viallon M, Delavelle J. Pathology of the trigeminal nerve. Neuroimaging Clin N Am 2008; 18: 283–307.

Bigal ME. Diagnostic evaluation and treatment of trigeminal neuralgia. Curr Pain Headache Rep 2009; 13: 256–7.

Blanchet PJ, Popovici R, Guitard F, et al. Pain and denture condition in edentulous orodyskinesia: comparisons with tardive dyskinesia and control subjects. Mov Disord 2008; 23: 1837–42.

Blanchet PJ, Rompré PH, Lavigne GJ, Lamarche C. Oral dyskinesia: a clinical overview. Int J Prosthodont 2005; 18: 10–19.

Boban M, Brinar VV, Habek M, Radoš M. Isolated hypoglossal nerve palsy: a diagnostic challenge. Eur Neurol 2007; 58: 177–81.

de Bree R, van der Waal I, Leemans CR. Management of Frey syndrome. Head Neck 2007; 29: 773–8.

de Bree R, Duyndam JE, Kuik DJ, Leemans CR. Repeated botulinum toxin type A injections to treat patients with Frey syndrome. Arch Otolaryngol Head Neck Surg 2009; 135: 287–90.

Butler J, Fleming P, Webb D. Congenital insensitivity to pain—review and report of a case with dental implications. Oral Surg Oral Med Oral Pathol Oral Radiol Endod 2006; 101: 58–62. [Epub 2005 Nov 11].

Colella G, Cannavale R, Vicidomini A, Lanza A. Neurosensory disturbance of the inferior alveolar nerve after bilateral sagittal split osteotomy: a systematic review. J Oral Maxillofac Surg 2007; 65: 1707–15.

Erdem TL, Ozcan I, Ilgüy D, Sirin S. Hereditary sensory and autonomic neuropathy: review and a case report with dental implications. J Oral Rehabil 2000; 27: 180–3.

Fabbrini G, Defazio G, Colosimo C, Thompson PD, Berardelli A. Cranial movement disorders: clinical features, pathophysiology, differential diagnosis and treatment. Nat Clin Pract Neurol 2009; 5: 93–105.

Fatahzadeh M, Glick M. Stroke: epidemiology, classification, risk factors, complications, diagnosis, prevention, and medical and dental management. Oral Surg Oral Med Oral Pathol Oral Radiol Endod 2006; 102: 180–91.

Felicio AC, Bichuetti DB, Marin LF, dos Santos WA, Godeiro-Junior C. Bilateral horizontal gaze palsy with unilateral peripheral facial paralysis caused by pontine tegmentum infarction. J Stroke Cerebrovasc Dis 2009; 18: 244–6.

Gardiner J, Barton D, Vanslambrouck JM, et al. Defects in tongue papillae and taste sensation indicate a problem with neurotrophic support in various neurological diseases. Neuroscientist 2008; 14: 240–50.

Gilden DH. Clinical practice. Bell's palsy. N Engl J Med 2004; 351: 1323–31.

Gonella MC, Fischbein NJ, So YT. Disorders of the trigeminal system. Semin Neurol 2009; 29: 36–44.

Goto F. The long lasting effects of peripheral nerve blocks for trigeminal neuralgia using a high concentration of tetracaine dissolved in bupivacaine. Pain 1999; 79: 101–3.

Graff-Radford SB. Facial pain. Neurologist 2009; 15: 171–7.

Graham RM, Baldwin AJ. An unusual cause of Frey syndrome. Br J Oral Maxillofac Surg 2009; 47: 146–7.

Gregg JM. Neuropathic complications of mandibular implant surgery: review and case presentations. Ann R Australas Coll Dent Surg 2000; 15: 176–80.

Hagemann G, Aroyo IM. Bilateral facial palsy in neuroborreliosis. Arch Neurol 2009; 66: 534–5.

Harris MK, Shneyder N, Borazanci A, et al. Movement disorders. Med Clin North Am 2009; 93: 371–88, viii.

Hegedus F, Diecidue RJ. Trigeminal nerve injuries after mandibular implant placement—practical knowledge for clinicians. Int J Oral Maxillofac Implants 2006; 21: 111–16.

Keane J. Twelfth-nerve palsy: analysis of 100 cases. Arch Neurol 1996; 53: 561–6.

van Kleef M, van Genderen WE, Narouze S, et al. Trigeminal neuralgia. Pain Pract 2009; 9: 252–9.

Klein CM, Vernino S, Lennon VA, et al. The spectrum of autoimmune autonomic neuropathies. Ann Neurol 2003; 53: 752–8.

Klimacka-Nawrot E, Suchecka W. Methods of taste sensitivity examination. Wiad Lek 2008; 61: 207–10.

Komolafe MA, Fatusi OA, Alatise OI, et al. The role of human immunodeficiency virus infection in infranuclear facial paralysis. J Natl Med Assoc 2009; 101: 361–6.

Koopman JS, Dieleman JP, Huygen FJ, et al. Incidence of facial pain in the general population. Pain 2009; Sep 25. [Epub ahead of print].

Kovo M, Sagi Y, Lampl Y, Golan A. Simultaneous bilateral Bell's palsy during pregnancy. J Matern Fetal Neonatal Med 2009; 22: 1211–13.

Laurencet FM, Anchisi S, Tullen E, Dietrich PY. Mental neuropathy: report of five cases and review of the literature. Crit Rev Oncol Hematol 2000; 34: 71–9.

Lee C. Perineural spread of tumor along the fifth and seventh cranial nerves. Available from: [http://emedicine.medscape.com/article/875786-overview].

Lockhart P, Daly F, Pitkethly M, Comerford N, Sullivan F. Antiviral treatment for Bell's palsy (idiopathic facial paralysis). Cochrane Database Syst Rev 2009; CD001869.

Mackowiak A, Stojkovic T, Hurtevent JF, Maurage CA, Vermersch P. Late onset of type I familial amyloid neuropathy: results of biopsy from accessory salivary glands. Rev Neurol (Paris) 1999; 155: 155–7.

Madland G, Feinmann C. Chronic facial pain: a multidisciplinary problem. J Neurol Neurosurg Psychiatry 2001; 71: 716–19.

Maillefert JF, Gazet-Maillefert MP, Tavernier C, Farge P. Numb chin syndrome. Joint Bone Spine 2000; 67: 86–93.

Mohr JP, Choi DW, Grotta JC, Weir B, Wolf P A. Stroke: Pathophysiology, Diagnosis, and Management, 4th edn. London: Churchill Livingstone, 2004.

Mori K, Iijima M, Koike H, et al. The wide spectrum of clinical manifestations in Sjögren's syndrome-associated neuropathy. Brain 2005; 128(Pt 11): 2518–34.

Newton-John T, Madland G, Feinmann C. Chronic idiopathic orofacial pain. II. What can the general dental practitioner do? Br Dent J 2001; 191: 72–3 .

Obermann M, Katsarava Z. Update on trigeminal neuralgia. Expert Rev Neurother 2009; 9: 323–9.

Paduano S, Iodice G, Farella M, Silva R, Michelotti A. Orthodontic treatment and management of limited mouth opening and oral lesions in a patient with congenital insensitivity to pain: case report. J Oral Rehabil 2009; 36: 71–8.

Panconesi A, Bartolozzi ML, Guidi L. SUNCT syndrome or first division trigeminal neuralgia associated with cerebellar hypoplasia. J Headache Pain 2009; Sep 16. [Epub ahead of print].

Pearce JMS. Palatal myoclonus (syn. palatal tremor). Eur Neurol 2008; 60: 312–15.

Peñarrocha M, Cervelló MA, Martí E, Bagán JV .Trigeminal neuropathy. Oral Dis 2007; 13: 141–50.

Persu A, Băicuş A, Stavri S, Combiescu M. Non-polio enteroviruses associated with acute flaccid paralysis (AFP) and facial paralysis (FP) cases in Romania, 2001–2008. Roum Arch Microbiol Immunol 2009; 68: 20–6.

Quant EC, Jeste SS, Muni RH, et al. The benefits of steroids versus steroids plus antivirals for treatment of Bell's palsy: a meta-analysis. BMJ 2009; Sep 7; 339:b3354; doi: 10.1136/bmj.b3354.

Ram S, Teruel A, Kumar SK, Clark G. Clinical characteristics and diagnosis of atypical odontalgia: implications for dentists. J Am Dent Assoc 2009; 140: 223–8.

Robinson CM, Addy L, Wylie M, et al. A study of the clinical characteristics of benign trigeminal sensory neuropathy. J Oral Maxillofac Surg 2003; 61: 325–32.

Romero M, Simón R, García-Recuero JI, Romance A. Dental management of oral self-mutilation in neurological patients: a case of congenital insensitivity to pain with anhidrosis. Med Oral Patol Oral Cir Bucal 2008; 13: E644–7.

Rustemeyer J, Eufinger H, Bremerich A. The incidence of Frey's syndrome. J Craniomaxillofac Surg 2008; 36: 34–7.

Shiva Prasad BN, Balasubramanian R. Chronic otitis media and facial paralysis as a presenting feature of Wegener's granulomatosis. Singapore Med J 2009; 50: e155–7.

Shotts RH, Porter SR, Kumar N, Scully C. Longstanding trigeminal sensory neuropathy of nontraumatic cause. Oral Surg Oral Med Oral Pathol Oral Radiol Endod 1999; 87: 572–6.

Singla S, Marwah N, Dutta S. Congenital insensitivity to pain (hereditary sensory and autonomic neuropathy type V): a rare case report. J Dent Child (Chic) 2008; 75: 207–11.

Siqueira SR, Okada M, Lino AM, Teixeira MJ, Siqueira JT. Proposal for a standardized protocol for the systematic orofacial examination of patients with hereditary sensory radicular neuropathy. Int Endod J 2006; 39: 905–15.

Thompson AL, Bharatha A, Aviv RI, et al. Chondromyxoid fibroma of the mastoid facial nerve canal mimicking a facial nerve schwannoma. Laryngoscope 2009; 119: 1380–3.

Thompson EO, Smoker WR. Hypoglossal nerve palsy: a segmental approach. RadioGraphics 1994; 14: 939–58.

Vucic S, Tian D, Chong PS, et al. Facial onset sensory and motor neuronopathy (FOSMN syndrome): a novel syndrome in neurology. Brain 2006; 129(Pt 12): 3384–90. [Epub 2006 Sep 29].

Watt-Smith S, Mehta K, Scully C. Mefloquine-induced trigeminal sensory neuropathy. Oral Surg Oral Med Oral Pathol Oral Radiol Endod 2001; 92: 163–5.

Zaghi S, DaSilva AF, Acar M, Lopes M, Fregni F. One-year rTMS treatment for refractory trigeminal neuralgia. J Pain Symptom Manage 2009; 38: e1–5.

Zakrzewska JM. Classification issues related to neuropathic trigeminal pain. J Orofac Pain 2004; 18: 325–31.

Zakrzewska JM. Facial pain: an update. Curr Opin Support Palliat Care 2009; 3: 125–30.

Zakrzewska JM, Linskey ME. Trigeminal neuralgia. Clin Evid (Online) 2009; pii: 1207.

# 3 DIFFERENTIAL DIAGNOSES AND MANAGEMENT

3.1 Differential diagnoses by symptoms or signs
3.2 Differential diagnoses by site
3.3 Guide to the diagnosis and management of orofacial diseases
3.4 Guide to drugs used in the management of orofacial diseases
3.5 Guide to the orofacial adverse effects of drug treatment

## Anaesthesia or hypo-aesthesia

Numbness over the chin (numb chin syndrome) may indicate a lesion involving the mental or inferior alveolar nerves or may have more sinister implications

### Traumatic

Iatrogenic (e.g. nerve block anaesthesia, cancer surgery or osteotomy)
Jaw fracture
Direct trauma to trigeminal nerve or branches

### Idiopathic

Benign trigeminal sensory neuropathy
Hysteria

### Neoplasms

Disseminated malignancy in the absence of identifiable jaw deposits
Intracranial neoplasia
Jaw metastases
Pharyngeal neoplasia (Trotter syndrome)
Wegener granulomatosis

### Systemic non-malignant disease

Amyloidosis
Cerebrovascular disease and anomalies
Connective tissue disorders
Demyelinating diseases
Diabetes mellitus
Infections (sinusitis, osteomyelitis, syphilis and Whipple disease)
Sarcoidosis
Sickle cell disease
Vasculitides

### Drugs and poisons

Bisphosphonate-related osteonecrosis of the jaw
Osteochemonecrosis (denosumab, bevacizamab)
Others (see Section 3.5 and Chapter 1.6)

## Blisters

### Burns

### Angina bullosa haemorrhagica (localized oral purpura)

### Mucocutaneous diseases

Dermatitis herpetiformis
Epidermolysis bullosa (congenita and acquisita)
Erythema multiforme
Erythema multiforme and Stevens–Johnson syndrome
Intra-epidermal IgA pustulosis
Lichen planus (bullous)
Linear IgA disease
Pemphigoid (usually mucous membrane pemphigoid)
Pemphigus (usually pemphigus vulgaris)
Sweet syndrome

### Infections

Enteroviruses
Herpes simplex
Herpes varicella zoster

### Drugs (see Section 3.5 and Chapter 1.6)

### Paraneoplastic disorders

### Amyloidosis

### False blisters

Cysts
Superficial mucoceles

### Abscesses

## Burning mouth

### Psychogenic

Anxiety states
Cancerophobia
Depression
Hypochondriasis

### Drugs

See Section 3.5 and Chapter 1.6

### Deficiency states

B-complex deficiency
Folate deficiency

*(Continued)*

**Burning mouth**
*(Continued)*

Iron deficiency
Vitamin B$_{12}$ deficiency

*Neuropathic*

Various

*Infections*

Candidosis (rare)

*Others*

Diabetes mellitus
Erythema migrans (geographic tongue)
Xerostomia

**Cacogeusia**

*Oral disease*

Acute necrotizing ulcerative gingivitis
Bisphosphonate-related osteonecrosis of
   the jaws (BRONJ)
Chronic dental abscesses
Chronic periodontitis
Dry socket
Food impaction
Neoplasms
Osteochemonecrosis (denosumab,
   bevacizamab)
Osteomyelitis
Osteoradionecrosis
Pericoronitis
Sialadenitis

*Xerostomia*

Drugs
Irradiation damage
Sarcoidosis
Sjögren syndrome

*Psychogenic causes*

Anxiety states
Depression
Hypochondriasis
Psychoses

*Drugs* (see also Section 3.5 and Chapter 1.6)

*Smoking*

*Starvation*

*Nasal or pharyngeal disease*

Chronic sinusitis
Nasal foreign body
Neoplasm
Neoplasm
Oroantral fistula
Pharyngeal disease
Tonsillitis

*Diabetes*

*Respiratory disease*

Bronchiectasis
Neoplasm

*Gastrointestinal disease*

Gastric regurgitation
Liver disease
Pharyngeal pouch

*Central nervous system disease*

Temporal lobe epilepsy
Temporal lobe tumours

*Renal disease*

Uraemia

*Liver failure*

**Discharges**

*Dental disease*

Chronic dental and parodontal abscesses
Cysts
Dry socket
Infection by foreign body
Oroantral fistula
*(Continued)* Osteomyelitis

*Osteonecrosis*

Osteoradionecrosis
Bisphosphonate-related osteonecrosis of
   the jaw
Osteochemonecrosis (denosumab,
   bevacizamab)

| Discharges *(Continued)* | *Salivary gland disorders* | *Psychogenic (imagined discharges)* |
|---|---|---|

**Salivary gland disorders**

Salivary fistulae
Sialadenitis

**Psychogenic (imagined discharges)**

Depression
Hypochondriasis
Psychosis

---

**Dry mouth (xerostomia)**

(See also Section 3.5 and Chapter 1.6)

*Drugs with anticholinergic or sympathomimetic effects*

*Dehydration*

Diabetes insipidus
Diabetes mellitus
Diarrhoea and vomiting
Hypercalcaemia
Severe haemorrhage

*Psychogenic*

Anxiety states
Bulimia nervosa
Depression
Hypochondriasis

*Salivary gland disorders*

Amyloidosis or other deposits
Bone marrow transplantation/chronic
   graft-versus-host disease
Cystic fibrosis
Ectodermal dysplasia
HCV infection
HIV infection
Irradiation or chemotherapy damage
Salivary gland aplasia
Sarcoidosis
Sjögren syndrome

*Cholinergic dysautonomia*

---

**Dysarthria**

*Oral disease*

Cleft palate (including submucous cleft)
Oral or oropharyngeal neoplasia
Painful lesions or loss of mobility of the
   tongue or palate
Severe scarring
Tongue piercing

*Neurological disorders*

Amyotrophic lateral sclerosis
Bulbar and pseudo-bulbar palsy
Cerebellar ataxia
Cerebral disease
Cerebral palsy
Cerebrovascular accident
Dyskinesias
Dystonias
Huntington disease
Hypoglossal nerve palsy (also VII, IX and X)
Meige syndrome

Motor neurone disease
Multiple sclerosis
Myopathies
Parkinson disease
Sphyngolipidoses
Wilson disease

*Toxicity*

Adverse drug events
Alcohol
Narcotics
Overdoses

*Drugs* (see also Section 3.5 and
Chapter 1.6)

*Severe xerostomia*

*Mechanical*

Poorly fitting oral prostheses
Restricted jaw movement

**Dysphagia**

### Oral or pharyngeal disease

Inflammatory, traumatic, surgical or
  neoplastic lesions of tongue, palate or
  pharynx
Xerostomia

### Oesophageal disease

Extrinsic compressive lesions
  (e.g. mediastinal lymphadenopathy,
  left atrial dilatation in mitral
  stenosis)
Foreign body
Inflammatory, traumatic, surgical or
  neoplastic lesions
Oesophageal web (Plummer–Vinson,
  Patterson–Kelly–Brown or sideropaenic
  dysphagia)
Oesophagitis
Pharyngeal pouch
Schatzki ring
Scleroderma
Stricture

### Psychogenic

Hysteria (globus hystericus)

### Neurological disorders

Achalasia of the cardia
Amyopathic lateral sclerosis
Bulbar and pseudo-bulbar
  palsy
Cerebellar ataxia
Cerebral palsy
Cerebrovascular accident
Dystonias
Huntington disease
Lateral medullary syndrome
Motor neurone disease
Multiple sclerosis
Myopathies (e.g. myasthenia gravis)
Parkinson disease
Sphyngolipidoses
Syringobulbia/syringomyelia
Wilson disease

**Facial palsy**

### Neurological

Amyotrophic lateral sclerosis
Bell palsy
Bacterial infections (otitis media, botulism,
  leprosy, lyme disease)
Cerebral palsy
Cerebral tumour
Cerebrovascular accident
Connective tissue disorders
Diabetes mellitus
Kawasaki disease
Moebius syndrome
Multiple sclerosis
Trauma to facial nerve or its branches
Viral infection (e.g. herpes viruses,
  retroviruses or Guillain–Barré
  syndrome)

### Middle ear disease

Cholesteatoma
Malignancy
Mastoiditis

### Parotid lesions

Parotid malignancy
Parotid trauma

### Others

Crohn disease
Melkersson–Rosenthal syndrome
Orofacial granulomatosis
Reiter syndrome
Sarcoidosis (Heerfordt syndrome)

### Myopathies

## Facial swelling

Facial swelling is commonly inflammatory in origin—caused by cutaneous or dental (odontogenic) infections or trauma

### Infective

Cutaneous infections
Insect bites
Oral infections, cellulitis, fascial space infections

### Traumatic

Post-operative oedema or haematoma
Surgical emphysema
Traumatic oedema or haematoma

### Immunological

Allergic angioedema
$C_1$ esterase inhibitor deficiency
Crohn disease (and orofacial granulomatosis)
Melkersson–Rosenthal syndrome
Sarcoidosis

### Endocrine and metabolic

Acromegaly
Cushing syndrome and disease

Myxoedema
Nephrotic syndrome
Obesity
Systemic corticosteroid therapy

### Superior vena cava syndrome

### Cysts

### Neoplasms

Congenital (e.g. lymphangioma)
Lymphoma
Oral and antral tumours

### Foreign bodies

### Bone disease

Fibrous dysplasia
Paget disease
Cherubism

## Fissured tongue

Fissured tongue is common and usually inconsequential, although erythema-migrans is often associated

### Isolated

Developmental

### With systemic disease

Down syndrome
Melkersson–Rosenthal syndrome

## Halitosis (oral malodour)

### Oral sepsis

Bisphosphonate-related osteonecrosis of the jaw
Dental or periodontal sepsis
Dry socket
Food impaction
Necrotizing ulcerative gingivitis
Osteochemonecrosis (denosumab, bevacizamab)
Osteomyelitis
Osteoradionecrosis
Pericoronitis
Ulceration
Xerostomia

*(Continued)*

### Oral malignancy

### Nasopharyngeal disease

Foreign body
Neoplasm
Oesophageal pouch
Oesophageal reflux
Sinusitis
Tonsillitis

### Habits

Alcohol
Amyl nitrites
Solvent misuse
Tobacco

## Halitosis (oral malodour)
*(Continued)*

**Volatile foodstuffs**

Durian
Garlic
Highly spiced foods
Onions

**Drugs** (see also Section 3.5 and Chapter 1.6)
nitrates, phenothiazine, amphetamines,
cytotoxic drugs, disulfiram, melatonin,
nicotine lozenges, mycophenolate sodium
and aztreonam

**Systemic disease**

Acute febrile illness
Diabetic ketoacidosis
Hepatic failure
Renal failure
Respiratory tract infections
Trimethylaminuria

**Psychogenic (delusional)**

Neuroses
Psychoses

## Hirsutism

Hirsutism—defined as
more facial and body
hair than is acceptable
to a woman living in a
particular culture

ANDROGEN-MEDIATED

**Drugs**

Anabolic steroids
Androgens
Contraceptive pill

**Ovarian**

Insulin resistance
Ovarian tumours
Polycystic ovaries
Stromal hyperthecosis

**Adrenal**

Androgen-producing tumours
Congenital adrenal hyperplasia
Cushing syndrome

**Others**

Abducted thumbs syndrome
De Lange syndrome
Familial insulin resistance (and acanthosis
   nigricans)
Hurler syndrome
Idiopathic/hereditary
Leprechaunism
Lipodystrophy
Obesity
Pituitary tumour (e.g. prolactinoma)

Porphyria
Schwartz–Jampel syndrome
Scotts syndrome
Seckel syndrome
Testicular feminization
Trisomy 18
Weaver syndrome
Winchester syndrome

ANDROGEN-INDEPENDENT

**Racial**

**Pregnancy**

**Drugs**

Calcium-channel blockers
Ciclosporin
Corticosteroids
Danazol
Diazoxide
Minoxidil
Phenytoin

**Endocrine**

Acromegaly
Hypothyroidism

## Hyper-pigmentation

See Pigmentation

**Loss of taste**

*Anosmia*

Maxillofacial or head injuries (tearing of olfactory nerves)

Upper respiratory tract infections and sinus disease

*Neurological disease*

Bell palsy
Cerebral metastases
Cerebrovascular disease
Fractured base of skull
Frontal lobe tumour
Lesions of chorda tympani
Multiple sclerosis
Posterior cranial fossa tumours
Trigeminal sensory neuropathy

*Psychogenic*

Anxiety states
Depression
Psychoses

*Drugs* (see also Section 3.5 and Chapter 1.6)

*Others*

Herpes zoster virus infection
Hypothyroidism
Irradiation and chemotherapy
Uveoparotid fever and sarcoidosis
Vitamin $B_{12}$ deficiency
Xerostomia
Zinc or copper deficiency

---

**Pain**

*Local diseases*

*Diseases of the teeth*
Dentine sensitivity
Periapical periodontitis
Pulpitis

*Diseases of the periodontium*
Lateral (periodontal) abscess
Necrotizing periodontitis
Necrotizing ulcerative gingivitis
Pericoronitis

*Diseases of the jaws*
Bisphosphonate-related osteonecrosis of the jaw
Dry socket
Fractures
Infected cysts
Malignant neoplasms
Neuralgia-inducing cavitational osteonecrosis (a controversial diagnosis with some practitioners)
Osteochemonecrosis (denosumab, bevacizamab)
Osteomyelitis
Osteoradionecrosis

*(Continued)*

*Diseases of the maxillary antrum*
Acute sinusitis
Malignant neoplasms

*Diseases of the salivary glands*
Acute sialadenitis
Calculi or other obstruction to duct
HIV disease
Malignant neoplasms
Sjögren syndrome

*Diseases of the temporomandibular joint*
Arthritis
Temporomandibular joint dysfunction (facial arthromyalgia)
Others

*Vascular disorders*

Giant-cell arteritis
Migraine
Migrainous neuralgia

*Neurological disorders*

Bell palsy (rarely)
Herpes zoster (including post-herpetic neuralgia)
HIV disease
Malignant neoplasms involving the trigeminal nerve
Multiple sclerosis
Severe unilateral neuralgia with conjunctival tearing (SUNCT syndrome)
Trigeminal neuralgia

## Pain *(Continued)*

### Psychogenic pain

Idiopathic (atypical) facial pain and other oral symptoms associated with anxiety or depression

### Referred pain

Angina, nasopharyngeal, ocular and aural disease
Chest disease (rarely)

### Others

Drugs (e.g. vinca alkaloids)

## Pigmentation

### Racial

### Pregnancy

Chloasma

### Food/drugs (see Section 3.5 and Chapter 1.6)

### Endocrinopathies

Addison disease
Ectopic ACTH production
Nelson syndrome

### Others

Acanthosis nigricans
Agyria
Albright syndrome
Beta-thalassaemia
Betel nut chewing
Biliary atresia
Ecchymoses
Ephelis

Epithelioid angiomatosis
Haemochromatosis/haemosiderosis
Heavy-metal poisoning (lead, bismuth and arsenic)
Kaposi sarcoma
Laugier–Hunziker syndrome
LEOPARD syndrome
Melanoacanthoma
Melanoma
Melanotic macule
Naevus
Permanganate or silver poisoning
Peutz–Jeghers syndrome
Pigmentary incontinence
Smoker's melanosis
Spotty pigmentation, myxoma, endocrine overactivity syndrome
Tattoos (amalgam, lead pencils, ink, dyes, carbon)
von Recklinghausen neurofibromatosis

## Purpura

### Trauma (including suction)

### Platelet and vascular disorders

'Senile' purpura
Chronic renal failure
Ehlers–Danlos syndrome
Hyperglobulinaemic purpura,
Malignant histiocytosis
Marfan syndrome
Scurvy
*(Continued)* Thrombasthenia

Thrombocytopenia (especially drugs and leukaemias)
Von Willebrand disease
Waldenstrom macroglobulinaemia

### Vasculitis

Henoch Schonlein Purpura
Polyarteritis nodosa

**Purpura**
*(Continued)*

*Infections*

HIV infection
Infectious mononucleosis
Rubella

*Localized oral purpura (angina bullosa haemorrhagica)*

*Amyloidosis*

*Mixed connective tissue disease*

---

**Red areas**

*Generalized redness*

Candidosis (erythematous, acute atrophic and denture-associated)
Mucosal atrophy (e.g. avitaminosis B)
Mucositis
Polycythaemia

*Localized red patches*

Amyloidosis
Angiomas (purple)
Avitaminosis B$_{12}$
Burns
Candidosis
Crohn disease
Deep mycoses
Denture-related stomatitis
Desquamative gingivitis
Drug allergies
Epithelioid angiomatosis
Erythroplasia

Fixed drug eruptions
Geographic tongue
Haemangiomata
Kaposi sarcoma
Lichen planus
Lichenoid reactions
Lupus erythematosus
Median rhomboid glossitis
Mucoepithelial dysplasia syndrome
Plasma cell gingivitis
Psoriasis
Purpura
Sarcoidosis
Sprue and coeliac disease
Telangiectases
Wegener granulomatosis

*Vasculitis*

Henoch Schonlein Purpura
Polyarteritis nodosa

---

**Sialorrhoea (hypersalivation)**

*Psychogenic (usually)*

*Painful lesions in the mouth*

*Foreign bodies in the mouth*

*Drugs* (see also Section 3.5 and Chapter 1.6)

*Poor neuromuscular coordination*

Facial palsy
Other physical disability
Parkinsonism

*Poisoning*

Copper sulphate
Heavy metals
Insecticides
Mercury
Nerve agents

*Others*

Learning impairment
Obstructions
Oesophageal or pharyngeal
Oesophagitis
Pellagra (niacin deficiency)
Rabies (rarely)
Toxins
Viral labyrinthitis

**Taste Changes**

*Old Age*

*Upper respiratory conditions*

Tumors
Infections

*Trauma*

To cranial nerves

*CMS disorders*

Alzheimer disease
Brain tumors
Epilepsy
Parkinsonism

*Drugs*

Cytotoxic agents
Others (Section 3.5)

*Psychiatric disorders*

---

**Telangiectasia**

Ataxia telangiectasia
Carcinoid
Chronic liver disease
Hereditary haemorrhagic telangiectasia

Oestrogens
Post-irradiation
Pregnancy
Scleroderma

---

**Trismus**

*Extra-articular causes*

BRONJ
Coronoid hypertrophy or fusion to
  zygomatic arch
Fibrosis (including scars, scleroderma,
  radiotherapy and submucous fibrosis)
Fractured condylar neck
Hysteria
Infection, haematoma or inflammation in
  or near masticatory muscles or joint
Invading neoplasm
Lipoid proteinosis
Myositis ossificans
Strychnine poisoning
Submasseteric abscess

Temporomandibular joint dysfunction
  syndrome (facial arthromyalgia)
Tetanus
Tetany

*Intra-articular causes*

Ankylosis
Arthritides
Dislocation or subluxation
Intracapsular fracture
In contrast, some drugs such as
  metoclopramide and phenothiazines
  may cause facial muscle spasm inhibiting
  the patient from *closing* his or her mouth

---

**Ulcers**

*Local causes*

Traumatic (may be artefactual)
Chemical, electrical, thermal, radiation burns

*Neoplastic*

Carcinoma and other malignant tumours

*Recurrent aphthous stomatitis*

[Including aphthous-like ulcers as seen in
  Behçet's syndrome/MAGIC syndrome,
  Sweet's syndrome and auto-inflammatory
  syndromes (e.g. PFAPA: periodic fever,
  aphthae, pharyngitis, adenitis)]

Blood or vascular disorders: Anaemia,
  sideropenia, neutropenias, leukaemias,
  myelofibrosis, myelodysplasia, multiple
  myeloma, giant-cell arteritis, periarteritis
  nodosa
Gastrointestinal: Coeliac disease, Crohn's
  disease, orofacial granulomatosis
  ulcerative colitis
Connective tissue disease: Lupus
  erythematosus, Reiter disease, mixed
  connective tissue disease, Felty syndrome
Infective: Herpes simplex, chickenpox,
  herpes zoster, hand, foot and mouth
  disease, herpangina, infectious

*(Continued)*

**Ulcers**
*(Continued)*

### Systemic disease

Cutaneous disease: Erosive lichen planus, pemphigus, pemphigoid, erythema multiforme, dermatitis herpetiformis and linear IgA disease, epidermolysis bullosa, epidermolysis bullosa acquisita, IgA intraepithelial pustular dermatosis, chronic ulcerative stomatitis, graft-versus-host disease, osteomyelitis, BRONJ, osteochemonecrosis (denosumab, bevacizamab)

Others: Wegener granulomatosis, midline lethal granuloma, Langerhans cell histiocytoses, angiolymphoid hyperplasia with eosinophilia, necrotizing sialometaplasia, noma, hypereosinophilic syndrome

mononucleosis, cytomegalovirus infection, necrotizing ulcerative gingivitis, tuberculosis, atypical mycobacterial infections, syphilis, aspergillosis, cryptococcosis, leishmaniasis, tularaemia, lepromatous leprosy, mucormycosis, paracoccidioidomycosis, histoplasmosis, coccidioidomycosis, blastomycosis, HIV infection, Gram-negative bacteria, BRONJ

Drugs: Cytotoxics, many others (see Section 3.5 and Chapter 1.6)

**White lesions**

### Congenital

Darier disease
Dyskeratosis congenita
Hereditary benign intraepithelial dyskeratosis
Leukoedema
Pachyonychia congenita
Tylosis
White sponge naevus

### Acquired

*Inflammatory*
Infective: Candidosis, hairy leukoplakia, syphilitic leukoplakia, Koplik spots, papillomas

Non-infective: Lichen planus, lichen sclerosis, lupus erythematosus, pyostomatitis vegetans, xanthomatosis, dermatomyositis

*Neoplastic and possibly pre-neoplastic*
Keratoses (leukoplakias)
Carcinoma

*Others*
Drug burns
Grafts

**Table 3.1.1** MAIN ISOLATED HYPERPIGMENTED ORAL LESIONS

| Lesion | Usual age of presentation | Morphology | Colour | Main locations | Approximate size | Other comments |
|---|---|---|---|---|---|---|
| Amalgam tattoo | >5 years | Macular | Greyish or black | Floor of mouth mandibular gingivae | <1 cm | May be revealed by radiography |
| Graphite tattoo | >5 years | Macular | Greyish or black | Palate | <0.5 cm | May be revealed by radiography |
| Kaposi sarcoma | >Puberty | Macular becoming nodular | Purple or brown | Palate; gingivae | Any | Mainly in HIV/AIDS |
| Melanoma | Any | Macular becoming nodular | Brown, grey or black | Palate | Any | Rare |
| Melanotic macules | Any | Macular | Brown or black | Lips; gingivae | <1 cm | Mostly in Caucasians |
| Naevi | 3rd–4th decade | Raised | Blue or brown | Palate | <1 cm | |
| Purpura | Any | Macular | Red, purple or brown | Palate; buccal or lingual mucosa | Any | Usually traumatic |

**The lips**

## Angular stomatitis (cheilitis, cheilosis)

Acrodermatitis enteropathica
Anaemia
Ariboflavinosis (rarely), iron, folate or B12
    deficiency
Candidosis (denture-related stomatitis or
    other types)
Crohn disease and orofacial granulomatosis
Diabetes
HIV infection
Staphylococcal, streptococcal or mixed
    infections

## Bleeding

Angiomas
Arteriovenous malformations
Cracked lips
Erythema multiforme
Trauma
Underlying haemorrhagic disease
    aggravates tendency to bleed

## Blisters

Actinic cheilitis
Allergic cheilitis
Burns
Epidermolysis bullosa
Erythema multiforme
Herpes labialis
Herpes zoster
Impetigo
Mucoceles
Paraneoplastic pemphigus
Pemphigus vulgaris

## Desquamation and crusting

Actinic cheilitis
Acute febrile illness
Allergic cheilitis
Candidal cheilitis
Chemical cheilitisor
Dehydration
Drugs
Erythema multiforme
Exfoliative cheilitis
Exposure to hot dry winds
Mouth-breathing
Psychogenic (self-induced)

*(Continued)*

## Swellings

There is a wide individual and racial
    variation in the size of the lips

### Diffuse swellings

Allergic angioedema
Ascher syndrome
$C_1$ esterase inhibitor deficiency
Cheilitis glandularis
Cheilitis granulomatosa
Crohn disease
Haemangioma
Lymphangioma
Macrocheilia
Melkersson–Rosenthal syndrome
Oedema (trauma or infection or insect bite)
Orofacial granulomatosis
Sarcoidosis

### Localized swellings

Abscesses
Amyloid
Angioma
Anthrax
Basal cell carcinoma
Chancre
Crohn disease and orofacial
    granulomatosis
Cysts
Fibrous lumps
Foreign bodies
Haematomas
Infections
Insect bites
Keratoacanthoma
Leprosy
Lymphangioma
Lymphoma
Mucoceles
Mycoses
Pyogenic granuloma
Rhinoscleroma
Salivary adenoma
Sarcoidosis
Squamous cell carcinoma
Trauma
Trichiniasis
Tuberculosis
Ulceration
Warts

**The lips**
*(Continued)*

### Ulceration

*Infective*
Herpes labialis
Herpes zoster
Impetigo
Leishmaniasis
Mycoses
Syphilis

*Tumours*
Basal cell carcinoma
Keratoacanthoma
Others
Squamous cell carcinoma

*Burns*
*Mucocutaneous disease*
Erythema multiforme
Lichen planus

Lupus erythematosus
Pemphigoid
Pemphigus
Trauma

### White lesions

Actinic keratosis
Carcinoma
Fordyce spots
Keratoses
Leukoplakias
Lichen planus
Lupus erythematosus
Scars
White sponge naevus

---

**The gingivae**

### Red areas

Redness is usually a sign of chronic
gingivitis or periodontitis, but is then
restricted to the gingival margins. Other
red lesions, which may affect the gingiva
include:

*Congenital*
Angiomas
Cyclic neutropenia
Hereditary haemorrhagic telangiectasia
Mucoepithelial dysplasia
syndrome

*Acquired*
Dermatomyositis
Desquamative gingivitis: lichen planus,
pemphigoid, pemphigus, dermatitis
herpetiformis, linear IgA disease, lupus
erythematosus, pyostomatitis vegetans,
psoriasis
Drugs: e.g. chlorhexidine, cinnamonaldehyde
Epithelioid angiomatosis
Leukaemia(s)
Mycoses: candidosis, *Geotrichum candidum*,
deep mycoses
Neoplasms (carcinoma, Kaposi sarcoma,
lymphoma)
Neutropenias
Plasma cell gingivitis (gingivostomatitis)
*(Continued)* Potential malignancy (e.g. erythroplasia)

Primary biliary cirrhosis
Sarcoidosis
Scleroderma
Trauma: physical, chemical, radiation,
thermal
Wegener's granulomatosis

### Bleeding

*Periodontal disease*
Acute ulcerative gingivitis
Aggressive periodontitis
Chronic gingivitis
Chronic periodontitis
HIV gingivitis
HIV periodontitis

*Haemorrhagic disease*
Angiomas
Arteriovenous malformations
Bleeding tendencies
Chronic renal failure Ehlers–Danlos
syndrome
Haemophilias
Hepatobiliary disease
Hereditary haemorrhagic telangiectasia
Idiopathic thrombocytopenic purpura
Lymphoproliferative disorders
Myelodysplastic disorders
Myelofibrosis
Myeloproliferative disorders
Primary platelet disorders

**The gingivae**
*(Continued)*

Scurvy
Von Willebrand disease

*Drugs*
Anticoagulants
Cytotoxics
Non-steroidal anti-inflammatory drugs
Sodium valproate

### Gingival swelling

*Generalized and congenital*
Amyloidosis
Aspartylglucosaminuria
Cross syndrome
Fucosidosis
Gingival fibromatosis
Gingival fibromatosis with growth hormone
  deficiency (Byars–Jurkiewicz syndrome)
Hypoplasminogenaemia
Infantile systemic hyalinosis
Jones' syndrome
Leprechaunism (Donohue syndrome)
Lipoid proteinosis
Mucolipidosis (I-cell disease)
Mucopolysaccharidosis 1-H
Murray–Puretic–Drescher syndrome
Pfeiffer syndrome
Ramon syndrome
Rutherfurd syndrome
Zimmermann–Laband syndrome

*Generalized and acquired*
Acute myeloid leukaemia
Aplastic anaemia
Drugs (phenytoin, ciclosporin, calcium
  channel blockers, others)
Preleukaemic leukaemia
Vitamin C deficiency

*Localized and congenital*
Congenital gingival granular cell tumour
Cowden syndrome (multiple hamartoma
  and neoplasia syndrome)
Fabry syndrome (angiokeratoma corporis
  diffusum universale)
Focal dermal hypoplasia
Hypoplasminogenaemia
Lipoid proteinosis
Sturge–Weber angiomatosis
Tuberous sclerosis

*Localized and acquired*
Crohn disease
Epithelioid angiomatosis
Fibroepithelial epulis
Giant cell epulis
Heck disease
Langerhans cell tumours
Lymphomas
Multiple myeloma
Neoplasms (e.g. papillomas, squamous cell
  carcinoma, Kaposi sarcoma)
Orofacial granulomatosis
Plasmacytomas
Pregnancy epulis
Pyogenic granuloma
Sarcoidosis
Wegener granulomatosis

### Ulcers

Ulcers that affect predominantly the gingivae
  are usually traumatic, acute ulcerative
  gingivitis or occasionally results of
  immunodeficiency, especially acute leukaemia, neutropenias or HIV disease. The
  gingivae can, however, be affected by most
  other causes of mouth ulcers (see page 420)

### Enhanced periodontal destruction

The association between inflammatory
  periodontal disease and candidate gene
  polymorphisms is controversial but
  interleukin-1 (IL-1), IL-6, IL-10, IL-12, IL-16
  and vitamin D receptor may be involved.
  A range of immunodeficiencies or other
  defects or lifestyle choices may underlie
  accelerated or aggressive periodontitis

*Secondary immunodeficiencies*
Crohn disease
Diabetes mellitus
HIV disease
Leukaemias
Malnutrition
Pregnancy

*Primary immunodeficiencies*
Acatalasia
Benign familial neutropenias
Chediak–Higashi syndrome
Chronic granulomatous disease

**The gingivae**
*(Continued)*

Cyclic neutropenia
Defective neutrophil function
Down syndrome
Fanconi anaemia
Hyperimmunoglobulinaemia E (Job syndrome)
Kartagener syndrome
Leukocyte adhesion deficiency
Severe combined immunodeficiency (SCID)

*Other congenital disorders*
Acro-osteolysis (Hajdu–Cheney syndrome)

Dyskeratosis benigna intraepithelialis mucosae et cutis hereditara
Ehlers–Danlos syndrome type VIII
Haim–Munk syndrome
Hypophosphatasia
Oxalosis
Papillon–Lefèvre syndrome
Type 1b glycogen storage disease

*Other acquired causes*
Tobacco use
Vitamin C deficiency

---

**The palate**

*Lumps*

*Developmental*
Angiomas
Cysts
Torus palatinus
Unerupted teeth

*Inflammatory*
Abscesses
Adenomatoid hyperplasia
Cysts
Franklin heavy chain disease
Necrotizing sialometaplasia
Papillary hyperplasia
Sarcoidosis

*Neoplasms*
Fibrous overgrowths
Kaposi sarcoma
Lymphomas
Oral or antral carcinoma
Papillomas and condylomas
Salivary tumours

*Redness*

Redness restricted to the denture-bearing area of the palate is almost invariably denture-related stomatitis (candidosis), although erythematous candidosis of HIV disease can commonly occur as a red patch of the palate. Other red lesions may be erythroplasia, Kaposi sarcoma or other lesions

*Ulceration*

Burns
Infections (e.g. herpesviruses, enteroviruses)
Lichen planus
Lupus
Necrotizing sialometaplasia
Neoplasms
Osteonecrosis
Pemphigoid
Pemphigus
Trauma

---

**The tongue**

*Swellings or lumps*

*Localized*
Congenital: lingual thyroid, haemangioma, lymphangioma, lingual choristoma
Inflammatory: infection, abscess, median rhomboid glossitis, granuloma, foliate papillitis, insect bite
Traumatic: oedema, haematoma
Neoplastic: fibrous lump, papilloma, neurofibroma, carcinoma, sarcoma, granular cell tumour (granular cell myoblastoma)
Others: foreign body, cysts, warts, condylomas

*Diffuse*
Congenital: Down syndrome, cretinism, mucopolysaccharidoses, lymphangioma, haemangioma
Inflammatory: infection, insect bite, Ludwig angina
Traumatic: oedema, haematoma
Others: multiple endocrine adenomatosis type 3; angioedema; amyloidosis; cyst; acromegaly; muscular (Beckwith–Wiedeman syndrome); deposits (glycogen storage disease, I cell disease, mucopolysaccharidoses)

*(Continued)*

## The tongue
*(Continued)*

### Sore tongue

*With obvious localized lesions*
Any cause of oral ulceration
  (see page 420)
Foliate papillitis
Geographic tongue
Median rhomboid glossitis

*Glossitis (generalized redness and depapillation)*
Anaemias
Avitaminosis B

Candidosis
Chemotherapy
Graft-versus-host disease
Post-irradiation mucositis

*With no identifiable physical abnormality*
Anaemia/sideropenia
Depression or cancerophobia
Diabetes
Glossodynia
Hypothyroidism

## The major salivary glands

### Swellings

*Inflammatory*
Actinomycosis
Ascending (acute suppurative)
  sialadenitis
HCV infection
HIV salivary gland disease
Lymphadenitis
Mumps
Recurrent parotitis
Recurrent sialadenitis
Sarcoidosis
Sjögren syndrome

*Neoplasms*
*Others*
Amyloidosis
Duct obstruction
Haemochromatosis
HIV disease

Mikulicz disease (lymphoepithelial lesion
  and syndrome)
Sialosis (sialadenosis)

*Drug-associated*
See also Section 3.5 and Chapter 1.6

### Salivary gland pain

*Inflammatory*
Acute sialadenitis
HIV sialadenitis
Mumps
Recurrent sialadenitis
Sjögren syndrome
Stones or other causes of obstruction

*Neoplastic*
Salivary gland malignant tumours

*Drug-associated*
See also Section 3.5 and Chapter 1.6

## The neck

### Swellings in the neck

*Cervical lymph nodes*
Inflammatory: lymphadenitis
  (nasopharyngeal, antral, dental, tonsillar,
  aural, facial or scalp infections),
  glandular fever syndromes (EBV, CMV,
  Brucella, Toxoplasma, HIV, HHV-6),
  tuberculosis or other mycobacterial
  infections, other infections (rubella, cat
  scratch, syphilis)
Neoplasms: secondary carcinoma (oral,
  nasopharyngeal or thyroid primary),
  lymphoma, leukaemia

*(Continued)*

Others: connective tissue disease, drugs
  (e.g. phenytoin), mucocutaneous lymph
  node syndrome (Kawasaki syndrome),
  sarcoidosis

*Salivary glands*
Mumps
Tumours
Sjögren syndrome
Sarcoidosis
Sialadenitis
Sialosis

*Side of the neck*
Actinomycosis

**The neck**
*(Continued)*

Branchial cyst
Parapharyngeal cellulitis
Pharyngeal pouch
Cystic hygroma
Carotid body tumours or aneurysms

*Muscle or other soft tissue neoplasm*
Focal myositis
Myositis ossificans
Proliferative myositis
Nodular pseudosarcomatous fasciitis

*Midline of the neck*
Submental lymphadenopathy
Thyroglossal cyst
Ectopic thyroid
Thyroid tumours or goitre
'Plunging' ranula
Ludwig angina
Dermoid cyst
Other skin lesions

**The teeth**

### Abnormalities of shape

Connation (double)
Dilaceration; bent root/tooth
Enamel clefts
Macrodontia; all teeth enlarged
Microdontia; all teeth small
Taurodontism

### Causes of Staining

*Extrinsic causes*
*Brown stain*
Cetylpyridinium chloride rinse
Chlorhexidine rinse
Dental plaque
Doxycycline
Iodine
Khat leaf
Liquorice and other coloured foods
Metals
Stannous fluoride
Tea, coffee, wine and other beverages
Tobacco products
*Black stain*
Betel nut
Certain foods
Chromogenic bacteria
Dental plaque
Iron medications
Metals
Tea, coffee, wine and other beverages
Tobacco products
*Green stain*
Chromogenic bacteria
Metals
Tea

*(Continued)*

*Orange stain*
Chromogenic bacteria
Doxycycline
Metals

*Intrinsic causes*
*Localized colour changes (in one or two
   adjacent teeth)*
*White (opaque) stain*
Incipient caries (primary or secondary teeth)
Mild trauma to teeth during enamel
   formationamelogenesis (secondary teeth),
   e.g. turner tooth
Periapical infection of primary tooth
   predecessor
Traumatic injury to primary developing
   tooth or teeth
*Yellow stain*
Caries (active)
Composites or glass ionomer or acrylic
   restorations
Focal tooth abrasion
Moderate trauma to teeth during enamel
   formation amelogenesis (secondary
   teeth), e.g. turner tooth
Periapical infection of primary tooth
   predecessor
Trauma without haemorrhage
Traumatic injury to primary tooth or teeth
*Brown stain*
Severe trauma to teeth during amelogenesis
   (secondary teeth), e.g. turner tooth
Periapical infection of primary predecessor
Traumatic injury to primary tooth or teeth
Composite, glass ionomer or acrylic
   restoration
Caries (active or remineralized)
Pulpal trauma with haemorrhage

**The teeth**
*(Continued)*

*Blue, grey or black stain*
Amalgam restoration
Glass ionomer or acrylic restoration
Metal crown margin associated with porcelain fused to metal crown
Pulpal trauma with haemorrhage

*Regional colour changes*
*White (opaque) stain*
Infection (maternal or childhood) during enamel formation
Mild fluorosis (short-term exposure)
Nutritional deficiency
Trauma to multiple teeth during enamel formation
*Yellow stain*
Epidermolysis bullosa
Hyperbilirubinaemia
Infection (maternal or childhood) during enamel formation
Moderate fluorosis (short-term exposure)
Nutritional deficiency
Regional tooth abrasion or erosion
Trauma to multiple teeth during enamel formation
*Brown stain*
Infection (maternal or childhood) during enamel formation
Severe fluorosis (short-term exposure)
Trauma to multiple teeth during enamel formation

Adapted from Kerr R.

*Blue, grey or black stain*—tetracycline therapy (short-term exposure)
*Green stain*—hyperbilirubinaemia (e.g. haemolytic disease of newborn (HDN) biliary atresia)

*Generalized changes (involving primary and/or permanent dentitions)*
*White (opaque) stain*
Amelogenesis imperfecta
Mild fluorosis
*Yellow stain*
Amelogenesis imperfecta
Dentinal dysplasia
Dentinogenesis imperfecta
Diseases causing hyperbilirubinemia
Epidermolysis bullosa
Haemolytic diseases
Moderate fluorosis
Tooth surface loss (attrition, abrasion or erosion)
*Brown stain*
Porphyria
Tetracycline therapy (long-term exposure)
*Blue, grey or black stain*
Minocycline therapy
Tetracycline therapy (long-term exposure)
*Green stain*—hyperbilirubinaemia (e.g. HDN, biliary atresia)

---

**Oral complaints frequently associated with psychogenic factors[a]**

[a]Organic causes should first be excluded.

Atypical facial pain
Atypical odontalgia
Bad or disturbed taste
Dry mouth
Gripping dentures
Non-existent discharges
Non-existent lumps or spots

Sore or burning mouth
Supposed anaesthesias and dysaesthesias
Supposed sialorrhoea
Temporomandibular joint dysfunction
Vomiting or nausea caused by dentures

# 3.3 GUIDE TO THE DIAGNOSIS AND MANAGEMENT OF OROFACIAL DISEASES

| Condition | Typical main clinical features | Investigations that may be indicated for diagnosis in addition to history and examination | Management |
|---|---|---|---|
| **Abscess (dental)** | Pain ± swelling | Radiography ± vitality test | Drain either by incision if pointing, or through tooth. Analgesics; antimicrobials |
| **Acanthosis nigricans** | Hyperpigmented confluent papillomas mainly in groin/axillae | Biopsy, gastroscopy, barium studies | Treat underlying cause. Exclude diabetes mellitus and malignancy |
| **AIDS** | Opportunistic infections (especially fungal and viral), Kaposi sarcoma, lymphomas, encephalopathy | HIV antibodies and viral load, CD4 lymphocyte count | Anti-retroviral therapy (ART). Prophylaxis/ treatment of infections |
| **Acromegaly** | Increasing prognathism and hand size, enlarging pituitary fossa, headaches, tunnel vision, lethargy, weight gain | Lateral skull radiography, growth hormone assays, visual fields, CT/MRI | Treat pituitary adenoma |
| **Actinomycosis** | Purplish indurated swelling(s) over mandible or neck | Pus for microscopy and culture 'sulphur granules' | Antimicrobial: penicillin for 4 weeks |
| **Acute bacterial sialadenitis** | Painful salivary swellings ± fever and/or trismus | Pus for culture and sensitivity | Antimicrobial: flucloxacillin |
| **Acute necrotizing ulcerative gingivitis** | Interdental papillary ulceration and bleeding, halitosis, pain | Smear may help | Antimicrobial: penicillin or metronidazole. Consider excluding HIV. Oral hygiene improvement. Mechanical debridement |
| **Addison disease** | Weakness, lassitude, loss of weight, hyperpigmentation | Blood pressure, electrolytes, 24-hour cortisol Synacthen test | Corticosteroids |
| **Adenoid cystic carcinoma** | Firm salivary swelling | Biopsy and radiography | Surgery |
| **Agammaglobulinaemia** | Recurrent pyogenic infections, especially respiratory and cutaneous | Serum immunoglobulins | Immunoglobulin replacement Antimicrobials |
| **Albright's syndrome** | Fibrous dysplasia, precocious puberty, hyperpigmentation, endocrine disease | Radiography ± bone biopsy | ± Surgery ± calcitonin |
| **Alveolar osteitis (dry socket)** | Empty painful extraction socket, halitosis | Radiography to exclude fracture or foreign body | Debridement, obtundent dressing ± antimicrobial |

| Condition | Typical main clinical features | Investigations that may be indicated for diagnosis in addition to history and examination | Management |
| --- | --- | --- | --- |
| **Amalgam tattoo** | Grey to black pigmented area(s) usually over the mandible | ± Radiography. Biopsy if any doubt | Reassurance |
| **Ameloblastoma** | Slow growing swelling, usually in mandible | Imaging and biopsy | Surgery |
| **Angioedema** | Facial swelling (see also hereditary angioedema) | C1 esterase inhibitor, IgE, C3 and C4 levels | Antihistamines/corticosteroids |
| **Angular cheilitis** | See cheilitis | | |
| **Aphthae** | Recurrent oral ulcers only | Full blood picture, exclude underlying systemic disease (e.g. coeliac disease) | Corticosteroids topically, amlexanox, chlorhexidine, topical tetracycline (doxycycline) |
| **Atypical (idiopathic) facial pain** | Persistent dull ache typically in one maxilla in a female | Clinical and radiographic MRI exclusion of organic disease | Reassurance, cognitive behavioural therapy (CBT), tricyclic antidepressants, selective serotonin reuptake inhibitors (SSRIs) |
| **Bell palsy** | Lower motor neurone facial palsy only | Exclude middle ear lesion Lyme disease, cerebellopontine angle tumour, diabetes, hypertension, HIV | Corticosteroids systemically. Protect cornea |
| **Behçet syndrome** | Recurrent oral and genital ulceration, other systemic features | Full blood picture, white cell count and differential | Colchicine, thalidomide or azathioprine may be indicated |
| **Black hairy tongue** | Black hairy tongue | – | Reassurance. Brush tongue ± tretinoin |
| **Bourneville–Pringle disease (epiloia)** | Papules or nodules around nose/mouth, cerebral subungual fibromas, ash leaf patches | Skull radiography. Biopsy skin lesions | Anticonvulsants |
| **Bruton syndrome** | See agammaglobulinaemia | | |
| **Bruxism** | Attrition and sometimes masseteric hypertrophy | Full blood picture, electrolytes | Reassurance. Psychogenic care. Restoration of dental erosions |
| **Bulimia nervosa** | Recurrent self-induced vomiting | Radiography/sialography sialodendoscopy | Reassurance, CBT, tricyclic antidepressants, SSRIs. Surgery ± lithotripsy |

| Condition | Typical main clinical features | Investigations that may be indicated for diagnosis in addition to history and examination | Management |
|---|---|---|---|
| **Burning mouth syndrome** | See glossodynia | | |
| **Calculus, salivary** | Recurrent salivary swelling ± pain at mealtimes | | Debridement |
| **Cancrum oris** | Chronic ulceration | Consider biopsy, consider immune defect | Antimicrobial, improve nutrition |
| **Candidosis** | White or red persistent lesions | Smear plus culture, consider immune defect | Antifungal |
| **Carcinoma** | Ulcer, lump or red or white lesion | Biopsy. Chest radiography | Surgery ± radiotherapy |
| **Central papillary atrophy** | See median rhomboid glossitis (see candidosis) | | Antimicrobial: penicillin |
| **Chancre** | Single, painless indurated ulcer usually on lip or tongue | Syphilis serology ± biopsy | |
| **Cheek-chewing** | Shredded or keratotic lesions around occlusal line and/or on lower labial mucosa | | Avoid habit, occlusal splint, botulinum toxoid |
| **Cheilitis, actinic** | Soreness and/or keratosis on lower lip Sun exposure | Consider biopsy | Avoid exposure. Bland UV protecting creams. Laser excision Imiquimod, retinoids |
| **angular** | Commissures | Haematological screen Denture assessment | Denture modification/ replacement Oral and denture hygiene Antifungal: miconazole |
| **Cherubism** | Slowly enlarging swellings over mandible | Radiography biopsy | Reassurance |
| **Child abuse syndrome** | Various injuries inconsistent with history | Photographs radiography | Manage injuries. Protect child from further abuse |
| **Chronic granulomatous disease** | Recurrent pyogenic infections, cervical lymphadenopathy | Assay neutrophil phagocytosis and killing of bacteria | Antimicrobials Bone marrow transplantation |
| **Chronic mucocutaneous candidosis** | Persistent mucocutaneous candidosis | Assay T-cell function. Biopsy fungal culture | Antifungals |
| **Cicatricial pemphigoid** | See mucous membrane pemphigoid | | |

| Condition | Typical main clinical features | Investigations that may be indicated for diagnosis in addition to history and examination | Management |
|---|---|---|---|
| **Cleidocranial dysplasia** | Patent fontanelles, clavicles can approximate | Radiography of skull and clavicles | Remove supernumerary teeth/cysts |
| **Coeliac disease** | Loose stool, malabsorption, loss of weight/failure to thrive | Tissue transglutaminase small bowel biopsy | Gliadin or endomysial antibodies, gluten-free diet |
| **Condyloma acuminata (condylomas)** | Warts | Biopsy | Surgery, podophyllum or interferon or imiquimod |
| **CREST syndrome** | Raynaud phenomenon, changing facial appearance. Mucosal telangiectases Sjögren syndrome | Anti-centromere antibodies + radiographs | Immunosuppressives |
| **Crohn disease** | Loose stool, malabsorption, abdominal pain ± orofacial granulomatosis | Endoscopy, biopsy. Barium meal and follow-through | Sulphasalazine or corticosteroids or tacrolimus |
| **Cyclic neutropenia** | Recurrent pyogenic infections | Serial neutrophil counts | Antimicrobials, colony-stimulating factor |
| **Denture-induced hyperplasia** | Hyperplasia close to denture flange | Biopsy | Ease denture flange; excise hyperplasia |
| **Denture-related stomatitis** | Erythema in denture-bearing area | Fungal culture | Leave denture out at night stored in antifungal |
| **Dermatitis herpetiformis** | Pruritic rash | Small bowel biopsy, gliadin antibodies | Gluten-free diet Dapsone or sulphapyridine |
| **Dermatomyositis** | Proximal limb and trunk weakness plus heliotrope rash | Serum creatine kinase and aldolase Electro-myography Skin/muscle biopsy | Systemic corticosteroids, other systemic immunosuppressants and acetylsalicyclic acid |
| **Dermoid cyst** | Submental swelling | Radiography | Surgery |
| **Desquamative gingivitis** | Erythematous desquamating gingivae | Biopsy ± immunofluorescence | Topical corticosteroids or tacrolimus, improve oral hygiene |
| **Diabetes mellitus** | Polyuria, polydipsia | Blood sugar (fasting) Hyperglycaemia Glucose tolerance test | Diet or insulin ± oral hypoglycaemic agent |
| **Discoid lupus erythematosus** | See lupus | | |
| **Dry mouth** | See Sjögren syndrome | | |
| **Dry socket** | See alveolar osteitis | | |

| Condition | Typical main clinical features | Investigations that may be indicated for diagnosis in addition to history and examination | Management |
|---|---|---|---|
| **Ectodermal dysplasia** | Dry thin hair, dry skin, fever, hypodontia | Radiography for hypodontia | Restorative dentistry |
| **Ephelis** | See freckles | | |
| **Epidermolysis bullosa** | Blisters at sites of trauma | Biopsy | Protect against trauma Vitamin E ± phenytoin |
| **Epiloia** | See Bourneville–Pringle disease | | |
| **Epulis** | | | |
| congenital | Firm nodule on gingiva | — | Excise if no resolution |
| fibrous | Firm nodule on gingiva | — | Excise |
| fissuratum | Firm leaf-like swellings | — | Change denture. Excise |
| giant cell | Purplish swelling in premolar area | Exclude hyperparathyroidism | Surgery |
| in pregnancy | Soft swelling typically on anterior gingivae | Pregnancy test | Leave or excise |
| **Erythema** | | | |
| migrans | Desquamating patches on tongue | — | Reassurance |
| multiforme | Oral ulcers, swollen lips. Target lesions | Biopsy | Corticosteroids, aciclovir if herpes-induced |
| nodosum | Tender red lumps on shins | Biopsy ± serum for immune complexes | Treat underlying cause |
| **Erythroplakia (erythroplasia)** | Red velvety patch | Biopsy | Excise |
| **Facial arthromyalgia** | TMJ pain, click, limitation of movement | Rarely radiography ± arthroscopy | Reassurance, occlusal splint, anxiolytics or antidepressants |
| **Familial fibrous dysplasia** | See cherubism | | |
| **Familial white-folded gingivostomatitis** | White persistent lesions in mouth, rectum, vagina | Biopsy | Reassurance |
| **Felty syndrome** | Rheumatoid arthritis, splenomegaly, neutropenia | Full blood picture, rheumatoid factor, erythrocyte sedimentation rate | Salicylates |
| **Fibroepithelial polyp** | Firm pink polyp | | Excision |
| **Fibroma, leaf** | See fibroepithelial polyp | | |

| Condition | Typical main clinical features | Investigations that may be indicated for diagnosis in addition to history and examination | Management |
|---|---|---|---|
| **Fibromatosis, gingival** | Firm pink gingival swellings | — | Excision |
| **Fibrous dysplasia** | Bony swelling | Radiographs and biopsy | Excision or await resolution |
| **Fibrous lump** | See fibroepithelial polyp | | |
| **Foliate papillitis** | Painful swollen foliate papilla | — | Reassurance |
| **Fordyce spots** | Yellowish granules in buccal mucosae or lips | — | Reassurance |
| **Fragilitas ossium** | Spontaneous fractures, blue sclera | Radiography | Orthopaedic care |
| **Freckles (ephelides)** | Brown macules | | Reassurance |
| **Frey syndrome** | Gustatory sweating | Starch-iodine test | Glycopyrrolate |
| **Gardner syndrome** | Osteomas, desmoid tumours, colonic polyps | Radiography of jaws, colonoscopy | Excision of colonic polyps Genetic counselling |
| **Geographic tongue** | See erythema migrans | | |
| **German measles** | Macular rash, fever, occipital lymphadenopathy | — | Symptomatic |
| **Glandular fever** | Fever, sore throat, generalized lymphadenopathy | White cell count and differential, Paul Bunnell test, consider HIV and other serology | Symptomatic, corticosteroids systemically if airway threatened |
| **Glossitis** | | | |
| atrophic | Depapillated tongue | Full blood picture, haematinic assay | Treat underlying cause and deficiency |
| benign migratory | See erythema migrans | | |
| in iron deficiency | Depapillated tongue, angular stomatitis, ulcers | Full blood picture, serum ferritin | Treat underlying cause and deficiency |
| median rhomboid | See central papillary atrophy | | |
| **Moeller in vitamin B$_{12}$ deficiency** | Depapillated tongue angular stomatitis, ulcers | Full blood picture, serum B12 | Treat underlying cause and deficiency |
| **Glossodynia** | Burning normal-looking tongue | Full blood picture, haematinic assay, fasting blood glucose | Treat underlying cause where possible ± antidepressants |

| Condition | Typical main clinical features | Investigations that may be indicated for diagnosis in addition to history and examination | Management |
|---|---|---|---|
| Gorlin–Goltz syndrome (Gorlin syndrome) | Odontogenic keratocysts, basal cell naevi, skeletal anomalies | Radiography skull, jaws, chest | Remove cysts. ± Etretinate |
| Haemangioma | Blush or reddish swelling | Empties on pressure angiography | Leave or cryoprobe, laser, embolize or sclerose |
| Haemophilia | Haemarthroses, ecchymoses, severe bleeding after trauma | Haemostasis assays | Cover surgery with factor replacement antifibrinolytics |
| Hairy leukoplakia | White lesions on tongue | HIV serology ± biopsy | ART |
| Halitosis | Oral malodour | Oral/ENT examination and radiography | Treat underlying cause |
| Hand, foot and mouth disease | Oral ulcers, mild fever, vesicles on hands and/or feet | — | Symptomatic |
| Heck disease | Oral papules | Biopsy | Observe, interferon or remove |
| Heerfordt syndrome | Uveitis, parotitis, fever, facial palsy | Chest radiography. Biopsy, serum angiotensin-converting enzyme, calcium levels | Corticosteroids |
| Hereditary angioedema | Recurrent facial swellings | C1 esterase inhibitor, C3 and C4 assays | Danazol or stanazolol or C1 esterase inhibitor |
| Hereditary haemorrhagic telangiectasia | Telangiectasia on lips, mouth, hands | Full blood picture and haemoglobin | Laser or cryoprobe to bleeding Telangiectases |
| Herpangina | Oral ulcers, mild fever | — | Symptomatic |
| Herpetic stomatitis | Oral ulcers, gingivitis, fever | Sometimes smear or serology | Symptomatic ± aciclovir |
| Herpes labialis | Vesicles, pustules, scabs at mucocutaneous junction | Sometimes serology | Penciclovir or aciclovir cream |
| Herpes zoster | See shingles | | |
| Histiocytosis (Langerhans cell) | Osteolytic lesions | Biopsy, skeletal survey | Depends on type; from no treatment to chemotherapy and irradiation |
| Histoplasmosis | Cough, fever and weight loss | Biopsy ± chest radiography | Fluconazole |
| Hodgkin lymphoma | Chronic lymph node swelling ± fever | Biopsy ± lymphangiography | Radiotherapy/ chemotherapy |
| Horner syndrome | Bilateral pupil constriction, ptosis | Chest radiography | Identify cause |

| Condition | Typical main clinical features | Investigations that may be indicated for diagnosis in addition to history and examination | Management |
|---|---|---|---|
| **HIV** | See AIDS | | |
| **Human papillomavirus infections** | Warty lesions | Biopsy | Excise, podophyllum, imiquimod or topical or intralesional interferon |
| **Hyperparathyroidism** | Renal calculi, polyuria, abdominal pain<br>Brown tumour in jaws | MRI jaw ± skeletal radiography, plasma calcium, phosphate and parathyroid hormone, bone scan | Remove parathyroid adenoma |
| **Hypo-adrenocorticism** | See Addison disease | | |
| **Hypohidrotic ectodermal dysplasia** | See ectodermal dysplasia | | |
| **Hypoparathyroidism, congenital** | Tetany, cataracts, enamel hypoplasia (may be part of polyendocrinopathy syndrome) | Plasma parathormone, calcium phosphate levels | Calcium, vitamin D |
| **Hypophosphatasia** | Anorexia, bone pain, weakness | Plasma calcium phosphate and alkaline phosphatase levels | Calcium, vitamin D |
| **Idiopathic midfacial granuloma syndrome (T/NK lymphoma)** | Ulceration | Biopsy, anti-neutrophil cytoplasmic antibody | Chemotherapy; radiotherapy |
| **Impetigo** | Facial rash, blisters, often golden yellow | Culture and sensitivity | Antimicrobial: penicillin |
| **Infectious mononucleosis** | See glandular fever | | |
| **Kaposi sarcoma** | Purplish macules or nodules | Biopsy, HIV serology | Chemotherapy or radiotherapy, ART |
| **Kawasaki disease** | Lymphadenopathy, conjunctivitis, dry lips, strawberry tongue, desquamation, cardiomyopathy/myocarditis | Full blood picture, erythrocyte sedimentation rate, electrocardiogram | Symptomatic |
| **Keratoconjunctivitis sicca** | See Sjögren syndrome | | |
| **Keratosis** | | | |
| **frictional** | White lesion usually on alveolar ridge | | Try to eliminate cause |
| **smoker's** | White lesion in palate | | Try to eliminate cause |

| Condition | Typical main clinical features | Investigations that may be indicated for diagnosis in addition to history and examination | Management |
|---|---|---|---|
| **verrucous** | Raised or warty white lesion | Biopsy | Excise if dysplastic, stop tobacco use |
| **sublingual** | White lesion in floor of mouth and ventrum of tongue | Biopsy | Excise if dysplastic, stop tobacco use |
| **Langerhans cell histiocytoses** | See histiocytosis | | |
| **Leishmaniasis** | Mucocutaneous ulceration, lymphadenopathy | Biopsy | Pentamidine or stibogluconate |
| **Leprosy** | Hypo- or hyperpigmented patches, lymphadenopathy, neuropathy | Biopsy | Dapsone or clofazimine |
| **Letterer–Siwe disease** | See histiocytosis | | |
| **Leukaemia** | Anaemia, bleeding tendency, infections, lymphadenopathy | Full blood picture ± film, bone marrow biopsy | Chemotherapy; bone marrow transplantation |
| **Leukopenia** | Recurrent infections | Full blood picture, bone marrow biopsy | Antimicrobials; bone marrow transplantation |
| **Leukoplakia** | See keratosis and see hairy leukoplakia | | |
| **Lichen planus** | Mucosal white or other lesions. Polygonal purple pruritic papules on skin | Biopsy ± immunofluorescence | Corticosteroids or tacrolimus topically, stop tobacco use |
| **Lichenoid lesions: drug-induced** | Mucosal white lesions. Polygonal purple pruritic papules on skin | Biopsy | Corticosteroids topically, stop causative drug |
| **Linear IgA disease** | Mucosal vesicles or desquamative gingivitis | Biopsy ± immunofluorescence | Dapsone ± sulphapyridine, gluten-free diet |
| **Localized oral purpura** | Blood blisters only in mouth | Platelet count, biopsy may be needed to differentiate from pemphigoid | Reassurance ± deflate blisters |
| **Ludwig angina** | Tender brawny submandibular swelling, fever | Pus for culture and sensitivity | Drainage, antimicrobials: penicillin in high dose ± tracheostomy |
| **Lupus erythematosus** | Arthralgia, fever, rash, lymphadenopathy, lichenoid mucosal lesions | Antibodies to double-strand DNA | Corticosteroids, antimalarials |

| Condition | Typical main clinical features | Investigations that may be indicated for diagnosis in addition to history and examination | Management |
|---|---|---|---|
| **Lyme disease** | Acute arthritis—mainly knee, rash ± facial palsy | Serology | Antimicrobials |
| **Lymphadenitis** | | | |
| acute | Tender swollen lymph nodes | Temperature, examine drainage area<br>White cell count and differential | Treat cause |
| chronic | Chronically enlarged lymph nodes | Temperature, examine drainage area<br>White cell count and differential chest radiograph. Consider biopsy ± HIV testing | Treat cause |
| **Lymphangioma** | Swelling but empties on pressure | Imaging | Leave or surgery, cryotherapy, laser therapy or sclerosant |
| **Lymphoma** | Wide spectrum. Swollen lymph nodes, fever, weight loss | Biopsy<br>Radiography | Chemotherapy ± radiotherapy |
| **Lymphosarcoma** | See lymphomas | | |
| **McCune–Albright syndrome** | See Albright's syndrome | | |
| **Maffucci syndrome** | Enchondromatosis plus cavernous haemangiomas | Radiography | Reassurance |
| **MAGIC syndrome** | See Behçet syndrome | | |
| **Masseteric hypertrophy** | Masseter enlarged on both or occasionally one side | — | Symptomatic<br>Rarely surgery ± botulinum toxoid |
| **Measles** | Fever, lymphadenopathy, conjunctivitis, rhinitis, maculopapular rash | — | Symptomatic<br>Avoid aspirin |
| **Median rhomboid glossitis** | Rhomboidal red or nodular and depapillated or white, in midline of dorsum of tongue, just anterior to circumvallate papillae | Smear of lesion | Antifungals if *Candida* present<br>Stop smoking<br>Biopsy (wide excision) |
| **Melanoma** | Usually hyperpigmented papule in palate | Biopsy | Surgery |
| **Melanotic macules** | Hyperpigmented macule | | Reassurance |
| **Melkersson–Rosenthal syndrome** | Facial swelling, fissured tongue, facial palsy | Exclude Crohn disease and sarcoidosis | Reassurance ± salazopyrine ± dapsone ± intralesional steroids |

| Condition | Typical main clinical features | Investigations that may be indicated for diagnosis in addition to history and examination | Management |
|---|---|---|---|
| **Migrainous neuralgia** | Nocturnal unilateral retro-ocular pain | Imaging | H3 blockers, oxygen, analgesics |
| **Molluscum contagiosum** | Umbilicated papules | Consider HIV infection | Pierce with orangewood stick |
| **Morsicatio buccarum** | See cheek chewing | — | |
| **Mucocele** | Fluctuant swelling with clear or bluish contents | — | Surgery or cryotherapy |
| **Mucoepidermoid tumour** | Firm salivary swelling | Biopsy ± radiography | Surgery |
| **Mucormycosis** | Sinus pain and discharge plus fever and palatal ulceration | Biopsy. Radiography Full blood picture Exclude diabetes | Surgery. Antifungals |
| **Mucous membrane pemphigoid** | Blisters, mainly in mouth occasionally on conjunctivae, genitals or skin. Scarring | Biopsy ± immunostaining | Topical corticosteroids Dapsone Systemic steroids or immunosuppressives |
| **Multiple myeloma** | Bone pain, anaemia, nausea, infections, amyloidosis | Radiography. Serum and urine and electrophoresis. Bone marrow biopsy | Radiotherapy and chemotherapy. Bisphosphonates. Bone marrow transplantation |
| **Mumps** | Fever, painful swollen salivary gland(s) mainly but no pustular discharge from duct | Serology may be helpful | Symptomatic |
| **Mycosis fungoides** | Variable rash | Biopsy. Full blood picture bone marrow biopsy | Topical chemotherapy ± radiotherapy |
| **Myelodysplastic syndrome** | Ulcers, anaemia, neutropenia, thrombocytopenia | Full blood picture. Bone marrow biopsy | Chemotherapy, bone marrow transplantation |
| **Necrotizing sialometaplasia** | Ulceration, usually in palate | Biopsy may be indicated | Self-healing |
| **Neurofibromatosis** | Neurofibromas and skin pigmentation usually | Radiography and biopsy may help | Excise symptomatic tumours Genetic counselling |
| **Noma** | See cancrum oris | | |
| **North American blastomycosis** | Chronic oral ulceration, pulmonary involvement | Biopsy ± chest radiography | Antifungals: fluconazole, ketoconazole or amphotericin |
| **Oral dysaesthesia** | See burning mouth | | |

| Condition | Typical main clinical features | Investigations that may be indicated for diagnosis in addition to history and examination | Management |
|---|---|---|---|
| **Oral submucous fibrosis** | Firm fibrous bands in cheek and/or palate History of chilli use | Biopsy | Stretch Avoid chillis and pan Corticosteroids intralesionally |
| **Orf** | Umbilicated nodule | Electron microscopy ± biopsy | Spontaneous resolution |
| **Orofacial granulomatosis** | Facial swelling, mucosa cobblestoned, ulcers, angular stomatitis (see also Crohn disease) | Exclude Crohn's disease/ sarcoidosis Biopsy ± allergy testing | Avoid allergens. Reassurance Corticosteroids intralesionally Clofazimine, anti-tumour necrosis factor (TNF) agents |
| **Osler–Rendu–Weber syndrome** | See hereditary haemorrhagic telangiectasia | | |
| **Osteogenesis imperfecta** | See fragilitis ossium | | |
| **Osteomyelitis** | Pain, swelling, fever, sensory loss | Radiography. Pus for culture and sensitivity | Drainage. Antimicrobials |
| **Osteopetrosis** | Anaemia, cranial neuropathies Hepatosplenomegaly | Radiography | Bone marrow transplant |
| **Osteoradionecrosis** | See osteomyelitis | | |
| **Osteosarcoma** | Pain, swelling | Biopsy Radiography | Surgery ± chemotherapy |
| **Paget disease** | Pain, craniofacial neuropathies, cardiac failure | Biopsy Radiography, serum alkaline phosphatase, urinary hydroxyproline | Bisphosphonates, acetylsalicyclic acid, calcitonin |
| **Pain dysfunction syndrome** | See facial arthromyalgia | | |
| **Papillary hyperplasia** | Small papillae in palate | | Surgery or leave alone |
| **Paracoccidioidomycosis** | Chronic oral ulceration, pulmonary involvement. Time in Latin America | Biopsy ± chest radiography | Antifungals: fluconazole, ketoconazole or amphotericin |
| **Parodontal abscess** | Painful swelling alongside a periodontally involved tooth | Radiography, culture pus | Drain. Antimicrobial: penicillin |
| **Pemphigoid** | See mucous membrane pemphigoid membrane | | |

| Condition | Typical main clinical features | Investigations that may be indicated for diagnosis in addition to history and examination | Management |
|---|---|---|---|
| **Pemphigus** | Skin vesicles ± bullae, mouth<br>Mouth ulcers | Biopsy. Serology, immunostaining | Corticosteroids systemically and topically<br>Consider azathioprine, gold or mycophenolate |
| **Periadentitis mucosa necrotica recurrens (Sutton ulcers)** | See aphthae | | |
| **Periarteritis nodosa** | See polyarteritis nodosa | | |
| **Pericoronitis** | Painful swelling of operculum of partially erupted tooth ± trismus ± fever | Radiography | Debridement ± antimicrobial<br>Reduce occlusion. Consider extracting offending tooth |
| **Periodontitis (acute apical)** | Pain, tenderness on touching tooth | Radiography ± vitality test | Open tooth for drainage and relieve occlusion (or extract), analgesics ± antimicrobial |
| **Perleche** | See cheilitis, angular | | |
| **Phycomycosis** | See mucormycosis | | |
| **Pleomorphic salivary ademona** | Firm salivary swelling | Biopsy ± radiography | Surgery |
| **Polyarteritis nodosa** | Fever, weakness, arthralgia, myalgia, abdominal pain, hypertension | Full blood picture, erythrocyte sedimentation rate<br>Biopsy | Systemic corticosteroids |
| **Polycythaemia rubra vera** | Headache, thromboses, haemorrhage, splenomegaly | Haemoglobin, full blood picture, marrow biopsy | Phlebotomy ± chemotherapy |
| **Polyps—fibroepithelial** | See fibroepithelial polyp | | |
| **Pulpitis** | Toothache | Radiography ± vitality test | Open tooth (or extract). Extirpate pulp<br>Analgesics |
| **Pyogenic arthritis** | Pain, fever, limited jaw movement, swelling | Radiography, culture joint aspirate | Antimicrobial, analgesics |
| **Pyogenic granuloma** | Swelling, usually on lip, tongue or gingiva | Biopsy (excision) | Excise |
| **Pyostomatitis vegetans** | Irregular oral ulcers and pustules | Biopsy. Exclude Crohn disease and ulcerative colitis | Treat underlying condition |
| **Ranula** | See mucocele | | |

| Condition | Typical main clinical features | Investigations that may be indicated for diagnosis in addition to history and examination | Management |
|---|---|---|---|
| Recurrent aphthous stomatitis | See aphthae | | |
| Recurrent parotitis | Recurrent painful parotid swelling | Sialography. Exclude Sjögren syndrome | Consider duct dilatation Antimicrobials |
| Reiter syndrome | Arthritis, conjunctivitis, mucocutaneous lesions, urethritis | Full blood picture, erythrocyte sedimentation rate Radiography | Tetracycline. Non-steroidal anti inflammatory drugs |
| Rheumatoid arthritis | Painful swollen small joints ± deformities | Rheumatoid factor, full blood picture associated with Sjögren syndrome Check for xerostomia | Salicylates. Non-steroidal anti-inflammatory drugs. Biological response modifiers, e.g. anti-TNF |
| Rickets | Skeletal deformities, retarded growth, fractures | Radiography Blood calcium, phosphate, alkaline phosphatase | Vitamin D. Calcitonin |
| Rubella | See German measles | | |
| Rubeola | See measles | | |
| Sarcoidosis | Various—especially hilar lymphadenopathy and rashes | Radiography. Renal function tests Chest radiograph ± serum angiotensin-converting enzyme | Corticosteroids systemically |
| Scleroderma | Tightening facial and other skin Associated with Sjögren syndrome | Serology Scl-70 antibody white blood cell count | Systemic immunosuppressive agents Supportive |
| Scrotal tongue | Fissured tongue | — | Reassurance |
| Scurvy | Purplish chronically swollen gingivae | Vitamin C levels | Vitamin C |
| Shingles | Painful facial rash and oral ulcers if affecting maxillary or mandibular division of trigeminal nerve | Consider underlying immune defect | Analgesics, aciclovir, valaciclovir, protect cornea |
| Sialolithiasis | See calculus, salivary | | |
| Sialorrhoea | Excess salivation | Salivary flow rate | Avoid anticholinesterases, otherwise reassurance or consider atropinics |

| Condition | Typical main clinical features | Investigations that may be indicated for diagnosis in addition to history and examination | Management |
| --- | --- | --- | --- |
| **Sialosis** | Painless persistent bilateral salivary gland swelling | Exclude alcoholism, diabetes, bulimia, sarcoidosis, Sjögren syndrome, liver disease | Remove underlying cause |
| **Sinusitis (acute)** | Pain especially on moving head | Radiography Transillumination, endoscopy | Decongestants, analgesics and antimicrobial |
| **Sjögren syndrome** | Autoimmune exocrinopathy. Dry eyes, dry mouth and often a connective tissue disease | Serology—SS-A (Ro) and SS-B (La) antibodies. Exclude HCV, HIV. Consider labial gland biopsy ± salivary flow rate ± sialography ± scintiscan | Artificial tears and saliva. Preventive dentistry, pilocarpine, cevimeline |
| **Smoker's keratosis** | See keratosis | | |
| **South American blastomycosis** | See paracoccidioidomycosis | | |
| ***Staphylococcus aureus* lymphadenitis** | Painful swollen lymph node(s) ± fever | Pus for culture and sensitivity | Antimicrobials |
| **Stevens–Johnson syndrome** | See erythema multiforme | | |
| **Streptococcal tonsillitis** | Sore throat. Tonsillar exudate | Throat swab | Antimicrobials |
| **Stroke** | Hemiplegia usually ± facial palsy | | Physiotherapy, rehabilitation, oral hygiene, treatment of drooling |
| **Subluxation-temporo-mandibular joint** | Limited jaw movement ± pain, condyle palpably displaced | Radiography | Reduce. Consider use of sclerosant agent sodium tetradecyl sulphate or Dautrey operation |
| **Surgical emphysema** | Swelling which crackles on palpation | | Reassurance. Antimicrobials |
| **Tori** | Asymptomatic bony lumps | | Reassurance. Surgery if interfering with denture wear |
| **Toxoplasmosis** | Lymphadenopathy ± chorioretinitis | Serology | Sulphonamide ± pyrimethamine |

| Condition | Typical main clinical features | Investigations that may be indicated for diagnosis in addition to history and examination | Management |
|---|---|---|---|
| **Trigeminal neuralgia** | Severe lancinating pain often associated with trigger zone | Skull base CT, MRI | Avoid trigger zone. Carbamazepine, oxcarbazine, lamotrigine, phenytoin, gabapentin, baclofen or clonazepam. Neurosurgical procedures |
| **Tuberculosis** | Cough, cervical, lymphade-nopathy, weight loss, oral ulceration | Chest radiograph Sputum microscopy and culture. PCR | Antimicrobials: rifampicin, isoniazid, ethambutol, streptomycin |
| **White sponge naevus** | See familial white folded gingivostomatitis | Biopsy | |
| **Zygomycosis** | See mucormycosis | | |

# 3.4 GUIDE TO DRUGS USED IN THE MANAGEMENT OF OROFACIAL DISEASES

This section refers to agents most commonly used in routine oral medicine practice. Biological response modifiers and other drugs that are currently largely restricted to medical specialist practice are not included. Before using a drug always check doses, possible interactions, contraindications and adverse effects, with the British National Formulary, or Physician's Desk Reference or www.bnf.org, www.medsafe.govt.n2/profs/datasheet/dsform.asp, or www.nlm.nih.gov/medlineplus/druginformation.html. While every attempt has been made to include accurate data, the authors and publishers accept no liability.

**Table 3.4.1** ANALGESICS (including opioids)

| Drug | Type | Comments | Route | Adult dose |
|---|---|---|---|---|
| **Paracetamol** (Acetaminophen) | Non-opioid; not usually termed an NSAID | Mild analgesic: suitable for children<br>No anti-inflammatory action<br>Hepatotoxic in overdose or prolonged use or with alcohol<br>Contraindicated in liver or renal disease. Co-methiamole also contains methionine to reduce hepatotoxicity. Mixed analgesics are co-codamol which also contains codeine, and co-dydramol which also contains dihydocodeine | Oral | 500–1000 mg up to 6 times a day |
| **Nefopam** | Non-opioid | Analgesic for moderate pain<br>May cause nausea, dry mouth or urine retention<br>Contraindicated in epilepsy | Oral | 60 mg up to 3 times a day |
| **NSAIDS**[a] | | | | |
| **Aspirin** | NSAID | Mild analgesic:<br>Contraindicated in children, renal and liver disease, heart failure, bleeding tendency, asthma, peptic ulcer, pregnancy, breast feeding, allergies | Oral | 300–600 mg up to 6 times a day after meals; maximum 4 g daily (use soluble or dispersible or enteric-coated aspirin) |
| **Diclofenac** | NSAID | Analgesic for moderate pain: risk of thromboses<br>Contraindicated in renal and liver disease, heart failure, bleeding tendency, porphyria, peptic ulcer, pregnancy, breast feeding, allergies | Oral or IM | 25–75 mg up to twice daily |
| **Ibuprofen** | NSAID | Mild analgesic: risk of thromboses. Lowest risk of NSAIDs from gastric irritation<br>Contraindicated in renal and liver disease, heart failure, bleeding tendency, asthma, peptic ulcer, pregnancy, breast feeding, allergies | Oral | 300–400 mg up to 4 times a day |

*(Continued)*

**Table 3.4.1** ANALGESICS (INCLUDING OPIOIDS) (*Continued*)

| Drug | Type | Comments | Route | Adult dose |
|---|---|---|---|---|
| **Mefenamic acid** | NSAID | Mild analgesic<br>May be contraindicated in asthma, gastro-intestinal, liver and renal disease and pregnancy<br>May cause diarrhoea or haemolytic anaemia | Oral | 250–500 mg up to 3 times a day |
| **OPIOIDS**[b] | | | | |
| **Codeine phosphate** | Opioid | Analgesic for moderate pain<br>Contraindicated in liver disease, head injuries and late pregnancy<br>Avoid alcohol<br>May cause sedation and constipation<br>Reduces cough reflex | Oral | 10–60 mg up to 6 times a day (or 30 mg IM) |
| **Dextropropoxy-phene** | Opioid | Analgesic for moderate pain<br>Risk of respiratory depression in overdose, especially if taken with alcohol<br>Occasional hepatotoxicity or cardiotoxicity<br>No more effective and longer-acting than paracetamol or aspirin alone | Oral | 65 mg up to 4 times a day |
| **Dihydrocodeine tartrate** | Opioid | Analgesic for moderate pain<br>May cause nausea, drowsiness and constipation a day<br>Contraindicated in children, asthma, hypothyroidism and renal disease<br>May *increase* post-operative dental pain | Oral | 30 mg up to 4 times (or 50 mg IM) |
| **Pentazocine** | Opioid | Analgesic for moderate pain<br>May produce hallucinations or provoke withdrawal symptoms in narcotic addicts<br>Contraindicated in pregnancy, children, right-sided heart failure, hypertension, respiratory depression, head injuries or raised intracranial pressure | Oral | 50 mg up to 4 times (or 30 mg IM or IV) a day |
| **Buprenorphine** | Opioid | Potent analgesic<br>More potent than pentazocine and longer action than morphine<br>No hallucinations<br>May cause salivation, sweating, dizziness and vomiting<br>Respiratory depression in overdose<br>Contraindicated in pregnancy, children, with MAOIs, liver or respiratory disease | Sub-lingual | 0.2–0.4 mg up to 4 times a day (or 0.3 mg IM) |

(*Continued*)

**Table 3.4.1** ANALGESICS (INCLUDING OPIOIDS) (*Continued*)

| Drug | Type | Comments | Route | Adult dose |
|---|---|---|---|---|
| **Meptazinol** | Opioid | Potent analgesic<br>Side-effects as buprenorphine<br>Contraindicated in myocardial infarction | IM or IV | 75–100 mg up to 6 times a day |
| **Pethidine** | Opioid | Potent analgesic<br>Less potent than morphine. May cause neurotoxicity and restlessness<br>Contraindicated with MAOI | SC or IM | 25–100 mg up to 4 times a day |
| **Morphine** | Opioid | Potent analgesic<br>Often causes nausea and vomiting<br>Reduces cough reflex, causes pupil constriction | SC or IM or oral | 5–10 mg as required |
| **Diamorphine** | Opioid | Potent analgesic<br>More potent than pethidine and morphine but more dependence | SC or IM or oral | 2.5 mg by injection; 5–10 mg orally |

[a]NSAID, non-steroidal anti-inflammatory drug—all can cause gastric irritation (especially in older people) and a bleeding tendency; use lowest dose for shortest time possible.
[b]Opioids can cause dependence and respiratory depression.
*Abbreviations*: IM, intramuscular; IV, intravenous; SC, subcutaneous; MAOI, monoamine oxidase inhibitor.

**Table 3.4.2** ANTIFUNGALS FOR THE TREATMENT OF ORAL CANDIDOSIS

| Drug | Dose (oral) | Comments | Contraindications |
|---|---|---|---|
| **POLYENES** | | | |
| **Amphotericin** | 10–100 mg 6-hourly | Dissolve in mouth slowly<br>Active topically | Negligible absorption from gastro-intestinal tract. Intravenous amphotericin is cardiotoxic and can cause anaphylaxis |
| **Nystatin** | 500,000 unit lozenge, dissolve in mouth slowly<br>100,000 unit pastille, or<br>100,000 unit per millilitre of suspension 6-hourly | Active topically<br>May contain sugar | Negligible absorption from gastro-intestinal tract. Contraindicated in pregnancy and breast feeding and hepatic disease |
| **IMIDAZOLE** | | | |
| **Miconazole** | Dissolve in mouth slowly 250 mg tablet<br>6-hourly or<br>25 mg/ml gel used as 5 ml 6-hourly | Active topically<br>Also has antibacterial activity. Theoretically best antifungal to treat angular cheilitis[a] | Low absorption from gastro-intestinal tract but potentiates statins and warfarin and can cause nausea |

(Continued)

**Table 3.4.2** ANTIFUNGALS FOR THE TREATMENT OF ORAL CANDIDOSIS (*Continued*)

| Drug | Dose (oral) | Comments | Contraindications |
|---|---|---|---|
| **TRIAZOLES** | | | |
| **Fluconazole** | 50–100 mg once daily (capsules or 50 mg/5 ml suspension) | Less toxic than ketoconazole[b] | Well absorbed from gastro-intestinal tract Contraindicated in pregnancy, infants and renal disease May cause nausea and abdominal pain |
| **Itraconazole** | 100 mg once daily | May be indicated for fluconazole-resistant infections but is hepatotoxic | May precipitate congestive cardiac failure; avoid in older people, those on calcium channel blockers and avoid high doses or prolonged use |

[a]Fusidic acid is an alternative therapy for angular stomatitis (page 435).
[b]Ketoconazole is hepatotoxic.

**Table 3.4.3** ANTIVIRAL THERAPY OF OROFACIAL HERPETIC INFECTIONS

| Virus | Disease | Otherwise healthy patient | Immunocompromised patient |
|---|---|---|---|
| **Herpes simplex** | Primary herpetic gingivostomatitis | Consider oral aciclovir[a,b] 100–200 mg, five times daily as suspension or tablets | Aciclovir 250 mg/m$^2$ IV[b] every 8 hours |
| | Recurrent herpetic infection, e.g. herpes labialis | 1% penciclovir or 5% aciclovir cream | Consider systemic aciclovir[b] as above depending on risk to patient of infection |
| **Herpes varicella zoster** | Chickenpox | — (unless neonate) | Aciclovir 250 mg/m$^2$ IV[b] every 8 hours |
| | Zoster (shingles) | Consider oral aciclovir[a] 800 mg, five times daily | Aciclovir 250 mg/m$^2$ IV[b] every 8 hours |

[a]In neonate, treat as if immunocompromised.
[b]Systemic aciclovir: caution in renal disease and pregnancy; occasional increase in liver enzymes and urea, rashes. Famciclovir 250 mg three times per day or valaciclovir 500–1000 mg three times per day are other choices.
*Abbreviation*: IV, intravenous.

**Table 3.4.4** ANTIBACTERIALS

| Drug | Comments[a] | Route | Dose |
|---|---|---|---|
| **PENICILLINS** | Most oral bacterial infections respond well to drainage ± penicillin such as:<br>• phenoxymethyl penicillin—usually effective and cheap<br>• amoxicillin—often used and is usually effective, but almost four times as expensive<br>• ampicillin—also often effective<br>Micro-organisms that produce beta-lactamases are resistant to many penicillins | | |
| **Amoxicillin** | Orally effective (absorption better than ampicillin)<br>Broad-spectrum penicillin derivative<br>*Staphylococcus aureus* often resistant<br>Not resistant to penicillinase<br>Contraindicated in penicillin hypersensitivity<br>Rashes in infectious mononucleosis, cytomegalovirus infection, lymphoid leukaemia, allopurinol<br>May cause diarrhoea | Oral, IM or IV | 250–500 mg 8-hourly |
| **Ampicillin** | Broad-spectrum penicillin derivative<br>Less oral absorption than amoxicillin<br>Not resistant to penicillinase (there are many analogues but these have few, if any, advantages)<br>Contraindicated in penicillin hypersensitivity<br>Rashes in infectious mononucleosis, cytomegalovirus infection, lymphoid leukaemia, allopurinol<br>May cause diarrhoea | Oral, IM or IV | 250–500 mg 6-hourly |
| **Co-amoxiclav (Augmentin or co-amoxiclav)** | Mixture of amoxicillin and potassium clavulanate<br>Inhibits some penicillinases and, therefore, active against *Staphylococcus aureus*<br>Inhibits some lactamases and is, therefore, active against some Gram-negative and penicillin-resistant bacteria<br>Contraindicated in penicillin hypersensitivity<br>Beware of diarrhoea and hepatobiliary events | Oral | 125/250 mg 8-hourly |
| **Benzylpenicillin** | Not orally active<br>Most effective penicillin where organism sensitive<br>Not resistant to penicillinase<br>Contraindicated in penicillin hypersensitivity<br>Large doses may cause K$^+$ to fall and Na$^+$ to rise | IM | 2–4 g 6-hourly |
| **Flucloxacillin** | Orally active penicillin derivative<br>Effective against most, but not all, penicillin-resistant Staphylococci<br>Contraindicated in penicillin hypersensitivity<br>May induce cholestatic jaundice especially in older people on treatment for >2 weeks, or where there is liver disease or hypersensitivity to beta lactams | Oral or IM | 250 mg 6-hourly |

*(Continued)*

**Table 3.4.4** ANTIBACTERIALS (*Continued*)

| Drug | Comments[a] | Route | Dose |
|------|-------------|-------|------|
| **Phenoxymethyl penicillin (penicillin V)** | Orally active<br>Best taken on empty stomach<br>Not resistant to penicillinase<br>Contraindicated in penicillin hypersensitivity | Oral | 250–500 mg 6-hourly |
| **Benethamine penicillin (triplopen)** | Depot penicillin penicillins<br>Not resistant to penicillinase<br>Contraindicated in penicillin hypersensitivity<br>Contains benzyl (300 mg), procaine (250 mg) and benethamine (475 mg) | IM | 1 vial every 2–3 days |
| **SULPHONAMIDES** | Contraindicated in pregnancy and in renal disease<br>In other patients, adequate hydration must be ensured to prevent the (rare) occurrence of crystalluria<br>Other adverse reactions include erythema multiforme, rashes and blood dyscrasias<br>Co-trimoxazole may be used to treat sinusitis but now reserved largely for pneumocystis infections | | |
| **Co-trimoxazole** | Broad spectrum<br>Combination of trimethoprim and sulphamethoxazole<br>Orally active<br>Occasional rashes or blood dyscrasias<br>Contraindicated in pregnancy, liver disease<br>May increase the effect of protein-bound drugs | Oral or IV | 960 mg twice daily |
| **TETRACYCLINES** | Orally active<br>Broad-spectrum antibacterial and active against MRSA<br>There is little to choose between the many preparations, but doxycycline is useful since a single dose is adequate, and minocycline is effective against meningococci; and both are safer in renal failure than most of the tetracyclines, which are nephrotoxic<br>Tetracyclines cause discolouration of developing teeth and have absorption impaired by iron, antacids, milk, etc.<br>Use of tetracyclines may predispose to candidosis, and to nausea and gastro-intestinal disturbance<br>Contraindicated in pregnancy and children at least up to 8 years<br>Reduced dose indicated in renal failure, liver disease, older patients | Oral | 250–500 mg 6-hourly |
| **Doxycycline** | Orally active<br>Broad spectrum<br>Single daily dose<br>Contraindicated in pregnancy and children up to at least 8 years<br>Safer than tetracycline in renal failure (excreted in faeces)<br>Reduce dose in liver disease and older people<br>Mild gastro-intestinal effects | Oral | 100 mg once daily |

*(Continued)*

**Table 3.4.4** ANTIBACTERIALS (*Continued*)

| Drug | Comments[a] | Route | Dose |
|---|---|---|---|
| **Minocycline** | Orally active<br>Broad spectrum: active against meningococci<br>Safer than tetracycline in renal disease (excreted in faeces)<br>May cause dizziness and vertigo<br>Absorption not reduced by milk<br>Contraindicated in pregnancy and children up to at least 8 years<br>May also cause mild hepatic dysfunction, or oral pigmentation in adults | Oral | 100 mg twice daily |
| **CEPHALOSPORINS AND CEPHAMYCINS** | Beta lactam antibiotics<br>Broad spectrum, expensive and bactericidal with few absolute indications for use in orofacial infections as they are less active against anaerobes than are penicillins, although they may be effective against *Staphylococcus aureus*<br>They produce false-positive results for glycosuria with 'Clinitest'<br>Hypersensitivity is the main adverse effect<br>Some cause a bleeding tendency<br>Some are nephrotoxic<br>Cefuroxime is less affected by penicillinases than other cephalosporins and is currently the preferred drug of the many available | | |
| **Cefotaxime and ceftazidime** | Not orally active<br>Broad spectrum; third generation cephalosporins<br>Contraindicated if history of anaphylaxis to penicillin<br>Expensive | IM or IV | 1 g 12-hourly |
| **Cefuroxime** | Not orally active<br>Broad spectrum; second generation cephalosporin<br>Contraindicated if history of anaphylaxis to penicillin | IM or IV | 250–750 mg 8-hourly |
| **Ceftriaxone** | Not orally active; third generation cephalosporin<br>Longer action than most cephalosporins<br>Contraindicated in liver disease or history of anaphylaxis to penicillin | IM or IV | 1 g daily as single dose |
| **Meropenem** | Beta lactam<br>Not orally active<br>Similar to imipenem but not inactivated by the renal enzyme that degrades imipenem<br>Caution in pregnancy, breast feeding, renal disease | IV | 500 mg three times per day |
| **MACROLIDES** | | | |
| **Erythromycin** | Similar antibacterial spectrum to penicillin and is therefore used in penicillin-allergic patients<br>Active against most staphylococci, *Mycoplasma* and *Legionella*, but not always against oral *Bacteroides*<br>Do not use erythromycin estolate, which may cause liver disease | | |

*(Continued)*

**Table 3.4.4** ANTIBACTERIALS (*Continued*)

| Drug | Comments[a] | Route | Dose |
|---|---|---|---|
| **Erythromycin stearate** | Orally active<br>Useful in those hypersensitive to penicillin<br>Effective against most staphylococci and streptococci<br>May cause nausea<br>Rapid development of resistance<br>Reduced dose indicated in liver disease<br>Can increase ciclosporin absorption and toxicity | Oral | 250–500 mg 6-hourly |
| **Erythromycin lactobionate** | Used where parenteral erythromycin indicated<br>Comments as above | IV | 2 g daily<br>Give by infusion |
| **Azithromycin** | Orally active<br>Useful in those hypersensitive to penicillin. Caution in liver disease, pregnancy and breast-feeding | Oral | 500 mg daily |
| **Clarithromycin** | Orally active<br>Useful in those hypersensitive to penicillin<br>Caution in renal disease, pregnancy and breast-feeding | Oral | 250 mg daily |
| **OTHERS** | | | |
| **Clindamycin** | Effective against *Staphylococcus aureus* (including MRSA), streptococci and *Bacteroides fragilis* and is well concentrated in bone. Should, however, only be used for the treatment of orofacial infections that have failed to respond to metronidazole or penicillin.<br>May induce antibiotic-associated colitis due to *Clostridium difficile* | Oral, IM or IV | 150–300 mg four times per day |
| **Fusidic acid** | Effective against staphylococcal infections | Topical | 2% ointment applied three times per day |
| **Gentamicin** | Reserved for serious infections<br>Can cause vestibular and renal damage, especially if given with furosemide (frusemide)<br>Contraindicated in pregnancy and myasthenia gravis<br>Reduce dose in renal disease | IM or IV | Up to 5 mg/kg daily |
| **Metronidazole** | Orally active<br>Effective against anaerobes<br>Avoid alcohol (disulfiram-type reaction)<br>May increase warfarin effect<br>May cause tiredness<br>IV preparation available but expensive<br>Suppositories effective<br>Contraindicated in pregnancy<br>Use only for 7 days (or peripheral neuropathy may develop, particularly in liver-disease patients) | Oral or IV | 200–400 mg 8-hourly (take with meals) |

*(Continued)*

**Table 3.4.4** ANTIBACTERIALS (*Continued*)

| Drug | Comments[a] | Route | Dose |
|---|---|---|---|
| **Rifampicin** | Reserved mainly for treatment of tuberculosis but can be used for prophylaxis against post-traumatic meningitis<br>Safe and effective but resistance rapidly occurs<br>Body secretions turn red<br>May interfere with oral contraception<br>Occasional rashes, jaundice or blood dyscrasias | Oral or IV | 0.6–1.2 g daily in 2–4 divided doses |
| **Vancomycin** | Reserved for serious infections<br>Extravenous extravasation causes necrosis and phlebitis<br>May cause nausea, rashes, tinnitus, deafness<br>Rapid injection may cause 'red neck' syndrome<br>Contraindicated in renal disease, deafness<br>Expensive | Oral or IV | 500 mg 6-hourly for pseudomembranous colitis |

This is a small selection of the antibacterials that are in use in maxillofacial surgery and medicine.
[a]It should be noted that some antibacterials impair the activity of oral contraceptives.
*Abbreviations*: IM, intramuscular; IV, intravenous; MRSA, meticillin-resistant *Staphylococcus aureus*.

**Table 3.4.5** SOME TOPICAL CORTICOSTEROIDS (many more potent preparations are available)

| Drug | Dose 6-hourly | Comments |
|---|---|---|
| **LOW POTENCY** | | |
| **Hydrocortisone hemisuccinate pellets** | 2.5 mg | Dissolve in mouth close to lesions<br>Use at early stage |
| **Triamcinolone acetonide in carmellose gelatin paste** | Apply thin layer | Adheres best to dry mucosa<br>Affords mechanical protection<br>Of little value on tongue or palate<br>Discontinued in the United Kingdom—2009 |
| **MODERATE POTENCY** | | |
| **Betamethasone phosphate tablets**<br>Unlicensed use | 0.5 mg as a mouth wash | More potent than preparations above but at least theoretically may produce adrenal suppression |
| **Beclometasone dipropionate (inhaler)**<br>Unlicensed use | Spray on oral lesion, 50–200 μg | |
| **Clobetasol**<br>Unlicensed use | 0.05% cream | |

**Table 3.4.6** SOME INTRALESIONAL CORTICOSTEROIDS

| Drug | Dose | Comments |
|------|------|----------|
| **Prednisolone sodium phosphate** | Up to 24 mg | Short acting |
| **Methylprednisolone acetate** | 4–80 mg every 1–5 weeks | Also available with lidocaine (lignocaine) |
| **Triamcinolone acetonide** | 2–3 mg every 1–2 weeks | – |
| **Triamcinolone hexacetonide** | Up to 5 mg every 3–4 weeks | – |

**Table 3.4.7** SOME INTRA-ARTICULAR CORTICOSTEROIDS

| Drug | Dose | Comments |
|------|------|----------|
| **Dexamethasone sodium phosphate** | 0.4–5 mg at intervals of 3–21 days | More expensive than hydrocortisone acetate |
| **Hydrocortisone acetate** | 5–50 mg | Usual preparation used |

Also used are those listed in Table 3.4.6 under intralesional corticosteroids.

**Table 3.4.8** SYSTEMIC IMMUNOMODULATORY DRUGS

| Drug | Comments | Adult dose |
|------|----------|-----------|
| **CORTICOSTEROIDS**[a] | | |
| **Betametasone** | May be useful to reduce post-surgical oedema after minor oral surgery | 1 mg orally the night before operation<br>1 mg orally with premedication<br>1 mg orally every 6 hours for 2 days post-operatively |
| **Dexamethasone** | May be used to reduce post-surgical oedema after minor oral surgery | 5 mg IV with premedication followed by 0.5–1.0 mg daily for 5 days, orally if possible |
| **Methylprednisolone** | May be useful to reduce post-surgical oedema after major surgery | Methylprednisolone succinate 1 g IV at operation, 500 mg on evening of operation followed by 125 mg IV every 6 hours for 24 hours. Then methylprednisolone acetate orally 80 mg every 12 hours for 24 hours |
| **Prednisolone** | May be indicated systemically for pemphigus and Bell palsy, and occasionally other disorders | Initially 40–80 mg orally each day in divided doses, reducing as soon as possible to 10 mg daily<br>Give enteric-coated prednisolone with meals |

(Continued)

**Table 3.4.8** SYSTEMIC IMMUNOMODULATORY DRUGS (*Continued*)

| Drug | Comments | Adult dose |
|---|---|---|
| **STEROID-SPARING AGENTS** | | |
| **Azathioprine** Unlicensed use | Steroid-sparing for immuno-suppression<br>Myelosuppressive and hepato-toxic, and long-term may predispose to neoplasms<br>Contraindicated in pregnancy | Use only in patients who are thiopurine methyl transferase positive<br>Orally 2–2.5 mg/kg daily |
| **Colchicine** Unlicensed use | May be used in severe oral ulceration<br>Occasional nausea, abdominal pain or blood dyscrasia<br>Contraindicated in pregnancy, renal or gastro-intestinal disease | Orally up to 500 µg 4 times daily |
| **Dapsone** Unlicensed use | May be used in some derma-toses<br>Occasional neuropathy, head-ache, haemolytic anaemia, rashes<br>Contraindicated in glucose-6-phosphate dehydrogenase deficiency, pregnancy, anae-mia, cardiorespiratory disease | Orally up to 1–2 mg/kg daily |
| **Mycophenolate mofetil** | Blocks T- and B-cell prolifera-tion and leukocyte recruit-ment<br>No liver or kidney damage<br>More gastrointestinal, haemato-logical effects and infections than with azathioprine | Orally up to 2 g per day |
| **Thalidomide** Unlicensed use | May be used in severe oral ulceration<br>Peripheral neuropathy in prolonged use<br>Contraindicated in women of child-bearing potential | Orally 50–200 mg preferably on alternate days (dose <75 mg usually avoids neuropathy)<br>Strict rules for prescribing apply in most countries |

aMultiple potential adverse effects including: hypertension, diabetes, psychoses, osteoporosis, fat redistribution, immunosuppression.
*Abbreviation*: IV, intravenous.

**Table 3.4.9** SOME DRUGS USED IN THE MANAGEMENT OF TRIGEMINAL NEURALGIA

| Drug | Comments | Route | Adult dose |
|---|---|---|---|
| **Baclofen** | Skeletal muscle relaxant. Cautions in psychiatric disorders, parkinsonism, cerebrovascular accident, peptic ulcer, diabetes, renal disease or older people | Oral (tablets or oral solution) | 5 mg three times per day with or after food |
| **ANTICONVULSANTS** | | | |
| **Gabapentin** | Anticonvulsant[a], prophylactic for trigeminal neuralgia—not analgesic<br>Cautions in pregnancy, breast feeding, diabetes, renal disease or older people. Avoid abrupt withdrawal. Can cause dry mouth | Oral | 300 mg on day 1, then 300 mg twice daily on day 2, then 300 mg three times per day |
| **Carbamazepine** | Anticonvulsant[a], prophylactic for trigeminal neuralgia—not analgesic<br>Occasional dizziness, diplopia, liver dysfunction and blood dyscrasia, usually with a rash and usually in the first 3 months of treatment<br>Potentiated by cimetidine, dextropropoxyphene and isoniazid potentiates lithium<br>Interferes with oral contraceptives. Test for HLA-B[a]1502 in people of Han or Hong Kong chinese or Thai origin who are liable to Stevens–Johnson syndrome | Oral | Initially 100 mg once or twice daily. Many patients need about 200 mg 8-hourly. Do not exceed 1800 mg daily |
| **Lamotrigine**<br>Unlicensed indication | Anticonvulsant[a], prophylactic for trigeminal neuralgia—not analgesic. Can cause bone marrow depression or hypersensitivity. Erythema multiforme and Stevens–Johnson syndrome may occur especially in children | Oral | 25 mg daily |
| **Oxcarbazepine**<br>Unlicensed indication | Anticonvulsant[a], prophylactic for trigeminal neuralgia—not analgesic. Occasional dizziness, diplopia, liver dysfunction and blood dyscrasia, usually with a rash and usually in the first 3 months of treatment | Oral | 300 mg twice daily |
| **Phenytoin** | Anticonvulsant[a], prophylactic for trigeminal neuralgia—not analgesic<br>Occasional dizziness, diplopia, liver dysfunction and blood dyscrasia. Can cause gingival swelling | Oral | 150–300 mg daily |
| **Pregabalin** | Anticonvulsant[a], prophylactic for trigeminal neuralgia—not analgesic<br>Cautions in pregnancy, breast feeding. Can cause dry mouth | Oral | 50 mg three times per day on day 1 increasing if needed to 100 mg three times per day |

Local nerve injections, e.g. with glycerol may be effective.

[a] Anticonvulsants may be teratogenic, cause drowsiness and interfere with driving, induce depression/suicidal behaviour and may enhance hepatic drug-metabolizing enzymes; abrupt withdrawal should be avoided. Caution in pregnancy, breast-feeding and liver disease. Avoid abrupt withdrawal.

**Table 3.4.10** SOME TRICYCLIC ANTIDEPRESSANTS

| Drug | Comments | Route | Adult dose |
|---|---|---|---|
| **Amitriptyline** | Antidepressant effect may not be seen until up to 30 days after start<br>Sedative effect also<br>When treatment established, use single dose at night<br>Contraindicated for arrhythmias and ischaemic heart disease and breastfeeding | Oral | 25–75 mg daily in divided dose |
| **Dosulepin** | Anxiolytic effect also useful in atypical facial pain<br>When treatment established, use single dose at night | Oral | 25 mg three times a day or 75 mg at night |
| **Clomipramine** | Equally effective as amitriptyline but less sedative effect<br>Useful in phobia or obsessional states | Oral | 10–100 mg daily in divided doses |

May cause dry mouth, precipitate glaucoma, constipation and urinary retention; may impair performance of skilled tasks (e.g. driving) and should not be taken with alcohol. May be cardiotoxic especially in overdose. Should not be withdrawn abruptly. Antidepressants may sometimes cause suicidal behaviour.

**Table 3.4.11** SOME OTHER ANTIDEPRESSANTS

| Drug | Type | Comments | Route | Adult dose |
|---|---|---|---|---|
| **Fluoxetine** | SSRI | Less sedative or cardiotoxic than tricyclics<br>Contraindicated in cardiovascular, hepatic or renal disease, pregnancy, diabetes and epilepsy. Possibly causes self-harm behaviour | Oral | 20 mg daily |
| **Flupentixol** | Thioxanthene | Fewer adverse effects than tricyclics<br>Contraindicated in cardiovascular, hepatic or renal disease, parkinsonism or overexcitable/over-active patients | Oral | 1–3 mg in the morning |
| **Mianserin** | Tricyclic-related | Fewer adverse effects than tricyclics<br>May depress bone marrow | Oral | 30–40 mg daily at night |
| **Moclobemide** | Reversible monoamine oxidase inhibitor | May interact with tyramine-containing foods (e.g. cheese, yeast, soya) and sympathomimetics. Avoid in agitated or manic-depressive patients, pregnancy or breast-feeding | Oral | 100 mg three times per day |
| **Venlafaxine** | Serotonin and noradrenaline re-uptake inhibitor | Also anxiolytic. Contraindicated in pregnancy, cardiac arrhythmias and uncontrolled hypertension<br>Caution in glaucoma, bleeding disorders, breast feeding, hepatic or renal disease, and epilepsy. Avoid abrupt withdrawal | Oral | 37.5 mg twice daily |

May impair performance of skilled tasks (e.g. driving) and should not be taken with alcohol. Hyponatraemia may be seen in older patients especially with SSRIs. Antidepressants may sometimes cause suicidal behaviour.
*Abbreviation*: SSRI, selective serotonin re-uptake inhibitor.

**Table 3.4.12** SOME HYPNOTICS/ANXIOLYTICS

| Drug | Comments | Preparations | Route | Adult dose |
|---|---|---|---|---|
| **Chlormethiazole** | Useful in older people<br>Contraindicated in liver disease, acute pulmonary disease and alcohol dependent subjects<br>May cause dependence | 192 mg capsule<br>250 mg/5 ml syrup | Oral | 500 mg |
| **Dichloralphenazone** (chloral betaine) | Derivative of chloral hydrate<br>Useful in older people<br>Contraindicated in porphyria, and patients on oral anticoagulants | 707 mg | Oral | 1300 mg |
| **Propranolol** | Useful anxiolytic which does not cause amnesia, but reduces tremor and palpitations<br>Contraindicated in asthma, cardiac failure, pregnancy, breast feeding | 10 or 40 mg | Oral | 10–40 mg |
| **BENZODIAZEPINES**[a] | | | | |
| **Diazepam** | Useful hypnotic<br>Reduce dose in older people. Contraindicated in respiratory disease and muscle weakness | 5 or 10 mg | Oral | 5–10 mg |
| **Lorazepam** | Useful hypnotic<br>Reduce dose in older people | 1 mg | Oral | 1–2 mg |
| **Nitrazepam** | No more useful than diazepam but longer effect and with hangover effect<br>Avoid in older people | 5 mg | Oral | 5–10 mg |
| **Temazepam** | Useful in older people<br>Less hangover effect than nitrazepam | 10 mg | Oral | 10–20 mg |

Any may interfere with driving and decision-making, and respiration and should not be taken with alcohol.
[a]May cause amnesia, dependence or paradoxical reactions.

**Table 3.4.13** SOME SEDATIVES AND TRANQUILLIZERS

| Drug | Comments | Preparations | Route | Adult dose |
|---|---|---|---|---|
| **ANXIOLYTICS** | | | | |
| **Chlordiazepoxide** | Reduce dose in older people | 5 or 10 mg | Oral | 5–10 mg 8-hourly |
| **Diazepam** | Reduce dose in older people | 2, 5 or 10 mg | Oral, IM or IV | 2–30 mg daily in divided doses |

*(Continued)*

**Table 3.4.13** SOME SEDATIVES AND TRANQUILLIZERS (*Continued*)

| Drug | Comments | Preparations | Route | Adult dose |
|------|----------|--------------|-------|------------|
| **MAJOR TRANQUILLIZERS**[a] | | | | |
| **Chlorpromazine** | Phenothiazine<br>May cause dyskinesia, photosensitivity, eye defects and jaundice<br>Contraindicated in epilepsy. IM use causes pain and may cause postural hypotension | 25 mg tablet<br>25 mg/ml syrup<br>50 mg/2 ml injection | Oral or IM | 25 mg 8-hourly |
| **Haloperidol** | Butyrophenone<br>Useful in older people, and for patients with agitation, severe anxiety and intractable hiccups | 500 μg | Oral | 500 μg 12-hourly |
| **Thioridazine** | Phenothiazine with fewer adverse effects than chlorpromazine<br>Rare retinopathy | 10 or 25 mg | Oral | 10–50 mg 8-hourly |

Any may interfere with driving and decision-making, and respiration and should not be taken with alcohol.
[a]Extrapyramidal reactions and neuroleptic malignant syndrome may be precipitated by major tranquillizers.
*Abbreviations*: IM, intramuscular; IV, intravenous.

# 3.5 GUIDE TO THE OROFACIAL ADVERSE EFFECTS OF DRUG TREATMENT

Most orofacial adverse effects to drug treatment are rare but the more common causes are indicated in **bold** in the following section. Some relate to single case reports. Some of the drugs mentioned are now unavailable in the developed world but sometimes obtainable from other sources.

Opportunistic infections may be secondary to cytotoxic chemotherapy and the prevalence of dysplastic and malignant lip and oral lesions has increased in immunosuppressed patients. Tobacco, alcohol and betel are risk factors for leukoplakia and oral epithelial dysplasia.

For further details of adverse reactions outlined in the following tables, the reader is referred to the Physicians Desk Reference or British National Formulary.

## ANGIOEDEMA
(see also FACIAL SWELLING)

Acetylsalicylic acid
Aldesleukin (human recombinant IL-2)
Angiotensin-converting enzyme (ACE) inhibitors
**Asparaginase**
**Captopril**
Carbamazepine
Cephalosporin derivatives
Clindamycin
Clonidine
**Co-trimoxazole**
Disulphite sodium
**Droperidol**
Enalapril
Epoetin alpha
Ibruprofen
Indometacin
IFN-alpha
**Iodine and iodides**
**Ketoconazole**
Local anaesthetic agents
Mianserin
Miconazole
Naproxen
Nitrofurantoin
Penicillamine
**Penicillin derivatives**
Pyrazolone derivatives
Quinine
Streptomycin
Sulphonamides
Thiouracil

## BLACK HAIRY TONGUE

**Antibiotics (broad spectrum and griseofulvin)**

Antidepressants (MAOI or tricyclics)
**Bismuth-containing preparations**
**Chlorhexidine**
Corticosteroids
Hormone replacement therapy
**Iron salts**
Methyldopa
Perborates
Peroxides
Phenothiazines
Proton pump inhibitors

## BRUXISM

**Amfetamines**
**Ecstasy**

## BURNING MOUTH SENSATION

**Angiotensin-converting enzyme inhibitors**
**Protease inhibitors**

## CANDIDOSIS

**Broad spectrum antimicrobials**
**Corticosteroids**
**Drugs causing xerostomia**
**Immunosuppressives**

## CERVICAL LYMPHADENOPATHY

Cervical lymphadenopathy (drug-induced hypersensitivity syndrome)
Abacavir
Allopurinol
Atenolol
Azathioprine
Captopril
Carbamazepine
Clomipramine

Dapsone
Diltiazem
Gold salts
Isoniazid
Lamotrogine
Mexiletine
Minocycline
Nevirapine
Oxicam
Phenobarbitone
**Phenytoin**
Sulphasalazine
Sulphonamides
Trimethoprim

## CHEILITIS

**Actinomycin**
**Atorvastatin**
**Busulphan**
Clofazimine
Clomipramine
Cyancobalamin
**Cytotoxic agents**
Ethyl alcohol
**Etretinate**
Gold
**Indinavir**
Isoniazid
**Isotretinoin**
Lithium
**Menthol**
**Methyldopa**
Penicillamine
**Phenothiazines**
**Selegiline**
Streptomycin
Psoralens
Sulphasalazine
Tetracycline
**Vitamin A**

## DRY MOUTH

Alfuzosin
Amiloride
Amitriptyline
Amoxapine
**Antidepressants**
**Antihistamines**
**Antimuscarinics** (anticholinergics)
**Baclofen**
Benzhexol
Benztropine
**Beta blockers**
Biperiden
Bupropion
Buspirone
**Calcium channel blockers**
Cannabis
Cetirizine
Chlormezanone
Chlorpromazine
Citalopram
Clemastine
Clomipramine
Clonidine
Clozapine
**Cyclizine**
Cyclobenzaprine
**Desipramine**
Dexamphetamine
Diazepam
Dicyclomine
**Dideoxyinosine**
Dihydrocodeine
Disopyramide
**Diuretics**
Donopezil
**Dosulepin**
**Doxepin**
**Duloxetine**
Ecstasy
Elliptinium
Ephedrine
Fenfluramine
Fluoxetine
Furosemide
Guanfacine
5HT agonists
Hyoscine
**Imipramine**
Indoramine

Inteferon (IFN) alpha
Inteleukin (IL-2)
Ipratropium
Iprindole
Isocarboxazid
Isotretinoin
Ketorolac
Ketotifen
**Lansoprazole**
L-dopa
Lithium
Lofepramine
Lofexidine
Loratadine
Maprotiline
Mepenzolate
Methyldopa
Mianserine
Mirtazapine
Monoamine oxidase inhibitors
Morphine
Morphine
Moxonidine
Nabilone
Nefopam
**Nortriptyline**
**Olanzapine**
**Omeprazole**
**Opioids**
Orphenadrine
Oxitropium
**Oxybutynin**
Paroxetine
Phenelzine
Pipamperone
Pipenzolate
Pirenzipine
Poldine
**Protease inhibitors**
Pratropium
Procyclidine
Propafenone
**Propantheline**
Propiverine
Pseudoephedrine
Quetiapine
Reboxetine
Rilmenidine
Risperidone
Rizatriptan
Selegiline

Sertraline
Sibutramine
**SSRIs**
Sucralfate
Tamsulosin
Terazosin
Thiabendazole
Tiapride
Tiotropium
Tizamidine
Tolterodine
Tramadol
Tranylcypromine
Trazodone
Trepium chloride
Triamterene
**Tricyclics**
Trimipramine
**Trospium**
Venlafaxine
Viloxazine
Zopiclone

### ERYTHEMA MULTIFORME

Erythema multiforme (and
    Stevens–Johnson syndrome and
    toxic epidermal necrolysis).
Acetylsalicylic acid
Allopurinol
Amlodipine
Antimicrobials (antimalarials,
    penicillins, sulphonamides,
    tetracyclines)
Arsenic
Atropine
**Barbiturates**
Busulphan
**Carbamazepine**
**Cephalosporins**
Chloral hydrate
Chlorpropamide
Clindamycin
Codeine
**Co-trimoxazole**
Diclofenac
Diflunisal
Digitalis
Diltiazem
Ethambutol
Ethyl alcohol
Fluconazole

Fluorouracil
Furosemide
Gold
Griseofulvin
**Hydantoin**
Hydrochlorothiazide
Indapamide
Lamotrigine
Measles/mumps/rubella vaccine
Meclofenamic acid
Mercury
Mesterolone
Minoxidil
Nifedipine
NSAIDs
Omeprazole
Oseltamivir phosphate
Oxyphenbutazone
**Penicillin derivatives**
Phenolphthalein
**Phenylbutazone**
Phenytoin
Piroxicam
Progesterone
Protease inhibitors
Pyrazolone derivatives
Quinine
Retinol
Rifampicin
Streptomycin
Sulindac
Sulphasalazine
**Sulphonamides**
Tenoxicam
Tetracyclines
Theophylline
Tocainide
Tolbutamide
Trimethadione
Vancomycin
Verapamil
Zidovudine

## FACIAL HIRSUTISM

**Ciclosporin**
**Cyproterone acetate**
**Formestane**
**Medroxyprogesterone**
**Minoxidil**
**Nandrolone decanoate**
**Norethisterone**

**Oxemetholone**
**Phenytoin**
**Testosterone**
**Tibolone**

## FACIAL FLUSHING

Adenosine
Alprostadil
Buserelin
Calcitonin
**Calcium channel blockers**
Caroprost
Chlorpropamide
**Clomifene**
Co-dergocrine
Danazol
**L-Dopa**
Flumazenil
**Formestane**
Loxapine
Morphine
Nicotinic acid
Pentoxifylline (Oxpentifylline)
Pentamidine
Protirelin
Quinine
Rifampicin
Ritodrine
Sermorelin
Tamoxifen
Thymoxamine
Thyroxine
Trilostane

## FACIAL INVOLUNTARY MOVEMENTS

Butyrophenones
Carbamazepine
L-dopa
Lithium
Methyldopa
**Metoclopramide**
Metirosine
**Phenothiazines**
Phenytoin
Tetrabenazine
**Tricyclic antidepressants**
Trifluoroperazine

## FACIAL SWELLING

Facial swelling
  (see also ANGIOEDEMA)

Ciclosporin
Cinoxacin
**Corticosteroids**
Trilostane

## GINGIVAL SWELLING

**Drugs most commonly
  implicated**
**Amlodipine**
Calcium channel blockers
  (amlodipine, bepridil, diltiazem,
  felodipine, isradipine, nicardipine,
  nifedipine, nimodipine,
  nisoldipine, nitrendipine,
  oxidipine, verapamil)
**Ciclosporin**
**Diltiazem**
**Felodipine**
**Lacidipine**
**Nifedipine**
Oral contraceptives
**Phenytoin**
Verapamil
**Drugs occasionally implicated**
  Amphetamine
  Bleomycin
  Co-trimoxazole
  Erythromycin
  Diphenoxylate
  Ethosuximide
  IFN-alpha
  Ketoconazole
  Lamotrigine
  Lithium
  Mephenytoin
  Nitrendipine
  Norethisterone + mestranol
  Phenobarbitone
  Primidone
  Sertraline
  Topiramate
  Valproate
  Vigabatrin

## GLOSSITIS

Captopril
Chloramphenicol
Cytotoxics
Enalapril
Ergot alkaloids
Flunisolide

Gold
Griseofulvin
Isoniazid
Methyldopa
Metronidazole
**Phenelzine**
Phenothiazine derivatives
**Streptomycin**
Sulindac
Tetracycline
Tricyclic antidepressants
Zidovudine

**HALITOSIS**

Halitosis (also medications that
  reduce salivary flow, such as
  antihistamines, diuretics,
  narcotics, antidepressants,
  decongestants, antihypertensives
  and antipsychotics)
Amphetamines
Amyl nitrites
Azeotrenam
Cytotoxic drugs
Dimethyl sulphoxide
Disulfiram
Isorbide dinitrate
Melatonin
Mycophenolate sodium
Nicotine lozenges
Nitrates
Phenothiazine
Solvent misuse

**HYPERPIGMENTATION OF MUCOSAE**

ACTH
Amiodarone
Amodiaquine
Anticonvulsants
Antimalarials (chloroquine,
  hydroxychloroquine,
  quinacrine, quinidine)
Arsenic
Betel
Bismuth
Bromine
Busulphan
Chlorhexidine
Chloroquine
Clofazimine
Copper

Chlorpromazine
Cyclophosphamide
Doxorubicin
Gold
Heroin
Iron
Ketoconazole
Lead
Manganese
Mepacrine
Methyldopa
Minocycline
Oestrogens
Phenolphthalein
Phenothiazines
Quinacrine
Quinidine
Silver
Thallium
Tin
Vanadium
Zidovudine
*Blue*
Amiodarone
Antimalarials
Bismuth
Mepacrine
Minocycline
Phenazopyridine
Quinidine
Silver
Sulphasalazine
*Brown (hypermelanosis)*
Aminophenazone
Betel nut
Bismuth
Busulphan
Clofazimine
Contraceptives
Cyclophosphamide
Diethylstilbestrol
Doxorubicin
Doxycycline
Fluorouracil
Heroin
Hormone-replacement therapy
Ketoconazole
Menthol
Methaqualone
Minocycline
Phenolphthalein

Propranolol
Smoking
Zidovudine
*Black*
Amiodiaquine
Betel nut
Bismuth
Methyldopa
Minocycline
*Grey*
Amiodiaquine
Chloroquine
Fluoxetine
Hydroxychloroquinine
Lead
Silver
Tin/zinc
*Green*
Copper

**HYPERSALIVATION**

Alprazolam
Amiodarone
**Anticholinesterases**
Buprenorphine
Buspirone
Clonazepam
Clozapine
Diazoxide
Ethionamide
Gentamicin
Guanethidine
Haloperidol
Imipenem/cilastatin
Iodides
Kanamycin
Ketamine
Lamotrigine
L-Dopa
Mefenamic acid
Mercurials
Neostigmine
Nicardipine
Niridazole
Pentoxifylline
Remoxipride
Risperidone
Rivastigmine
Tacrine
Tobramycin
Triptorelin

Venlafaxine
Zaleplon

**LICHENOID REACTIONS**

Allopurinol
Amiphenazole
**Antimalarials**
Barbiturate
**Beta blockers**
Bismuth
Captopril
Carbamazepine
Carbimazole
Chloral hydrate
Chloroquine
Chlorpropamide
Chlorothiazide
Cholera vaccine
Cimetidine
Cinnarizine
Clofibrate
Colchicine
Cyanamide
Dapsone
Dipyridamole
Ethionamide
Fenclofenac
Flunarizine
Furosemide
Gaunoclor
Gold
Griseofulvin
Hepatitis B vaccine
Hydroxychloroquine
IFN-alpha
Isoniazid
Ketoconazole
Labetalol
Levamisole
Levopromazine
Lincomycin
Lithium
Lorazepam
Mepacrine
Mercury (amalgam)
Metformin
Methyldopa
Methopromazine
Metronidazole
Niridazole
NSAIDs

Oral contraceptives
Oxprenolol
Palladium
Para-aminosalicylate
Penicillamine
Penicillins
Phenindione
Phenothiazines
Phenylbutazone
Phenytoin
Piroxicam
Practolol
Prazosin
Procainamide
Propranolol
Propylthiouracil
Prothionamide
Pyrimethamine
Quinidine
Quinine
Rifampicin
Spironolactone
**Sulphonamides**
Streptomycin
Tetracycline
Tocainide
Tolbutamide
**Triprolidine**

**LUPOID REACTIONS**

Carbamazepine
Chlorpromazine
Ethosuximide
Gold
Griseofulvin
**Hydantoins**
**Hydralazine**
**Isoniazid**
Lithium
Methyldopa
Para-aminosalicylate
Penicillin
Penicillamine
Phenytoin
Phenothiazines
Primidone
Procainamide
Quinidine
Reserpine
Streptomycin
Sulphonamides

Tetracyclines
Thiouracils
Trimethadione

**OSTEONECROSIS**

Bevacizamab
**Bisphosphonates**
Denosumab

**PAIN**

Benztropine
Biperidin
Griseofulvin
Lithium
Penicillins
Phenothiazines
Stilbamidine
Ticarcillin
**Vinca alkaloids**
Vitamin A

**PEMPHIGOID-LIKE REACTIONS**

Amoxicillin
Antibiotics (penicillins,
    sulphonamides)
Antirheumatics (penicillamine,
    ibuprofen, phenacetin)
Azapropazone
Cardiovascular drugs (furosemide,
    captopril, clonidine)
Clonidine
Furosemide
Ibuprofen
Isoniazid
Mefenamic acid
Nadolol
Penicillin v
Penicillamine
Phenacetin
Practolol
**Salicylic acid**
Sulphasalazine
Sulphonamides

**PEMPHIGUS-LIKE REACTIONS**

Ampicillin
Arsenic
Benzylpenicillin
Captopril
Cefadroxil
Cefalexin

Cilazapril
Diclofenac
Dipyrone
Enalapril
Ethambutol
**Glibenclamide**
Gold
Heroin
Ibuprofen
**IFN-beta**
IL-2
Nifedipine
Norfloxacin
Oxyphenbutazone
Penicillamine
Penicillin
Phenobarbotal
Phenylbutazone
Piroxicam
Practolol
Propranolol
Pyritinol chlorohydrate
Probenecid
Procaine penicillin
Quinapril
Rifampicin
Theobromine
Typhoid and influenza vaccination

## PETECHIAE

Acetylsalicylic acid
Ampicillin
Chloramphenicol
Heparin
Lamotrigine
Penicillin
Phenylbutazone
Quinidine
Quinine
Rifampicines
Sedormid
Sulphonamides
Thiazides
Trimethoprine
Valproate
Warfarin

## SALIVA DISCOLOURATION

Clofazimine
L-dopa
Rifabutin

Rifampicin

## SALIVARY GLAND PAIN OR SWELLING

**Antithyroid drugs**
Bethanidine
Bretylium
Cimetidine
Clonidine
Clozapine
Deoxycycline
Famotidine
Guanethidine
Insulin
IFN
**Iodides**
Isoprenaline
Methyldopa
Naproxen
Nicardipine
Nifedipine
Nitrofurantoin
Oxyphenbutazone
**Phenothiazines**
Phenylbutazone
Phenytoin
Ranitidine
Ritodrine
**Sulphonamides**
Trimepramine
Vinca alkaloids

## TASTE DISTURBANCE

Acarbose
Acetazolamide
Alcohol
Allopurinol
**Amiloride**
Amiodarone
Amitryptiline
Amphetamines
Amphotericin
Amrinone
Aspirin
Atorvastatin
Auranofin
Aurothiomalate
Azathioprine
Azelastine
Aztreonam
Baclofen
Biguanides

Bleomycin
Bretylium
Calcitonin
Captopril
Carbamazepine
Carbimazole
Carboplatin
Ceftirizine
Cephamandole
Chlormezanone
Cholestyramine
Choline magnesium trisalicylate
Cilazapril
Cisplatin
Clarithromycin
Clidinium
Clofibrate
Clomipramine
Cocaine
Cytotoxic agents
Diazoxide
Dicyclomine
Diltiazem
Dipyridamole
EDTA
Enalapril
Ethambutol
Ethionamide
Etidronate
Flunisolide
Fluoxetine
Flurazepam
5-Fluorouracil
Fluvoxamine
Glycopyrrolate
Gold
Griseofulvin
Hexetidine
Hydrochorothiazide
Hydrocortisone
Hyoscyamine
Imipenem
Indometacin
IFN gamma
Iodine
Isotretinoin
L-dopa
Levamisole
Levodopa
Lincomycin
Lisinopril

Lithium
Lomefloxacin
Losartan
Lovastatin
Metformin
Methimazole
Methotrexate
Methyl methacrylate
Methylthiouracil
Metronidazole
Nifedipine
Niridazole
Nitroglycerin
Ofloxacin
Omeprazole
Penicillamine
Pentamidine
Pergolide
Perindopril
Phenformin
Phenindione
Phenylbutazone
Phenytoin
Procaine penicillin
Propafenone
Propantheline
Propranolol
Propylthiouracil
Protease inhibitors
Quinapril
Ramipril
Rifabutin
Rivastigmine
Selegiline
Sodium lauryl sulphate
Spironolactone
Sulphasalazine
Terbinafine
Tetracycline
Thiamazole
Tocainide
Topiramate
Trandolapril
Triazolam
**Venlafaxine**
Zopiclone

## TOOTH DAMAGE

**Abnormal odontogenesis**[a]
Anticonvulsants
Cytotoxic drugs

*Caries*
Sugar containing paediatric (liquid)
    medications
**Erosion**
Anti-asthmatic drugs such as
    beclomethasone diproprionate,
    fluticasone, salmeterol and
    terbutaline sulphate powders
    have a pH lower than 5.5
Aspirin
Carbonated drinks
Drugs that cause
    gastro-oesophageal reflux
Fruit juices
Alcoholic drinks
Mouthwashes
**Attrition from bruxism**
Amphetamine
Ecstacy

## TOOTH DISCOLOURATION

*Intrinsic tooth discolouration*
Ciprofloxacin
Enalapril
Etidronate
Fluorides
Fosinopril
Lisinopril
Pentamidine
Perindopril
Propafenone
Quinapril
Ramipril
Terbinafine
Tetracyclines
Trandolopril
Zopiclone
*Extrinsic tooth discolouration*
Betel
Chlorhexidine
Co-amoxiclav
Essential oils
Iron salts
Khat
Linezolid
Tobacco

## TRIGEMINAL PARAESTHESIA OR HYPOAESTHESIA

Acetazolamide
Amitryptiline

Articaine
Chlorpropamide
Colistin
Ergotamine
Gonadotropin-releasing
    hormone analogues
Hydralazine
IFN alpha
Isoniazid
Labetalol
Mefloquine
Methysergide
Monoamine oxidase inhibitors
Nalidixic acid
Nicotinic acid
Nitrofurantoin
Pentamidine
Phenytoin
Prilocaine
Propofol
Propranolol
Protease inhibitors
Prothionamide
Stilbamidine
Streptomycin
Sulphonylureas
**Sulthiame**
Tolbutamide
Tricyclics
Trilostane
Vincristine
Streptomycin

## ULCERATION[b]

Alendronate
Allopurinol
Aurothiomalate
Aztreonam
Barbiturates
Bortezomib
Captopril
Carbamazepine
Clarithromycin
**Cytotoxic drugs**
Dapsone
Desloratadine
Diclofenac
Dideoxycytidine
Emepromium
Flunisolide
Gold

Imatinib mesylate
Indometacin
IFNs
IL-2
Isoprenaline
Ketorolac
Losartan
Meprobamate
Methyldopa
Molgramostim
Naproxen

**Nicorandil**

**NSAIDs**
Olanzapine
Pancreatin
Penicillamine
Phenindione
Phenylbutazone
Phenytoin
Potassium chloride
Proguanil
Propranolol

Sertraline
Sirolimus
Spironolactone
Sulindac
Sulphonamides
Tacrolimus
Tetracyclines
Thiazides
Tiotropium
Tolbutamide
Vancomycin

[a]Abnormal dental development, including tooth agenesis, disturbed root formation, arrested tooth development, microdontia and disturbances affecting enamel, dentine and cementum.
[b]Also from direct contact with compounds containing aspirin, hydrogen peroxide, or phenol.
*Abbreviations*: IL, interleukin; IFN, interferon; NSAIDs, nonsteroidal anti-inflammatory drugs; MAOI, monoamine oxidase inhibitor; ACTH, adrenocorticotropic hormone; EDTA, ethylenediaminetetraacetic acid.

## Further Reading

Scully C, Bagan JV. Adverse drug reactions. Crit Rev Oral Biol Med 2004; 15: 221–39.

Tredwin C, Scully C, Bagan JV. Drug-induced dental disorders. Adverse Drug React Bull 2005; 232: 891–94.

Tredwin C, Scully C, Bagan JV. Drug-induced disorders of teeth. J Dent Res 2005; 84: 596–602.

# INDEX

Page numbers in *italics* represent figures or tables.

Printed and bound by CPI Group (UK) Ltd, Croydon, CR0 4YY

23/10/2024

01778226-0018